Manual of Cardiac Care in Children

AF887397

Anne I. Dipchand · David J. Barron ·
Alejandro A. Floh
Editors

Manual of Cardiac Care in Children

Springer

Editors
Anne I. Dipchand
Hospital for Sick Children
Toronto, Canada

David J. Barron
Hospital for Sick Children
Toronto, Canada

Alejandro A. Floh
Hospital for Sick Children
Toronto, Canada

ISBN 978-3-031-70975-3 ISBN 978-3-031-70973-9 (eBook)
https://doi.org/10.1007/978-3-031-70973-9

© The Editor(s) (if applicable) and The Author(s), under exclusive license to Springer Nature Switzerland AG 2024, corrected publication 2025

This work is subject to copyright. All rights are solely and exclusively licensed by the Publisher, whether the whole or part of the material is concerned, specifically the rights of translation, reprinting, reuse of illustrations, recitation, broadcasting, reproduction on microfilms or in any other physical way, and transmission or information storage and retrieval, electronic adaptation, computer software, or by similar or dissimilar methodology now known or hereafter developed.
The use of general descriptive names, registered names, trademarks, service marks, etc. in this publication does not imply, even in the absence of a specific statement, that such names are exempt from the relevant protective laws and regulations and therefore free for general use.
The publisher, the authors and the editors are safe to assume that the advice and information in this book are believed to be true and accurate at the date of publication. Neither the publisher nor the authors or the editors give a warranty, expressed or implied, with respect to the material contained herein or for any errors or omissions that may have been made. The publisher remains neutral with regard to jurisdictional claims in published maps and institutional affiliations.

This Springer imprint is published by the registered company Springer Nature Switzerland AG
The registered company address is: Gewerbestrasse 11, 6330 Cham, Switzerland

If disposing of this product, please recycle the paper.

Acknowledgements

The editors would like to express their special thanks to Jacqueline Moonsammy for the time and efforts she provided throughout the development of this handbook. Her diligence and dedication were invaluable to achieving the project's completion. We would also like to thank Jacqueline Carillo for her excellent support in formatting the handbook chapters.

Contents

Contributors

Jose Carlos Aldana-Aguirre Division of Neonatology, Department of Paediatrics, The Hospital for Sick Children, Toronto, ON, Canada

Osman O. Al-Radi Cardiac Surgery, Department of Surgery, King Abdulaziz University, Jeddah, Saudi Arabia

Bahaaldin Alsoufi Department of Cardiothoracic Surgery, University of Louisville, Louisville, KY, USA

Meredith Ames Department of Pharmacy, The 'Hospital for Sick Children, Toronto, ON, Canada

Cory Anderson Division of Critical Care Medicine, Department of Paediatrics, London Health Sciences Centre, University of Western Ontario, London, Canada

Kathryn R. Armstrong Division of Cardiology, Department of Paediatrics, University of British Columbia, British Columbia Children's Hospital, Vancouver, BC, Canada

David J. Barron Division of Cardiovascular Surgery, Department of Surgery, Labatt Family Heart Centre, The Hospital for Sick Children, University of Toronto, Toronto, ON, Canada

Lee Benson Division of Pediatric Cardiology, Department of Paediatrics, Labatt Family Heart Centre, The Hospital for Sick Children, University of Toronto, Toronto, ON, Canada

Timothy J. Bradley Department of Paediatrics, University of Saskatchewan, Jim Pattison Children's Hospital, Saskatchewan Health Authority, Saskatoon, SK, Canada

Leonardo R. Brandao Division of Haematology/Oncology, Department of Paediatrics, Hospital for Sick Children, University of Toronto, Toronto, ON, Canada

Colm Breatnach Children's Health Ireland at Crumlin, Dublin, Ireland

Anica Bulic Division of Pediatric Cardiology, Hospital for Sick Children, University of Toronto, Toronto, ON, Canada

Devin Chetan Division of Cardiology, Labatt Family Heart Centre, The Hospital for Sick Children, Toronto, ON, Canada

Vannessa Chin Division of Paediatric Cardiac Anaesthesia, Department of Anaesthesia and Pain Medicine, The Hospital for Sick Children, University of Toronto, Toronto, ON, Canada

Haley Christian Department of Critical Care Medicine and Labatt Family Heart Centre, Hospital for Sick Children, University of Toronto, Toronto, ON, Canada; Department of Paediatrics, Hospital for Sick Children, University of Toronto, Toronto, ON, Canada

Lynn Crawford-Lean Perfusion Services, Labatt Family Heart Centre, Hospital for Sick Children, Toronto, Ontario, Canada

Mimi Xiaoming Deng Department of Cardiovascular Surgery, Labatt Family Heart Centre, Hospital for Sick Children, University of Toronto, Toronto, ON, Canada

Anne I. Dipchand Division of Paediatric Cardiology, Department of Paediatrics, Labatt Family Heart Centre, Hospital for Sick Children, University of Toronto, Toronto, ON, Canada

Andreea Dragulescu Department of Paediatrics, Division of Cardiology, Labatt Family Heart Centre, Hospital for Sick Children, University of Toronto, Toronto, ON, Canada

Daniel E. Ehrmann Department of Paediatrics, University of Michigan Medical School, Ann Arbor, MI, USA

Alejandro A. Floh Department of Critical Care Medicine, Division of Cardiac Critical Care Unit, Labatt Family Heart Centre, The Hospital for Sick Children, University of Toronto, Toronto, ON, Canada

Celeste Foreman Perfusion Services, Labatt Family Heart Centre, Hospital for Sick Children, Toronto, Ontario, Canada

Lindsay R. Freud Division of Cardiology, Department of Paediatrics, Labatt Family Heart Centre, The Hospital for Sick Children, University of Toronto, Toronto, ON, Canada

Michael D. Fridman Section of Paediatric Cardiology, Department of Paediatrics, Alberta Children's Hospital, University of Calgary, Calgary, AB, Canada

Michael Grattan Department of Paediatrics, Children's Hospital at London Health Sciences Centre, London, ON, Canada

Seth B. Gray Department of Critical Care Medicine, Division of Cardiac Critical Care Medicine, The Hospital for Sick Children, Toronto, ON, Canada

Lars Grosse-Wortmann Division of Cardiology, Department of Paediatrics, Oregon Health and Science University, CDRC, St. Portland, OR, USA

Luciana Rodriguez Guerineau Cardiac Critical, Department of Critical Care Medicine, Labatt Family Heart Centre, Hospital for Sick Children, Toronto, ON, Canada

Christoph Haller Division of Cardiovascular Surgery, Labatt Family Heart Centre, Department of Surgery, The Hospital for Sick Children, University of Toronto, Toronto, ON, Canada

Robert Hamilton Division of Cardiology, Department of Paediatrics, Labatt Family Heart Centre, Hospital for Sick Children, University of Toronto, Toronto, ON, Canada

Joann Herridge Clinical Dietetics, Hospital for Sick Children, Toronto, ON, Canada

Osami Honjo Division of Cardiovascular Surgery, Department of Surgery, Labatt Family Heart Centre, The Hospital for Sick Children, University of Toronto, Toronto, ON, Canada

Emilie Jean-St-Michel University Hospital for Northern British Columbia, Prince George, BC, Canada

Aamir Jeewa Department of Paediatrics, Division of Cardiology, Labatt Family Heart Centre, The Hospital for Sick Children, University of Toronto, Toronto, ON, Canada

Anusha Jegatheeswaran Great Ormond Street Hospital for Children, London, UK

Michael Khoury Division of Pediatric Cardiology, Department of Paediatrics, University of Alberta, Stollery Children's Hospital, Edmonton, AB, Canada

Bhavikkumar D. Langanecha Division of Cardiac Critical Care, Department of Critical Care Medicine, Labatt Family Heart Centre, The Hospital for Sick Children, University of Toronto, Toronto, ON, Canada

Myunghyun M. Lee Division of Cardiovascular Surgery, Labatt Family Heart Centre, Hospital for Sick Children, Toronto, ON, Canada

Shuhua Luo Department of Cardiovascular Surgery, West China Hospital, Sichuan University, Chengdu, Sichuan, China

Áine Lynch Columbia University Vagelos College of Physicians and Surgeons, Morgan Stanley Children's Hospital of New York Presbyterian, New York, NY, USA

Andrea Maurich Division of Cardiology, Labatt Family Heart Centre, Hospital for Sick Children, Toronto, ON, Canada

Amine Mazine Division of Cardiovascular Surgery, University of Toronto, Toronto, ON, Canada

Brian McCrindle Division of Cardiology, Department of Paediatrics, Labatt Family Heart Centre, The Hospital of Sick Children, Toronto, ON, Canada

Luc Mertens Division of Cardiology, Department of Paediatrics, Labatt Family Heart Centre, The Hospital for Sick Children, Toronto, ON, Canada

Seema Mital Labatt Family Heart Centre, Department of Paediatrics, Hospital for Sick Children, University of Toronto, Toronto, ON, Canada

Conall Morgan Division of Cardiology, Department of Paediatrics, Labatt Family Heart Centre, The Hospital for Sick Children, University of Toronto, Toronto, ON, Canada

Komail Nadeem Department of Pharmacy, The Hospital for Sick Children, Toronto, ON, Canada

Constanza Jimenez Navia Cardiac Critical Care Unit, Hospital de Niños Dr. Luis Calvo Mackenna, Santiago, Chile

Fiona Perelini Starship Children's Hospital, Auckland, New Zealand

Alyssa Power Division of Cardiology, Labatt Family Heart Centre, Hospital for Sick Children, Toronto, ON, Canada

Evan J. Propst Department of Otolaryngology, The Hospital for Sick Children, Otolaryngology, University of Toronto, Toronto, ON, Canada

Jennifer L. Russell Division of Cardiology, Labatt Family Heart Centre, The Hospital for Sick Children, Toronto, ON, Canada

Mike Seed Division Head, Cardiology, The Hospital for Sick Children, University of Toronto, Toronto, ON, Canada

Winnie Seto Department of Pharmacy, The Hospital for Sick Children, Toronto, ON, Canada

Anna Tedesco-Bruce Clinical Dietetics, Hospital for Sick Children, Toronto, ON, Canada

Angie Thiessen Department of Pharmacy, The Hospital for Sick Children, Toronto, ON, Canada

Mark Todd Department of Critical Care Medicine, Hospital for Sick Children, Toronto, ON, Canada;
Department of Respiratory Medicine, Hospital for Sick Children, Toronto, ON, Canada

Rachel D. Vanderlaan Division of Cardiovascular Surgery, Department of Surgery, Labatt Family Heart Centre, The Hospital for Sick Children, University of Toronto, Toronto, ON, Canada

Karen Wong Department of Pharmacy, The Hospital for Sick Children, Toronto, ON, Canada

Shi-Joon Yoo Department of Diagnostic Imaging, The Hospital for Sick Children, University of Toronto, Toronto, ON, Canada

Laura Zahavich Department of Genetic Counselling, Labatt Family Heart Centre, Hospital for Sick Children, University of Toronto, Toronto, ON, Canada; Department of Molecular Genetics, Labatt Family Heart Centre, Hospital for Sick Children, University of Toronto, Toronto, ON, Canada

Oshri Zaulan Cardiac Critical, Department of Critical Care Medicine, Labatt Family Heart Centre, Hospital for Sick Children, Toronto, ON, Canada

Abbreviations

1.5VR	One and a half ventricle repair
AA	Aortic atresia
AAo	Ascending aortic
AAOCA	Anomalous aortic origin of a coronary artery
ABO-i	ABO-incompatible
ACC	American College of Cardiology
ACD	Alveolar capillary dysplasia
ACE	Angiotensin-converting enzyme
ACR	Acute cellular rejection
ACT	Activated coagulation time
ADHF	Acute decompensated heart failure
ADL	Activity of daily living
AHA	American Heart Association
AI	Aortic insufficiency
AIS	Arterial ischemic stroke
AKI	Acute kidney injury
ALCAPA	Anomalous left coronary artery from the pulmonary artery
AMR	Antibody-mediated rejection
AoD	Aortic dissection
AoR	Aortic root
AoRz	Aortic root Z-score
AoV	Aortic valve
AP	Aortopulmonary
APCs	Aortopulmonary collaterals
APLA	Antiphospholipid antibody
aPTT	Activated partial thromboplastin time
ARB	Angiotensin receptor blocker
ARCAPA	Anomalous right coronary from the pulmonary artery
ARNI	Angiotensin receptor-neprilysin inhibitor
AS	Aortic stenosis
ASA	Aspirin/acetasalicylic acid

ASD	Atrial septal defect
ASO	Arterial switch operation
ASPEN	American Society of Parenteral and Enteral Nutrition
AT	Antithrombin
ATS	Arterial tortuosity syndrome
AV	Atrioventricular
AVC	Arrhythmogenic cardiomyopathy
AVM	Arteriovenous malformation
AVRT	Atrioventricular re-entrant tachycardiac
AVSD	Atrioventricular septal defect
AVV	Atrioventricular valve
AVVR	Atrioventricular valve regurgitation
BAS	Balloon atrial septostomy
BAV	Bicuspid aortic valve
BB	Beta blocker
BCPS	Bidirectional cavopulmonary shunt
BID	Twice a day
BIPAP	Bilevel positive airway pressure
BiV	Biventricular
BIVAD	Biventricular assist device
BMR	Basal Metabolic Rate
BNP	B-type natriuretic peptide
BP	Blood pressure
BPEG	British Pacing and Electrophysiology Group
BSA	Body surface area
BTT	Blalock–Taussig–Thomas
CaCl	Calcium chloride
CAPD	Cornell Assessment of Pediatric Delerium
CAV	Cardiac allograft vasculopathy
CCB	Calcium channel blocker
CCCU	Cardiac critical care unit
CCHB	Congenital complete heart block
ccTGA	Congenitally corrected transposition of the great arteries
CFM	Cerebral function monitoring
CHB	Complete heart block
CHD	Congenital heart disease
CHF	Congestive heart failure
CHSS	Congenital Heart Surgeon Society
CIED	Cardiac implantable electronic device
CKD	Chronic kidney disease
CLABSI	Central line-associated bloodstream infection
CM	Cardiomyopathy
CMA	Chromosome microarray analysis
CMRI	Cardiac magnetic resonance imaging
CMV	Cytomegalovirus

CNI	Calcineurin inhibitor
CNS	Central nervous system
CNV	Copy number variants
CO	Cardiac output
CoA	Coarctation of the aorta
CPAP	Continuous positive airway pressure
CPB	Cardiopulmonary bypass
CPET	Cardiopulmonary exercise test
CPR	Cardiopulmonary resuscitation
CPS	Cardioplegia solution
CRP	C reactive protein
CRT	Cardiac resynchronization therapy
CRT-D	Cardiac resynchronization therapy—defibrillator
CRT-P	Cardiac resynchronization therapy—pacemaker
CSVT	Cerebral sinus venous thrombosis
CTA	Computed tomography angiography
CUF	Conventional ultrafiltration
CVL	Central venous line
CVP	Central venous pressure
Cx	Circumflex
CXR	Chest X-ray
DA	Ductus arteriosus
DAA	Double aortic arch
DCD	Donation after cardiac death
DCM	Dilated cardiomyopathy
DDD	Dual paced, dual sensed, dual response (pacemaker mode)
DHCA	Deep hypothermic circulatory arrest
DILV	Double inlet left ventricle
DKS	Damus–Kaye–Stansel
DO2	Oxygen delivery
DOAC	Direct oral anticoagulant
DOLV	Double outlet left ventricle
DORV	Double outlet right ventricle
DRI	Dietary reference intakes
DSA	Donor specific antibody
DTI	Direct thrombin inhibitor
DVT	Deep vein thrombosis
EBV	Epstein–Barr virus
ECG	Electrocardiogram
ECLS	Extracorporeal life support
ECMO	Extracorporeal membrane oxygenation
ECPR	ECMO cardiopulmonary resuscitation
EER	Estimated energy requirements
EF	Ejection fraction
EFE	Endocardial fibroelastosis

EL	Ectopia lentis
EN	Enteral nutrition
EP	Electrophysiology
ERS	European Respirology Society
ESC	European Cardiology Society
ESPNIC	European Society of Pediatric and Neonatal Intensive Care
ETT	Endotracheal tube
FALD	Fontan-associated liver disease
FBN1	Fibrillin-1 gene
FCF	Fontan circulatory failure
FFP	Fresh frozen plasma
FISH	Fluorescent in situ hybridization
FP	Frozen plasma
FRC	Functional residual capacity
FTAAD	Familial thoracic aortic aneurysm and dissection
GA	Gestational age
GDMT	Guideline-directed medical therapy
GIR	Glucose infusion rate
HCM	Hypertrophic cardiomyopathy
HCT	Hematocrit
HF	Heart failure
HFpEF	Heart failure with preserved ejection fraction
HFrEF	Heart failure with reduced ejection fraction
HIT	Heparin-induced thrombocytopenia
HLA	Human leukocyte antigen
HLHS	Hypoplastic left heart syndrome
HLM	Heart-lung machine
HR	Heart rate
HRS	Heart Rhythm Society
hsPDA	Hemodynamically significant persistent ductus arteriosus
HTx	Heart transplant
IAA	Interrupted aortic arch
iCal	Ionized calcium
ICD	Implantable cardiac defibrillator
ICH	Intracranial hemorrhage
IDU	Injection drug users
IE	Infective endocarditis
ILR	Implantable loop recorder
iNO	Inhaled nitric oxide
INR	International normalized ratio
IS	Immunosuppression
ISHLT	International Society of Heart and Lung Transplantation
IVC	Inferior vena cava
JET	Junctional ectopic tachycardia
JVP	Jugular venous pulsation

LA	Left atrium
LAA	Left atrial appendage
LAD	Left anterior descending
LAVV	Left atrioventricular valve
LAVVR	Left atrioventricular valve regurgitation
LAVVS	Left atrioventricualar valve stenosis
LCA	Left coronary artery
LCOS	Low cardiac output syndrome
LCT	Long chain triglycerides
LDS	Loeys–Dietz syndrome
LGE	Late gadolinium enhancement
LIJV	Left internal jugular vein
LMCA	Left main coronary artery
LMWH	Low molecular weight heparin
LPA	Left pulmonary artery
LSCA	Left subclavian artery
LSVC	Left SVC
LV	Left ventricle
LVAD	Left ventricular assist device
LVEDP	Left ventricular end diastolic pressure
LVEDV	Left ventricular end diastolic volume
LVH	Left ventricular hypertrophy
LVOT	Left ventricular outflow tract
LVOTO	Left ventricular outflow tract obstruction
MA	Mitral atresia
MAPCAs	Major aortopulmonary collaterals
MCS	Mechanical support
MCT	Medium chain triglycerides
MFS	Marfan syndrome
MIS-C	Multisystem inflammatory syndrome
mLV	Morphologic left ventricle
MMF	Mycophenolate mofetil
MPA	Main pulmonary artery
MPA	Mycophenolic acid
mPAP	Mean pulmonary artery pressure
MR	Mitral regurgitation
MRA	Magnetic resonance angiography
MRI	Magnetic resonance imaging
MRSA	Methicillin-resistant staphylococcus aureus
mRV	Morphologic right ventricle
MS	Mitral stenosis
mTORi	Mammalian target of rapamycin inhibitors
MUF	Modified ultrafiltration
MV	Mitral valve
MVO2	Mixed venous oxygen saturation

MVP	Mitral valve prolapse
NASPE	North American Society for Pacing and Electrophysiology
NBTE	Nonbacterial thrombotic endocarditis
NEC	Necrotizing enterocolitis
NG	Nasogastric
NiBP	Non-invasive blood pressure
NIRS	Near-infrared spectroscopy
NPO	Nil per os
NPPV	Non-invasive positive pressure ventilation
NSAIDs	Non-steroidal anti-inflammatory drugs
NSVT	Non-sustained ventricular tachycardia
NT-proBNP	N-terminal prohormone of brain natriuretic peptide
NYHA	New York Heart Association
OR	Operating room
OVKA	Oral vitamin K antagonist
PA	Pulmonary artery
PA/IVS	Pulmonary atresia/intact ventricular septum
PA/VSD	Pulmonary atresia/ventricular septal defect
PA/VSD/MAPCAs	Pulmonary atresia/ventricular septal defect with major aortopulmonary collateral arteries
PAB	Pulmonary artery band
PACES	Pediatric and Congenital Electrophysiology Society
PAH	Pulmonary arterial hypertension
PAP	Pulmonary artery pressure
PAPVC	Partial anomalous pulmonary venous connection
PAWP	Pulmonary arterial wedge pressure
PBF	Pulmonary blood flow
pCO_2	Carbon dioxide
PCR	Polymerase chain reaction
PDA	Persistent ductus arteriosus
PE	Pulmonary embolism
PEEP	Positive end expiratory pressure
PFO	Persistent foramen ovale
PGE	Prostaglandin
PH	Pulmonary hypertension
PI	Pulmonary insufficiency
PI	Pulsatility index
PICC	Peripherally inserted central catheter
PIP	Peak inspiratory pressure
PLA A	Plasmalyte A
PLE	Protein-losing enteropathy
PM	Pacemaker
PMT	Pacemaker mediated tachycardia
PN	Parenteral nutrition
POD	Post-operative day

PPAS	Peripheral pulmonary artery stenosis
PRBC	Packed red blood cells
PS	Pulmonary stenosis
PTLD	Post-transplant lymphoproliferative disorder
PTS	Post-thrombotic syndrome
PTT	Prothrombin time
PVARP	Post-ventricular atrial refractory period
PVOD	Pulmonary veno-occlusive disease
PVR	Pulmonary vascular resistance
PVRi	Pulmonary vascular resistance indexed
PVS	Pulmonary vein stenosis
QOL	Quality of life
Qp	Pulmonary blood flow
Qs	Systemic blood flow
RA	Right atrium
RAA	Right aortic arch
RAAS	Renin-angiotensin-aldosterone system
RAVVR	Right atrioventricular valve regurgitation
RCA	Right coronary artery
RCM	Restrictive cardiomyopathy
RDA	Recommended Daily Allowance
REV	Reparation à l'étage ventriculaire
ROTEM	Rotational thromboelastometry
RPA	Right pulmonary artery
RPM	Revolutions per minute
RRT	Renal replacement therapy
RV	Right ventricle
RVAD	Right ventricular assist device
RVDCC	Right ventricle coronary circulation
RVEDP	Right ventricular end diastolic pressure
RVEF	Right ventricular ejection fraction
RVH	Right ventricular hypertrophy
rVIIa	Recombinant factor VIIa
RVOT	Right ventricular outflow tract
RVOTO	Right ventricular outflow tract obstruction
RVSP	Right ventricular systolic pressure
S. aureus	Staphylococcus aureus
SA	Sinoatrial
SAM	Systolic anterior motion
SaO_2	Systemic arterial oxygen saturation
SAS	Subaortic stenosis
SC	Subcutaneous
SCD	Sudden cardiac death
SGLT2i	Sodium-glucose cotransporter-2 inhibitor
SSI	Surgical site infection

SV	Single ventricle
SVAD	Systemic ventricular assist device
SVASD	Sinus venosus atrial septal defect
SVC	Superior vena cava
SvO_2	Systemic venous oxygen saturation
SVR	Systemic vascular resistance
SVT	Supraventricular tachycardia
T21	Trisomy 21
TA	Truncus arteriosus
TAA	Thoracic aortic aneurysm
TAAD	Thoracic aortic aneurysm and dissection
TAH	Total artificial heart
TAPVC	Total anomalous pulmonary venous connection
TCPC	Total cavopulmonary connection
TDM	Therapeutic drug monitoring
TEE	Total energy expenditure
TEE	Transesophageal echocardiogram
TEG	Thromboelastography
TGA	Transposition of the great arteries
TGA/IVS	Transposition of the great arteries/intact ventricular septum
TGA/VSD	Transposition of the great arteries/ventricular septal defect
TGF-β	Transforming growth factor-beta
THAA	Tubular hypoplasia of the aortic arch
TID	Three times a day
TOF	Tetralogy of Fallot
TOF/PA	Tetralogy of Fallot/pulmonary atresia
TR	Tricuspid regurgitation
TV	Tricuspid valve
TVP	Tricuspid valve prolapse
UFH	Unfractionated heparin
UTI	Urinary tract infection
V/Q	Ventilation/perfusion
VA ECMO	Venous arterial extracorporeal membrane oxygenation
VA	Ventriculo-arterial
VAC	Vacuum-assisted closure
VAD	Ventricular assist device
VAP	Ventilator acquired pneumonia
vEDS	Vascular Ehlers-Danlos syndrome
VO_2	Oxygen consumption
VSD	Ventricular septal defect
VT	Ventricular tachycardia
VTE	Venous thrombotic events
WES	Whole exome sequencing
WGS	Whole genome sequencing
WHO	World Health Organization

WPW	Wolff-Parkinson-White
WU	Woods units
ΔAVO2	Arterial-venous oxygen saturation difference

Nomenclature and Segmental Analysis of the Heart

Mike Seed and Shi-Joon Yoo

Abstract A uniform approach to the terminology used to describe the morphology of congenital heart disease allows clear communication between clinicians. There are two main schools of nomenclature being used in major centers in North America and Europe. These two approaches devised by Van Praagh and Anderson share the principle of categorizing hearts into three major components, the atria, ventricles, and great vessels. Cardiac anatomy is described according to the individual anatomical segments and the connections they form. Although certain patterns of cardiac morphology are common, an important principle is that virtually any combination of segments and connections is possible. SickKids uses the approach defined by Anderson and colleagues and the rest of this chapter will refer to this classification system.

Keywords Nomenclature · Segmental analysis · Morphology · Atria · Ventricles · Great vessels · Situs · Ventricular topology

Abbreviations

AV	Atrioventricular
DOLV	Double outlet left ventricle
DORV	Double outlet right ventricle
IVC	Inferior vena cava
LA	Left atrium
LV	Left ventricle
RA	Right atrium

M. Seed (✉)
Division Head, Cardiology, The Hospital for Sick Children, University of Toronto, Toronto, ON, Canada
e-mail: mike.seed@sickkids.ca

S.-J. Yoo
Department of Diagnostic Imaging, The Hospital for Sick Children, University of Toronto, Toronto, ON, Canada

© The Author(s), under exclusive license to Springer Nature Switzerland AG 2024

A. I. Dipchand et al. (eds.), *Manual of Cardiac Care in Children*,
https://doi.org/10.1007/978-3-031-70973-9_1

RV	Right ventricle
VA	Ventriculo-arterial

1 Nomenclature

- A uniform approach to the terminology used to describe the morphology of congenital heart disease allows for clear communication between clinicians.
- Two main schools of nomenclature : Van Praagh and Anderson.
- Hearts are categorized into 3 major components / segments: the atria, ventricles, and great vessels (Fig. 1).
- Segments are attributed sidedness based on anatomical characteristics rather than their position in the chest or their relationship to other segments.
- The 3 segments of the heart should be listed in sequence with the connections between atria and ventricles, and ventricles and great vessels also defined.
- Systemic and pulmonary venous connections to the heart are then described as well as any associated lesions such as atrial and ventricular septal defects and the presence or absence of a patent ductus arteriosus.
- Coronary artery anatomy is described.
- SickKids uses the approach defined by Anderson and colleagues and the rest of this chapter will refer to this classification system.
- The Van Praagh system consists of a three-part abbreviation of letters in brackets separated by commas used to describe the visceroatrial situs, the orientation of the ventricular loop, and the position and relation of the great vessels. For example, {S, D, S} represents normal anatomic configuration.

2 Segmental Sequential Analysis

- SickKids uses the approach defined by Anderson and colleagues.
- Although certain patterns of cardiac morphology are common, an important principle is that virtually any combination of segments and connections is possible.
- A full segmental sequential analysis begins with definition of the position of the heart in the chest: right, left or center of the chest.
- The position of the cardiac apex should be described as to the left, right or center of the chest.

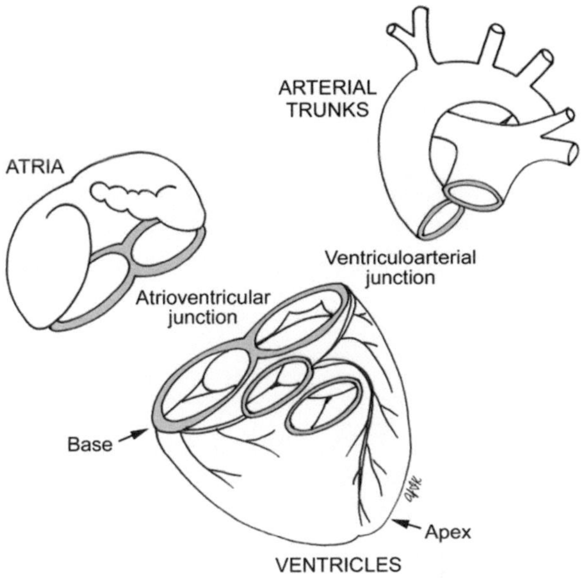

Fig. 1 The 3 primary cardiac segments

2.1 *Atrial Arrangement*

- 4 possible patterns: usual atrial arrangement (situs solitus), mirror image atrial arrangement (situs inversus), right isomerism and left isomerism (Fig. 2).
- Atrial morphology cannot be determined using the venous connections to the atria; right and left atria differentiate by the appearances of the atrial appendages and pectinate muscles.
  - Right atrial appendage: broad base and triangular shape with its pectinate muscles extending over the internal wall of the right atrial body as far as the crista terminalis and right atrial vestibule.
  - Left atrial appendage has a more slender, finger-like form with pectinate muscles which do not extend beyond its narrow orifice.

2.2 *Isomerism (Fig. 3)*

- In right or left isomerism, both of the atria have of the same type of appendage and pectinate muscle morphology.
- Isomerism patients usually have abnormalities of the morphology and position of other organs.
  - Bronchial anatomy: most consistent association
  - Visceral heterotaxy: abdominal viscera frequently abnormally arranged.

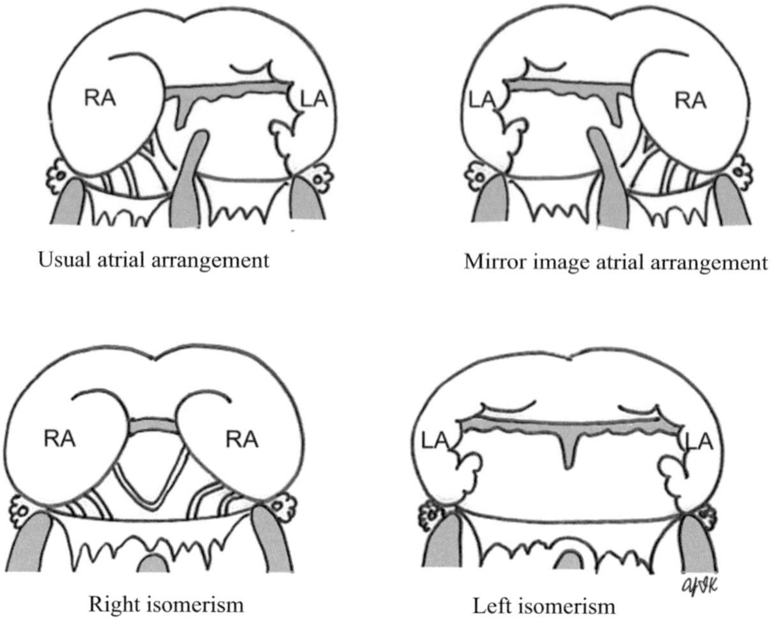

Fig. 2 The four possible atrial arrangements showing appendage and pectinate muscle morphology

  - Abnormalities of bowel rotation are common with both forms of isomerism.

- Right isomerism
  - The trachea bifurcates into symmetrical short main bronchi with bilateral trilobed lungs.
  - Pulmonary arteries pass into the lungs anterior to the bronchi
  - Frequently associated with absence of the spleen and a midline liver

- Left isomerism
  - The major bronchi are of left main bronchial type with a more distal origin of the upper lobar bronchus.
  - Main pulmonary arteries pass over the major bronchi before entering the lungs
  - Polysplenia
  - Biliary atresia in 20%

- Atrial appendage morphology that defines the morphology of the atria cannot usually be seen using echocardiography.
- Bronchial branching pattern may be seen clearly with other imaging modalities, and this may be used to define atrial morphology in the majority of patients.
- Echocardiography can also be used to define the atrial arrangement because the arrangement of the descending aorta, inferior vena cava and azygous vein in the upper abdomen are fairly consistent in each of the 4 atrial arrangements.

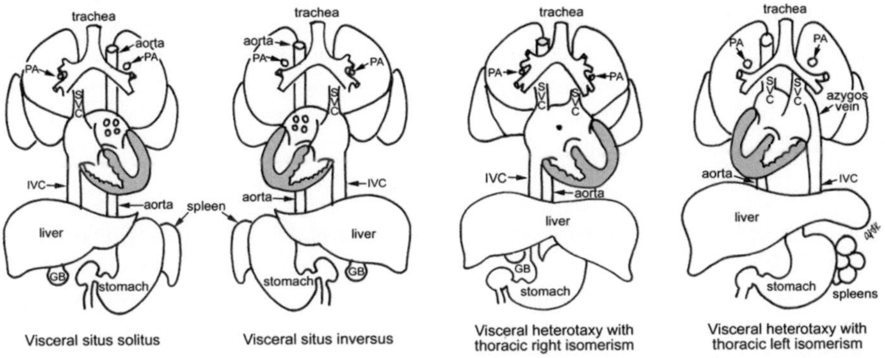

Fig. 3 Typical bronchial, vascular and visceral anatomy for each atrial arrangement

  - Usual atrial arrangement: the IVC enters the thorax on the right of the spine and the descending aorta passes into the abdomen on the left of the spine.
  - Mirror image atrial arrangement: the IVC and descending aortic positions are reversed, with the aorta on the right and IVC on the left.
  - In these arrangements the IVC is usually anterior to the aorta
  - Left isomerism: usually associated with azygous continuation of the IVC and so the major vein entering the chest is posteriorly located compared with the aorta.
  - Right isomerism: the descending aorta and IVC are usually positioned on the same side of the spine with the IVC anterior to the aorta.

- The other useful echocardiographic feature differentiating between right and left atria is the limbus of the foramen ovale, which is always found on the right atrial side of the interatrial septum.

2.3 *Ventricular Morphology*

- Must first consider ventricular morphology: the vast majority of hearts have 2 ventricles, a morphological right ventricle and a morphological left ventricle.
- Right ventricle (RV)
  - Most consistent differentiating feature is thicker apical trabeculations
  - Moderator band: a stout trabeculation giving rise to the antero-superior papillary muscle of the tricuspid valve.
  - Tri-leaflet tricuspid valve with its attachment to the interventricular septum usually opens into the RV.
- Left ventricle (LV)

  - Has much finer trabeculations
  - The mitral valve has 2 leaflets and 2 papillary muscles with no septal connection

2.4 Ventricular Topology

- Morphological RV is usually positioned anterior and to the right of the morphological LV.
- Exceptions occur, e.g. heart in the right chest, apex to the right and mirror image atrial arrangement – in which the RV is frequently on the left side of the LV.
- Ventricular topology distinguishes between right hand topology and left hand topology of the right ventricle.
  - Place right or left palm on the RV surface of the interventricular septum with the extended thumb pointing towards the inlet valve and the fingers pointing towards the RV outlet (Fig. 4)
- When this is possible with the right hand there is right hand topology of the RV which is usually the case in the normal heart.
- In hearts with incomplete ventricles, it may not be possible to attribute right or left hand topology to the RV; it is necessary to describe the spatial relationship of the two ventricles.
- If a hypoplastic ventricle is postero-inferiorly located in relation to the larger ventricle it is likely to be of LV morphology; superior and anterior it is likely to be an RV, although it may be positioned more leftward or rightward with respect to the larger LV (Fig. 5).

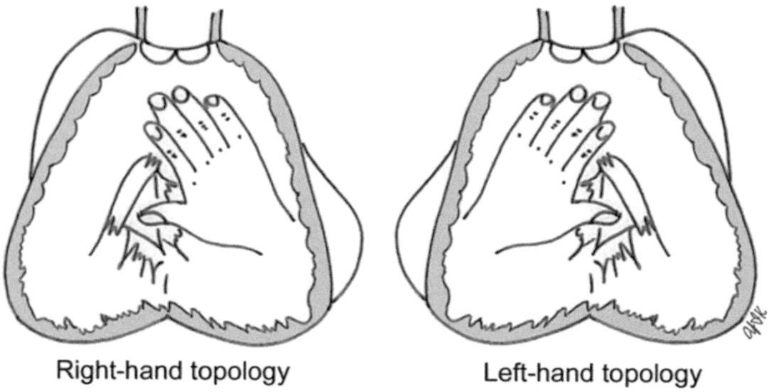

Fig. 4 Ventricular topology

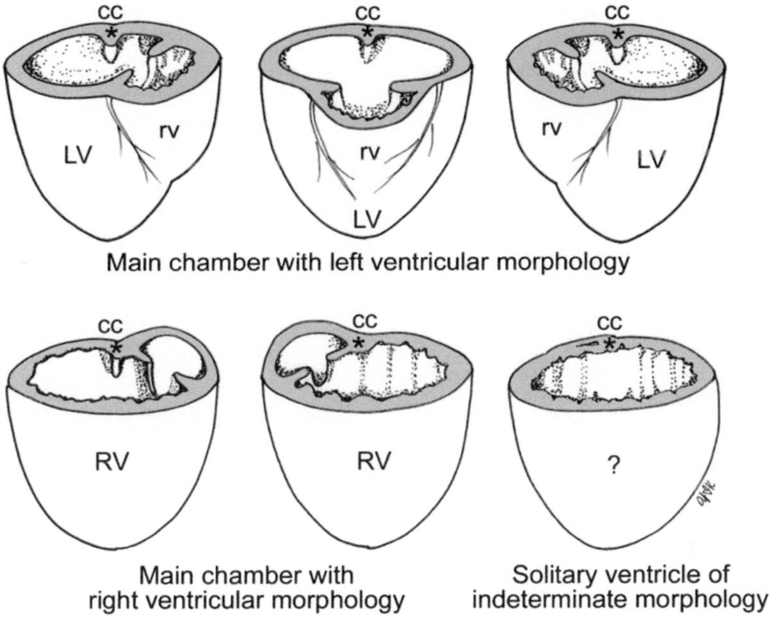

Fig. 5 Defining ventricular morphology in the setting of ventricular hypoplasia

2.5 *Atrio-Ventricular (AV) Connection*

- 2 common types of atrio-ventricular connections: biventricular and univentricular (Fig. 6)
- A third and very rare type is uni-atrial and biventricular with absence of the one AV connection and an AV valve which overrides both ventricles.
- Biventricular connections are either concordant, discordant or mixed (Fig. 7).
  - Concordant AV connections: the RA is connected to the RV and the LA to the LV.
  - Discordant AV connections: the RA is connected to the LV and the LA to the RV.
  - Mixed atrio-ventricular communication: right or left isomerism and biventricular connections.
- Univentricular connection: absence of the right or left AV connection (Fig. 8).
  - On the right or left side of the heart (with respect to the chest) the atrial and ventricular myocardium invaginate to touch the central fibrous body of the heart with no potential passage between the two chambers.

    Must be distinguished from a right or left imperforate AV valve which is a type of biventricular connection.

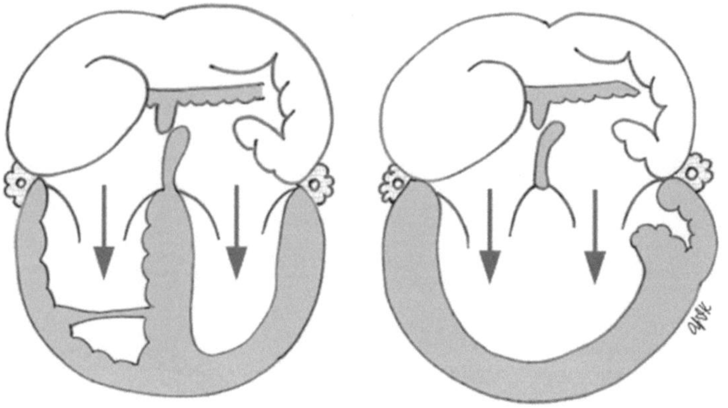

Fig. 6 The two forms of atrioventricular connection

- Double inlet AV connection: both atria are connected to the RV or LV.
  - 50% rule: when parts of one or both atria are connected to both ventricles, a double inlet connection is present when more than 50% of both atria are committed to one ventricle (Fig. 9). DILV is most common with DIRV being exceptionally rare
- AV connections are further defined by the mode of connection which describes the morphology of the AV valves.
  - AV valvar anatomy may be comprised by separate valves or by the common AV valve seen in an atrio-ventricular septal defect.
  - Valvar annulus: may be exclusively committed to its underlying ventricle, or may be overriding, where part of the valve is positioned over the other ventricle.
  - Straddling: present when chordal apparatus of an AV valve crosses the ventricular septum via a ventricular septal defect and inserts in the contralateral ventricle.
  - Straddling and overriding often occur together.
  - AV valves can also be imperforate, stenotic or regurgitant.

2.6 Ventriculo-Arterial (VA) Connection

- VA connections with 2 great arteries arising from the ventricular mass may be concordant, discordant or double outlet (Fig. 10).
- The aorta and pulmonary artery can be identified in terms of their branches.
  - Aorta: coronary arteries and head and neck arteries

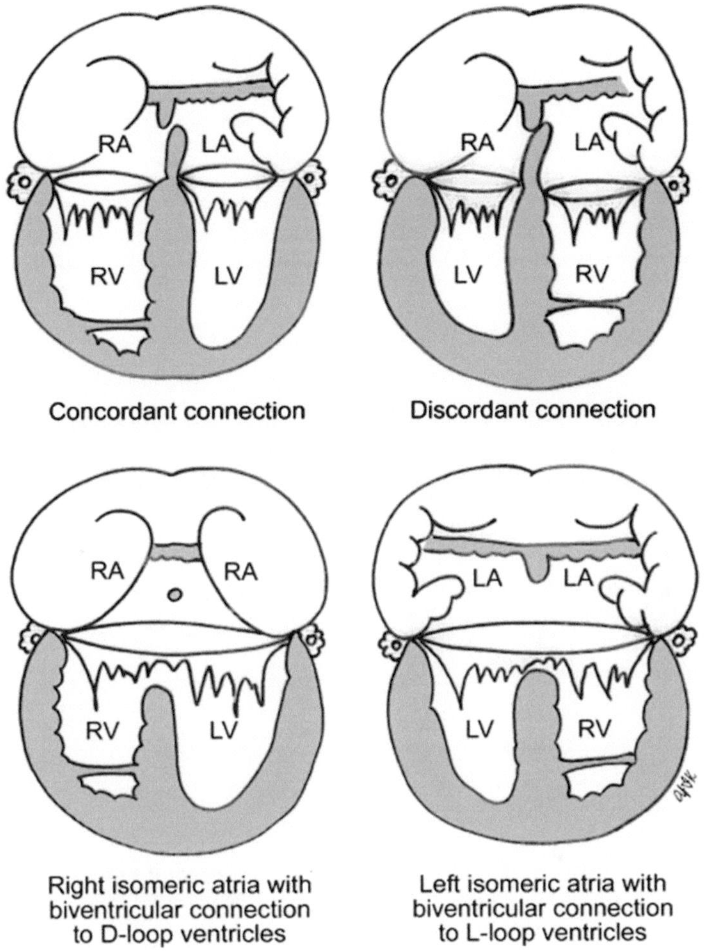

Fig. 7 The four types of biventricular atrioventricular connections

   - Pulmonary artery: usually bifurcates into right and left pulmonary arteries.

- Concordant VA connections: the LV gives rise to the aorta and RV gives rise to the pulmonary artery.
- Double outlet right and left ventricles: the great arteries are both committed to one ventricle; when one great vessel is overriding the ventricular septum, the type of connection is determined using the 50% rule. DORV is most common with DOLV being extremely rare.
- Single outlet: when only 1 vessel arises from the ventricular mass:
   - Common arterial trunk (or truncus arteriosus): usually overrides both ventricles; gives rise to the coronary arteries, at least one pulmonary artery and the majority of the systemic arterial supply

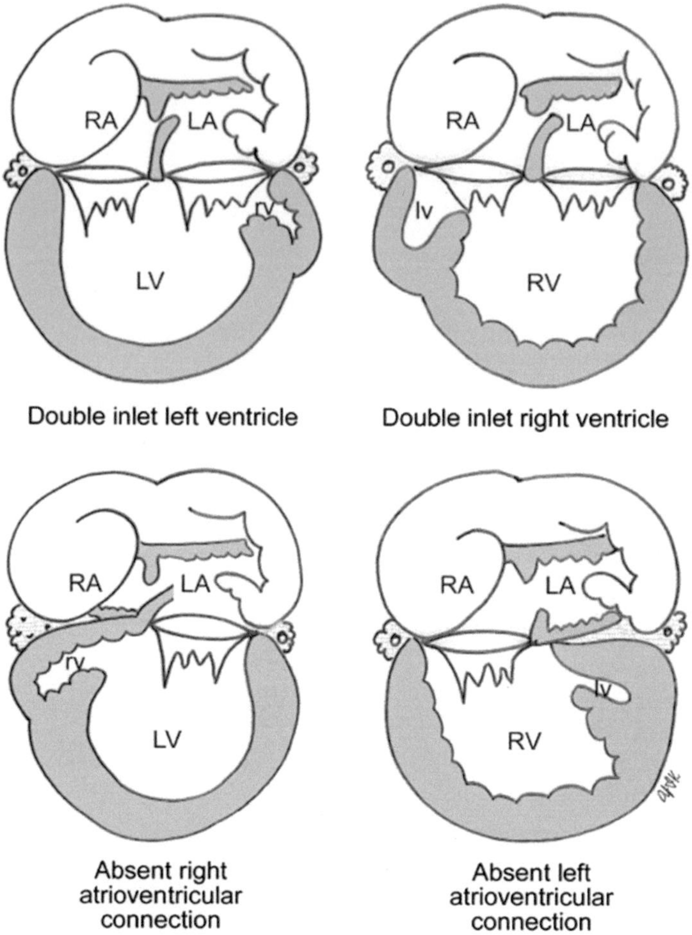

Fig. 8 Absent and double inlet atrioventricular connections

- Solitary arterial trunk: usually overrides both ventricles; present when it is not possible to identify any remnant of an intra-pericardial main pulmonary trunk.
- Other 2 types of single outlet hearts occur in the uncommon situation where aortic atresia or pulmonary atresia are present but it is not possible to determine the position of the connection of the diminutive aorta or pulmonary artery to the ventricular mass.

  If it is possible to attribute the diminutive vessels to its respective ventricle, the type of VA connection is concordant, discordant or double outlet with an imperforate pulmonary or aortic valve.

- Sometimes necessary to describe the ventricular outlet regions and to detail the arrangement of the great vessels in relation to each other.

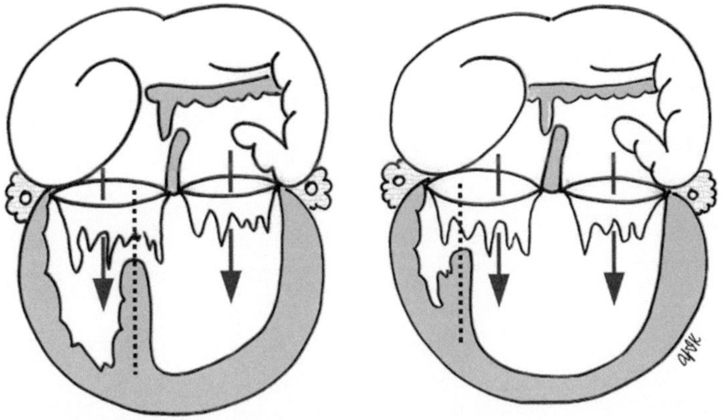

Fig. 9 Examples of biventricular and univentricular atrioventricular connections according to the 50% rule

- Normal hearts

  RV: gives rise to a complete muscular ring of tissue supporting the pulmonary trunk
  LV: fibrous continuity between the mitral and aortic valves with no muscular infundibulum.

- Hearts with malformations of the VA connection

  Variation of the normal arrangement which may result in muscular obstruction beneath the semi-lunar valves
  Convention to describe the position of the aorta with relation to the pulmonary artery at the level of the semi-lunar valves.

3 Important Remaining Anatomic Descriptors

- Arch-sidedness: defined by the position of the aortic arch in relation to the trachea
  - Left aortic arch: most common (70%), arch runs to the left of the trachea; most commonly gives rise to the right brachiocephalic artery, left common carotid artery and left subclavian artery (in that order) which is referred to as "normal branching".

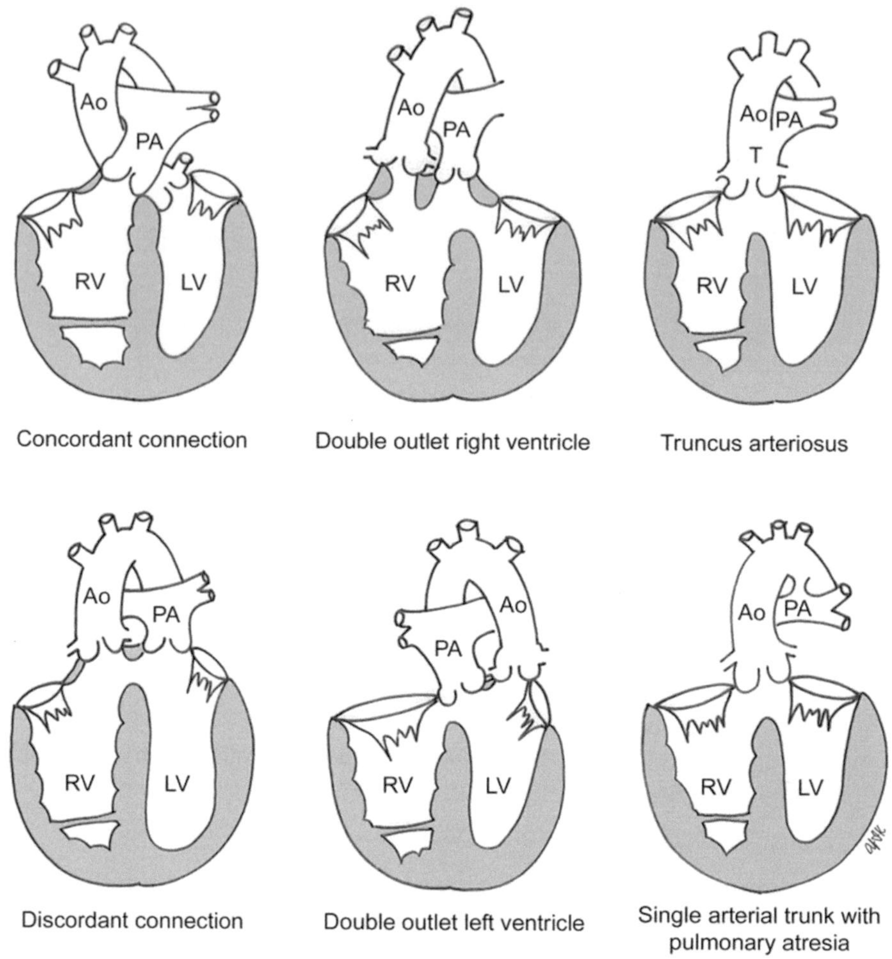

Fig. 10 Types of ventriculo-arterial connections

  - Right aortic arch: arch runs to the right of the trachea; most commonly gives rise to right brachiocephalic artery, right common carotid artery and right subclavian artery which is referred to as “mirror image branching”.
- Systemic and pulmonary venous connections.
  - Normal systemic venous connections: the caval veins are connected to the RA. A left superior vena cava connected to the coronary sinus may be considered a normal variant.

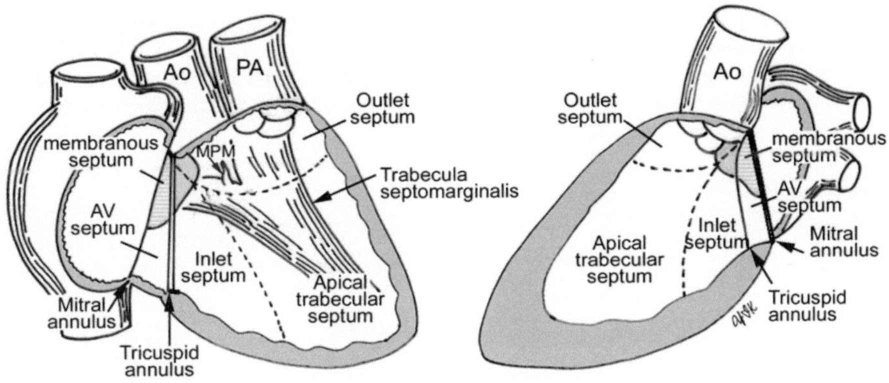

Fig. 11 Regions of the ventricular septum

- All 4 pulmonary veins are normally connected to the LA. Virtually any combinations of abnormal pulmonary venous connections are possible with connections to the systemic venous return, coronary sinus or directly to the right atrium.

- Inter-atrial and interventricular communications (Fig. 11).
- Patent ductus arteriosus.
- Coronary artery anatomy. The Leiden Convention provides a simple an unequivocal approach that is applicable in the setting of transposed or malposed great vessels whereby the examiner imagines the surgeon standing in the non-coronary aortic valve cusp, facing the pulmonary trunk. To their right is sinus 1 and to their left is sinus 2.
  - Normally related great arteries:

    Left aortic valve sinus (sinus 2) usually gives rise to the left main coronary artery which bifurcates into the left anterior descending and circumflex coronary arteries
    Right aortic sinus (sinus 1): usually give rise to the right coronary artery

  - Describe the positions of the ostia and the course of the proximal coronary arteries.

Bibliography

1. Ed. Wernovsky G, Anderson RH, Krishna K, Redington A, Twedell JS, Tretter J. Anderson's Pediatric cardiology, 4th ed. Philadelphia PA: Elsevier; 2020.
2. Gittenberger-de Groot AC, Sauer U, Oppenheimer-Dekker A, Quaegebeur J. Coronary arterial anatomy in transposition of the great arteries: a morphologic study. Pediatr Cardiol. 1983;4:15–24.

3. Jacobs JP, Franklin RCG, Beland MJ, et al. Nomenclature for pediatric and congenital cardiac care: unification of clinical and administrative nomenclature—The 2021 international paediatric and congenital cardiac code (IPCCC) and the eleventh revision of the international classification of diseases (ICD-11). World J Pediatric Congenital Heart Surgery. 2021;12(5):E1–18.

Atrial Septal Defects (ASD)

Shuhua Luo and Christoph Haller

Abstract Interatrial communications are common congenital cardiac defects that range from clinically insignificant to hemodynamically important lesions with symptoms of right heart overload which are life-shortening if not closed. There are four main anatomical types (in order of frequency): secundum ASD, sinus venosus defect, primum defect and undroofed coronary sinus. ASDs commonly occur in association with other cardiac defects. Surgery is indicated if the resulting Qp/Qs is > 1.5 or there is progressive RV volume loading. If the anatomy is suitable, device closure by interventional catheter is preferred – but is mainly limited to secundum defects. Most other significant defects require surgical repair involving different patching techniques that ensure adequate separation of left and right atrium and rerouting of venous return, as well as correcting any associated lesions. Defects in older patients need careful evaluation to assess a patient's operability. Surgical risk is very low and returns life expectancy to that of the normal population.

Keywords Atrial septal defect · ASD · Primum · Secundum · Sinus venosus · Unroofed coronary sinus · Common atrium

Abbreviations

ASD	Atrial septal defect
AV	Atrioventricular
CT	Computed tomography
CXR	Chest X-ray
ECG	Electrocardiogram

S. Luo
Department of Cardiovascular Surgery, West China Hospital, Sichuan University, Chengdu, Sichuan, China

C. Haller (✉)
Division of Cardiovascular Surgery, Labatt Family Heart Centre, Department of Surgery, The Hospital for Sick Children, University of Toronto, Toronto, ON, Canada
e-mail: christoph.haller@sickkids.ca

© The Author(s), under exclusive license to Springer Nature Switzerland AG 2024

A. I. Dipchand et al. (eds.), *Manual of Cardiac Care in Children*,
https://doi.org/10.1007/978-3-031-70973-9_2

IVC	Inferior vena cava
LSVC	Left SVC
MRI	Magnetic resonance imaging
PAPVD	Partial anomalous pulmonary venous drainage
PFO	Persistent foramen ovale
Qp	Pulmonary blood flow
Qs	Systemic blood flow
RA	Right atrium
SVC	Superior vena cava

Key Points

- Common congenital heart lesion. Incidence 1 to 2 per thousand live births.
- ASD with $Qp/Qs > 1.5$ is indicated to undergo repair
- Elective repair at 3–5 years of life, earlier if important symptoms are present
- Primarily diagnosed by echocardiography.
- Associated pulmonary venous anomalies can be further evaluated by MRI, CT, or catheterization.
- Sinus venosus defect, primum defect, and unroofed coronary sinus need surgical closure. Many Secundum defects may be suitable for catheter-based repair
- Results of ASD closure in the modern era are excellent

1 Nomenclature

An atrial septal defect (ASD) is defined as an opening, or hole, in the interatrial septum. In a broader sense, defects that lead to shunting at the atrial level may be referred to as atrial septal defects, although they do not necessarily involve the anatomic atrial septum (e.g. sinus venosus defects or unroofed coronary sinus) and should more appropriately be termed interatrial communications.

There are 6 types of interatrial communications (Fig. 1):

- Secundum ASD
- Vestibular ASD
- Sinus venosus defect
- Primum defect (also called partial atrio-ventricular septal defect, see Chapter "Partial Atrioventricular Septal Defect")
- Coronary sinus defect
- Common atrium

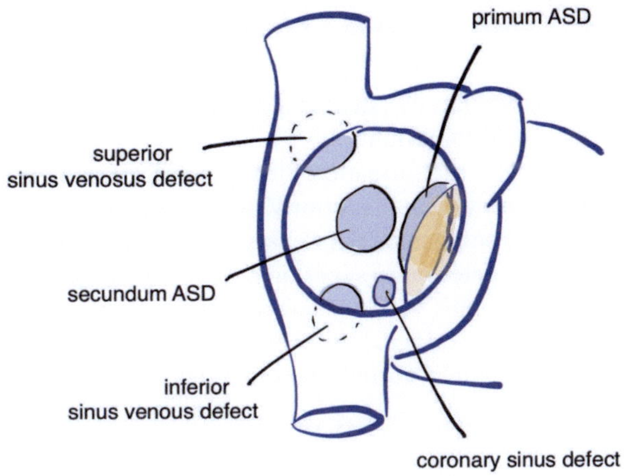

Fig. 1 Anatomic locations of various types of defects resulting in atrial level shunting

2 Anatomy

2.1 Persistent Foramen Ovale

- The lack of fusion between the septum primum and septum secundum.
- A PFO is usually a flap valve and so not usually associated with left-to-right shunting unless the opening becomes stretched. PFOs are not generally classified as true ASDs.

2.2 Secundum ASD

- One or several defects within the fossa ovalis (i.e. septum primum).
- May vary in size from a miniscule perforation to large opening with essentially no inferior rim.

2.3 Vestibular ASD

- Vestibular defects are located in the muscular antero-inferior rim of the fossa ovalis.

2.4 *Sinus Venosus Defect*

- Most commonly situated at the junction between the superior vena cava (SVC) and the right atrium.
- Complex malformation involving displacement of some of the right-sided pulmonary veins anteriorly, and superiorly, allowing for left to right shunting (partial anomalous pulmonary venous drainage). Often drain into the distal SVC but can enter more superiorly.
- Inferior sinus venosus defects are very rare - occur adjacent to the inferior vena cava (IVC) orifice. IVC override and anomalous pulmonary venous drainage may be an effect of normal anatomic relations rather than true abnormal connections.

2.5 *Unroofed Coronary Sinus*

- Deficiency of the tissue separating the coronary sinus from the left atrium (unroofed coronary sinus). Thus, the coronary sinus opening becomes a communication between left and right atria.
- The coronary sinus blood drains into the left atrium, but this is not usually sufficient volume to create any detectable desaturation.
- However, if associated with persistence of a left-sided superior vena cava then there will be a large right-to-left shunt created by this large volume of systemic venous blood entering the left atrium, causing clinical cyanosis.

2.6 *Common Atrium*

- Completely absent atrial septum creating a large common chamber.

3 Embryology

- Septum primum begins to develop at the roof of the atrium, growing toward the endocardial cushions of the developing atrioventricular valves.
- While the septum primum closes, new perforations form in its superior part giving rise to the foramen secundum (i.e. foramen ovale).
- To the right of the septum primum, the septum secundum forms as an invagination of the atrial wall.
- Secundum ASD results from excessive apoptosis of the cephalic portion of the septum primum or incomplete development of the septum secundum.

4 Epidemiology

4.1 Incidence/Prevalence

- Interatrial communications are the second most common type of congenital heart defect, with an estimated incidence 100 per 100,000 livebirths.
- Secundum defects account for 80–90% of ASDs.(2)
- The other types of interatrial communications occur far less frequently: sinus venosus defects (5–10% of interatrial communications), primum ASDs (3–4%) and coronary sinus defects (1%).
- Interatrial communications can also occur in conjunction with more significant congenital heart defects.

4.2 Population at Risk, Inheritance

- Usually sporadically occurring, but autosomal dominant inheritance has rarely been reported.
- Secundum ASDs are more frequent in female patients (2–3:1 female:male ratio).

5 Clinical Physiology and Presentation

The direction and magnitude of shunting at the atrial level is determined by the size of the defect and by the compliance of the ventricles. Shunting across the septum is mainly diastolic and a consequence of the lesser compliance of the left ventricle if there are no associated lesions.

- In children, interatrial communications are usually diagnosed incidentally.
- Symptoms may be absent throughout childhood.
- Exercise intolerance is uncommon in young children. The frequency of exercise intolerance increases insidiously with age.
- Palpitations from atrial flutter or atrial fibrillation may occur later in life, incidences of which increase with age.
- A subtle systolic ejection murmur audible over the pulmonary artery reflecting high flow across the pulmonary valve.
- Wide and fixed splitting of the second heart sound, because pulmonary valve closure is delayed.
- Shunting may increase with age due to decreasing compliance of the left ventricle.
- Large, longstanding interatrial communications with relatively low Qp/Qs should raise concerns of associated pulmonary hypertension.

5.1 Natural History

- Patients with interatrial communications are at risk of right ventricular volume overload with eventual dysfunction and congestive heart failure. They do not usually cause raised pulmonary vascular resistance (pulmonary hypertension), but the two conditions can co-exist, in which case cyanosis can eventually occur.
- Untreated large secundum defects are associated with a reduced lifespan.
- Progression is slow. Patients remain asymptomatic until late in the disease's course.
- Spontaneous closure occurs frequently in small defects (4–5 mm), but seldom in defects larger than 10 mm. Defects very rarely close after the first year of life.

6 Associated Lesions

6.1 Common

- PAPVD
- Left superior vena cava

6.2 Less Common Associations

- Ventricular septal defect
- Patent ductus arteriosus
- Coarctation of aorta

7 Diagnostic Studies

7.1 ECG

- Can be within normal limits.
- Tall P wave indicative of right atrial enlargement.
- Incomplete right bundle branch block pattern, and right axis deviation.
- The rhythm is typically sinus, but in adult patients can be atrial flutter or fibrillation

7.2 CXR

- Enlarged main pulmonary artery and right atrium.

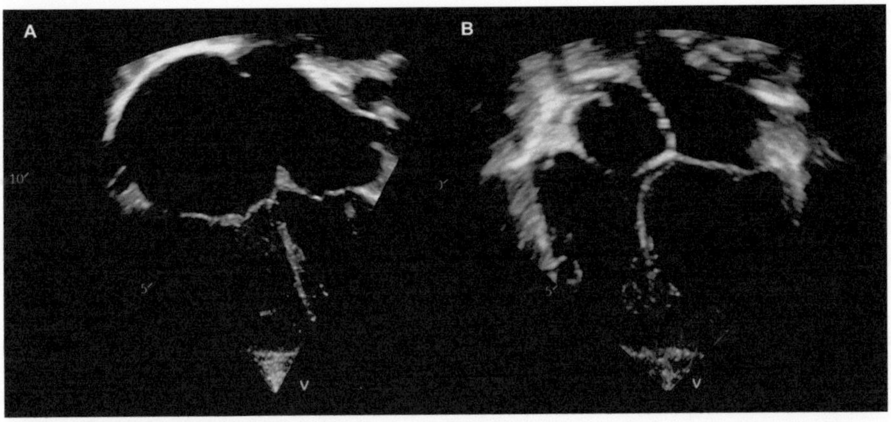

Fig. 2 Echocardiographic image of a large secundum ASD before (A) and after (B) surgical patch closure

- The lung fields are plethoric.

7.3 *Echocardiography*

- The most common and widely used diagnostic technique.
- Two-dimensional imaging with color Doppler flow mapping depicts the location and size of the defect and the direction of flow.
- Delineation of degree of right ventricular volume overload.
- Degree of tricuspid valve regurgitation.
- Assessment of right-sided pressures (i.e. right ventricular systolic pressure).
- Fig. 2 shows echocardiographic images before and after surgical repair of a secundum ASD.

7.4 *MRI*

- Anatomic detailing of PAPVD if necessary.
- Calculation of Qp/Qs.

7.5 *CT*

- Diagnostic value limited – may help with unusual anomalous veins
- CT is 2nd choice for cross-sectional imaging.

7.6 Cardiac Catheterization

- Performed if there is a question of operability of patients with associated pulmonary hypertension.
- Calculations of Qp/Qs in patients with isolated PAPVD of only parts of one lung.

8 Indications for Intervention / Surgery

- Interatrial communications with Qp/Qs > 1.5 or presence of enlargement of right heart structures.
- If anatomically suitable, catheter intervention with device closure preferred.
- Surgical patch closure if large defect, associated lesions necessitating repair, or anatomic characteristics prohibitive for interventional closure.
- Minimally invasive closure possible in majority of surgical candidates.

9 Timing of Intervention and Management Strategy

- Elective repair at 3–5 years of life.
- Repair earlier if important symptoms are present.

10 Surgical/Interventional Strategy

10.1 Secundum ASD (Fig. 2)

- Transcatheter ASD device closure can be performed safely with a high success rate and low morbidity. It has become the standard approach to ASD closure in patients with suitable anatomy (see Fig. 3).
- Deficient rims or very large defects may be unsuitable for catheter-based approaches.
- Small to moderately sized ASDs with a septum primum flap can be closed by direct suture.
- Large ASDs with a deficient rim of the fossa ovalis can be closed with an autologous pericardial patch, which avoids distortion or undue tension on the margins. Other patch materials such as xenograft pericardium is an alternative.

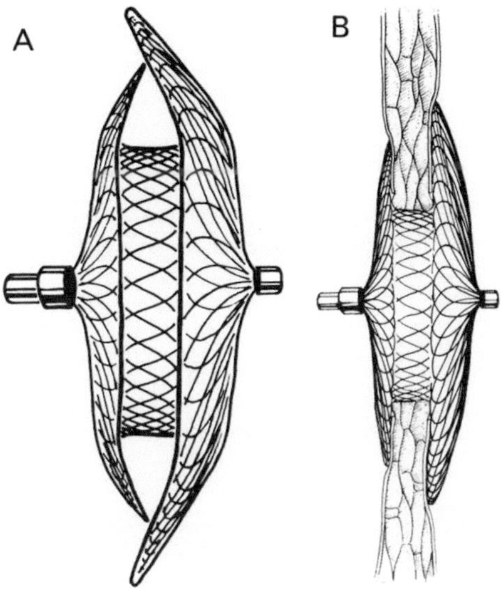

Fig. 3 Original Amplatzer transcatheter device for secundum ASD. A. Inward angulation of retention discs and smaller right atrial disc. B. Direct stenting with the central waist and Dacron-augmented secondary thrombosis accomplish closure

10.2 Sinus Venosus Defect (Fig. 4)

- If no PAPVD to SVC, single patch technique similar to standard ASD closures is employed.
- If PAPVD coexists with the sinus venosus defect, the atrial incision is extended up into the root of the SVC. The veins are rerouted with an autologous pericardial patch to the defect, thereby separating left atrium and pulmonary veins from the right atrium. A second patch on the outer aspect of the SVC-RA junction is commonly used to ensure unobstructed flow. An alternative is to perform a V–Y plasty in closing the incision to widen the RA/SVC junction.
- If anomalous pulmonary veins enter the SVC distant to the SVC-RA junction, the Warden operation (division of the SVC superiorly to the pulmonary vein inflow and reconnection with the right atrial appendage) may be used because of concerns about the potential for sinus node dysfunction and SVC obstruction (Fig. 4).

10.3 Unroofed Coronary sinus

- Because unroofed coronary sinus defects are close to the AV node, patch closure is suggested.
- If there is an LSVC then the repair must also ensure LSVC drainage back to the RA. This can be achieved by creating a baffle to reconstruct a roof of the coronary sinus. An alternative approach is to disconnect the LSVC and connect it directly to the RA appendage if this can be achieved without tension.

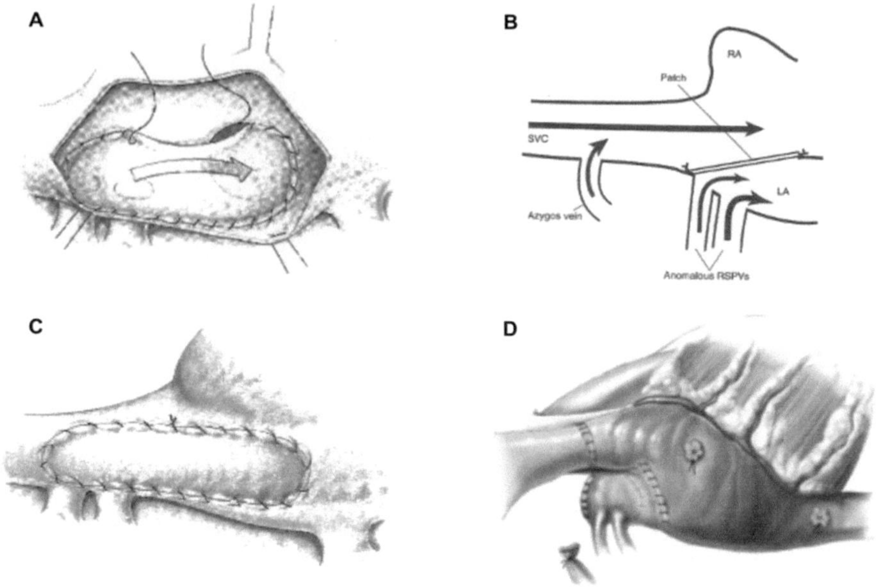

Fig. 4 Surgical correction of sinus venosus defect. A. Pericardial baffle to reroute associated anomalous pulmonary veins and close the interatrial communication. Reprinted from Stark et al., with permission from Wiley. B. Cross-sectional view of systemic and pulmonary venous drainage after placement of the atrial septal baffle. Reprinted from Backer et al., with permission from Wiley. C. Patch enlargement of SVC-RA junction. Reprinted from Stark et al., with permission from Wiley. D. Warden repair. Reprinted from Cardiac Surgery, Alexi-Meskhishvili et al. with permission from Springer Nature

11 Intensive Care Physiology and Management

- Most patients can be extubated in the operating room or shortly thereafter.
- No need for intensive care management postoperatively except for a short monitoring period with a subsequent return to an inpatient ward in 4–6 h.
- Usually suitable for early discharge (often within 48 h).

12 Outcome

- Early mortality for repair of interatrial communications has approached 0%.
- Post cardiotomy syndrome is a rare but relevant cause for postoperative morbidity in isolated patients and necessitates echocardiographic follow-up (1, 3 and 6 weeks postoperatively).
- Long-term survival of patients with interatrial communications or PAPVD repaired during the first few years of life is that of the matched general population.

13 Alternative Strategies and Controversies

13.1 Alternative Approaches

The traditional surgical technique for interatrial communications closure is through a median sternotomy approach. Minimally invasive techniques are commonly used.

- Transcatheter ASD closure can be performed safely with a high success rate and low morbidity. It has become the standard approach to secundum ASD closure in patients with suitable anatomy.
- Limited lower sternotomy, anterolateral thoracotomy, or lateral thoracotomy can be used as more cosmetic strategies.
- Full minimally invasive techniques with or without peripheral cannulation and small axillary incisions are also now being used.

13.2 Controversies

- The role of interatrial communication closure in the setting of pulmonary hypertension. If Qp:Qs is still raised then closure may still be indicated but a fenestrated patch closure is recommended.
- The benefit in older adults needs to be carefully assessed pre-operatively.

Bibliography

1. Alexi-Meskhishvili V, Unbehaun A, Hetzer R. Aanomalous pulmonary venous connections and congenital defects of the atria, the atrioventricular septum and the atrioventricular valves. 2017. P. 299–423
2. Backer CL, Mavroudis C, Idriss RF. Pediatric, 4th ed. 2012.
3. Gupta S, McEwen C, Eqbal A, Haller C. Minimally invasive surgery for congenital heart disease. Ann Thorac Surg. 2024;118(4):953–62.
4. Jozef M, Gavora P, Podnar T. Long-term outcome of transcatheter secundum-type atrial septal defect closure using amplatzer septal occluders. J Am Coll Cardiol. 2005;45(4):505–7.
5. Rojas CA, El-Sherief A, Medina HM, et al. Embryology and developmental defects of the interatrial septum. Am J Roentgenol. 2010;195(5):1100–4.
6. Stark JF, de Leval MR, Courtney M, Tsang VT. Surgery for congenital heart defects, 3rd ed. 2006
7. Yoo SJ, Lee S, de la Mora R, et al. New insights into sinus venosus defects from cross-sectional imaging. Congenit Heart Dis. 2022;17(1):5–23.
8. Webb G, Gatzoulis M. Atrial septal defects in the adult: recent progress and overview. Circulation. 2006;114(15):1645–53.

Partially Anomalous Pulmonary Venous Connection (PAPVC)

Shuhua Luo and Christoph Haller

Abstract Partially anomalous pulmonary venous connection (PAPVC) comprises any abnormal drainage of the pulmonary veins to either a systemic vein or the right atrium while at least one pulmonary vein drains normally to the left atrium. Surgical correction is advocated if resulting Qp/Qs is > 1.8, if all pulmonary venous return of one lung drains anomalously, or if the pulmonary venous pathway is obstructed or at risk (as in scimitar syndrome). Right-sided anomalous pulmonary veins are commonly rerouted with intracardiac baffles across the atrial septum. Left-sided anomalous pulmonary veins are usually directly anastomosed to an incision in the left atrial appendage. Surgical mortality and morbidity are low but the procedure carries the risk of anastomotic stenosis (including SVC stenosis) or complete occlusion. Lifelong follow-up is recommended.

Keywords Partial anomalous pulmonary venous drainage · PAPVD · Partial anomalous pulmonary venous connection · PAPVC · Partial anomalous pulmonary venous return · PAPVR · Scimitar syndrome

Abbreviations

ASD	Atrial septal defect
CT	Computed tomography
IVC	Inferior vena cava
LA	Left atrium
MRI	Magnetic resonance imaging
PAPVC	Partial anomalous pulmonary venous connection

S. Luo
Department of Cardiovascular Surgery, West China Hospital, Sichuan University, Chengdu, Sichuan, China

C. Haller (✉)
Division of Cardiovascular Surgery, Labatt Family Heart Centre, Department of Surgery, The Hospital for Sick Children, University of Toronto, Toronto, ON, Canada
e-mail: christoph.haller@sickkids.ca

© The Author(s), under exclusive license to Springer Nature Switzerland AG 2024

A. I. Dipchand et al. (eds.), *Manual of Cardiac Care in Children*,
https://doi.org/10.1007/978-3-031-70973-9_3

PFO	Persistent foramen ovale
Qp	Pulmonary blood flow
Qs	Systemic blood flow
RA	Right atrium
RV	Right ventricle
SVASD	Sinus venosus atrial septal defect
SVC	Superior vena cava

Key Points

- Rare congenital heart defect.
- PAPVD with Qp/Qs > 1.8 is indicated to undergo repair if low procedural risk.
- Elective repair at 3–5 years of life.
- Primarily diagnosed by echocardiography.
- CT or MRI may be necessary if high entrance of pulmonary veins into superior caval veins, in anomalously draining left pulmonary veins, and for scimitar syndrome.
- Anomalously draining right-sided pulmonary veins are commonly routed across the atrial septum within the right atrium with or without additional patch enlargement of the systemic venous pathway.
- Anomalously draining left-sided pulmonary veins are commonly directly anastomosed to the left atrial appendage.
- Surgical results are very good but are mixed for scimitar syndrome.
- Postoperative risk of pulmonary vein stenosis necessitates long-term follow-up.

1 Nomenclature

- Partially anomalous pulmonary venous connection (PAPVC) comprises any abnormal drainage of the pulmonary veins to either a systemic vein or the right atrium (RA) while at least one pulmonary vein drains normally to the left atrium (LA).
- Many variations are possible ranging from isolated anomalous drainage of a single pulmonary vein to a mixed pattern of pulmonary venous drainage to different systemic venous components.

2 Anatomy

2.1 Isolated Right-Sided PAPVC

- Can affect one or all right-sided pulmonary veins.
- Drainage most commonly to SVC with variable distance to RA, but direct connection to RA can occur (commonly occurs in association with sinus venous defect, see Chapter 2)
- Drainage to IVC is referred to as scimitar syndrome.

2.2 Scimitar Syndrome

- All or part of right-sided pulmonary veins drain to subdiaphragmatic portion of IVC. The dilated channel creates a characteristic curved shadow on CXR next to the RA said to resemble a scimitar.
- Associated with sequestration of segments and hypoplasia of the right lung (and right pulmonary artery) as well as abnormal arterial supply to the right lung.

2.3 Isolated Left-Sided PAPVC

- Very rare. Can affect one or all left-sided pulmonary veins.
- Drainage most commonly to innominate vein via vertical vein or remnant left persistent SVC but can also drain to coronary sinus.

2.4 Mixed PAPVC

- Although rare, any combination of anomalous pulmonary venous return may occur (Fig. 1).

2.5 Embryology

- Incomplete connection of the common pulmonary vein to splanchnic plexus leaves parts of the intraparenchymal pulmonary venous plexus disconnected.
- These parts of the intraparenchymal pulmonary venous plexus retain their communication with the systemic venous plexus.

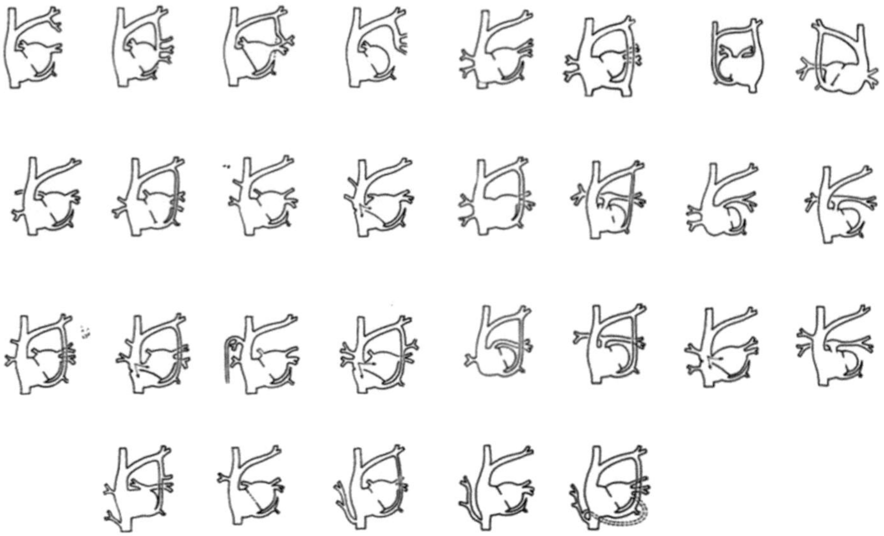

Fig. 1 Various types of partial anomalous pulmonary venous drainage. Reprinted from Snellen et al.

3 Epidemiology

3.1 Incidence/Prevalence

- Rare congenital cardiac defect (0.4–0.7%)
- Right-sided anomalous connections most common.
- Mixed bilateral partial anomalous connections are very rare.

3.2 Population at Risk, Inheritance

- Usually sporadically occurring, but associations with genetic syndromes have been found.
- Associate with heterotaxy / isomerism.

4 Clinical Physiology and Presentation

- Magnitude of left–right shunting is proportional to the lung segments draining incorrectly.
- Variability is introduced if an interatrial septal communication is present.

- In isolated PAPVD, shunting is not expected to change as a reflection of changes in ventricular compliance (as seen in ASDs).
- PAPVD is usually diagnosed incidentally.
- Most patients are asymptomatic, but longstanding disease or large shunt volume can present with general signs of heart failure. Scimitar may present with recurrent fevers or chest infections related to abnormal or sequestered segments.
- Atrial arrhythmia can occur with increasing enlargement of the right-sided chambers.
- Pulmonary hypertension is rare but has been reported even in isolated PAPVD.

5 Natural History

- Disease course relatively constant. Q_p:Q_s to remain stable over time.
- Patients can develop pulmonary hypertension even in isolated PAPVD.
- Risk of death if one lung is abnormally draining entirely if the normally connected lung is compromised.
- Scimitar syndrome is associated with significant mortality in infants, especially if associated with stenosis of the left sided veins to the LA. The course is much milder in older patients.

6 Associated Lesions

6.1 Common

- ASD / PFO
- SVASD

6.2 Less Common Associations

- Mitral valve abnormalities

7 Diagnostic Studies

7.1 ECG

- Can be within normal limits.
- Tall P wave indicative of right atrial enlargement if larger shunt.

7.2 CXR

- Depending on amount of shunting, signs of right heart enlargement and increased pulmonary vascularity.

7.3 Echocardiography

- Mainstay of diagnostic workup.
- High entrance of pulmonary veins into SVC or innominate vein may be difficult to visualize.
- Delineation of degree of RV volume overload.
- Degree of tricuspid valve regurgitation.
- Assessment of right-sided pressures (i.e., right ventricular systolic pressure).

7.4 MRI

- Anatomic details, especially if the exact position and course of pulmonary veins is unclear (Fig. 2)
- Calculation of Qp/Qs.

7.5 CT

- Diagnostic value limited.
- CT is 2nd choice for cross-sectional imaging.

7.6 Cardiac Catheterization

- Rarely indicated. May be helpful in scimitar syndrome to measure pulmonary venous saturations, and occasionally to embolize redundant aorta-pulmonary arterial connections.

8 Indications for Intervention/Surgery

- Q_p:Q_s > 1.5 (some centres accept > 1.8)
- Isolated uncomplicated PAPVD with Q_p:Q_s < 1.5 not indicated for correction.

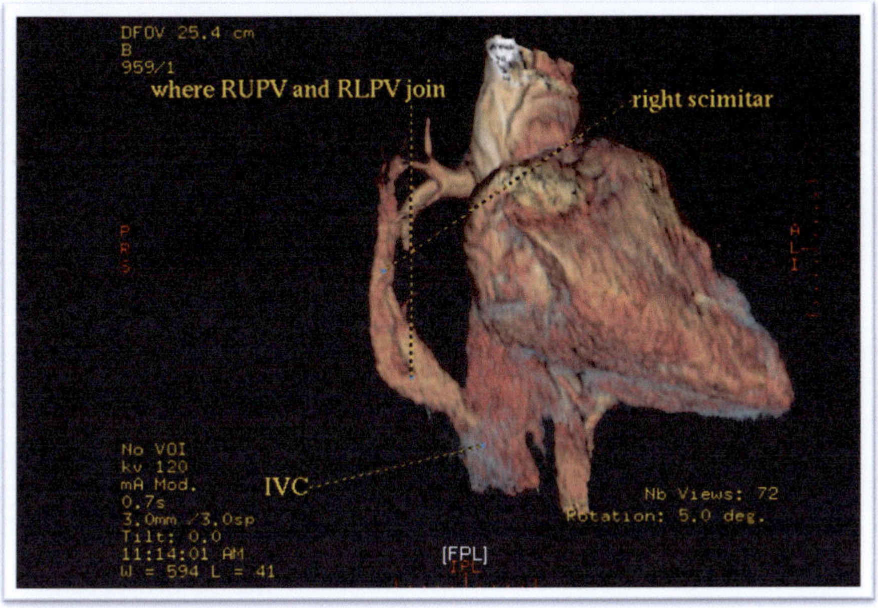

Fig. 2 MRI Image showing Scimitar Syndrome

- Scimitar syndrome needs careful assessment, including Q_p:Q_s, any obstruction of the draining vein as well as associated abnormalities in the right lung (sequestration) and arterial supply.
- Abnormal drainage of one entire lung is usually an indication for correction irrespective of calculated Q_p:Q_s.

9 Timing of Intervention and Management Strategy

- Elective repair at 3–5 years of life or once diagnosed.
- Repair earlier if important symptoms are present.

10 Surgical Strategy

10.1 Right-Sided PAPVD

- Anomalous veins commonly rerouted by an autologous pericardial patch across a preexisting or intentionally created ASD (Fig. 3).

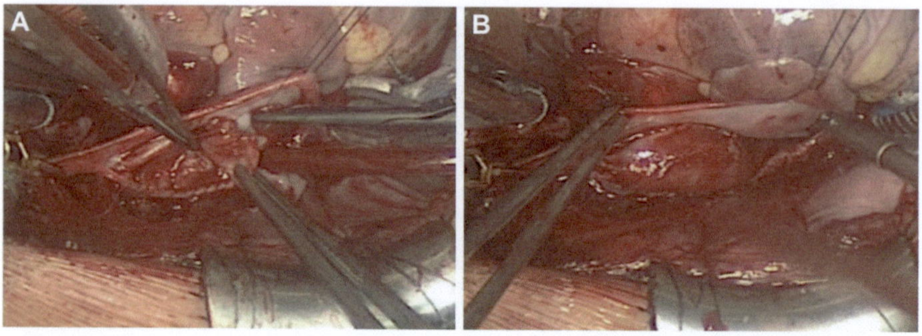

Fig. 3 Rerouting of PAPVD of the right upper pulmonary veins with an autologous pericardial patch. A. Pericardial patch placement. B. Distended patch after deairing of the left heart

- Additional patching of the RA or SVC-RA junction may be necessary to ensure unobstructed systemic venous return.
- As described for sinus venosus defects, high entrance into the SVC may be addressed with a Warden procedure (see Chapter 2).

10.2 Left-Sided PAPVD

- Vein is divided at the level of the vertical draining vein, leaving enough length to connect without tension to the left atrium.
- Wide direct anastomosis of the pulmonary vein to the broadly incised left atrial appendage.
- Risk of anastomotic stenosis. In older/adult patients, use of a Goretex graft may reduce risk of anastomotic stricture.
- If draining to the coronary sinus, techniques used in unroofed coronary sinus corrections may be applicable.

10.3 Scimitar Syndrome

- Baffle within IVC across the atrial septum
- Direct anastomosis with LA or interposition grafts have been used and may reduce risk of creating an obstructed baffled pathway.
- High risk of obstruction post repair.
- Resection of lung sequester may be necessary.
- Important to assess left sided pulmonary veins as associated stenosis of these veins carries a very bad prognosis.

11 Intensive Care Physiology and Management

- Extubation in the operating room feasible in most patients.
- No need for intensive care management postoperatively except for a short monitoring period.
- Usually short hospital stay (a few days).

12 Outcome

- Early mortality for uncomplicated PAPVD approaches 0%.
- Scimitar syndrome, if addressed in infancy, is associated with high mortality after repair (~30%). Elective repair in older age groups has better prognosis but risk of baffle obstruction.
- Long-term survival is good.
- Increased risk of pulmonary venous obstruction if direct anastomosis to left atrium or Scimitar syndrome.
- Simple PAPVD has excellent late outcomes. Scimitar or complex baffles to the vena cavae have risk of obstruction and need repeated imaging

13 Alternative Strategies and Controversies

Most right-sided PAPVD can be addressed minimally invasively.

Bibliography

1. Bahaaldin A, Cai S, Van Arsdell G, et al. Outcomes after surgical treatment of children with partial anomalous pulmonary venous connection. Ann Thorac Surg. 2007;84(6):2020–6. https://doi.org/10.1016/j.athoracsur.2007.05.046.
2. Gupta S, McEwen C, Eqbal A, Haller C. Minimally invasive surgery for congenital heart disease. Ann Thor Surg. 2024;118(4):953–962. https://doi.org/10.1016/j.athoracsur.2023.11.032
3. Hanjay W, Kalfa D, Rosenbaum M, et al. Scimitar syndrome in children and adults: natural history, outcomes, and risk analysis. Ann Thorac Surg. 2018;105(2):592–8. https://doi.org/10.1016/j.athoracsur.2017.06.061.
4. Snellen HA, Ingen HC, Hoefsmit EChM. Patterns of Anomalous Pulmonary Venous Drainage. Circulation. 1968;38(1):45–63. https://doi.org/10.1161/01.CIR.38.1.45.

Ventricular Septal Defects (VSD)

Bahaaldin Alsoufi

Abstract Ventricular septal defect (VSD) is the most common congenital cardiac defect, found in 25–30% of all congenital heart disease. VSDs vary in location, size and number, and can be associated with additional intra and extra cardiac anomalies. Muscular VSDs are commonest, but perimembranous VSDs are the commonest variant needing surgical closure. The need for intervention depends on the size and location of the VSD. Small VSDs that might close spontaneously are treated conservatively. Large VSDs usually require closure in the first 6 months of life to manage heart failure. Moderate size VSDs are closed if associated with significant increased pulmonary blood flow, complications such as aortic insufficiency or double chambered right ventricle. Untreated large VSDs can lead to development of pulmonary hypertension. Outcomes of surgical VSD closure are generally good with low perioperative mortality and excellent long-term survival. Hybrid and interventional therapies are available in selected cases.

Keywords VSD · Ventricular septal defect · Perimembranous VSD · Inlet VSD · Outlet VSD · Doubly committed VSD · Muscular VSD · Subpulmonary VSD · Subaortic VSD

Abbreviations

AI	Aortic insufficiency
AoV	Aortic valve
AVSD	Atrioventricular septal defect
DORV	Double outlet right ventricle
IAA	Interrupted aortic arch
iNO	Inhaled nitric oxide
PDA	Persistent ductus arteriosus

B. Alsoufi (✉)
Department of Cardiothoracic Surgery, University of Louisville, Louisville, KY, USA
e-mail: balsoufi@hotmail.com

© The Author(s), under exclusive license to Springer Nature Switzerland AG 2024

A. I. Dipchand et al. (eds.), *Manual of Cardiac Care in Children*,
https://doi.org/10.1007/978-3-031-70973-9_4

Qp	Pulmonary blood flow
Qs	Systemic blood flow
TGA	Transposition of the great arteries
TOF	Tetralogy of Fallot
VSD	Ventricular septal defect

Key Points

- Ventricular septal defect (VSD) is the most common congenital cardiac defect.
- Variable in position, size and number
- VSD closure is mandated if
  - Unlikely to close spontaneously (size, location, age)
  - Signs of heart failure
  - Significantly increased pulmonary blood flow (Qp/Qs > 2.0)
  - Associated Aortic valve insufficiency
- Low perioperative mortality and excellent long-term survival.
- Hybrid and interventional therapies are available in selected cases.

1 Embryology

- Septation of the ventricles starts around 5th week and ends around 7th week of gestation.
- The septum is formed from endocardial cushions, the infolding of the ventricular muscle (muscular septum), and the bulbar ridges septating the arterial trunk.
- Failure of the formation or interaction of those components results in VSD formation.
- The interventricular septum is a complex non-planar structure that has can be divided into three components when viewed from the right ventricle:
  - Inlet septum
  - Apical trabecular septum
  - Outlet septum
- The membranous septum is found at the crux of the heart where the inlet and outlet components meet, in direct continuity with the tricuspid and aortic valves, Any VSD that involves the membranous septum is called ‘perimembranous’.

2 Anatomy (Fig. 1)

- The definition of a ventricular septal defect (VSD) is an opening in the interventricular septum connecting the two ventricles.
- There are variations in:
  - Size.
  - Location in the septum.
  - Number (single or multiple).
  - Associated lesions (intracardiac or extracardiac).
- Several terminologies have been used to categorize VSD types according to anatomic location.
- Various classification schemes were developed and traditionally assigned the VSD into one of four anatomic types as used in the Society of Thoracic Surgeons unified nomenclature system: (Percentages refer to the distribution within VSDs undergoing surgical closure)
  - Type I VSD Doubly-Committed (5–10%)

    Also called juxtaarterial, conal, supracristal or infundibular VSD.
    Located in the infundibular portion of the right ventricular outflow tract, above the crista supraventricularis, underneath the pulmonary valve and adjacent to the right coronary cusp of the aortic valve. (Thus, the aortic and pulmonary valves are in direct fibrous continuity)
    Higher incidence in Asians (approximately 30%).
  - Type II VSD Perimembranous VSD (65–70%)

Fig. 1 Types of VSDs

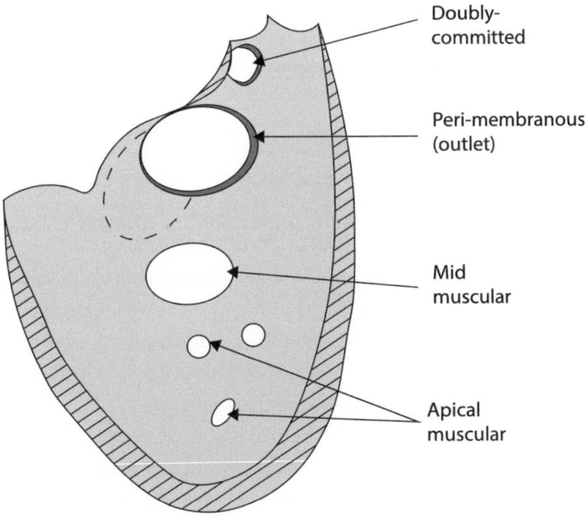

Also called perimembranous, conoventricular or paramembranous VSD.
Located contiguous to the membranous portion of the ventricular septum, below the crista supraventricularis, adjacent to the aortic valve and the septal leaflet of the tricuspid valve.

- Type III VSD Atrio-ventricular Septal Defect (5%)

  Also called inlet or atrioventricular canal VSD.
  Located posteriorly at the inlet portion of the ventricular septum, adjacent to the septal leaflet of the tricuspid valve.

- Type IV VSD Muscular VSD (10–20%)

  Also called muscular VSD.
  Can include a variety of single and multiple defects that are located in the muscular septum (categorized as anterior, posterior, midventricular or apical). These VSDs can be in the inlet or outlet and are characterized by having a perimeter which is entirely muscular.
  Swiss cheese septum is vaguely defined as the presence of 4 or more muscular VSDs, usually predominantly in the apical trabecular septum.

3 Epidemiology

- Isolated VSD (not part of another major congenital cardiac anomaly) occurs in approximately 2/1000 live births and constitutes > 25% of all congenital cardiac defects.
- Most common congenital cardiac anomaly.

4 Associated Lesions

- VSDs are often part of a more complex cardiac lesion such as TOF, TGA, truncus arteriosus, IAA, AVSD, DORV, single ventricles.
- Additional sites for left to right shunt such as PDA and ASDs might be present in more than 25% of infants with VSD.
- Coarctation of the aorta with or without hypoplasia of the aortic arch is present in 5–10% of patients.
- The VSDs in some of these lesions (e.g. TOF or coarctation/VSD) can have malalignment of the edges of the defect, which leads to the possibility of outflow tract obstruction with closure.
- Additional left sided lesions such as aortic stenosis, mitral valve hypoplasia can be present in about 2% of patients for each.

5 Clinical Physiology and Presentation

- Significant left to right shunt is uncommon in first 4–6 weeks of life due to elevated pulmonary vascular resistance.
- As the pulmonary vascular resistance drops, left to right shunt increases.
- Infants with significant left to right shunt develop symptoms and signs of congestive heart failure (e.g. tachypnea, tachycardia, indrawing, sweatiness, difficulty feeding, failure to thrive etc.).
- Small VSDs tend to get smaller (especially type II or IV) and with small shunt across the defect, they might be identifiable by murmur only.
- A significant left to right shunt that is not repaired can lead to pulmonary vascular disease. Over years, this may become irreversible and can reverse flow across the VSD resulting in cyanosis and development of Eisenmenger syndrome.
- Prolapse of the aortic cusps into the VSD may decrease shunting but result in aortic regurgitation. In type II VSDs, about 12% develop aortic cusp prolapse and 7% develop aortic regurgitation. In type I VSDs, almost 40% of VSDs will develop aortic prolapse with some aortic regurgitation.
- The chronic left to right shunt can lead to ventricular hypertrophy in the right ventricular outflow tract with infundibular stenosis (right ventricular muscle bundles) in 5–10% of patients, and in the extreme cases, development of double chamber right ventricle.

6 Natural History

- Spontaneous closure depends on the age, size and type of VSD.
  - 80% of VSDs detected at 1 month of age close.
  - 60% at 3 months.
  - 25% at 12 months.
  - 50% at 6 months.
  - Type IV (muscular) VSDs are most likely to spontaneously close.
  - Type I, III and malalignment VSDs are less likely to close.
- The development of Eisenmenger syndrome increases the risk of death by 10–12 fold and carries a 25-year survival of only 42%, although modern pulmonary hypertension therapy might prove to offer better survival to these patients.
- Increased risk of infective endocarditis.
- 25-year survival of 82.3% if untreated.

7 Diagnostic Studies

7.1 ECG

- Can be within normal limits.
- May show evidence of left, right or biventricular hypertrophy.

7.2 CXR

- Cardiomegaly.
- Increased pulmonary vascular markings.
- Pulmonary edema in severe cases.

7.3 Echocardiography

- Size, location and number of VSDs.
- Presence of associated lesions such as PDA or ASD.
- Presence of left sided obstructive lesions such as mitral hypoplasia, left ventricular outflow tract obstruction, coarctation of the aorta and hypoplasia of the aortic arch.
- Presence of atrioventricular valve straddling that might complicate repair.
- Development of complications such as double chamber right ventricle or aortic valve prolapse and regurgitation.
- Assessment of right-sided pressures (i.e. right ventricular systolic pressure).
- non-invasive estimation of Qp/Qs, but MRI/catheterization preferable due to higher accuracy.

7.4 MRI

- Rarely warranted for an uncomplicated VSD. May help define three-dimensional anatomy in cases associated with DORV or outflow obstruction.
- Calculation of Qp/Qs.

7.5 CT

- Diagnostic value limited. Only usually required if additional arch or great vessel anomalies.
- 2nd choice for cross-sectional imaging.

7.6 *Cardiac Catheterization*

- Rarely needed in infants and young children.
- Performed if there is a question of operability of patients with pulmonary hypertension.
- Determination of response of the pulmonary artery pressure to pulmonary vasodilators
- Calculations of Qp/Qs.

8 Indications for Intervention/Surgery

The division of VSD into large, moderate, and small VSD is mostly arbitrary (Table 1).

8.1 *Indication by Size*

- Large VSD
  - VSD closure is usually performed before 6 months of age.
  - Surgery earlier in those with intractable heart failure failing to respond to medical therapy.
- Moderate VSD
  - Surgery can be delayed till after 12 months of age and is indicated when Qp/Qs is > 2.0 or pulmonary vascular resistance is > 4WU × m^2.
- Small VSD
  - Treated medically with surgery indicated for history of endocarditis, aortic valve prolapse and regurgitation, double chamber right ventricle or left ventricular dilatation. If Qp:Qs remains > 1.5 then closure should be considered.

Table 1 VSD categories by size

Size	Relative Size to the aortic annulus	RV pressure	Qp/Qs
Large	Same or larger	Systemic	>2.5
Medium	≥ Half	≥ half systemic	≥ 2.0
Small	< Half	< half systemic	≥1.5

8.2 Indication by Type

- Type I are almost all surgically closed due to lack of spontaneous closure and the risk of prolapse of right aortic coronary cusp and development of aortic regurgitation.
- Type IV have higher possibility of spontaneous closure and more difficult access to close so more commonly observed.

8.3 Contraindications to Close

- Closure is contraindicated in patients with predominant right to left shunt and pulmonary vascular resistance > 8WU × m^2 with no response to pulmonary vasodilators.

9 Timing of Intervention and Management Strategy

- Infants and young children with congestive heart failure are managed with diuretics and fortification of feeds. Some infants require enteral tube feeding. Medical management is continued until either a decision is made to operate or the left-to-right shunt restricts enough such that surgery is not necessary.
- If large or signs of heart failure persist, VSDs are usually closed at 3–6 months of age.
- If moderate in size, closure can be delayed to determine if further restriction will occur and mitigate the need for surgery; otherwise, surgical closure is indicated with evidence of an increased Qp/Qs.
- If small in size, patients are usually asymptomatic and can be managed expectantly.

10 Surgical Strategy

- Right atrial approach
  - The most commonly applied approach for type II, III and IV VSDs.
  - Most surgical VSDs are closed with the use of patch material.
  - Occasionally, detachment of the septal leaflet of the tricuspid valve might facilitate VSD exposure but may risk causing TV dysfunction.
  - In order to avoid injury to the conduction system, the sutures should be placed superficially on the right ventricular aspect of the postero-inferior margin of the VSD and also passed through the septal leaflet of the tricuspid valve near the apex of the triangle of Koch where the atrioventricular node is located.

- Care should be taken to avoid injury to the tricuspid or aortic valve.

- Transpulmonary approach
  - Commonly applied approach for type I VSDs through a transverse pulmonary artery incision.
  - At the superior aspect of the patch, the sutures are usually anchored at the base of the pulmonary valve cusps.
- Transaortic approach
  - Very rarely used.
  - Oblique incision directed towards the noncoronary sinus, mainly in patients with type I VSDs associated with significant aortic valve prolapse and regurgitation.
- Right ventricular approach
  - Vertical infundibular incision is rarely required to close type I, II or IV defects that are hard to expose through the right atrium, typically those associated with DORV where the aorta is more anterior.
  - Vertical apical right ventricular incision is rarely used for apical type IV VSD.
- Left ventricular approach (very rarely used and should be avoided if possible)
  - Vertical apical incision.
  - Rarely used for closure of apical type IV VSD.
- Transatrial or perventricular hybrid device closure
  - Has been described for closure of apical and other trabecular type IV VSDs, sometimes with the help of preoperative localization with a wire and epicardial echo.
- Closure of multiple muscular VSDs
  - Can be challenging due to poor access and exposure.
  - The usual approach is transatrial although additional right ventricular, perventricular or hybrid approach might be necessary for adequate exposure.
  - Closure of the VSDs can be with the use of a patch to seal off the apex, a device, or direct closure.
  - Reendocardialization technique comprises double-layered closure of septal trabeculations in all four compartments of the muscular septum.
- Aortic valve repair
  - Might be necessary in patients with moderate to severe aortic regurgitation while the majority of patients with less severe degrees of aortic regurgitation have stabilization or improvement of the regurgitation with patch closure alone.
  - Usually, the right coronary cusp is affected in type I VSDs while the noncoronary cusp is affected in type II VSDs.

- Several techniques have been described for aortic valve repair such as:
  - Commissural suspension and commissural plication (Trusler technique).
  - Central Plication of the prolapsed cusp
  - Reefing of the redundant cusp.
  - Use of the cusp to close the VSD (Yacoub technique).
  - Various aortic repair techniques can be employed.
- In neonates with VSD and duct dependent coarctation of the aorta: the repair strategies can include:
  - Single stage, single incision repair of both VSD and coarctation (commonest approach).
  - Single stage, two incision repair of both VSD and coarctation.
  - Two stage strategy with initial coarctation repair, with or without pulmonary artery band.
  - Single stage repair is preferred in all patients with a large VSD and coarctation. Initial coarctation repair alone is reserved to those with small VSDs (especially type IV).
- The pulmonary artery band can be useful in neonates with large VSD and concomitant comorbidities such as intracranial bleeding, multi-organ failure, and with difficult multiple VSDs

11 Intensive Care Physiology and Management

- Standard measures after cardiac surgery apply.
- Management focuses on pulmonary vascular reactivity with risk of pulmonary hypertension.
- Arrhythmia (e.g. AV-block) may be present and temporary pacing necessary.

12 Outcome

- Isolated VSD closure
  - Current operative mortality is less than 1%.
  - Most common complications include:

    Permanent heart block requiring pacemaker (1–2%).

  - Residual VSD requiring reoperation (1–2%).
  - Aortic valve or tricuspid valve regurgitation (rarely requiring reoperation).
- VSD closure and coarctation repair

  - Current operative mortality is 5–6% (comparable for different treatment strategies).
  - Freedom from reoperation for residual VSD following closure is around 98% at 10 years.
  - Freedom from reoperation for recurrent arch obstruction is 90–95% at 10 years.
  - Freedom from surgery for left-sided obstructive lesions is 80–90% at 10 years.

- VSD and aortic insufficiency (AI)
  - The degree of residual AI depends on patients age, timing of surgery and the severity of preoperative AI.
  - For the majority of patients with mild to moderate AI, the degree of regurgitation is stabilized or improved following VSD closure.
  - Freedom from aortic valve reoperation is around 80% at 10–20 years.
  - If AI > mild consider concomitant AoV repair – usually leaflet plication/resuspension
  - Some patients need aortic valve replacement.

- Closure of multiple VSDs:
  - Current mortality is 5%, (in the past 10–20%).
  - Common complications include:

    Heart block requiring pacemaker (5–15%).
    Ventricular dysfunction due to ventriculotomy, division of the moderator band or right ventricle trabeculae for exposure.
    Residual VSDs.
    Septal dysfunction as a result of deep suturing in the septum, division of major trabeculae, or application of multiple devices.

13 Alternative Strategies

- Interventional closure of VSD
  - Specific devices available to close perimembranous VSDs – usually in older patients with smaller defects. Conduction injury and aortic valve injury have been reported and careful patient selection is important.
  - Not suitable for all VSDs.

- Hybrid closure:
  - Intraoperative, echo guided device closure.
  - Can be used as an adjunct for apical VSDs that are not amenable to surgical closure.

- Flap-valve VSD closure:

- Used in patients with high pulmonary vascular resistance, who are not responding to medical treatment (e.g. oxygen, iNO, endothelin receptor antagonists).
- Allows for intermittent right-to-left shunting if necessary.

- Single vs two stage repair of VSD and ductal dependent coarctation of the aorta.
  - Single stage, single incision repair of both VSD and coarctation.

    Advantages:

    Single stage management of arch obstruction and elimination of shunt.
    Ability to augment the aortic arch.
    Ability to address other lesions such as left ventricular outflow tract obstruction.

    Disadvantages:

    Two incisions.
    Inability to augment the arch in patients with proximal arch hypoplasia or to address additional left sided obstructive lesions.

  - Two stage strategy with initial coarctation repair, with or without pulmonary artery band:

    Advantages:

    Avoidance of cardiopulmonary bypass or circulatory arrest in neonates.
    Might be the only surgery needed in patients with small to moderate size VSDs that eventually close of decrease in size.

    Disadvantages:

    Problems related to persistent left to right shunt in children with large VSDs.
    Problems related to pulmonary artery band if used.
    The need for a second operation for second stage VSD closure, with or without pulmonary artery debanding or augmentation
    Inability to address proximal arch hypoplasia or left sided obstructive lesions at time of initial surgery.

Bibliography

1. Alsoufi B, Cai S, Coles JG, et al. Outcomes of different surgical strategies in the treatment of neonates with aortic coarctation and associated ventricular septal defects. Ann Thorac Surg. 2007;84:1331–6.
2. Bacha EA, Cao QL, Galantowicz ME, et al. Multicenter experience with perventricular device closure of muscular ventricular septal defects. Pediatr Cardiol. 2005;26:169–75.

3. Gaynor JW, Wernovsky G, Rychik J, et al. Outcome following single-stage repair of coarctation with ventricular septal defect. Eur J Cardiothorac Surg. 2000;18:62–7.
4. Kidd L, Driscoll DJ, Gersony WM, et al. Second natural history study of congenital heart defects. Results of treatment of patients with ventricular septal defects. Circulation 1993;87(2 Suppl):I38–51
5. Seddio F, Reddy VM, McElhinney DB, et al. Multiple ventricular septal defects: how and when should they be repaired? J Thorac Cardiovasc Surg. 1999;117:134–9.
6. Tweddell JS, Pelech AN, Frommelt PC. Ventricular septal defect and aortic valve regurgitation: pathophysiology and indications for surgery. Semin Thorac Cardiovasc Surg Pediatr Card Surg Ann. 2006;9:147–52.
7. Van Praagh R, Geva AT, Kreutzer J. Ventricular septal defects: how shall we describe, name and classify them? J Am Coll Cardiol. 1989;14:1298–9.
8. Wilcox BR, Anderson RH. Surgical anatomy of the heart, 2nd edn. Gower Medical Publishing, London p 7–24 (1992).

Double Outlet Right Ventricle (DORV)

Christoph Haller

Abstract Double outlet right ventricle (DORV) encompasses a whole family of lesions characterised by both great arteries arising predominantly from the right ventricle in the presence of a ventricular septal defect (VSD). The aorta often overrides the VSD but at least 50% of the aorta must be committed to the RV in order to classify as a DORV. Instead of forming a distinct cardiac lesion, DORV is a large group of congenital defects with highly variable anatomy and physiology. The spectrum ranges from VSD-like or TOF-type physiology to TGA/VSD or complex single ventricle disease. Driven by the respective physiology, anatomic characteristics, and associated defects, clinical management and surgical strategy can include primary repair, staged procedures, complex biventricular reconstructions, and single ventricle pathways. Outcome across the spectrum is good, but worse in subgroups with outflow tract obstructions, associated arch hypoplasia, and in single ventricle patients.

Keywords DORV · Double outlet · VSD · Interventricular communication · Aortic override

Abbreviations

AV	Atrioventricular
AVV	Atrioventricular valve
BTT	Blalock Taussig Thomas
ccTGA	congenitally corrected transposition of the great arteries
CoA	Coarctation of the aorta
DORV	Double outlet right ventricle
LV	Left ventricle

C. Haller (✉)
Division of Cardiovascular Surgery, Labatt Family Heart Centre, Department of Surgery, The Hospital for Sick Children, University of Toronto, 555 University Avenue, Toronto, ON M5G 1X8, Canada
e-mail: christoph.haller@sickkids.ca

© The Author(s), under exclusive license to Springer Nature Switzerland AG 2024

A. I. Dipchand et al. (eds.), *Manual of Cardiac Care in Children*,
https://doi.org/10.1007/978-3-031-70973-9_5

LVOTO	Left ventricular outflow tract obstruction
PA	Pulmonary artery
REV	Reparation à l'étage ventriculaire
RV	Right ventricle
TAPVD	Total anomalous pulmonary venous drainage
TGA	Transposition of the great arteries
TOF	Tetralogy of Fallot
TV	Tricuspid valve
VSD	Ventricular septal defect

Key Points

- DORV presents with variable anatomy/physiology. Some resemble that of TOF, of TGA, or that of a simple VSD.
- Physiology may include
  - decreased pulmonary artery (PA) flow
  - left–right shunting
  - complete mixing
  - non-mixing
- Complexity of the repair ranges from straightforward to complex biventricular and single ventricle strategies
- Arch obstruction may coexist
- DORV has the possibility of defects at 4 anatomical levels
  - VSD (subpulmonary, subaortic, doubly committed, remote)
  - position of the great vessels
  - pulmonary/sub-pulmonary obstruction
  - aortic arch obstruction (not in TOF-types)

1 Nomenclature

- Definition varies and may often be controversially discussed between different observers. Absence of aorto-mitral continuity may be more accurate from a morphological standpoint.
- In cases of override, more than 50% of the aorta being committed to the right ventricle is frequently used in clinical practice to define DORV.
- Variable ventriculo-arterial relationship. Position of the great vessels is a key consideration.
- Ventricular septal defect (subpulmonary, subaortic, doubly committed, or remote)
- Aortic override (normal relations of the great arteries are most common)

- Possible pulmonary valvar/infundibular stenosis
- Possible aortic obstruction

2 Anatomy

- Position of the great vessels to each other and their relationship to the ventricular cavity and the VSD is variable.
- Normal relations (aorta posterior and to the right of the pulmonary artery) are most common.
- Position of the VSD in relation to the great arteries is of particular importance as it influences the physiology and operative strategy.
- VSDs are usually large.
- Position of the infundibular septum determines position of the VSD
- VSDs can be (Lev classification) (see Fig. 1):
  - Subaortic (most common)
  - infundibular septum attached to the anterior limb of the septomarginal trabecula
  - Subpulmonary
  - infundibular septum attached to the posterior limb of the septomarginal trabecula
  - doubly committed
  - absent infundibular septum
  - remote.
- Taussig-Bing malformation is a variant of DORV with a subpulmonary VSD (see Fig. 2).
- The international nomenclature recognises four types of DORV: VSD-type, TOF-type, TGA-type and Non-Committed-type.

2.1 Embryology

- All cardiac development begins with a DORV-like anatomy. The truncus arteriosus is initially connected to the bulbus cordis, which in turn is the precursor of the right ventricle.
- DORV can occur by inadequate torsion and rotation of the truncus, and insufficient absorption of the distal posterior bulbar segment. Nevertheless, morphogenesis is multifactorial and not completely clarified.

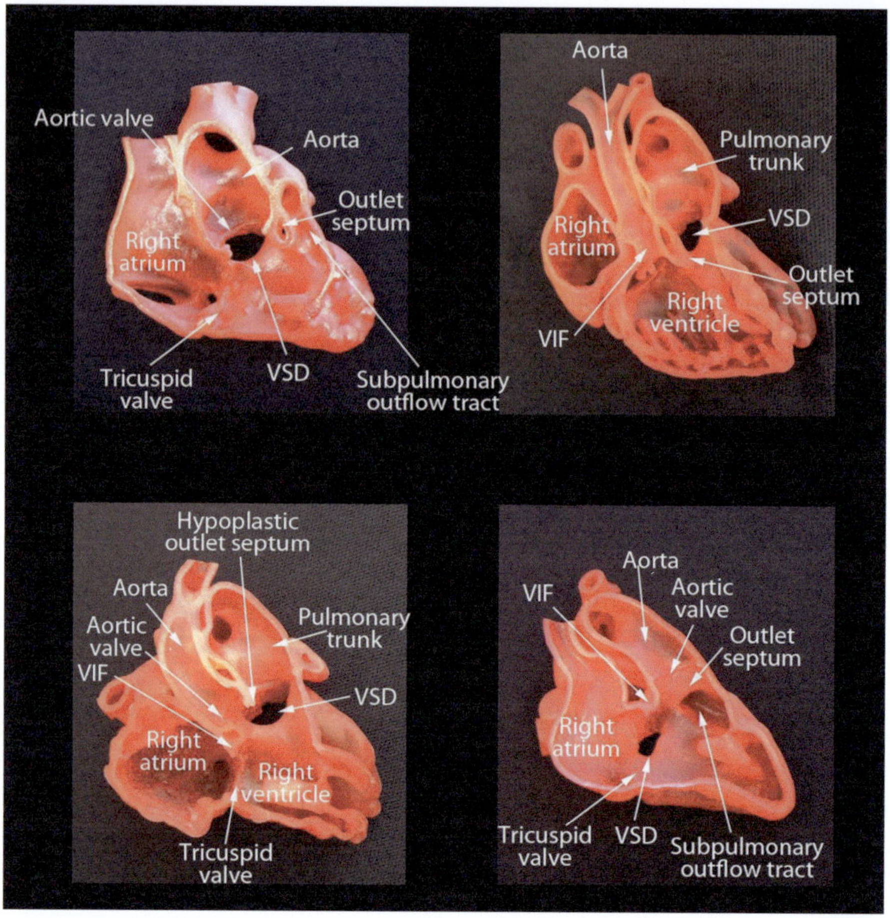

Fig. 1 3D models of subtypes of DORV, view of a longitudinal transection of the RV. A) subaortic VSD, B) subpulmonary VSD, C) doubly committed VSD, D) remote VSD. Reprinted from Haller et al.

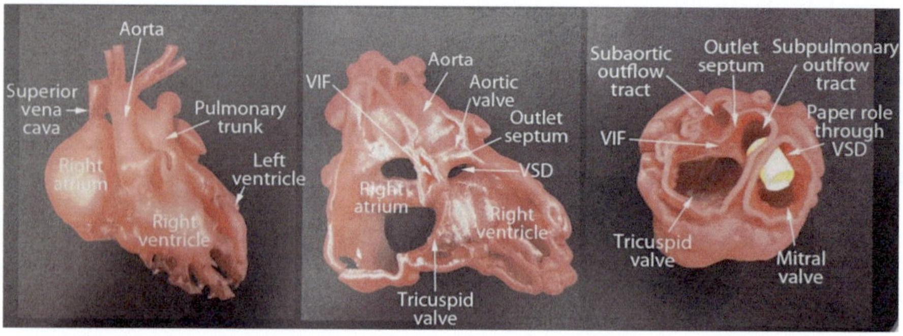

Fig. 2 Taussig-Bing malformation. Reprinted from Haller et al.

3 Epidemiology

3.1 Incidence/prevalence

- ~ 1% of all congenital cardiac defects.
- 3–24/100.000 live births.
- Exact incidence may be underestimated by variable assignment of borderline cases to other diagnostic groups.

3.2 Population at Risk, Inheritance

- More common in male than female patients.
- Complex inheritance pattern with multiple genes playing a role in neural crest cell migration and looping.
- Genetic abnormalities (trisomy 23, trisomy 18, 22q11 deletion) have been associated.

4 Clinical Physiology and Presentation

- Clinical signs and symptoms depend on the individual patient's anatomic characteristics.
- In uncomplicated DORV, with malposed great arteries and a subaortic VSD, clinical presentation is similar to patients with an unrestrictive VSD (i.e. increased pulmonary blood flow, no cyanosis).
- Doubly committed and remote VSDs can present with varying degrees of mixing.
- In a Taussig-Bing heart, the left-to-right shunt through the subpulmonary VSD is preferentially streamed to the pulmonary artery, while the aorta receives deoxygenated blood from the RV Thereby, Taussig-Bing anomaly may present with a TGA-like clinical picture (Fig. 3).
- Great vessesls are typically side-by-side and 60% have unusual coronary patterns (retropulmonary circumflex most common)
- Patients with subpulmonary stenosis show signs similar to TOF.

4.1 Natural History

Similar to the clinical presentation, the natural history of patients with DORV parallels that of patients with VSD, TGA or TOF, respectively.

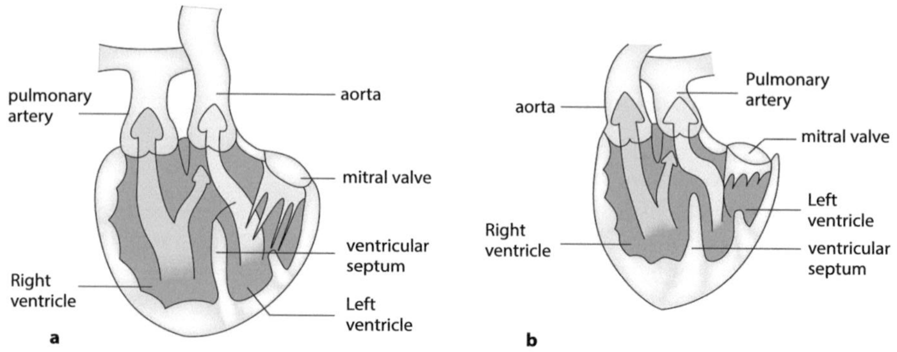

Fig. 3 Streaming effects depending on relationship between VSD and great arteries. A. Preferential streaming of oxygenated blood to aorta. B. Preferential streaming of deoxygenated blood to aorta. Reprinted from Haller et al.

5 Associated Lesions

- Hypoplastic ventricle (functional single ventricle)
- Atrioventricular discordance
- ccTGA
- Pulmonary atresia
- Right atrial isomerism
- TAPVD
- AVSD
- CoA and arch hypoplasia (esp. in Taussig-Bing)

Some morphologic subtypes may be classified as DORV but are functional single ventricle lesions following a single ventricle pathway (see Chap. 33 on ‘Other Single Ventricle Conditions’).

6 Diagnostic Studies

6.1 ECG

- Non-characteristic and variable.
- Signs of atrial enlargement.
- Right ventricular hypertrophy (right-axis deviation, V1 R-wave dominance, V5 S-wave dominance) and enlargement.
- Right bundle branch block.
- Signs of left ventricular changes in some forms of DORV.

6.2 CXR

- Reflects characteristics of the underlying physiology.
- Variable based on underlying physiology (e.g., enlarged cardiac silhouette, pulmonary plethora, etc.).
- Alteration of aortic/pulmonary shadow, depending on the relationship of the great arteries.

6.3 Echocardiography

- Echocardiography is usually diagnostic.
- Segmental anatomy.
- Relationship of aortic and pulmonary valves to both ventricles
- Relationship of great vessels to each other
- Outflow tract obstruction
- Size and position of VSD, direction of shunting
- AVV attachments/override/straddling
- Coronary artery origins/course
- Associated defects
  - Although most of the surgically important aspects can be detected on echocardiography, surgical decision-making may need additional imaging to assess options for intraventricular tunneling or other strategies (see CT-Angiography or 3D-Printing).

6.4 MRI

- Diagnostic tool for right ventricular function/volume or valve regurgitation (if replaced) during follow-up after corrective surgery.
- Feed and sleep protocol may avoid need for general anesthesia.

6.5 CT

- May add more/better information on spatial position and relationships of valves and VSD compared to echocardiography alone.
- Allows for 3D-reconstruction and 3D-Printing (see 3D-Printing).

6.6 Cardiac Catheterization

- Rarely used unless suspicion of associated lesions that are not adequately assessed with the other diagnostic techniques.

6.7 3D-Printing

- 3D-Models provide more information on spatial relationships (i.e., size and position of VSD, distance of PA to TV, great arterial relationship).

7 Indications for Intervention / Surgery

- Corrective single-stage surgery is preferred. Staged repair may be required if multiple associated lesions or concern about ability to achieve biventricular repair.
- Palliative (single ventricle repair strategy) may be necessary in some cases, usually where intracardiac anatomy precludes separation of the ventricles.

8 Timing of Intervention and Management Strategy

- 2–4 months if
  - hemodynamically stable
  - simple DORV (subaortic VSD, no obstruction of outflow tracts)
  - Treatment algorithm used for TOF applies in those with simple DORV and pulmonary stenosis.
- Neonatal repair (up to 14 days of age)
  - DORV with a TGA-like pattern, if amenable for VSD closure and arterial switch operation.
  - Aortic arch obstruction
- In more complex situations, that necessitate surgery for LVOTO, surgery may be delayed
  - 6–8 weeks for muscular LVOTO resection
  - 4–6 months in more complex repairs, such as REV, Nikaidoh, Rastelli
  - If there are signs of cyanosis, shunt placement or ductal stenting may be necessary
  - If signs of excess pulmonary blood flow, pulmonary artery banding should be considered in those with planned delayed repair.

- Decisions on the optimal type of procedure can sometimes be made only intraoperatively.

9 Surgical Strategy

9.1 General Aspects

- Position of the VSD and its relation to the great vessels are key aspects to consider.
- In VSD closure/rerouting, size of the VSD must be adequate to allow unobstructed flow.
- Enlargement may be necessary (anteriorly and leftward, away from conduction tissue).
- Ultimate goal is to achieve unobstructed concordant ventriculoarterial connection, although this may not always be possible.
- Complex patients may be palliated initially (BTT Shunt, ductal stenting or pulmonary trunk banding).

9.2 Simple DORV with Subaortic VSD

- VSD closure and rerouting to the aorta. Usually transatrial approach, but if the aorta is more anterior then a small right ventriculotomy may be necessary to access the top of the VSD.
- TOF-like resection is performed for a stenotic pulmonary component
- VSD enlargement may be necessary
- watch for inflow obstruction

9.3 DORV with Subpulmonary VSD (Taussig-Bing Anomaly)

- Corrected by VSD closure (which reroutes the pulmonary trunk to the LV) and Arterial Switch Operation.
- Aortic or coronary anomalies can be present further complicating the procedure.
- Intra-cardiac baffling has been described (Kawashima Procedure) in older children initially palliated first with PA band, but very rarely performed.

9.4 DORV and Outflow Tract Obstruction

Patients who are unsuitable for a conventional intraventricular repair (with or without arterial switch), may be amenable for one of the following:

- Rastelli
  - VSD tunneling to aorta. Closure of proximal pulmonary trunk. RV to PA conduit via anterior ventriculotomy.
  - High rate of recurrent LVOTO. Non-anatomic position of RV outflow.
- Reparation à l'étage ventriculaire (REV/Lecompte)
  - Wide resection of septal tissue for VSD enlargement and generous tunneling of VSD to aorta. Proximal pulmonary trunk is oversewn. Distal pulmonary trunk is reconnected to a right ventriculotomy with transannular patch after an initial Lecompte maneuver.
  - Residual risk of LVOTO.
- Nikaidoh
  - Mobilization of aorta + coronaries. Longitudinal pulmonary trunk and if necessary septal incision to open LV outflow. Aorta is shifted into the widened LV outflow tract. Septum is reconstructed. RV to PA connection either with wide patching or conduit implantation.
  - Complex procedure. Approach may be limited by coronary anatomy. Problematic in side-by-side configuration (may cause TV inflow obstruction)

9.5 Non-committed VSD

- Can sometimes be rerouted intraventricularly.
- May be repaired with the Rastelli or Nikaidoh procedure.
- Remote non-committed VSDs or multiple VSDs, straddling AV valves or hypoplastic development of the LV may challenge biventricular repair strategies. Univentricular palliation may be preferable.

10 Intensive Care Physiology and Management

- Physiologic changes are highly dependent on the respective surgical approach.
- Management can be that of patients after VSD closure, TOF repair, or TGA, respectively (see respective chapters).
- Focus should be set on potential systemic outflow (tunnel) obstruction, reduced LV function, pulmonary hypertension, and arrhythmia.
- Neonates should have both pleural spaces and peritoneum drained.
- Delayed sternal closure may be considered if complex repair.

11 Outcome

- Reports on outcome in DORV are biased by the inconsistent classification of the disease and its wide spectrum.
- Overall outcome has improved in recent years, even in complex cases.
- Association with heterotaxy is a risk factor for unfavorable outcome.
- DORV, irrespective of the underlying anatomy has a 10-year survival rate of approximately 86%.
- Simple DORV has generally a good outcome with low early mortality rates of approximately 2% and 15-year survival of 95.8%.
- Biventricular repair of Taussig-Bing anomaly has been reported with relatively low mortality in the more recent years but may still reach 5–10%. 1- and 5-year survival among patients treated between 1979–2005 was reported to be 72%, with 100% survival in those treated after 1998. Additional arch obstruction and abnormal coronary patterns account for increased risk.
- As the Nikaidoh procedure is used in various settings, outcomes do not relate to DORV only. In general, outcome is good, with low mortality and low risk of residual/recurrent LVOTO. Use of a transannular patch compared to a valved conduit showed a tendency to lower rate of reoperations.
- The risk of residual or recurrent LVOT/tunnel obstruction is one of the main concerns after repair.

12 Alternative Strategies and Controversies

- Choosing the most appropriate surgical strategy remains controversial in extreme cases.
- Intraventricular tunnel in subpulmonary VSD with short distance between pulmonary and tricuspid valve, has been described (Kawashima Procedure). The course of the tunnel is complex and prone to obstruction. Most of the time, direct rerouting of the VSD to the pulmonary valve, combined with an arterial switch procedure may be a more reliable approach.
- Atrial switch procedures have been used for treatment of DORV with remote VSD. However, keeping the morphological LV in the systemic circulation is preferable. In the rare case of atrioventricular discordance, an atrial switch procedure, combined with the appropriate approach to correct DORV itself, may still be appropriate.

Bibliography

1. Backer, CL, Mavroudis C. The Rastelli operation. In: Operative techniques in thoracic and cardiovascular surgery, vol. 8, no. 3. 2003. p. 121–30. https://doi.org/10.1053/S1522-2942(03)00034-7
2. Fricke TA, Konstantinov IE, Buratto E, Brizard CP. Surgery for Taussig-Bing anomaly with aortic arch obstruction. Oper Tech Thorac Cardiovasc Surg. 2021;26(4):647–55. https://doi.org/10.1053/j.optechstcvs.2021.08.007.
3. Haller C, Van Arsdell GS, Yoo S-J, George-Hyslop CST, Spicer DE, Anderson RH. Chapter 39 Double-outlet ventricle. In: Anderson's pediatric cardiology, 4th edn. Philadelphia PA: Elsevier; 2019. p. 715–40.
4. Lecompte Y, Vouhé P. Réparation à l'Etage Ventriculaire (REV Procedure): not a Rastelli procedure without conduit. Oper Tech Thorac Cardiovasc Surg. 2003;8(3):150–9. https://doi.org/10.1053/S1522-9042(03)00036-0.
5. Yim D, Dragulescu A, Ide H, Seed M, Grosse-Wortmann L, van Arsdell G, Yoo S-J (2018) Essential modifiers of double outlet right ventricle: revisit with endocardial surface images and 3-dimensional print models. In: Circulation: cardiovascular imaging, vol. 11, no. 3; 2018. p. e006891. https://doi.org/10.1161/CIRCIMAGING.117.006891

Persistent Ductus Arteriosus (PDA)

Jose Carlos Aldana-Aguirre and Luc Mertens

Abstract The ductus arteriosus (DA) is a normal vascular structure that typically connects the descending thoracic aorta to the pulmonary artery near the origin of the left pulmonary artery (LPA) and has an important physiological role in fetal life. Post birth, the DA is expected to close during the first week after birth. Persistence of the ductus arteriosus (PDA) is common in preterm infants especially in those born below 26 weeks' gestation but can occur also in term infants. Clinical manifestations of a PDA are determined by the degree of shunting and the latter is largely determined by PDA resistance and the ratio of systemic and pulmonary vascular resistance. A large left–right shunt can lead to pulmonary overcirculation, left atrial (LA) and left ventricular (LV) dilatation, and heart failure. When not closed, large PDAs can cause progressive pulmonary vascular disease and obstructive pulmonary hypertension. A PDA is also associated with an increased risk for endocarditis, albeit low. Clinical evaluation and echocardiography are used to assess the hemodynamic significance of a PDA. The presence of a hemodynamically significant PDA (hsPDA) is an indication for intervention. The therapeutic options for PDA include pharmacological treatment for premature infants, percutaneous closure by catheterization, and surgical ligation.

Keywords Persistent ductus arteriosus · PDA · Pulmonary hypertension · Prematurity · Transcatheter ductal closure · Duct ligation

Abbreviations

CHD Congenital heart disease

J. C. Aldana-Aguirre
Division of Neonatology, Department of Paediatrics, The Hospital for Sick Children, Toronto, ON, Canada
e-mail: Jose.aldana@sickkids.ca

L. Mertens (✉)
Division of Cardiology, Department of Paediatrics, Labatt Family Heart Centre, The Hospital for Sick Children, Toronto, ON, Canada
e-mail: luc.mertens@sickkids.ca

© The Author(s), under exclusive license to Springer Nature Switzerland AG 2024

A. I. Dipchand et al. (eds.), *Manual of Cardiac Care in Children*,
https://doi.org/10.1007/978-3-031-70973-9_6

DA	Ductus arteriosus
hsPDA	Hemodynamically significant persistant ductus arteriosus
GA	Gestational age
GI	Gastrointestinal
HLHS	Hypoplastic left heart syndrome
IVH	Intraventricular hemmorhage
LA	Left atrium
LPA	Left pulmonary artery
LV	Left ventricle
MPA	Main pulmonary artery
MV	Mitral valve
NEC	Necrotizing enterocolitis
NSAIDs	Non-steroidal anti-inflammatory drugs
PA	Pulmonary artery
PDA	Persistent ductus arteriosus
PVR	Pulmonary vascular resistance
RCT	Randomized control trial
RV	Right ventricle
RPA	Right pulmonary artery
SVR	Systemic vascular resistance
WU	Woods units

Key Points

- In healthy term neonates the DA usually closes by the fourth day after birth.
- The incidence of PDA is inversely related to the gestational age (GA) at birth and is high in infants < 26 weeks GA.
- In preterm infants, PDA is related to a developmental immaturity. In term infants, PDA can be related to genetic factors and environmental exposures.
- Major determinants of shunt volume are:
  - Intrinsic ductal resistance (determined by PDA diameter and length)
  - Ratio of the pulmonary vascular resistance (PVR) to the systemic vascular resistance (SVR)
- The diagnosis of a hemodynamically significant (hs) PDA requires integration of clinical and echocardiographic information.
- A large unrestrictive PDA exposes the pulmonary vascular bed to systemic pressure which can cause obstructive pulmonary vascular disease resulting in Eisenmenger syndrome.
- Indications for PDA closure include a hsPDA and large unrestrictive PDA.
- The indications for closure of a small and non-hemodynamically significant PDA are variable and controversial.

- Therapeutic approach in preterm infants includes pharmacological treatment (indomethacin, ibuprofen, acetaminophen), percutaneous closure, or surgical ligation, and in term infants includes percutaneous closure and surgical ligation.
- Stenting of the DA might be required in the context of congenital heart disease.

1 Anatomy

- Normal left DA in the presence of left aortic arch connects the MPA with the isthmus in the descending aorta, just distal to the origin of the left subclavian artery.
- Anatomic variations include:
  - Right PDA in the presence of right aortic arch originating close to the origin of the right subclavian artery and draining close to the RPA. It can be associated with other vascular anomalies such as a vascular ring.
  - PDA originating from the brachiocephalic artery, typically from the left brachiocephalic in the presence of right aortic arch.
  - Bilateral ducts: right and left sided PDA, typically associated with intracardiac anomalies such as Tetralogy of Fallot.
- Persistent ductus arteriosus (PDA): present after the time of expected closure.
- Steps in physiologic PDA closure:

- Functional: occurs within 72 h after birth in response to high oxygen tension and a drop in circulating prostaglandin.
- Anatomical: intima necrosis and fibrous remodeling of the vessel wall.

- Morphological PDA classification: original description in the 1980s by the Hospital for Sick Children in Toronto included 5 morphologies (A-E). Further description of the PDA in preterm infants (type F) was described by Philip et al. (Fig. 1)

2 Embryology

- The distal left sixth embryonic aortic arch forms the DA within the first 8 weeks of development.
- The proximal part of the sixth arches persists as the proximal branch pulmonary arteries.
- Normally the right distal sixth arch regresses.

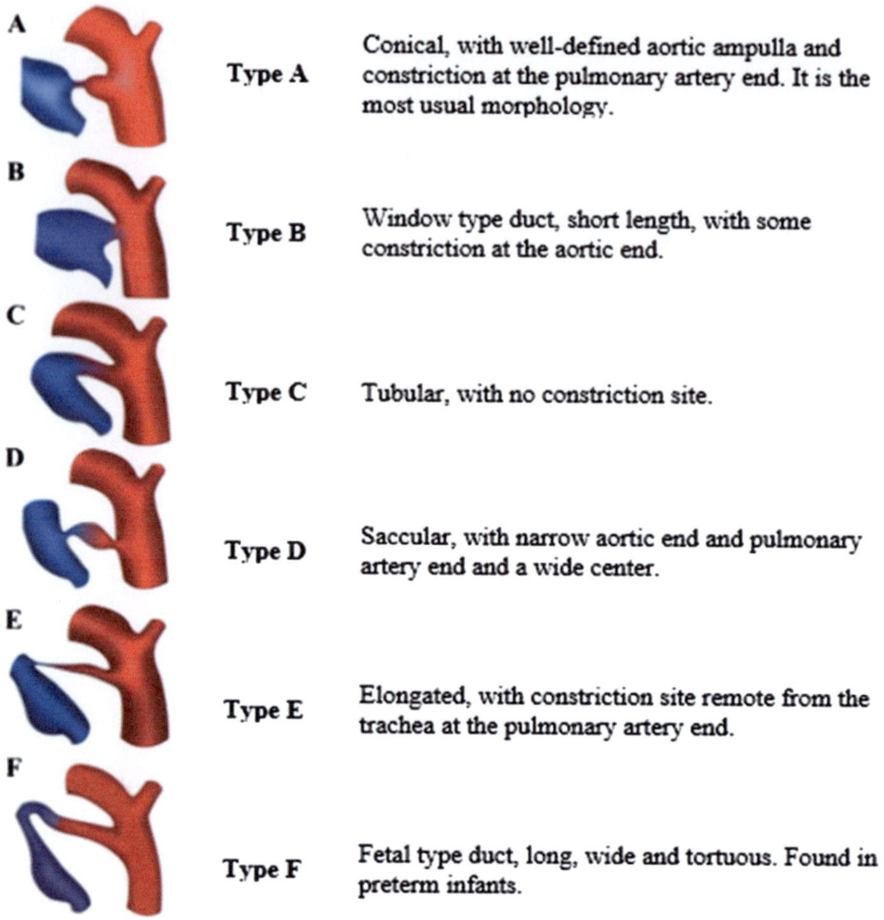

Fig. 1 Proposed classification of PDA. Reprinted from Catheterization and Cardiovascular Interventions, Vol 87, Philip R, Rush W, Agrawal V, et al., Morphologic characterization of the patent ductus arteriosus in the premature infant and the choice of transcatheter occlusion device, pages 310–317, 2016, with permission from Wiley

3 Epidemiology

- Incidence varies significantly dependent on GA at birth and postnatal age.
- Term infants:
  - Estimated incidence is ~ 1:2000 births, ~ 10% of all congenital heart disease (CHD).

- Associated with genetic abnormalities (e.g., trisomy 21, deletion 14-q, 4-p syndromes, 22q11.2 deletion, Holt-Oram, and Char syndrome) and environmental factors (e.g., fetal exposure to Zika, rubella virus, tetrahydrocannabinol, valproate, thalidomide).

- Preterm infants:
  - Present in > 50% of infants born < 26 weeks GA and is due to physiological immaturity.

4 Physiology and Clinical Presentation

- Major determinants of the PDA flow:
  - Intrinsic ductal resistance (determined by PDA diameter and length).
  - Ratio of the PVR to the SVR.
- Normal PVR with large left-to-right shunt:
  - Pulmonary overcirculation, left heart dilation and heart failure symptoms. Left-sided volume loading results in higher left filling pressure contributing to pulmonary congestion.
  - Low diastolic arterial blood pressure due to the "run off" into the pulmonary circulation leading to decreased coronary perfusion pressure.

    In preterm infants a diastolic flow reversal in abdominal aorta has been associated with decreased abdominal blood flow and altered brain perfusion.
- Unrestrictive PDA exposes the pulmonary vessels to systemic pressure which may lead to irreversible pulmonary vascular changes.
- Elevated PVR:
  - Ductal shunt is either bidirectional (with right-to-left in systole) or exclusively right-to-left shunt.
- In the context of CHD, the PDA can be essential as a source for pulmonary blood flow or systemic blood flow.

4.1 Defining a Hemodynamically Significant PDA (hsPDA)

- Preterm infants:

- Requires integration of clinical and echocardiographic parameters (Table 1).

Table 1 Echocardiographic and clinical markers for a hemodynamically significant PDA in preterm infants

Echocardiogram markers of hsPDA	
Ductal characteristics	Size > 1.5–2 mm (size can also be indexed to weight, and LPA) Doppler pattern: restrictive vs unrestrictive (max velocity < 2 m/s) Note areas of constriction
Pulmonary over-circulation and left-sided cardiac volume load	End-diastolic flow velocity in LPA (>50 cm/s) Increased PV diastolic velocity (>50 cm/s) LA and LV dilation MV regurgitation Others: MV inflows, LV IVRT, LVO
Systemic steal	Diastolic retrograde flow in abdominal aorta Diastolic retrograde flow in middle cerebral arteries
Ventricular function	Assess for systolic and diastolic ventricular function
Clinical markers of at-risk infants	
	Lower gestational age, particularly < 26 weeks
	Evolving BPD
	Growth restriction
	Unexpected high level and chronic need of respiratory support
	Pulmonary edema and cardiomegaly on chest x-ray Feeding intolerance

Abbreviations: *BPD* Bronchopulmonary dysplasia, *hsPDA* Hemodynamic significant persistent ductus arteriosus, PDA Persistent ductus arteriosus (PDA), *IVRT* Isovolumic relaxation time, *LA* Left atrium, *LPA* Left pulmonary artery, *LVO*, *LV* Output, *LV* Left ventricle, *MV* mitral valve, PV, XE "Pulmonary veins"

- Term infants and older children: determined by signs of heart failure and/or echocardiographic evidence of LA or LV enlargement. A small restrictive PDA is generally clinically well tolerated during childhood.

4.2 Clinical Presentation

- Typical presentation with large left-to-right shunt: active precordium with leftward apex shifted, wide pulse pressure, failure to thrive, heart failure, recurrent respiratory infections, continuous murmur in the left infraclavicular area that can radiate to the back.

- Preterm infants: In addition to heart failure symptoms, a hsPDA is associated with necrotizing enterocolitis, intraventricular hemorrhage, and bronchopulmonary dysplasia.

5 Natural History

- A long-standing unrestrictive PDA may lead to Eisenmenger syndrome with eventual reversal of shunt direction (to right-to-left) and differential cyanosis.
- A pressure restrictive PDA with a large L-R shunt may produce heart failure and elevated pulmonary artery pressures.
- Endocarditis:
  - Small PDA: very low risk of endocarditis with an annual incidence of 0.14%.
  - Very small/silent PDA: risk is extremely low.
  - Latest guidelines do not recommend antibiotic prophylaxis for PDAs.

6 Associated Lesions

- Any type of congenital defect can be associated with a PDA.
- Need to rule out CHD before proceeding to close the PDA.

7 Diagnostic Studies

7.1 ECG

- Small PDA: usually normal.
- Moderate to large PDA: LA enlargement and LV hypertrophy.
- If pulmonary hypertension develops, right axis deviation and RV hypertrophy.

7.2 Chest X-Ray (CXR)

- Small PDA: normal.
- Moderate to large PDA: cardiomegaly, dilated MPA, increased pulmonary vascular markings, and pulmonary edema.
- With pulmonary arterial hypertension: dilated MPA, decreased peripheral vascular markings.

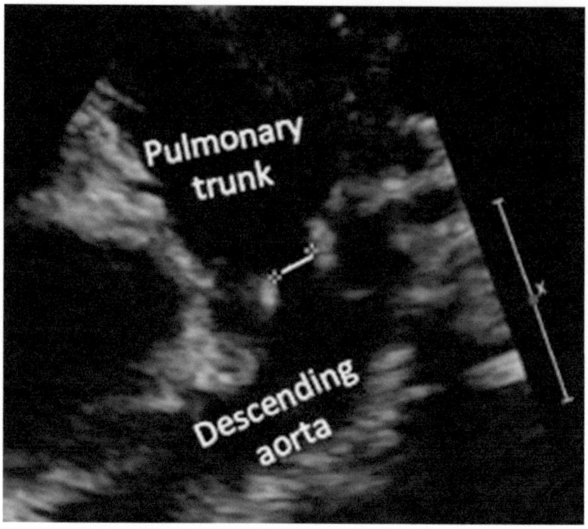

Fig. 2 Ductal view from a high left parasternal view of a left-sided PDA

7.3 *Echocardiography*

- Gold standard test for diagnosis and hemodynamic assessment.
- Approach includes:
  - Assessment to rule out associated CHD.
  - Evaluate PDA anatomy and hemodynamic significance.

- Table 1 summarizes the echocardiographic markers of hsPDA in preterm infants.
- Best echocardiographic view to image a left PDA is the ductal view (Fig. 2)

7.4 *Doppler Examination*

- Timing in the cardiac cycle and direction of ductal flow provides important information on pressure difference between the systemic and pulmonary circulations.
- Three different Doppler flow patterns can be distinguished
  - Dominant left-to-right shunt: present in isolated PDA with PVR < SVR.
  - Bidirectional shunt: right-to-left flow in systole and left-to-right flow in diastole. Physiologic neonatal transition or secondary either to significant left sided obstruction or pulmonary hypertension.
  - Dominant right-to-left shunt: significant left sided lesion or severe pulmonary hypertension (where PVR is equal to or greater than SVR).

  (Figs. 3, 4, 5):

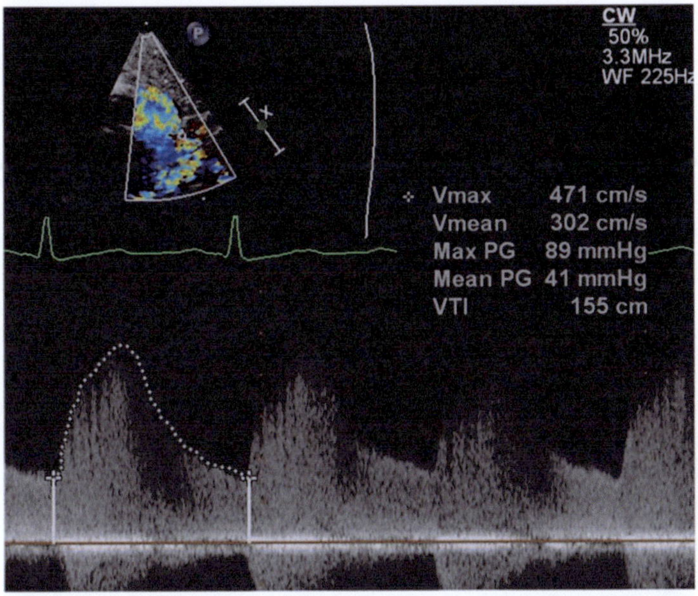

Fig. 3 PDA with left-to-right shunt and high max and mean velocities from which pressure gradients between the aorta and the pulmonary trunk are derived by the modified Bernoulli equation. This suggests low pulmonary artery pressure and pulmonary vascular resistance

7.5 *Cardiac Catheterization*

- Indications:
  - Device closure of the PDA.
  - PDA stenting for maintenance of pulmonary or systemic blood flow (see section Intervention/surgery).
  - Diagnostic catheterization in patients with pulmonary hypertension.

7.6 *MRI and CT*

- Useful in the presence of limited echocardiography windows. CT is useful to delineate complicated vascular anatomical variations.
- Phase contrast MRI is useful to quantify Qp and Qs.

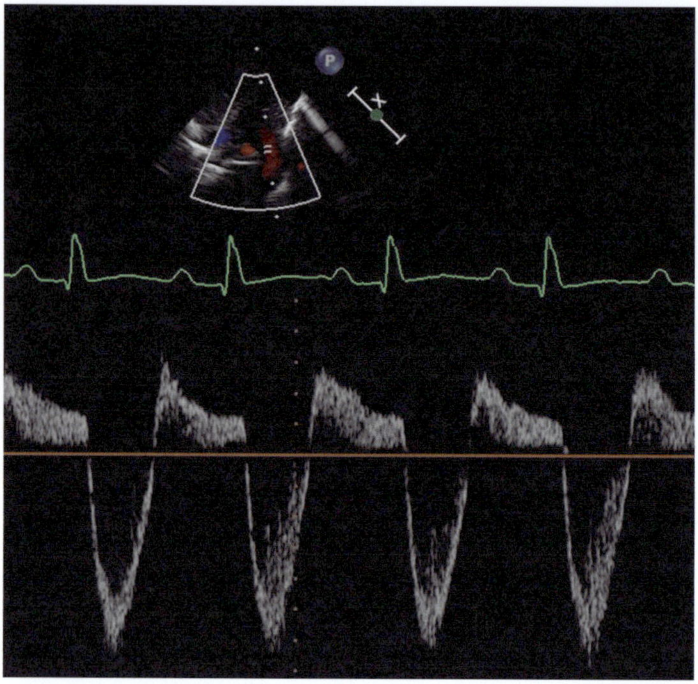

Fig. 4 Spectral Doppler tracing of PDA with bidirectional shunt, left-to-right in diastole and right-to-left in systole. This suggests that pulmonary artery pressure in systole is higher than the aortic pressure and the presence of increased PVR

(a) (b)

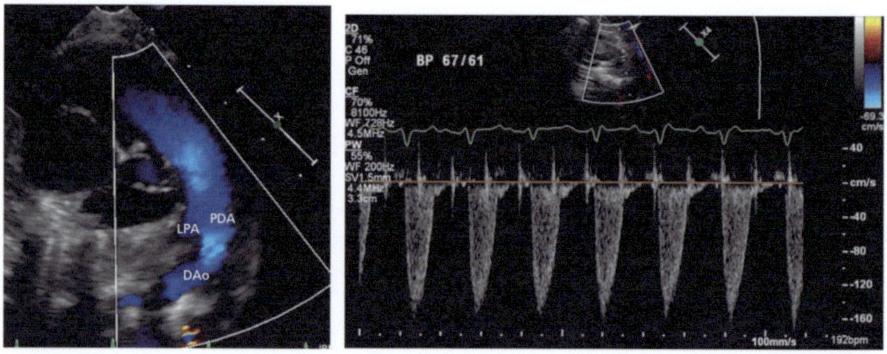

Fig. 5 **(a)** Color Doppler image in high left parasternal view of a large PDA with right-to-left shunt. **(b)** Spectral Doppler with all right-to-left shunt. DAo, descending aorta; LPA, left pulmonary artery. Reprinted from Echocardiography in pediatric and congenital heart disease: from fetus to adult. Third edition, Chapter 19, Lai, WW, Mertens LL, Cohen MS, Geva T, Abnormalities of the ductus arteriosus and pulmonary arteries page 365, 2022 ISBN: 9,781,119,612,803, with permission from Wiley

8 Symptomatic Medical Treatment

- Patients with heart failure are commonly treated with diuretics and calorie-intake optimization.

9 Indications for PDA Closure

- Term infants and children:
  - Large shunt resulting in clinical signs of heart failure.
  - Increased pulmonary artery pressures related to an unrestrictive PDA beyond the first 6 months of life.
  - Moderate to large duct with no significant pulmonary arterial hypertension generally will undergo duct closure if there is evidence of LA and/or LV volume loading.
- Closure is not recommended in severe pulmonary hypertension (PVR $\geq$ 5–6 WU) or Eisenmenger syndrome.
- There is no strong evidence to recommend closure of silent and small PDAs but practice varies widely.
- Preterm infants:
  - Interventions to close the PDA convey risks, thus adequate selection and timing is essential. However, selection criteria have not been well established despite multiple studies and trials on the subject (see section on Controversies).
  - When decision has been made that a PDA warrants closure in preterm infants, the sequential approach is:
- Pharmacologic treatment. Four strategies based on timing. See Table 2.
- Non-steroidal anti-inflammatory drugs (cyclooxygenase inhibitors, NSAIDs) and acetaminophen (peroxidase inhibitor).
- Relative contraindications: NSAIDs are not used if there are concerns for bowel disease (e.g., NEC), renal injury or high-risk of hemorrhage.
- If pharmacological treatment fails, transcatheter or surgical closure is attempted.

10 Transcatheter or Surgical Closure

10.1 PDA Occlusion by Transcatheter Device Closure

- First-line approach in patients $\geq$ 6 kg.
- Newer devices for preterm infants are available.

Table 2 Pharmacologic strategies for PDA closure in preterm infants. Choice of medication varies among centers

Timing of treatment	Commonly used medication	Pros	Cons	Comments
Prophylaxis in selected infants (6-24 h after birth)	Indomethacin	Decreased IVH and pulmonary hemorrhage	Oliguria, increase in creatinine, associated with bowel perforation when used in conjunction with post-natal steroids	Unnecessary treatment of many infants
Early targeted (<6 days after birth)	Indomethacin	Decreased pulmonary hemorrhage	Same as prophylactic indomethacin	
	Ibuprofen	Less negative effects on end-organ perfusion compared to indomethacin	Use during first 24 h was associated with risk of renal failure, GI hemorrhage	Oral route is considered more effective than IV
Symptomatic treatment with hsPDA $\geq$ 6 days after birth	Ibuprofen	Same as above	Risk of oliguria, increase in creatinine, GI side-effects	
Rescue treatment	Acetaminophen	No known renal or GI side-effects	Possibly less effective in PDA closure vs other medications	In general, used if NSAIDs failed or if there is contraindication for NSAIDs

GI Gastrointestinal; *IVH* Intraventricular hemorrhage; *NSAIDs* Nonsteroidal anti-inflammatory drugs

- Balloon test occlusion can be useful in determining hemodynamic suitability for closure particularly in patients with pulmonary hypertension.
- Different devices are available for different PDA morphologies, thus need to consider the PDA anatomic characteristics (ductal length, size, ampulla size, etc.).
  - Favorable duct anatomy: long duct with large ampulla.
- Complications are rare, include: device embolization, obstruction to LPA or aorta, hemolysis from high velocity residual shunt, thrombosis related to femoral access.
- Patients require infective endocarditis prophylaxis for 6 months following closure.

10.2 *Surgical Ligation of Duct Through Left thoracotomy*

- Surgical approach is reserved for those patients with unfavorable ductal morphology for transcatheter closure.
- Procedure is performed via a left-sided thoracotomy or in older patients with video-assisted thoracoscopy.
- Surgical options include:
  - PDA ligation
  - Vascular clip occlusion
- Surgical complications are rare and include:
  - Recurrent laryngeal nerve injury with subsequent vocal cord dysfunction.
  - Phrenic nerve injury resulting in diaphragmatic paralysis.
  - LPA or descending aorta ligation (extremely rare, prematurity is a risk factor).
  - Leaks: hemorrhage, pneumothorax, chylothorax.
  - In preterm infants, cardiovascular instability termed post-ligation syndrome related to development of LV dysfunction early after PDA closure.
- Ligation in older patients can be difficult, as the duct tends to be shorter, thicker and the aortic end calcified.

11 Ductal Stenting

- Can be done in small neonates (>2.5 kg)
- To provide pulmonary blood-flow in cyanotic lesions and duct-dependent pulmonary circulation (e.g., pulmonary atresia with intact ventricular septum) instead of a surgical shunt.
  - Has less periprocedural morbidity compared to a surgical shunt and similar outcomes related to death and unplanned interventions.
  - Duct morphology is very relevant as duct tortuosity, length and origin can make procedure more difficult.
  - Patients are started on anticoagulation after stent placement.
  - Complications:
    - Acute: ductal dissection, ductal spasm, stent thrombosis, stent migration, ductal stenosis (particularly if whole ductal length is not covered by stent)
    - Long-term: heart failure due to pulmonary overcirculation.
- To provide systemic flow in hypoplastic left heart syndrome (HLHS) or other duct-dependent systemic circulation:

- Part of the hybrid procedure as an alternative for stage I palliation in high-risk Norwood candidates (low birthweight, prematurity, ventricular dysfunction, tricuspid regurgitation, extracardiac malformations). Hybrid procedure includes ductal stenting and bilateral PA banding.
- Complications in Hybrid procedure:
  - Acute: stent thrombosis, malposition, embolization.
  - Long-term: retrograde aortic arch obstruction, ductal in-stent stenosis, restriction of atrial septum, PA growth.

12 Intensive Care Physiology and Management

- Term infants and older patients otherwise healthy:
  - Pre-procedure: typically, do not require intensive care.
  - Post-procedure: typically have stable hemodynamics; routine post procedure recovery.
- Situations where intensive care may be necessary:
  - Prematurity: at risk of developing "post-ligation syndrome" with cardiorespiratory deterioration within hours following procedure mostly attributed to changes in loading conditions (decreased LV volume load and increased LV afterload from excluding the low resistance pulmonary circulation).
  - High pulmonary vascular resistance.
  - Heart failure requiring advanced respiratory support.
- Intensive care management may be necessary for associated cardiac or non-cardiac diseases.

13 Outcome

- Transcatheter occlusion outcomes are excellent: complete closure rates are more than 98%.
- Surgical duct closure has excellent outcomes with mortality < 0.2%.
- Intermittent long-term follow-up:
  - Small PDA
  - Successful PDA device closure
  - Residual DA shunt post-procedure

14 Alternative Strategies and Controversies

- Optimal management of PDA in preterm infants is controversial for several reasons:
  - PDA-treatment randomized controlled trials (RCTs) to-date (over 60) have failed to establish improvement in outcomes.

    Possible reasons:

    - Failure to include the adequate population (e.g., extreme preterm infants with hsPDA)
    - Relying solely on PDA diameter as a criterion for intervention
    - Lack of medical treatment efficacy (failure to achieve ductal closure)
    - High rate of contamination in placebo groups with open label treatment and spontaneous ductal closure
  - Determining the point where PDA transitions from being an expected condition in prematurity to a pathological entity is challenging.
  - Factors that can help clarifying the controversy:

    Identification of the high-risk population who would benefit from intervention (e.g., preterm infants <26 weeks gestational age).
    Comprehensive assessment of PDA rather than relying solely on diameter.
    Investigate more effective therapeutic approaches.
    Long-term follow-up of patients who were chronically exposed to a large shunt.

- Centre-specific rationale for not closing small PDAs is related to the low long-term risks. Estimated risk of infective endocarditis in small PDA, assuming no change in size or hemodynamic significance over time, is 0.01% per year for 85–90 years, or 0.1% lifetime risk. This is similar to the risk of a major adverse side effect following intervention for closing a small PDA. Benefits do not outweigh risks and costs of closing all small PDAs in the entire population.

Bibliography

1. Aggarwal V, Petit CJ, Glatz AC, et al. Stenting of the ductus arteriosus for ductal-dependent pulmonary blood flow-current techniques and procedural considerations. Congenit Heart Dis. 2019;14(1):110–5. https://doi.org/10.1111/chd.12709.
2. Backes CH, Hill KD, Shelton EL, et al. Patent ductus arteriosus: a contemporary perspective for the pediatric and adult cardiac care provider. J Am Heart Assoc. 2022;11(17): e025784. https://doi.org/10.1161/JAHA.122.025784.

3. Caris E and Arya B (2022) Abnormalities of the ductus arteriosus and pulmonary arteries. In: Lai WW., Mertens LL., Cohen MS, Geva T (ed) Echocardiography in pediatric and congenital heart disease: from fetus to adult. 3rd edn. Wiley Blackwell, p 360–381.
4. Fortescue EB, Lock JE, Galvin T, et al. To close or not to close: the very small patent ductus arteriosus. Congenit Heart Dis. 2010;5(4):354–65. https://doi.org/10.1111/j.1747-0803.2010.00435.x.
5. Philip R, Waller BR 3rd, Agrawal V, et al. Morphologic characterization of the patent ductus arteriosus in the premature infant and the choice of transcatheter occlusion device. Catheter Cardiovasc Interv. 2016;87(2):310–7. https://doi.org/10.1002/ccd.26287.
6. Shepherd JL, Noori S. What is a hemodynamically significant PDA in preterm infants? Congenit Heart Dis. 2019;14(1):21–6. https://doi.org/10.1111/chd.12727.
7. Smith A, El-Khuffash A. Patent ductus arteriosus clinical trials: lessons learned and future directions. Children (Basel). 2021;8(1):47. https://doi.org/10.3390/children8010047.
8. Taggart NW, Anderson JH, Yasir Qureshi M, et al. Patent ductus arteriosus and aortopulmonary window. In: Shaddy RE, Penny DJ, Feltes TF, et al., editors. Moss and Adams' heart disease in infants, children, and adolescents : including the fetus and young adult. 10th ed. Philadelphia: Wolters Kluwer; 2022. p. 765–81.
9. Ungerleider GD, Williams DA, Ungerleider RM, et al. Patent Ductus Arteriosus. In: Ungerleider R, Nelson K, Cooper D, et al., editors. Critical Heart Disease in Infants and Children. 3rd ed. Elsevier; 2019. p. 536–43.
10. Valdeomillos E, Jalal Z, Boudjemline Y. Transcatheter ductus arteriosus stenting in paediatric cardiology: Indications, results and perspectives. Arch Cardiovasc Dis. 2020;113(2):129–41. https://doi.org/10.1016/j.acvd.2019.10.004.

Aortopulmonary Window

Conall Morgan and Anne I. Dipchand

Abstract Aortopulmonary window is a rare congenital heart lesion that presents in infancy with symptoms of congestive heart failure due to a large left to right shunt. It is an abnormal communication between the intrapericardial components of the ascending aorta and pulmonary trunk in the presence of two patent semilunar valves. It often occurs in isolation but can be associated with interruption of the aortic arch Type A and anomalous origin of a coronary artery or right pulmonary artery. Surgical correction is indicated at diagnosis and long-term outcomes are excellent.

Keywords Aortopulmonary window · Left to right shunt · Congestive heart failure · Anomalous origin of coronary artery · Aortic origin of right pulmonary artery

Abbreviations

AP	Aortopulmonary
CXR	Chest X-ray
ECG	Electrocardiogram
LA	Left atrium
LV	Left ventricle
IAA	Interrupted aortic arch
PA	Pulmonary artery
RPA	Right pulmonary artery
TGA	Transposition of the great arteries
VSD	Ventricular septal defect

C. Morgan · A. I. Dipchand (✉)
Division of Cardiology, Department of Paediatrics, Labatt Family Heart Centre, The Hospital for Sick Children, University of Toronto, Toronto, ON, Canada
e-mail: Anne.dipchand@sickkids.ca

C. Morgan
e-mail: Conallthomas.morgan@sickkids.ca

© The Author(s), under exclusive license to Springer Nature Switzerland AG 2024

A. I. Dipchand et al. (eds.), *Manual of Cardiac Care in Children*,
https://doi.org/10.1007/978-3-031-70973-9_7

Key Points

- An abnormal communication between the intrapericardial components of the ascending aorta and pulmonary trunk in the presence of two patent arterial valves.
- Defects are usually large and usually present with heart failure in infancy.
- Defects occur in isolation in only 50% so careful thought must be given to rule out coexisting cardiac anomalies, including IAA or anomalous origin of right coronary artery or pulmonary artery
- Early surgical repair is associated with excellent long-term outcome and a low complication rate.

1 Nomenclature

- Abdominal situs solitus, levocardia, atrioventricular concordance, ventriculoarterial concordance, left aortic arch. Communication between the ascending aorta and main pulmonary trunk.

2 Anatomy

- Abnormal communication between the intrapericardial components of the ascending aorta and pulmonary trunk in the presence of two patent arterial valves.
- Distinguished from common arterial trunk by the presence of two separate arterial valves arising from discrete subaortic and subpulmonary outflow tracts.
- The defect is usually located between the left lateral wall of the aorta and the right wall of the pulmonary trunk
- Its dimensions determine the amount of shunt and pulmonary arterial pressures
- The window is usually circular, helical or rarely tunnel-like and positioned proximal to the branching of the pulmonary arteries but distal to the arterial valves.
- Classification of AP windows is according to a system proposed by Mori et al. (Fig. 1).

3 Embryology

- Failure of closure of the embryonic aortopulmonary foramen during developmental separation of aorta and pulmonary trunk (fusion of proximal central cushions).

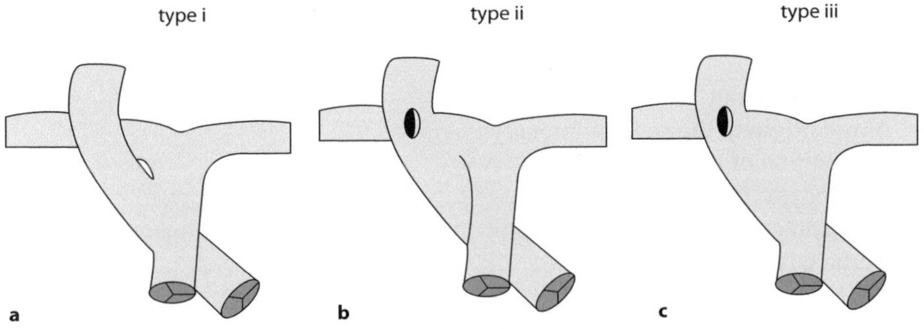

Fig. 1 Classification of aortopulmonary windows A Type 1 (proximal) defect: occurs in the proximal part of the aortopulmonary septum. B Type 2 (distal) defect: occurs in the distal part of the aortopulmonary septum adjacent to the origin of the right pulmonary artery. C Type 3 defect (total): is a combination of both type 1 and 2 defects

4 Epidemiology

- Rare; accounting for only 0.2–0.6% of all cases of congenital heart disease
- 1/600 (~0.2%) of surgical cases at SickKids

5 Clinical Physiology and Presentation

- Produces a left to right shunt which is haemodynamically similar to a common arterial trunk.
- Symptoms depend on the size of the defect.
- Most defects result in a large continuous left to right shunt.
- Cardiomegaly due to a volume loaded left atrium and ventricle.
- Branch pulmonary arteries are usually enlarged.
- Typically presents with heart failure which begins in the neonatal period as the pulmonary vascular resistance falls.
- Cyanosis does not occur unless there is bidirectional shunting in the setting of increase pulmonary vascular resistance.

6 Natural History

- Similar to other uncorrected large left to right shunts (e.g. VSD) with high mortality.
- Late presentation is usually accompanied by significant (or even fixed) pulmonary hypertension.

7 Associated Lesions

- Isolated in about 50% of patients
- Aortic origin of the right pulmonary artery
- Interruption of the aortic arch type A
- Tetralogy of Fallot
- Anomalous origin of the left or right coronary arteries from pulmonary trunk
- Aortic coarctation
- VSD

7.1 Rare

- Pulmonary or aortic atresia
- Tricuspid atresia
- TGA
- Not associated with DiGeorge syndrome
- Non cardiac abnormalities include VATER association, renal anomalies and hypospadius[4].

8 Diagnostic Studies

8.1 ECG

- Usually normal
- Left atrial enlargement or left ventricular hypertrophy can be sometimes seen.

8.2 CXR

- Cardiomegaly with prominent pulmonary vascular markings and hyperinflation.

8.3 Echocardiography

- Diagnostic imaging of choice.
- Antenatal diagnosis is possible; a dilated LA/LV may raise suspicion.
- Can usually be imaged directly and colour applied to see flow through the defect.

- Often ultrasonographic “dropout” in the area where the aorta and pulmonary arteries cross may give the impression of an AP window so careful examination of this area is required.
- Parasternal long and short axis views are used to demonstrate two arterial valves therefore ruling out common arterial trunk.
- Significant flow reversal in the abdominal aorta may be seen.
- Pulmonary hypertension should be ruled out as well as coexisting cardiac anomalies.

9 Indications for Intervention/Surgery

- Presence of the defect.

10 Timing of Intervention and Management Strategy

- Repair usually at presentation; preferably before age 3–6 months before irreversible pulmonary vascular changes occur.
- Preoperative management includes the medical treatment of heart failure.

11 Surgical Strategy

- Surgical repair usually involves division of the window with patch repair of both the aortic and pulmonary defects taking care to identify the position of the coronary ostia.
- Alternative is patch closure from a transaortic approach (still requiring median sternotomy and cardiopulmonary bypass).
- Important to locate the left coronary ostium which may be close to the edge of the aortopulmonary window.
- If the right pulmonary artery is anomalous, the patch can be tunneled to include the RPA in the repair.
- Transcatheter approach has been reported but is not the approach of choice.
- Potential residual lesions
  - Residual shunt
  - Narrowing of PA or Aorta
  - Pulmonary hypertension (especially if late repair)
  - Coronary ostial stenosis.

12 Intensive Care Physiology and Management

- Potential for postoperative pulmonary hypertension in patients with late presentation and/or cyanosis.
- Otherwise, good candidates for early extubation.
- Post-operative course is expected to be short and uncomplicated.

13 Outcome

- Long term outcome is excellent if surgical repair is performed early in life.
- Mortality < 2% for isolated defects. If in combination with other defects, then outcome is similar to that of the associated defect.
- Late complications are rare.

Bibliography

1. Anderson RH, Baker EJ, Penny D, et al. Paediatric Cardiology. 3rd ed. Churchill: Livingstone; 2010.
2. Balaji S, Burch M, Sullivan ID. Accuracy of cross-sectional echocardiography in diagnosis of aortopulmonary window. Am J Cardiol. 1991;67(7):650–3.
3. Kutsche LM. Van Mierop LH (1987) Anatomy and pathogenesis of aorticopulmonary septal defect. Am J Cardiol. 1987;59(5):443–7.
4. Marmon LM, Balsara RK, Chen R, et al. Congenital cardiac anomalies associated with the DiGeorge syndrome: a neonatal experience. Ann Thorac Surg. 1984;38(2):146–50.
5. Mori K, Ando M, Takao A, et al (1978). Distal type of aortopulmonary window. Report of 4 cases. Br Heart J 40(6):681–689.
6. Valsangiacomo ER, Smallhorn JF (2002) Images in cardiovascular medicine. Prenatal diagnosis of aortopulmonary window by fetal echocardiography. Circulation 105(24):E192.

Partial Atrioventricular Septal Defect

Michael Grattan

Abstract Partial atrioventricular septal defects (AVSD) are variants of AVSDs with no ventricular shunt. They occur when there is incomplete fusion of the primum septum and endocardial cushions in embryogenesis. The result is a single atrioventricular (AV) junction with two separate valve orifices and an interatrial shunt (primum defect). Partial AVSDs and secundum atrial septal defects (ASD) have similar hemodynamics with right-sided volume overload. However, partial AVSDs also have a high incidence of AV valve dysfunction and other associated lesions, which can dominate their clinical presentation. Patients are often asymptomatic at presentation and referred for a heart murmur. The diagnosis of an interatrial shunt is made clinically, with the diagnosis of a partial AVSD confirmed by echocardiography. Echocardiography demonstrates the defining features of an AVSD with a primum defect but no interventricular shunting. Echocardiography is used to determine the size of the defect, the degree of AV valve dysfunction and the presence of associated lesions. The great majority of patients diagnosed with partial AVSDs are recommended for surgical repair in childhood. Partial AVSDs have a high rate of reoperation, usually for AV valve dysfunction and (less commonly) left ventricular outflow tract obstruction. Morbidity and mortality are higher than secundum ASD repair, especially if reoperation is required.

Keywords Atrioventricular septal defect · AVSD · Endocardial cushion defect · Primum ASD · Primum defect · Partial AVSD · Transitional AVSD

Abbreviations

ASD	Atrial septal defect
AV	Atrioventricular
AVSD	Atrioventricular septal defect

M. Grattan (✉)
Department of Paediatrics, Children's Hospital at London Health Sciences Centre, London, ON, Canada
e-mail: michael.grattan@lhsc.on.ca

© The Author(s), under exclusive license to Springer Nature Switzerland AG 2024

A. I. Dipchand et al. (eds.), *Manual of Cardiac Care in Children*,
https://doi.org/10.1007/978-3-031-70973-9_8

AVVR	Atrioventricular valve regurgitation
CoA	Coarctation of the aorta
LAVV	Left atrioventricular valve
LAVVR	Left atrioventricular valve regurgitation
LV	Left ventricle
LVOTO	Left ventricular outflow tract obstruction
RAVVR	Right atrioventricular valve regurgitation
RV	Right ventricle
VA	Ventriculo-arterial
VSD	Ventricular septal defect

Key Points

- Partial atrioventricular septal defects are variants of AVSDs with no ventricular shunt.
- Pathophysiology mainly due to left-to-right atrial shunt, atrioventricular (AV) valve dysfunction and associated lesions.
- Earlier clinical presentation compared to secundum atrial septal defect (ASD) due to associated lesions and AV valve dysfunction.
- Most patients with partial AVSDs are recommended to have surgical repair in childhood.
- High reintervention rate due to AV valve dysfunction and left ventricular (LV) outflow tract obstruction (LVOTO).

1 Nomenclature

- Segmental anatomy: situs solitus (rarely situs ambiguous or inversus), concordant AV and ventriculo-arterial (VA) connections, usually left aortic arch
- Partial AVSD:
  - Common AV junction with two separate AV valve orifices. The bridging leaflets have become fused to the ventricular septum, creating two orifices to what is embryologically a common AV valve.
  - Presence of interatrial communication (defect anterior and inferior to the true primum atrial septum, between the primum septum and the endocardial cushions).
  - No ventricular septal defect (VSD) component
- Transitional AVSDs are similar to partial AVSDs but with a small, restrictive VSD component (usually of minimal hemodynamic significance), between the attachments of the superior and inferior bridging leaflets to the ventricular septum
- Common Alternative Nomenclature

- Primum defect
- Primum ASD
- Partial or incomplete AVSD / AV canal defect

2 Anatomy

2.1 *Defining Characteristics of AVSD (Fig. 1)*

- Common AV junction.
- Unwedged (sprung), anteriorly displaced aortic outflow tract and aortic valve with loss of fibrous continuity between aortic and left AV valves (LAVV)
- Elongated LV outflow tract with inlet–outlet disproportion.

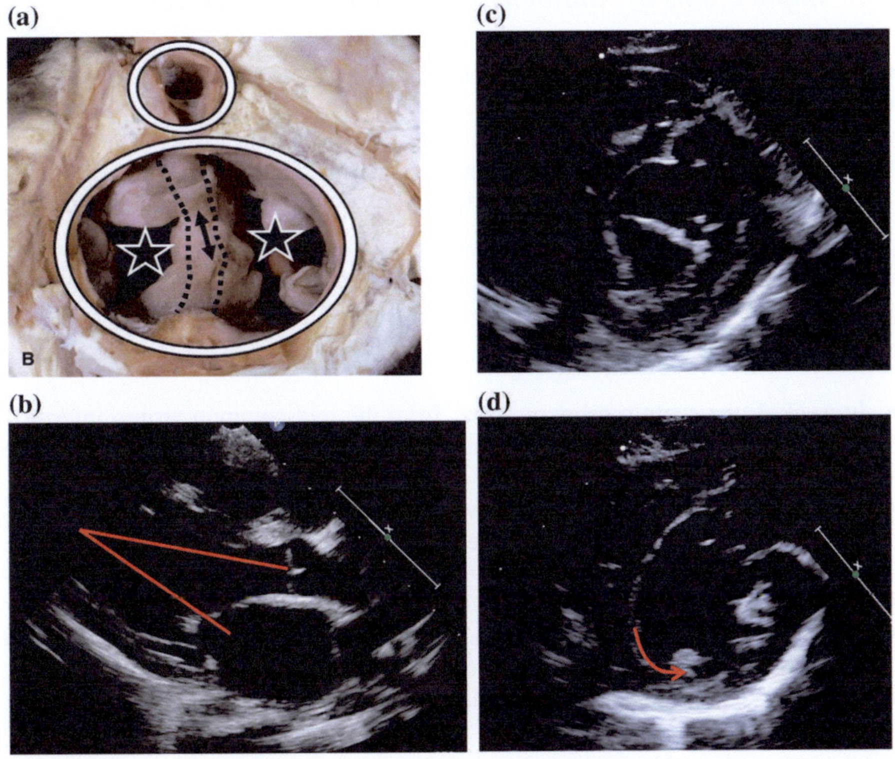

Fig. 1 A. Surgeon's view of the AV valves showing a common valve junction, two separate valve orifices and an unwedged aortic outflow tract. B. Echocardiographic parasternal long axis view showing inlet–outlet disproportion. C. Echocardiographic parasternal short axis view of the trileaflet left AV valve. D. Echocardiographic parasternal short axis view of the left AV valve papillary muscles showing rotation of the posterior-medial papillary muscle. Reprinted from Anderson et al.

- Counterclockwise rotated papillary muscles (especially posteromedial papillary muscle) and closely spaced papillary muscles.
- Trileaflet LAVV (zone of apposition between the superior and inferior bridging leaflets often referred to as a 'cleft' LAVV).

2.2 Additional Defining Characteristics of Partial AVSDs (Compared to Complete AVSDs)

- Two separate AV valve orifices.
- Interatrial communication antero-inferior to oval fossa.
- Scooped-out ventricular septum but no defect.

2.3 Implications of Anatomic Characteristics of AVSD

- Elongated aortic outflow tract with potential for LVOTO.
- Trifoliate LAVV with 'cleft' that is a potential source for AV valve regurgitation (AVVR).
- Increasing counterclockwise rotation of posteromedial papillary muscle results in smaller mural leaflet and increased risk for LAVV stenosis, or inability to fully close 'cleft'

3 Embryology

- In week 4, the septum primum grows from the mid-common atrium inferiorly towards the endocardial cushions. The leading edge of the septum primum is the mesenchymal cap.
- The septum primum normally fuses with the endocardial cushions, with reabsorption of the superior portion to form the ostium secundum. Subsequent invagination of the atrial wall completes the formation of the atrial septum.
- Failure of endocardial cushion fusion leads to characteristic AV valve abnormality.
- AV valve tissue completely shrouds any potential ventricular communication and forms a bridge of tissue separating common AV junction into two valve orifices.
- True atrial septum remains intact (additional secundum ASD often present).

4 Epidemiology

- AVSD: 3–4% of congenital heart disease (0.4 per 1000 patients).

- Partial AVSD less common than complete AVSD (exact incidence unknown; ~ 20% of all AVSDs in various surgical congenital heart disease databases).
- 23% of patients with partial AVSDs have Trisomy 21 and 6% have other genetic syndromes.
- Increased risk of congenital heart disease if first degree relative with AVSD.

5 Clinical Physiology and Presentation

- Left to right inter-atrial shunt causing excessive pulmonary blood flow and right heart dilatation.
- Degree of shunt influenced by size of defect, ventricular compliance, and associated lesions/hemodynamic abnormalities that raise left atrial pressure (e.g. coarctation of the aorta (CoA) or patent ductus arteriosus).
- Transitional AVSDs have small but insignificant ventricular shunt that does not affect clinical symptoms.
- Infants and children usually asymptomatic, but symptoms of pulmonary congestion may occur earlier than isolated secundum ASD due to associated lesions.
- Physical exam:
  - Palpation: Right ventricular (RV) heave.
  - Auscultation:

    Soft systolic ejection murmur at left upper sternal border due to increased pulmonary blood flow
    Fixed, widely split S2
    ± mid-diastolic rumble at left lower sternal border or apex (flow-related).
    ± holosystolic murmur (AVVR)
  - ± dysmorphic features of Down Syndrome.

6 Natural History

- Arrhythmia most common long-term complication (20% by 25 years, significant increase in incidence after 30 years).
  - Atrial fibrillation, atrial flutter, rarely complete heart block.
  - AVVR risk factor for atrial arrhythmia.
  - Tachy- and brady-arrhythmias precipitate heart failure by increasing left to right shunting.
- Pulmonary hypertension uncommon but described (often after 4th decade or associated with Trisomy 21).
- Infective endocarditis involving AV valves.
- Progressive AVVR.

- Earlier presentation of congestive heart failure (early childhood) with premature death.

- Associated CoA or LVOTO.
  - More rapid progression of Left AVVR (LAVVR) and progression of congestive heart failure.
  - Initial presentation may be exclusively related to CoA

7 Associated Lesions

7.1 Common

- Secundum ASD or patent foramen ovale (44%).
- Significant AVVR (left 36%, right 18%).
- Anatomic abnormality of the LAVV (e.g. parachute or double orifice; 18%).
- Patent ductus arteriosus (18%).
- Left superior vena cava (4%).
- Heterotaxy (4%)
  - More likely left atrial isomerism (right atrial isomerism more associated with unbalanced, complete AVSDs).

7.2 Less Common Associations

- LVOTO (2.3%)
  - Common late post-operative complication. Higher pre-operative incidence compared to complete AVSD. Often progressive.
- Mechanism includes:
  - Accessory AV valve tissue
  - Subaortic ridge/membrane
  - Tunnel-like obstruction
  - Hypoplastic aortic valve annulus
- CoA (1.1%; may lead to neonatal presentation independently or by exacerbating congestive heart failure. If neonatal presentation, associated CoA must be ruled out).
- Anomalous pulmonary venous return (1.7%).
- Others
  - Muscular VSD(s)
  - Hypoplastic LV or RV with septal malalignment

- Malaligned atrial septum
- Common atrium
- Pulmonary stenosis
- Cor Triatriatum

8 Diagnostic Studies

8.1 ECG

- Normal sinus rhythm (atrial rhythm if left atrial isomerism albeit rare).
- First-degree heart block.
- Superior axis or left axis deviation.
  - Median QRS axis − 30° but range − 70 to + 70°.
  - 45% of patients can have normal axis.
- Atrial enlargement.
- RV hypertrophy (volume overload) with RSR' or rsR' pattern.

8.2 CXR

- Cardiomegaly.
- Increased pulmonary arterial blood flow.
- Right atrial and RV enlargement.

8.3 Echocardiography

- Usually adequate for complete diagnosis.
- Shunts.
  - Atrial communication

    Size of primum defect.
    Presence of secundum ASD or patent foramen ovale.
  - Define atrial septum position (relative to ventricular septum).
  - Rule out ventricular component of AVSD and ventricular-atrial shunts.
  - Rule out additional VSDs and patent ductus arteriosus.
- Assessment of AV valve.
  - Morphology: mural leaflet size, papillary muscle number and spacing.
  - Valve function: stenosis and regurgitation.

  - Valve support apparatus and potential for subaortic obstruction.
- Assessment of LV outflow tract.
  - Obstruction and potential for obstruction.
- Ventricular dominance and function.
- Rule out associated lesions including
  - CoA and hypoplastic aortic arch.
  - Left superior vena cava.
  - Findings of left atrial isomerism.

8.4 Other Imaging Modalities

- Not routinely required.
- MRI for quantification of ventricular volumes (if potentially unbalanced), shunts and AVVR.
- Cardiac catheterization not routinely required; indicated for late repairs for assessment of pulmonary vascular resistance and vascular reactivity.
- Genetic testing.

9 Indications for Intervention/Surgery

- Repair offered due to long-term risk for of AVVR, arrhythmia and pulmonary hypertension
- Congestive heart failure or significant right sided heart enlargement
- Significant AVVR
  - Associated LVOTO

10 Timing of Intervention and Management Strategy

- Children are usually asymptomatic but may require diuretics and supplemental calories for congestive symptoms.
- Partial AVSDs are not amenable to interventional device closure.
- Uncomplicated primum defect.
  - Complete repair in early childhood (median 1.5–2.6 years).
  - Worse outcome when repaired in infancy or adulthood
  - Earlier surgery if significant pulmonary congestion or evidence of pulmonary hypertension.

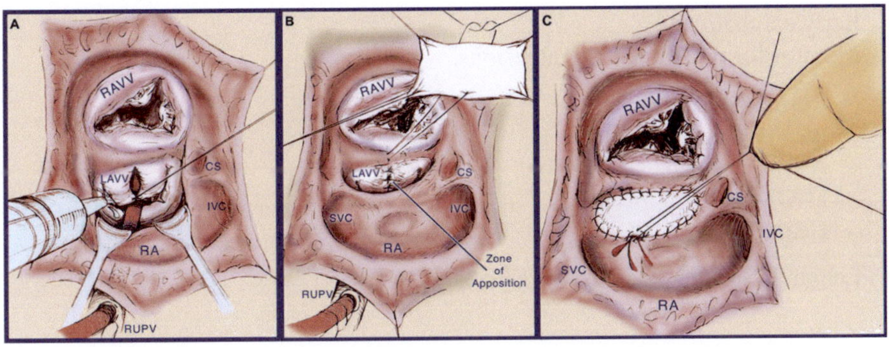

Fig. 2 Standard surgical repair involves a single patch of the primum defect and suture closure of the superior and inferior bridging leaflet commissure (cleft). Reprinted from Devlin et al.

- Associated lesions may necessitate earlier repair.
  - Moderate or greater AVVR.
  - LVOTO.
  - CoA (often neonatal repair of CoA with delayed complete repair).
- Other factors may necessitate alternative surgical approach.
  - Hypoplastic LV or RV.

11 Surgical Strategy (Fig. 2)

- Patch closure of ASD.
- Suture closure of 'cleft'.
  - Complete closure (versus partial- or non-closure) is protective against recurrent AVVR
  - Complete closure may not be possible if parachute LAVV or very small/ asymmetric mural leaflet.
  - Additional valve repair techniques such as commisurroplasty, edge-to-edge leaflet repairs and annuloplasty may be necessary
- Repair of associated lesions.
- Avoid conduction tissue
- Suitable for minimally invasive approach in experienced centres

12 Intensive Care Physiology and Management

- Usually uncomplicated in absence of residual lesions.

- Early extubation.
- Monitor for potential residual lesions.
  - Residual atrial shunt.
  - AVVR.
  - AV valve stenosis.
  - LVOTO.
  - Heart block.
- Length of hospitalization 3–4 days.

13 Outcome

13.1 Mortality

- < 1% early; 2–10% late (with residual lesions or complications); up to 98% 10-year survival.
- Risks for death
  - Grossly malformed LAVV.
  - Pre-operative pulmonary hypertension.
  - Residual lesions.
- Young age (less than 1 year) at repair does not increase mortality but is associated with increased hospital and intensive care unit stay
- Down's syndrome, weight and cardiac bypass/cross-clamp times do <u>not</u> increase mortality.

13.2 Reoperation

- High rate of reoperation(15–20%) at 10 years; higher rate of reoperation for LVOTO compared to complete AVSD (Fig. 3). Commonest reason is recurrent LAVVR
- Risk for reoperation:
  - Infant repair, non-Trisomy 21, heterotaxy, pre-existing LAVV anomaly
- Indications: LAVVR: 31–67%; LVOTO 25–38%, RAVVR 22%, ASD 11%.
- LAVVR.
  - Freedom from moderate + regurgitation: 89% at 5 years, 78% at 10 years.
  - Freedom from AV valve reintervention 91% at 10 years.

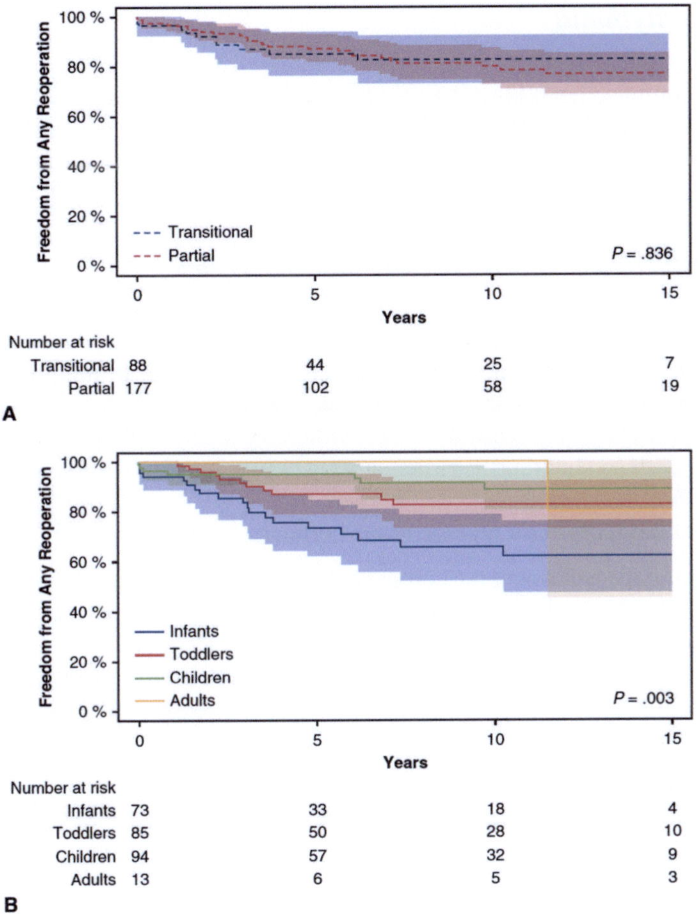

Fig. 3 Reoperation free survival following partial AVSD repair. Reprinted from Mery etal. [5]

 - Late regurgitation (moderate +) correlated with early postoperative regurgitation (moderate +) but not pre-operative regurgitation grade, method of cleft closure or age.

- LVOTO (second most common indication).
  - Reoperation negatively impacts on mortality.
  - Most likely subaortic membrane, tunnel-like obstruction or LAVV accessory tissue.
  - Recurrence rate of LVOTO if needing repair is high (35–45%), and often requiring more extensive reoperations.

13.3 Arrhythmia

- Early: complete heart block (0–2%; higher incidence compared to other ASDs).
- Late: atrial fibrillation/flutter (up to 25%, with no association with age at surgery), highest risk if atrial enlargement, and moderate + LAVVR

13.4 Alternative Strategies and Controversies

- Timing of surgery in standard partial AVSD – earlier surgery to minimize hemodynamic effects of lesion versus later surgery (>5 years) to minimize need for blood products and possibly decrease risk of reoperation.
- Timing for surgery in partial AVSDs with very small or absent primum defect (AVSD with no shunting) – earlier surgery to prevent AVVR versus later surgery only if AVVR develops.
- Route of atrial patch (in relation to the coronary sinus)
  - Routing the patch over the coronary sinus increases the distance of any sutures from the AV node. The coronary sinus drains to the left atrium (not feasible with left superior vena cava draining to the coronary sinus).
  - Routing the patch around the coronary sinus allows the coronary sinus to drain to the right atrium. This is more anatomic but may raise the risk of iatrogenic complete heart block.
- Increasing use of minimally invasive, endoscopic repairs.
- Borderline LV – single ventricle versus two ventricle repair (see Chap. 34).

Bibliography

1. Anderson RH, Wessels A, Vettukattil JJ. Morphology and morphogenesis of atrioventricular septal defect with common atrioventricular junction. World J Pediatr Congenit Heart Surg. 2010;1(1):59–67.
2. Anderson RH, Mohun TJ, Brown NA. Clarifying the morphology of the ostium primum defect. J Anat. 2015;226(3):244–57.
3. Devlin PJ, Backer CL, Eltayeb O, et al. Repair of partial atrioventricular septal defect: age and outcomes. Ann Thorac Surg. 2016;102(1):170–7.
4. Jacobs JP, Jacobs ML, Mavroudis C, et al. Atrioventricular septal defects: lessons learned about patterns of practice and outcomes from the congenital heart surgery database of the society of thoracic surgeons. World J Pediatr Congenit Heart Surg. 2010;1(1):68–77.
5. Jacquemart E, Bessiere F, Combes N, et al. Incidence, risk factors, and outcomes of atrial arrhythmias in adult patients with atrioventricular septal defect. JACC Clin Electrophysiol. 2022;8(3):331–40.
6. Hakacova N. Electrophysiologic and anatomical relationships studied in primum atrioventricular septal defect. J Electrocardiol. 2009;43(2):155–60.

7. Mery CM, Zea-Vera R, Chacon-Portillo MA, et al. Contemporary results after repair of partial and transitional atrioventricular septal defects. J Thorac Cardiovasc Surg. 2019;157(3):1117–27.
8. Smallhorn JF, Tommasini G, Anderson RH, et al. Assessment of atrioventricular septal defects by two dimensional echocardiography. Br Heart J. 1982;47(2):109–21.
9. Somerville J. Ostium primum defect: factors causing deterioration in the natural history. Br Heart J. 1965;27(3):413–9.
10. Tsao CW, Aday AW, Almarzooq ZI, et al. Heart disease and stroke statistics-2022 update: a report from the American heart association. Circulation. 2022;145(8):e153–639.

Complete Atrioventricular Septal Defect

Andreea Dragulescu

Abstract The complete atrioventricular septal defect (AVSD) is a variant of AVSD with significant atrial and ventricular components and a common atrioventricular valve (AVV). A high proportion of cases are detected prenatally. It is often associated with Trisomy 21 (Down syndrome). The patients usually develop symptoms of heart failure early in life. All patients with complete AVSD require surgical intervention, usually at 3–6 months of life, with low morbidity and mortality. Late referrals are at high risk of pulmonary vascular disease, especially if Trisomy 21. Complex forms of AVSD include associations with Tetralogy of Fallot and atrial isomerism. Main indications for reoperation are left atrioventricular valve regurgitation, left ventricular outflow tract obstruction, or residual shunt.

Keywords Atrioventricular septal defect · Common atrioventricular valve · Left/right atrioventricular valve · Cleft · Primum ASD · Inlet VSD · Bridging leaflet · Mural leaflet

Abbreviations

ASD	Atrial septal defect
AVSD	Atrioventricular septal defect
AVV	Atrioventricular valve
AVVR	Atrioventricular valve regurgitation
LVOTO	Left ventricular outflow tract obstruction
PDA	Persistent ductus arteriosus
PFO	Persistent foramen ovale
Qp	Pulmonary blood flow
Qs	Systemic blood flow
SVC	Superior vena cava

A. Dragulescu (✉)
Department of Paediatrics, Division of Cardiology, Labatt Family Heart Centre, Hospital for Sick Children, University of Toronto, Toronto, ON, Canada
e-mail: andreea.dragulescu@sickkids.ca

© The Author(s), under exclusive license to Springer Nature Switzerland AG 2024
A. I. Dipchand et al. (eds.), *Manual of Cardiac Care in Children*,
https://doi.org/10.1007/978-3-031-70973-9_9

T21	Trisomy 21
TOF	Tetralogy of fallot
VSD	Ventricular septal defect

Key Points

- Atrioventricular septal defect (AVSD) results from formation of a common fibrous ring connecting atria and ventricles, with associated atrial and ventricular septal defects.
- Primary repair at 3–6 months of age or earlier if signs and symptoms of heart failure.
- High incidence of Trisomy 21 (T21).
- High risk related to degree of atrioventricular valve regurgitation (AVVR) and morphology of the left atrioventricular valve (e.g., single papillary muscle).
- Postoperative management includes consideration for pulmonary hypertension or vascular reactivity, particularly in children with T21.
- Postoperative course may be complicated by residual lesions, including atrioventricular valve stenosis or regurgitation, or residual VSD).
- While in the majority of cases the ventricles and atrioventricular valve are balanced, there is a significant spectrum of ventricular dominance with implied hypoplasia of the other ventricle, that may result in a single-ventricle physiology.

1 Nomenclature

- Common atrioventricular junction with deficient atrioventricular septation.
- Primum ASD and inlet VSD under the bridging leaflets of the common AVV (Fig. 1).
- 30% in the setting of isomerism as part of a more complex anomaly.

2 Anatomy

- Common AVV is classically composed of two (superior and inferior) leaflets bridging across the ventricular septum, as well as a left lateral (mural) leaflet, a right antero-superior and a right inferior leaflet (Fig. 2).
- The Rastelli classification is based on the anatomy of the superior bridging leaflet: split, with multiple chordal attachments to the crest of the septum (type A), split, supported by a papillary muscle on the right side of the septum (type B) or a free floating superior leaflet (type C).

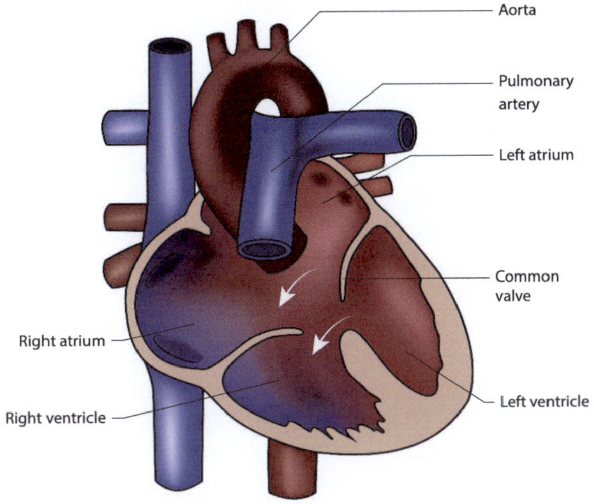

Fig. 1 Atrial and ventricular components (white arrows) of a complete atrioventricular septal defect, usually shunting left to right. Reproduced from Mayo Clinic Health Letter Diseases and Conditions, Atrioventricular canal defect-symptoms and causes—Mayo Clinic, Sept 13th, 2022, with permission from Mayo Foundation for Medical Education and Research, all rights reserved

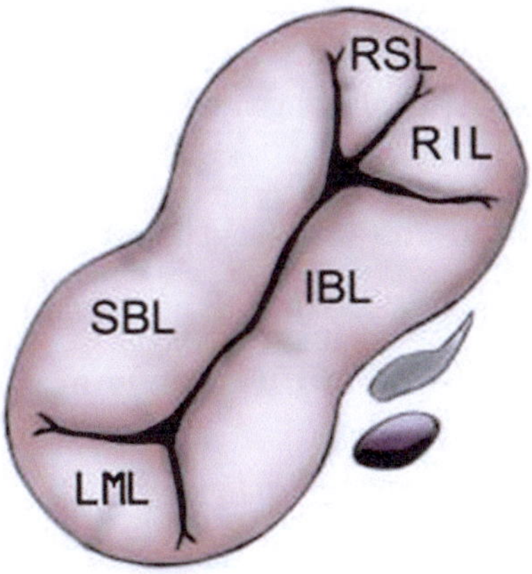

Fig. 2 Usual anatomy of the common atrioventricular valve. IBL—inferior bridging leaflet, LML—left mural leaflet, RIL—right inferior leaflet, RSL—right antero-superior leaflet, SBL—superior bridging leaflet

- Left mural leaflet may be absent or diminutive in cases with single or closely spaced papillary muscles.
- Ostium primum defect of the atrial septum. Non-restrictive defect in the inlet portion of the ventricular septum (variants with restrictive or absent ventricular component are discussed in Chap. 2; those with ventricular imbalance are discussed in Chap. 33).
- Aortic-mitral fibrous continuity is lost resulting in the aorta being "sprung" and elongation of the left ventricular outflow tract (goose neck).
- Atrioventricular valve dysplasia with significant regurgitation is more common in non-syndromic patients.
- Double orifice AVV is occasionally found (approximately 1 in 20 patients), especially if there are asymmetric papillary muscles.

3 Embryology

- The morphogenesis of AVSD is still not completely understood despite considerable research. Possibilities identified in mouse models include a defect in either endocardial cushion, mesenchymal cap, dorsal mesenchymal protrusion or a combination.
- In human embryos with AVSD no abnormal development of the endocardial cushions is described to date, whereas a diminished dorsal mesenchymal protrusion or vestibular spine development was observed in fetuses with T21 and an AVSD.
- In addition, abnormalities in fetal blood flow may affect septation and valve formation.
- Several genes have been identified to being involved in AVSD development: GATA4-6, TBX5, VEGF, amongst others.

4 Epidemiology

- Incidence 4–5.3 per 10.000 live births.
- 7% of all congenital heart diseases.
- Population at risk—genetic risk factors (i.e. T21), maternal risk factors (maternal diabetes, pregestational diabetes, obesity).
- 50–70% associated with T21; 25–30% of all T21 patients have a complete AVSD.

5 Clinical Physiology and Presentation

- The predominant presentation is congestive heart failure due to degree of shunting and atrioventricular valve regurgitation (AVVR).
- All babies with stigmata of T21 who have not had fetal echocardiography should undergo post-natal echocardiographic examination.
- The earliest presenting sign may be a heart murmur consistent with a VSD or AVVR.
- Complex forms may present with other symptoms such as cyanosis or even cardiogenic shock, depending on the associated lesions (TOF, obstructed pulmonary veins, duct dependent circulation).

6 Natural History

- If unoperated, progressive pulmonary vascular disease and Eisenmenger syndrome develop.
- This occurs earlier in T21 patients than in non-syndromic patients.

7 Associated Lesions

7.1 Common

- PFO or secundum ASD.
- PDA (more common in T21).

7.2 Less Common Associations

- Muscular VSDs (2–4%).
- TOF.
- Coarctation of the aorta.
- Bilateral SVC, unroofed coronary sinus.
- Isomerism (pulmonary stenosis/atresia, malposed great vessels, etc.).

8 Diagnostic Studies

8.1 ECG

- Superior axis, possible left or biventricular hypertrophy.

8.2 CXR

- Cardiomegaly.
- Increased pulmonary vascular markings.
- Pulmonary edema in severe cases.

8.3 Echocardiography

- Echocardiography adequately delineates the anatomy in over 99% of cases.
- Common atrioventricular valve; single vs. two left ventricular papillary muscles; size of left mural leaflet.
- Anatomy of the superior bridging leaflet (Rastelli classification).
- Location and degree of atrioventricular valve regurgitation.
- ASD size and shunting (primum, additional secundum ASD).
- VSD size and shunting (inlet, additional muscular VSD).
- Outflow tracts (e.g., obstruction).

- PDA.
- Aortic arch branching and flow.
- Pulmonary venous return.
- Systemic venous anatomy (e.g., left superior vena cava, unroofed coronary sinus).
- Assessment of valve commitment and balanced ventricles.
- Assessment for isomerism.

8.4 MRI or Cardiac Catheterization

- Rarely indicated; when late presentation and/or suspicion of pulmonary vascular disease.
- Calculation of Qp/Qs.
- Assessment of pulmonary vascular resistance.
- Assessment of ventricular volumes and flows in the setting of unbalanced ventricles.

9 Indications for Indication/Surgery

- Presence of the disease.

10 Timing of Intervention and Management Strategy

- Elective repair at 3–6 months of age.
- Repair earlier if intractable congestive heart failure despite medical treatment.
- A staged repair with initial pulmonary artery banding may be used in small babies, when neonatal arch repair is required or in cases with multiple VSDs.
- In cases with diminutive/absent mural leaflet, timing of repair will be dictated by severity of AVVR and/or clinical status.
- $>95\%$ are repaired electively.
- The association of AVSD – tetralogy of Fallot may require staged repair (e.g. right ventricular outflow tract stenting) as often presents with early cyanosis.
- Risk factors for mortality:
  - Weight < 3.5 kg
  - Age < 2.5 months

11 Surgical Strategy

- Surgical repair aims at complete repair of the septal defects and both atrioventricular valves.
- Different septation techniques have been described (single patch, two patch technique).
- Two patch repair is the most commonly used approach as it easily allows for individual customization.
- The single patch repair (also called Australian or Nunn technique) involves a single atrial patch, where the ventricular component is closed by the AVV leaflets being fixed to the crest of the septum (Fig. 3), is used mainly in cases with smaller VSD.
- Plane of septation of bridging leaflets needs to be found first. This is crucial, as it determines size, shape and level of left and right atrioventricular valve.
- VSD is closed first. Superior edge of patch runs underneath the atrioventricular valve bridging leaflets and the respective sutures separate these.
- The base of the ASD patch (autologous pericardium) sandwiches the bridging leaflets together with the superior edge of the VSD patch.
- Atrioventricular valve repair is crucial and may be limited by individual anatomic aspects (e.g., unbalanced AVSD, small mural leaflet, single papillary muscle).
- The left atrioventricular valve cleft is the “commissure” between superior and inferior bridging leaflet resulting from the septation procedure (zone of apposition).
- The cleft is usually closed completely (up to the insertion of primary chordae).

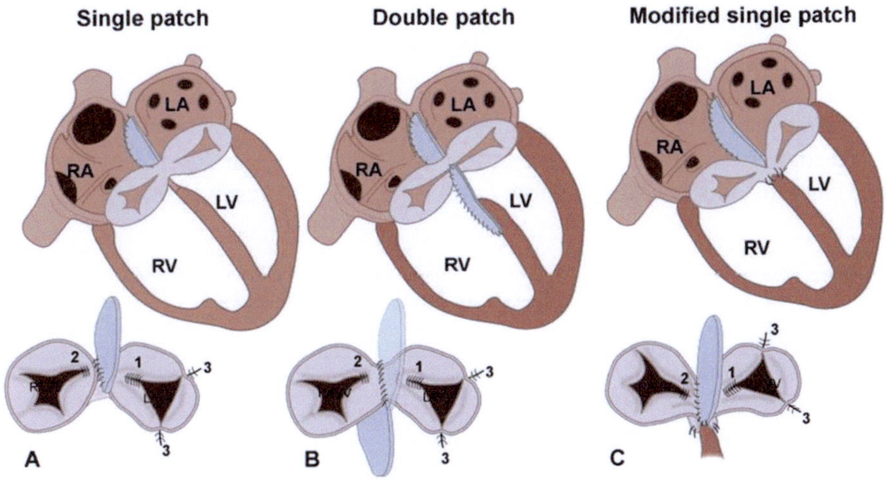

Fig. 3 Operative techniques. Reprinted from International Journal of Cardiology, Vol 202, Calkoen EE, Hazekamp MG, Blom NA, et al., Atrioventricular septal defect: From embryonic development to long-term follow-up, pp 784–795, 2016, with permission from Elsevier

- Additional procedures may be necessary to achieve valve competency (e.g., annuloplasty, commisuroplasty, papillary muscle splitting).
- Balance between residual regurgitation and inflow gradient needs to be found (target less than moderate regurgitation and less than 7–8 mmHg mean inflow gradient). This is highly depended on intraoperative judgment, especially because gradients are dependent on flow.
- ASD is closed with autologous pericardial patch or bovine pericardium.
- Great care needs to be taken to avoid impairment of conduction upon ASD closure. Patch suture usually runs at the very edge of the coronary sinus. Alternatively, the coronary sinus can be left on the left atrial side.
- More complex, staged interventions are required in complex cases depending on the associated lesions and clinical presentation.

12 Intensive Care Physiology and Management

- Early extubation possible following uncomplicated repair and stable hemodynamics—extubation in operating room rare given association with T21.
- Recognized risk of pulmonary vascular reactivity, especially in patients with T21 and if delayed closure.
- Risk of arrhythmia is low but can be associated with JET and atrial tachycardia.
- Systemic afterload reduction and avoidance of hypertension important consideration if residual left AVVR.

13 Outcome

- Perioperative mortality 2.9–3%.
- Overall survival 85% at 10y, 82% at 20y, 71% at 30y.
- Freedom from reoperation 88% at 10y, 83% at 20y, 78% at 30y.
- Main indications for reoperation: left AVVR, LVOTO, residual shunt.

14 Most Common Short-Term/long-Term Risks

- Early/late reoperation (~3/ ~ 12%).
- Significant ($\geq$ moderate) AVVR.
- Development of pulmonary hypertension.

Bibliography

1. Blom NA, Ottenkamp J, Wenink A, et al. Deficiency of the vestibular spine in atrioventricular septal defects in human fetuses with down syndrome. Am J Cardiol. 2003;91(2):180–4.
2. Calkoen EE, Hazekamp MG, Blom NA, et al. Atrioventricular septal defect: from embryonic development to long-term follow-up. Int J Cardiol. 2016;202:784–95.
3. Ginde S, Lam J, Hill GD, et al. Long-term outcomes after surgical repair of complete atrioventricular septal defect. J Thorac Cardiovasc Surg. 2015;150(2):369–74.
4. Hoffman JI, Kaplan S, Liberthson RR. Prevalence of congenital heart disease. Am Heart J. 2014;147(3):425–39.
5. Hove JR, Köster RW, Forouhar AS, et al. Intracardiac fluid forces are an essential epigenetic factor for embryonic cardiogenesis. Nature. 2003;421(6919):172–7.
6. Loffredo CA, Hirata J, Wilson PD, et al. Atrioventricular septal defects: possible etiologic differences between complete and partial defects. Teratology. 2001;63(2):87–93.
7. St Louis JD, Jodhka U, Jacobs JP, et al. Contemporary outcomes of complete atrioventricular septal defect repair: analysis of the Society of Thoracic Surgeons Congenital Heart Surgery Database. J Thorac Cardiovasc Surg. 2014;148(6):2526–31.
8. Ugaki S, Khoo NS, Ross DB, et al. Modified single-patch compared with two-patch repair of complete atrioventricular septal defect. Ann Thorac Surg. 2014;97(2):666–71.
9. Wenink AC, Zevallos JC. Developmental aspects of atrioventricular septal defects. Int J Cardiol. 1988;18(1):65–78.

Ebstein's Anomaly

Osami Honjo, Amine Mazine, and Lindsay R. Freud

Abstract Ebstein's anomaly is a rare congenital heart disease characterized by downward displacement and failure of delamination of the septal and posterior leaflets of the tricuspid valve. There is a wide spectrum of anatomy regarding the degree of downward displacement, severity of tricuspid regurgitation, size of the atrialized and functional portion of the right ventricle, and presence of right ventricular outflow tract obstruction. Physiology and clinical presentation vary substantially from neonatal presentation with profound low cardiac output, often in the context of circular shunting, to a stable biventricular circulation with minimal symptoms. Echocardiography is essential for diagnosis, and MRI is increasingly used in older patients. The natural history, indication for and type of surgical treatment strategy depend on the age and physiology at presentation. Neonatal management includes conservative medical management, ligation of the patent ductus arteriosus, or single ventricle palliation in the form of right ventricular exclusion (Starnes Procedure) depending on the severity of the lesion. Tricuspid valve repair (cone reconstruction) in later childhood or adult life is the mainstay of management in stable cases—but exact indications and timing for surgery are still controversial. Mortality is highest in the neonatal period at approximately 25%, with or without surgical intervention. The Starnes procedure and subsequent single ventricle palliation yields 10-year survival of approximately 80%. The cone reconstruction, which allows 360 degrees of tricuspid valve tissue in the anatomic, non-displaced tricuspid valve annulus, has become the first line surgical technique in childhood and young adults (beyond the neonatal period) and is associated with favorable short and medium-term clinical

O. Honjo
Division of Cardiovascular Surgery, Department of Surgery, Labatt Family Heart Centre, The Hospital for Sick Children, University of Toronto, Toronto, ON, Canada
e-mail: osami.honjo@sickkids.ca

A. Mazine
Division of Cardiovascular Surgery, University of Toronto, Toronto, ON, Canada
e-mail: amine.mazine@sickkids.ca

L. R. Freud (✉)
Division of Cardiology, Department of Paediatrics, Labatt Family Heart Centre, The Hospital for Sick Children, University of Toronto, Toronto, ON, Canada
e-mail: Lindsay.freud@sickkids.ca

© The Author(s), under exclusive license to Springer Nature Switzerland AG 2024
A. I. Dipchand et al. (eds.), *Manual of Cardiac Care in Children*,
https://doi.org/10.1007/978-3-031-70973-9_10

outcomes. The cone reconstruction can be done with very low operative mortality (< 2%) with 5-year freedom from tricuspid valve reoperation of 90–95%.

Keywords Ebstein's anomaly · Tricuspid valve · Tricuspid valve regurgitation · Cone reconstruction · Starnes procedure

Abbreviations

1.5VR	One and a half ventricle repair
ASD	Atrial septal defect
BCPS	Bidirectional cavopulmonary shunt
BTT	Blalock Taussig Thomas
CHD	Congenital heart disease
ECMO	Extracorporeal membrane oxygenation
LV	Left ventricle
iNO	Inhaled nitric oxide
PA	Pulmonary artery
PGE	Prostaglandin
PI	Pulmonary insufficiency
PVR	Pulmonary vascular resistance
Qp	Pulmonary blood flow
Qs	Systemic blood flow
RA	Right atrium
RCA	Right coronary artery
RV	Right ventricle
RVOTO	Right ventricular outflow tract obstruction
RVSP	Right ventricular systolic pressure
TR	Tricuspid regurgitation
TV	Tricuspid valve
VSD	Ventricular septal defect
WPW	Wolff-parkinson-white

Key Points

- Ebstein's anomaly is a rare congenital heart disease (CHD) that involves abnormalities of the tricuspid valve (TV) and right ventricle (RV) characterized by downward (apical) displacement and failure of delamination of the septal (and often posterior) leaflets.
- There is a wide spectrum of anatomy regarding the degree of downward displacement, severity of tricuspid regurgitation (TR), size of the atrialized and functional

portion of the RV, and presence of right ventricular outflow tract obstruction (RVOTO).

- Age, physiology and clinical presentation vary substantially from neonatal presentation with profound low cardiac output, often due to circular shunting, to a stable biventricular circulation with minimal TR in later childhood or adulthood.
- Indication and treatment strategy depend on the age and physiology at presentation and include conservative medical management or surgical intervention. Surgery can include: ligation of the persistent ductus arteriosus (PDA), or single ventricle palliation in the form of right ventricular exclusion (the Starnes Procedure) in the neonatal period or TV repair (cone reconstruction) in later childhood or adult life.
- The cone reconstruction, which allows 360 degrees of TV tissue in the anatomic, non-displaced TV annulus, has become the first line surgical technique in childhood and is associated with favorable short and medium-term clinical outcome.

1 Anatomy

- Tricuspid valve abnormalities
  - Downward (apical) displacement of the septal (and posterior) leaflet(s).
  - Failure of delamination of the septal (and posterior) leaflet(s) from the RV myocardium.
  - The anterior leaflet often has redundancy, multiple fenestrations, and tethering to the RV free wall, forming a sail-like curtain.
  - The true TV annulus in the right atrioventricular groove has various degrees of dilation, which often corresponds to the degree of TR.
- Right and left ventricular myocardium
  - Atrialized portion of the RV above the TV leaflets has abnormal thinning of the myocardium and disproportional dilation compared to the functional RV
  - Functional RV myocardium often has myopathic changes pathologically and clinically.
  - Anatomic RVOTO may exist, often in the form of anatomic pulmonary atresia. Functional pulmonary atresia refers to the inability of the RV to eject antegrade across the pulmonary valve.
  - Left ventricle (LV) and left side structures are often grossly normal, but the LV may be compressed by a hugely dilated RV and subjected to adverse ventriculo-ventricular interactions.
  - LV non-compaction co-exists in up to 20% of Ebstein's anomaly diagnosed in childhood (< 5% among adults with Ebstein's anomaly).
  - In the extreme form of fetal/neonatal Ebstein's anomaly, various degrees of lung hypoplasia may occur due to massive cardiomegaly (see Diagnostic Studies).

  - Right atrium (RA) is often hugely dilated. Atrial septal defects (ASD) are common (90%). Pre-excitation and accessory pathways in 30%.
- Charpentier Classification (Fig. 1): classification based on the severity of disease in 4 components, including septal/posterior leaflet displacement, anterior leaflet, atrialized ventricle, and functional RV. Type A is the mildest form with normal anterior leaflet and mild displacement through to Type D, the most severe with severe displacement resulting in a small functional RV limited to the outflow chamber.(Table 1).

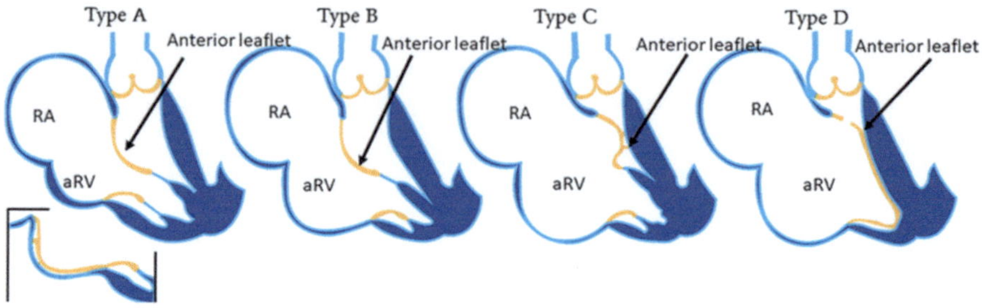

Fig. 1 Carpentier's classification of Ebstein's anomaly based on the severity of disease in 4 components: (1) septal/posterior leaflet displacement, (2) anterior leaflet, (3) atrialized ventricle (aRV), and (4) functional ventricle. Type A is mild septal leaflet displacement, normal anterior leaflet and normal RV size and function. Type B is moderate displacement with some reduced size or function of the RV and the anterior leaflet may have some tethering. Type C is severe septal leaflet displacement with small or reduced function RV and reduced anterior leaflet mobility. Type D is severe displacement with the RV only forming the outlet chamber and restriction of anterior leaflet. RA, right atrium. Reprinted from Pediatric Cardiology, Vol 44, Alsaied T, Christopher A, Adam B, et al., Multimodality imaging in Enstein Anomaly, pages 15–23, 1979, with permission from Springer Nature BV conveyed through Copyright Clearance Centre

Table 1 Charpentier classification

	Septal/posterior leaflet displacement	Anterior leaflet	Atrialized ventricle	Functional ventricle
Type A	Mild	Normal morphology and mobility	Small/ preserved function	Normal/ preserved function
Type B	Moderate	Abnormal attachment with normal mobility	Moderate/ reduced function	Reduced or preserved function
Type C	Severe	Abnormal adhesions to the ventricular free wall and restricted motion	Large/ reduced function	Small/reduced function
Type D	Extremely severe (tricuspid valve sac)	Severe adhesions to the ventricular wall	Very large/ minimal function	Infundibulum only/depressed function

2 Embryology

- TV leaflets develop from endocardial cushions and myocardium and delaminate from the interior surface of the ventricular myocardium.
- This process fails to occur in Ebstein's anomaly.
- The anterior leaflet is rarely affected because it originates from the supraventricular crest as opposed to the ventricular myocardium.

3 Epidemiology

- Incidence of 1/200,000 live births
  - Prenatal incidence is higher but many evolve to hydrops and fetal demise.
- 1% of all congenital heart defects.
- No specific etiologic factor; maternal exposure to lithium therapy is weakly associated.
- Rare cases of familial Ebstein's anomaly are reported.
- Trisomy 21, sarcomere gene MYH7 mutations (often in association with LV non-compaction), NKX2.5 mutations, 10p13-p14 deletion, and 1p34.3-p36.11 deletion have been reported.

4 Clinical Physiology and Presentation

- There are considerable differences in physiology and presentation from a critically unstable circulation in the neonatal period to a nearly normal circulation with minimal symptoms in children and adulthood.
- Physiology may be determined by the following factors:
  - Degree of displacement of TR.
  - Size and function of the functional RV, including the ability of the RV to generate pressure.
  - Presence of anatomic RVOTO or functional atresia (with or without pulmonary insufficiency (PI) /circular shunting).
- Presence and size of atrial septal defect (ASD) and direction of shunting.
- Extreme form (fetal/neonatal presentation).
  - Combination of severe TR and dysfunctional RV with poor pressure generation leads to minimal or no flow across the pulmonary valve (functional pulmonary atresia). Exacerbated by high PVR of the newborn.
  - Pulmonary blood flow depends on left to right shunting at the PDA

- If significant PI develops, then there is a circular shunt. In this circulation, there is ineffective cardiac output and steal from the systemic circulation. (Fig. 2).
  - Systemic blood flow diverted through PDA that, in turn, runs into to RV and subsequently to the RA through regurgitant TV, and shunts back to the left atrium (LA) resulting in very low output to the systemic circulation.
- Fetal demise with or without hydrops may ensue.
- Live-born neonates may present with low systemic perfusion (shock, lactic acidosis), cyanosis, and pulmonary overcirculation (respiratory distress, pulmonary edema). Lung hypoplasia (respiratory distress, inadequate oxygenation and carbon dioxide exchange) may exacerbate aberrant cardiac physiology.

• Moderate to severe form (neonatal presentation).
  - Duct-dependent pulmonary circulation at birth with or without antegrade blood flow through the pulmonary valve due to combination of sizable PDA, high pulmonary vascular resistance (PVR), moderate to severe TR, and/or RV dysfunction.
  - As PVR decreases and the PDA becomes smaller, more antegrade blood flow through the pulmonary valve may be generated by RV
  - Pulmonary circulation may subsequently be sufficiently maintained by the RV without a PDA or may remain duct-dependent.
  - Symptoms are mainly related to amount of pulmonary blood flow (cyanosis).

• Mild to moderate form (childhood presentation).
  - Three major modes of clinical presentation beyond the neonatal period are right-heart failure, cyanosis, and atrial arrhythmia.
  - The degree of right-heart failure symptoms such as exercise intolerance depends on the degree of TR and RV dysfunction.
  - Cyanosis at rest or exertion occurs when an ASD is present among patients with moderate or severe degree of TR and/or RV dysfunction and there is right to left shunting at this level.
  - Paradoxical embolization may occur.
  - Older children (> 10 years) and adults may present with arrhythmia, which may be atrial or ventricular and with or without pre-excitation.
  - Sudden cardiac death may rarely occur.
  - Many cases with mild disease remain completely asymptomatic in childhood.

5 Natural History

• The extreme form (fetal/neonatal presentation) is lethal without intensive treatment.

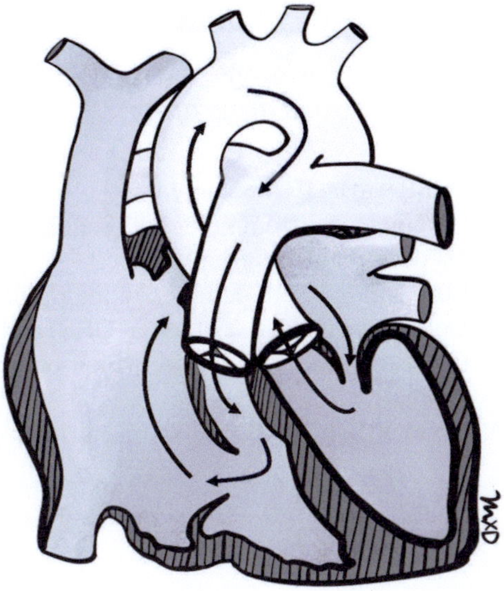

Fig. 2 Physiology of circular shunting. Blood flow from the aorta goes into the pulmonary artery via a large PDA as a left-to-right shunt. Due to significant pulmonary and tricuspid valve regurgitation and, often, severe RV dysfunction, blood flow in the pulmonary artery goes back into the right atrium, creating significant re-circulation and profound low systemic output. Reproduced with permission from Dr. Mimi Deng

- Even with intensive treatment, perinatal mortality is 45%, which is amongst the highest of all patients with CHD.
- Many infants, children, and adults will remain asymptomatic for years and even decades.
- RV dysfunction and arrhythmias will develop in most over time.
- Common causes of death are progressive right-heart failure and sudden cardiac death, which are presumed to be arrhythmia related.

6 Associated Lesions

- ASD (present in up to 90%).
- Pulmonary valve stenosis or atresia (anatomical or functional).
- Branch pulmonary artery (PA) stenosis or hypoplasia.
- PDA
- Ventricular septal defect (VSD). Rarely, the VSD can communicate above the septal leaflet causing an LV-RA shunt.
- LV non-compaction.
- Wolff-Parkinson-White (WPW) syndrome.
- Ebstein-like anomaly of the TV co-exists in patients with congenitally corrected transposition of the great arteries (Chapter 21).

7 Diagnostic Studies

7.1 *Electrocardiography*

- Tall P waves (RA enlargement).
- Complete or incomplete right bundle branch block.
- 1st degree atrioventricular block.
- Low-voltage QRS complex in the right/anterior precordial leads.
- Delta wave (slow rise of initial QRS) and QRS prolongation consistent with WPW (pre-excitation) syndrome, which occurs up to 30% of patients with Ebstein's anomaly
- Up to 30% have more than one atrial accessory pathways.

7.2 *Chest X Ray (Fig. 3)*

- Size of cardiac silhouette varies from massive in the extreme form (wall-to-wall heart, Fig. 3a) to mildly enlarged in asymptomatic patients (Fig. 3b).
- Globe-shaped heart with relatively narrow waist (Fig. 3b).
- Pulmonary vascular markings can be normal, increased in neonates with large PDA/circular shunting, or decreased in neonates with reduced pulmonary blood flow.
- Lung hypoplasia in the extreme form in neonates (Fig. 3a).

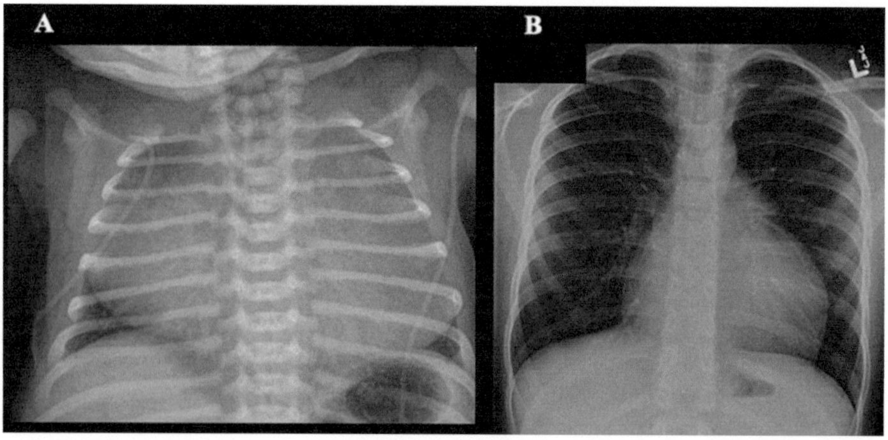

Fig. 3 A: chest X ray of a neonate with extreme form of Ebstein's anomaly. Massive cardiomegaly (wall-to-wall heart) leaves little room for lungs. B: Chest X ray of a 6-year-old child with severe Ebstein's anomaly with severe TR, demonstrating moderate to severe cardiomegaly with a globe-shaped heart and clear and well-expanded lung fields

7.3 *Echocardiography*

- Diagnostic modality of choice from fetus to adult.
- Detailed assessment of TV morphology and function should be performed:
  - Degree of downward displacement of the septal leaflet (Fig. 4); definition is downward displacement $\geq$ 8 mm/m^2.
  - Degree of dysplasia/morphology of the septal and posterior leaflets.
  - Redundancy of anterior leaflet and tethering to RV
  - Size of the TV annulus and severity of TR.
  - TR peak velocity as a measure of the ability of the RV to generate pressure.
- Size and function of the atrialized and functional RV
- Appearance of the pulmonary valve (normal, dysplastic, atretic) and degree of the flow (or regurgitation) across the pulmonary valve.
- PA size.
- Size and direction of shunting of the PDA (neonate).
- Size of the ASD and the amount and direction of shunt across the ASD
- Size, morphology, and function of the LV.
- Other associated cardiac lesions as mentioned above.
- Great Ormond Street Ebstein Score (GOSE score, Celermajer index) is an echocardiography-derived chamber size ratio that may be used to prognosticate neonatal Ebstein's anomaly.
  - GOSE score = area of RA + atrialized RV / area of functional RV + LV + LA [measured in diastole].
  - Grade 1: < 0.5, Grade 2: 0.5–0.99, Grade 3: 1–1.49. Grade 4: $\geq$ 1.5.
  - The higher the grade, the worse the clinical outcomes.
- Prognostication scores have also been developed based on fetal echocardiography:
  - SAS score (0–10): cardiothoracic ratio, GOSE score, pulmonary valve flow, PDA flow direction, right-left ventricular ratio.
  - SickKids score (0–10): cardiothoracic ratio, RA area index, pulmonary valve flow, TR, and PI.
  - Presence of PI is an independent risk factor for perinatal mortality as it signifies circular shunting.

7.4 *MRI*

- Cardiac MRI has become an increasingly-used modality for anatomic and functional assessment of the RV and for surgical planning.
- Quantification of the following should be performed:
  - Chamber volumes: RA, atrialized RV, functional RV, LV (Fig. 5).
  - RV and LV function (ejection fraction), TR regurgitant fraction.

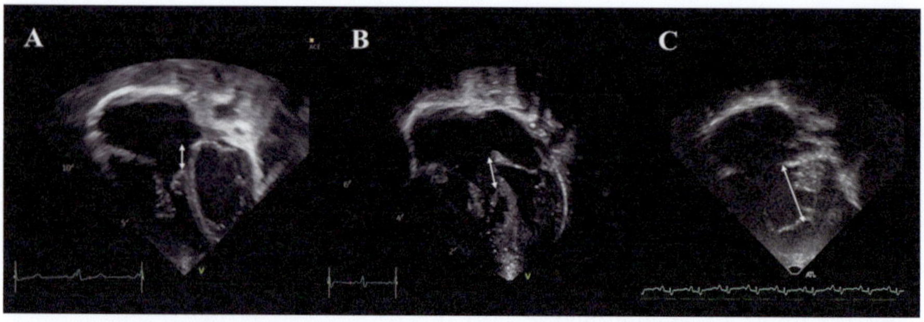

Fig. 4 4-chamber echocardiographic view of Ebstein's anomaly. **a** Mild form of Ebstein's anomaly with mild downward displacement of the septal leaflet. **b** Moderate degree of downward displacement of the septal leaflet with moderate-sized atrialized RV. **C** Severe downward displacement of the septal leaflet, very large atrialized RV, and extremely small functional RV.

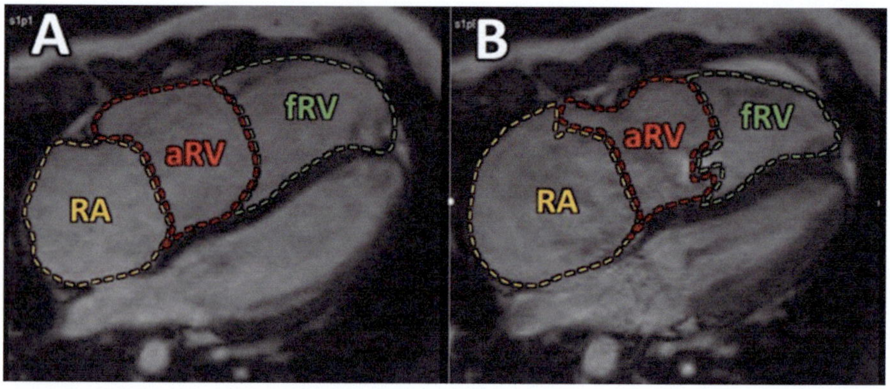

Fig. 5 Quantitative assessment of atrialized and functional right ventricle by cardiac MRI. **a** end-diastolic phase, **b** end-systolic phase. Reprinted with permission from Dr. Israel Valverde

– Pulmonary to systemic flow ratio (Qp:Qs).

7.5 Cardiac Catheterization

- Limited role for diagnostic or preoperative assessment PA pressure, PVR, visualization of peripheral branch PAs, and end-diastolic pressure measurements if patients require single ventricle palliation or 1.5 ventricle repair (1.5VR).

7.6 *Electrophysiology Study*

- Important role in diagnosis and management of patients with supraventricular and ventricular arrhythmias.
- Common arrhythmias that are diagnosed include WPW syndrome, other (concealed) accessory pathway mediated atrial tachycardias, ectopic atrial tachycardia, atrial flutter or fibrillation, and ventricular tachycardia.
- Accessory pathways may be mapped and ablated.
- Pre-operative studies are highly recommended for older patients (> 15 kg) since access for mapping and ablation may be affected by the nature of the surgical repair.

8 Indications for Intervention/Surgery and Management Strategies

8.1 *Severe to Extreme Form (Fetal/neonatal Presentation)*

- Neonates who have the extreme form of Ebstein's anomaly require immediate treatment after birth.
- Neonates with severe lung hypoplasia in the setting of extreme form of Ebstein's anomaly may be deemed untreatable, although the degree of lung expansion and maturation after cardiac surgical intervention is often difficult to predict.

8.2 *Sickkids Treatment Algorithm for Extreme Ebstein's Anomaly (Fig. 6)*

- Fetuses with significant circular shunting are treated with indomethacin to restrict the ductus arteriosus and stabilize hemodynamics.
- Fetuses with persistent poor prognostic signs despite indomethacin treatment may be delivered by Caesarean section to facilitate subsequent intervention in the delivery room, intensive care unit, or operating room.
- Immediate intensive treatment, including endotracheal intubation and mechanical ventilation, administration of prostaglandin (PGE), and/or inhaled nitric oxide (iNO) may be initiated.
- Immediate postnatal stabilization with extracorporeal membrane oxygenation (ECMO) may be required.
- Neonates with circular shunt and very low estimated RVSP by the TR jet (< 30–40 mmHg) are managed by Starnes procedure (or main PA ligation with maintenance of PGE in case of extreme prematurity).

- Neonates with high estimated RVSP (> 40 mmHg) who are hemodynamically stable are managed initially with medical intervention. The strategy is to conservatively manage for the first 48–72 h until PVR decreases, and to discontinue PGE to determine if the RV can generate sufficient forward flow to maintain oxygen saturations > 75% without the PDA.
- If the PDA remains large, then test occlusion of the PDA may be performed.
- If neonates are cyanotic, then intervention to secure pulmonary blood flow, such as PDA stenting or placement of Blalock-Thomas-Taussig (BTT) shunt, or the Starnes procedure is considered. The Starnes procedure is a safer choice amongst neonates with severe TR and borderline (or low) RV pressure.
- Neonatal biventricular repair is occasionally performed in the setting of high RV pressure.

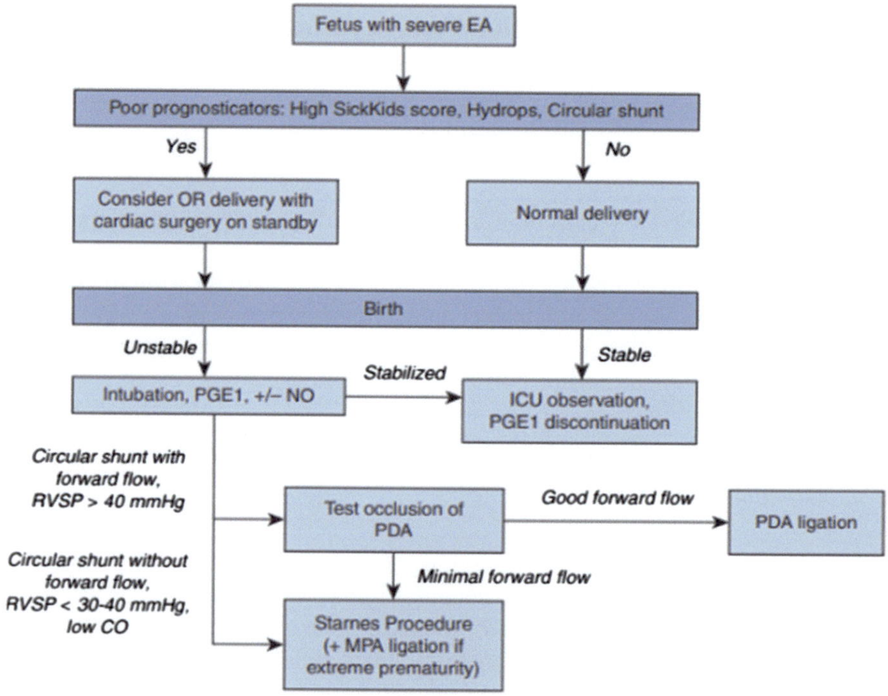

Fig. 6 SickKids decision-making and treatment algorithms for fetus and neonates with severe Ebstein's anomaly. EA, Ebstein's anomaly, NO, nitric oxide, RVSP, right ventricular systolic function. Reprinted from JTVCS Techniques, Vol 7, Deng MX, Kirsch R, Jaeggi E, Honjo O, Management of a premature low birth weight neonate with Ebstein anomaly and persistent circular shunt using modified Starnes procedure, pages 208–211, 2021, with permission from Elsevier

8.3 *Management Strategy Beyond Neonatal Period*

- Patients who do not need surgical intervention as a neonate are conservatively managed.
- Surgery in children, adolescents, and adults with mild to moderate TR may be considered when any of the following arise:
  - Progressive right-heart failure due to severe TR and/or RV dysfunction.
  - Progressive or persistent cyanosis due to right to left shunting at the ASD, either at rest or during exercise.
  - Evidence of progressive RV dilatation with severe TR. Repair at an earlier age (even 3–4 y) may reduce risks of late arrythmia and RV failure.
  - Development of significant atrial arrhythmia, which is often due to progressive dilatation of the RA.
- Serial assessment by echo, MRI, Holter, and exercise stress testing is recommended.

9 Surgical Strategy

9.1 *Neonates*

- The principles of neonatal Ebstein management are to choose an effective and less-invasive surgical option, and to avoid extensive open-heart surgery, particularly complex TV and biventricular repair for the following reasons:
  - RV may generate sufficient forward flow once PVR decreases despite significant TR.
  - Complex neonatal biventricular repair is associated with high mortality.
  - Much higher success rate of TV repair is expected if timing can be delayed beyond neonatal/infant period.
- Starnes procedure provides predictable single ventricle physiology and high survival rate, and does not exclude the possibility of future biventricular repair (See Alternative Strategies).
- PDA stenting or BTT shunt may be performed when right-heart failure is medically manageable and the RV pressure is high, but cyanosis persists. Our preference is PDA stenting over BTT shunt mainly based on the less-invasive nature of the procedure.
- Starnes procedure is indicated in the most critically ill neonates, often within the first 24 h of life. These patients require care coordination with the fetal cardiac and perinatal teams. The procedure includes the following components.
  - Closure of TV orifice typically with a GoreTex patch and a fenestration (typically 4 mm).

  - Atrial septectomy.
  - Ligation or division of the main PA.
  - Placement of BTT shunt (3 mm in neonates < 2.5 kg, 3.5 mm in neonates ≥ 2.5 kg).
  - RA reduction-plasty.
- Neonatal biventricular repair.
  - TV repair (various repair techniques reported such as Knott-Craig monocusp technique or the Cone Repair).
  - Right ventricular outflow tract reconstruction: (1) RV-PA valved conduit in cases of anatomic pulmonary atresia or hypoplastic pulmonary valve, (2) transannular patch (not ideal as it will load RV with significant PI, (3) no intervention when there is a normal pulmonary valve.
  - RA reduction and RV plication.
  - Downsizing ASD (typically leave a 3–4 mmresidual ASD to allow right-to-left shunt).
  - PDA ligation.

9.2 Tricuspid Valve Repair in Childhood or Adult Life

- Cone reconstruction (Fig. 7).
  - First-line surgical technique for repairing Ebstein TV in all age groups beyond the neonatal/infant period.
  - Provides 360 degrees of TV tissue in the anatomic, non-displaced TV annulus.
  - The key components of the procedure are:

    Detachment of most of the anterior leaflet from the TV annulus, including releasing abnormal attachments between the anterior leaflet and RV free wall.
    Surgical delamination and recruitment of the septal and posterior leaflets.
    Clockwise rotation of the mobilized anterior leaflet.
    Approximation of the mobilized three leaflets to create a 'cone', with an option to add a pericardial patch in the area of the posterior/septal leaflets if deficient. All fenestrations on leaflets will be closed in this process.
    Plication of the atrialized portion of the posterior/inferior RV free wall.
    Plication of the true tricuspid annulus.
    Reattachment of the reconstructed leaflet complex to the true TV annulus.
    The annulus can be reinforced by annuloplasty (ring or partial).
    Dilated atrial wall is reduced.
    A small ASD is typically left open (3–4 mm) allowing small amount of right-to-left shunting.

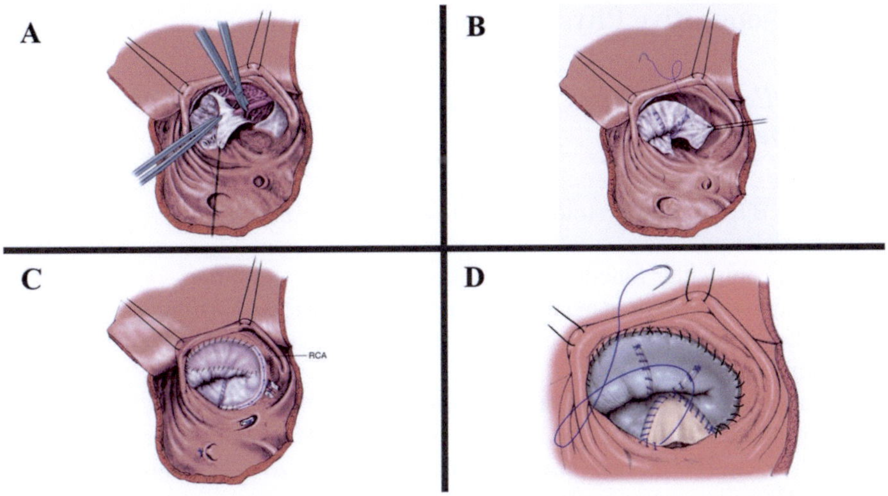

Fig. 7 Cone reconstruction. **a** Detachment of most of the anterior leaflet from the tricuspid valve annulus, including abnormal attachments between the anterior leaflet and RV free wall. **b** Approximation of the mobilized three leaflets to create a 'cone'. **c** Reattachment of the reconstructed leaflet complex to the true tricuspid valve annulus with partial annuloplasty. **d** Patch augmentation of the posterior leaflet by a fresh pericardial patch when the posterior leaflet is deficient. Reprinted from JTCVS Techniques, Vol 3, Dearani JA, Enstein repair: How I do it, pages 269–276, 2020, with permission from Elsevier

9.3 Other Surgical Techniques and Strategies

- Carpentier and Danielson TV repair techniques are rarely used in the current practice owing to excellent clinical outcomes of the Cone reconstruction.
  - Carpentier technique: longitudinal plication of RV and mobilization and rotation of the anterior leaflet.
  - Modified Danielson (Mayo clinic) technique: mobilization of anterior papillary muscle and plication of the posterior leaflet (monocuspitalization).
- TV replacement is performed when TV is not amenable to repair (rare) or there is significant residual or new TR after Cone reconstruction. A biosynthetic valve is used.
- Older adults with severe RV dysfunction may be better treated with primary TV replacement rather than attempted repair.
  - 1.5VR can be utilised, usually in the setting of severe RV dysfunction and dilatation. It unloads the RV by redirecting superior vena cava (SVC) blood flow to the pulmonary circulation directly, thereby reducing the volume load to the RV. There may be long-term complications such as SVC syndrome.
  - Right-sided Maze procedure or cavo-tricuspid isthmus surgical ablation is sometimes performed at the time of TV intervention.

10 Post-operative Physiology and Management

10.1 Following Starnes Procedure or Other Neonatal Operation

- Manage BTT shunt physiology: avoid excessive diastolic run off and pulmonary overcirculation.
- Support ventricular function with inotropes.
- Vasoactive support to manage Qp:Qs in single ventricle physiology.
- Tolerate saturations > 75% even with a biventricular repair due to right to left shunting at the atrial level.
- Recruit and support hypoplastic and often stiff lungs.
- Drain all cavities including bilateral pleura and abdomen (peritoneal dialysis catheter) to allow full expansion of lungs and minimize risks of fluid retention.
- Consider delayed sternal closure.
- Low threshold to use ECMO for 48–72 h to optimize cardiopulmonary physiology.

10.2 Following Cone Reconstruction

- RV dysfunction is expected after Cone reconstruction, although cardiac output is maintained in most cases.
- Desaturation (saturations in 80's) may occur due to right to left shunting across the ASD, which should be well tolerated and does not usually need any intervention.
- Early extubation is recommended as spontaneous negative pressure ventilation benefits dysfunctional RV
- Inotropic support (epinephrine, milrinone) and RV afterload reduction (iNO, PDE5 inhibitors) may be used to support RV function.
- Patients with severe, symptomatic postoperative RV dysfunction or cyanosis should be considered for a 1.5VR with a bidirectional cavopulmonary shunt (BCPS). If unexpected degree of RV dysfunction or arrythmias, coronary angiography may be indicated to exclude RCA distortion due to annuloplasty.

11 Outcomes

- Neonatal Presentation:
  - Large multi-centre study showed 75% survival to neonatal discharge.
  - 54% were managed with medical therapy only with 79% survival rate to discharge.
  - 46% had catheter-based or surgical intervention with the following survival:

  - 100% survival after Starnes procedure
  - 52% survival after BTT shunt, PA ligation, or PDA stenting.
- – 50–58% survival after biventricular repair (TV repair or RV-PA conduit).

- Starnes Procedure: 1-and 10-year survival rates of 84 ± 2% and 81 ± 4%.
- Cone reconstruction associated with operative mortality < 2% and freedom from TV reoperation of approximately 90–95%.
- Younger age at repair (< 4 years of age) may be related to higher rate of TV reoperation.

12 Alternative Strategies and Controversies

- There are wide practice variations in treating the extreme form of neonatal Ebstein patients, particularly the threshold to perform high-risk biventricular repair vs. Starnes procedure.
- Some centres advocate Cone reconstruction in neonates and infants, although this is not a common practice and overall outcomes are poor. Our preference is to perform Cone reconstruction after 3–4 years of age.
- There is no consensus on optimal timing of TV repair among children who have severe TR but remain asymptomatic or minimally symptomatic. In general, threshold to move forward with TV repair in asymptomatic patients is lower in recent years since surgical outcomes have improved with the Cone repair.
- There are institutional biases and preferences regarding the method of RV decompression, namely fenestrated ASD versus BCPS (1.5VR) among patients with severe RV dilatation and dysfunction who undergo TV repair or replacement and have persistent symptoms or desaturations. Our institutional bias is to leave a small ASD as a means of RV decompression.

Bibliography

1. Alsaied T, Christopher AB, Da Silva J, et al. Multimodality imaging in Ebstein anomaly. Pediatr Cardiol. 2023;44(1):15–23.
2. Attenhofer Jost CH, Connolly HM, Dearani JA, et al. Ebstein's anomaly. Circulation. 2007;115(2):277–85.
3. Carpentier A, Chauvaud S, Mace L, a,. A new reconstructive operation for Ebstein's anomaly of the tricuspid valve. J Thorac Cardiovasc Surg. 1988;96(1):92–101.
4. da Silva JP, Baumgratz JF, da Fonseca L, et al., The cone reconstruction of the tricuspid valve in Ebstein's anomaly. The operation: early and midterm results. J Thorac Cardiovasc Surg. 2007;133(1):215–223.
5. Dearani JA. Ebstein repair: how I do it. JTCVS Tech. 2020;3:269–76.
6. Deng MX, Kirsh R, Jaeggi E, Honjo O. Management of a premature low body weight neonate with Ebstein anomaly and persistent circular shunt using modified Starnes procedure. JTCVS Tech. 2021;7:208–11.

7. Freud LR, McElhinney DB, Kalish BT, et al. Risk factors for mortality and circulatory outcome among neonates prenatally diagnosed with Ebstein anomaly or tricuspid valve dysplasia: a multicenter study. J Am Heart Assoc. 2020;9(21): e016684.
8. Kumar SR, Kung G, Noh N, et al. Single-ventricle outcomes after neonatal palliation of severe Ebstein anomaly with modified Starnes procedure. Circulation. 2016;134(17):1257–64.
9. Schluz A, Marathe SP, Chavez M, et al. The association of age and repair modifications with outcome after cone repair for Ebstein's malformation. Semin Thorac Cardiovasc Surg. 2022;34(1):205–12.
10. Wertaschnigg D, Manlhoit C, Jeaggi M, et al. Contemporary outcomes and factors associated with mortality after a fetal or neonatal diagnosis of Ebstein anomaly and tricupid valve disease. Can J Cardiol. 2016;32(12):1500–6.

Pulmonary Stenosis

Michael Khoury and Lee Benson

Abstract Pulmonary stenosis is a common form of congenital heart disease. It often occurs in isolation or in association with genetic disease and identified syndromes, including Noonan syndrome, Williams or Alagille syndromes. The lesion exists along a spectrum of severity, from trivial to critical. As such, the clinical presentation and natural history are dependent on disease severity and associated lesions, such as the presence of an atrial-level communication. Echocardiography is the imaging modality of choice with more advanced imaging (e.g., cardiac magnetic resonance or cardiac catheterization) rarely required for diagnostic purposes. When indicated, the intervention of choice is balloon dilation, with surgical valvotomy reserved for specific circumstances such as multi-level obstruction or the presence of a significantly dysplastic pulmonary valve. The long-term prognosis for mild untreated disease or treated moderate or severe disease is generally excellent.

Keywords Pulmonary stenosis · Branch pulmonary arterial stenosis · Vavuloplasty · Noonan syndrome

Abbreviations

ASD	Atrial septal defect
JVP	Jugular venous pulsation
MPA	Main pulmonary artery
PDA	Persistent ductus arteriosus
PFO	Persistent foramen ovale

M. Khoury
Division of Pediatric Cardiology, Department of Pediatrics, University of Alberta, Stollery Children's Hospital, 8440-112th St. NW, Edmonton, AB T6G 2B7, Canada
e-mail: Khoury1@ualberta.ca

L. Benson (✉)
Division of Pediatric Cardiology, Department of Paediatrics, The Hospital for Sick Children, University of Toronto, 555 University Ave, Toronto, ON M5G 1X8, Canada
e-mail: lee.benson@sickkids.ca

© The Author(s), under exclusive license to Springer Nature Switzerland AG 2024

A. I. Dipchand et al. (eds.), *Manual of Cardiac Care in Children*,
https://doi.org/10.1007/978-3-031-70973-9_11

PGE1	Prostaglandin E1
PI	Pulmonary insufficiency
PPAS	Peripheral pulmonary artery stenosis
PS	Pulmonary stenosis
RVOT	Right ventricular outflow tract
RVOTO	Right ventricular outflow tract obstruction
RVSP	Right ventricular systolic pressure
RV	Right ventricle
RVH	Right ventricular hypertrophy
TGA	Transposition of the great arteries
TOF	Tetralogy of fallot

Key Points

- Pulmonary stenosis (PS) is characterized by right ventricular outflow tract (RVOT) obstruction and may be at multiple levels along the outflow tract: subvalvar, valvar or supravalvar or in combination.
- Presentation is dependent on severity, clinical symptoms and if it is associated with other cardiac lesions or syndromes.
- Clinical diagnosis is confirmed by echocardiography. The pressure gradient across the RVOT defines severity.
- Management for typical pulmonary valve stenosis is typically balloon dilation with timing dependent on severity of obstruction. Other forms may require surgery.
- The long-term outcomes of balloon therapies are excellent.

1 Nomenclature

- Isolated pulmonary valvar stenosis most commonly: situs solitus, levocardia, atrioventricular concordance, ventriculoarterial concordance.

2 Anatomy

- Stenosis of the pulmonary valve (typical).
  - Fusion of adjacent leaflets along the commissures, resulting in a narrow hemodynamic orifice.
- Post-stenotic dilation of the MPA often present with typical valve stenosis.
- Variable degrees of stenosis. Most severe form "critical" stenosis—ductal dependent pulmonary blood flow.

- A minority of children present with thickened, so-called dysplastic leaflets, with variable degrees of commissural fusion, and hypoplasia of the valve annulus with supravalvar leaflet tethering, a short main pulmonary artery and often small branch pulmonary arteries. This complex is often seen in children with Noonan syndrome.
- Right ventricular hypertropy (RVH).
- Normal size RV cavity may appear small due to free wall and apical trabecular hypertrophy.
- Peripheral pulmonary artery stenosis (PPAS) may be identified, involving the main pulmonary artery or either or both branches as well as smaller peripheral branches.

3 Epidemiology

- 2nd most common congenital cardiac malformation.
- ~ 0.08 to 0.1 per 1000 live births, but mild disease may be underestimated.
- Male-to-female ratio ~ 1:1.
- Typically sporadic, isolated.
- Familial transmission may occur (~4%).
- Occurs as isolated or contributing lesion in ~ 8-to-12% of congenitally malformed hearts.
- Associated with numerous syndromes (*See Associated Lesions*).
- May be acquired in congenital rubella syndrome.

4 Clinical Physiology and Presentation

- Obstruction at the RV outflow tract results in increased RV systolic pressure (RVSp).
- Increased RV mass to maintain stroke volume.
- Impaired diastolic properties (relaxation and filling).
- With time, the RV may eventually dilate and fail.
- Trivial obstruction (gradient $\leq$ 25 mmHg) tends to be non-progressive.
- In the fetus with significant obstruction, RV output is decreased. A larger than normal atrial level shunt maintains systemic cardiac output. RVH and decreased cavity size can mimic the clinical picture of pulmonary atresia with intact ventricular septum.
- In critical PS, pulmonary blood flow is contingent on L-R flow across the PDA; systemic desaturation from R-L shunt across the atrial septum with preserved systemic cardiac output.

4.1 Clinical Presentation

- Mild-to-moderate PS uncommonly diagnosed in fetal period.
- Clinical presentation depends on age, severity, and associated cardiac lesions.
- Neonates with severe stenosis: may present with cyanosis due to right-to-left atrial level shunting. Stenosis may be critical (i.e., dependent on a PDA).
- Most children with mild or moderate PS are asymptomatic and present with an incidentally found heart murmur.
- With more severe stenosis, symptoms may start in childhood or early adult life.
  - Exertional dyspnea.
  - Fatigue.
  - Chest pain, syncope, and sudden death may occur with strenuous exercise.
- During exercise the gradient across the stenosis increases due to increased blood flow.

5 Natural History

- Dependent on severity.
  - Mild: generally benign. Beyond 1 year of age, low risk of progression, particularly with trivial obstruction (gradient < 25 mmHg).
  - Moderate: variable course. May progress in some and result in symptoms from a fixed RV stroke volume (e.g., exercise intolerance).
  - Severe: often progressive during childhood. Irreversible RV dysfunction may occur.

6 Associated Lesions

- ASD/PFO in up to ¾ of cases.
- Muscular subpulmonary obstruction may be dynamic or fixed.
- Thickened tricuspid valve leaflets and chordal attachments. Tricuspid regurgitation often encountered.
- Post-stenotic dilation of the pulmonary artery.
- Some degree of pulmonary outflow tract obstruction is often a component in other cardiac lesions such as tricuspid atresia, Ebstein anomaly, TGA, TOF, or TGA/VSD.
- Genetic disorders and syndromes.
  - Noonan and LEOPARD Syndrome

    Cardiac examination often atypical and does not reflect the severity of the PS—ejection click usually absent and murmur is typically short and soft.

ECG typically shows superior axis.
Hypertrophic cardiomyopathy of the left ventricle in ~ 25% regardless of the presence of PS.

- Williams syndrome
- Alagille syndrome
- Neurofibromatosis.
- Glycogen storage diseases.
- PPAS commonly associated with congenital rubella syndrome, Williams syndrome, Noonan syndrome, Alagille syndrome, cutix laxa, Ehlers-Danlos syndrome, and Silver-Russell syndrome.

7 Diagnostic Studies

7.1 Physical Examination

- Assessment for findings of associated syndromes.
- Palpation: Severe stenosis—left parasternal RV systolic impulse and thrill (2nd–3rd intercostal space).
- Auscultation:
  - Wide splitting of the 2nd heart sound, proportional to PS severity.
  - Intensity of pulmonary component of 2nd heart sound decreases with increasing obstruction.
  - Severe stenosis—S4 often heard at the left lower sternal border.
  - Mild-to-moderate stenosis: normal S1 followed by pulmonary systolic ejection click. The more severe the stenosis, the earlier the click occurs until there is fusion with S1.

    Click decreases during inspiration and increases with expiration.
  - Typical murmur: systolic ejection at the left upper sternal border radiating to the back.
- The length of the murmur is related to the degree of stenosis.
  - Mild—short, peaks at/before mid-systole.
  - Moderate—murmur ends at/slight after aortic component of S2.
  - Severe—Murmur extends beyond aortic closure sound, which may become inaudible.
  - Critical PS—may have a deceptively soft murmur. Typically absent pulmonary closure sound.
- JVP.

- With increasingly severe obstruction, the "a" wave becomes progressively greater.

7.2 ECG

- Baseline ECG often normal with mild PS, or right axis deviation. In moderate or severe disease, there is almost always a right axis deviation and RVH (e.g., qR in V_1 with tall R waves in the right chest leads) in proportion to the severity of the RVOT obstruction. In infants older than 3-to-7 days, upright T-waves in the right chest leads is indicative of pathological RVH.
- RV conduction delay may be present.

7.3 CXR

- Heart size and vascularity usually normal in mild-to-moderate PS.
- Features of RVH—upturned cardiac apex.
- Post-stenotic dilation of the pulmonary trunk—prominence of the left upper heart border inferior to the aortic knuckle.
- Right atrial enlargement—pronounced convexity of the right lower border.
- With RV failure, cardiomegaly and decreased pulmonary vascularity is seen.

7.4 Echocardiography

- Diagnostic modality of choice.
- Severity can be easily assessed by transthoracic echocardiography. Peak-instantaneous pressure from echo-Doppler correlates well with invasively measured gradients (peak-to-peak gradient).
  - < 25 mmHg—trivial,
  - $25 < 40$ mmHg—mild
  - $40 < 60$ mmHg—moderate
  - ≥ 60 mmHg—severe.
- Assess for:
  - Site of obstruction: valvar, subvalvar, and/or supravalvar.

    Evidence of dynamic or fixed subpulmonary obstruction
  - Diameter of the pulmonary valve and annulus, valve thickness, leaflet motion, presence of leaflet doming, tethering of leaflet tips to the supra-annular ridge.
  - Post-stenotic dilation, presence of a ductus arteriosus.

- Branch PAs: proximal branch PAs typically delineated well but more peripheral branches often require CT, MRI, or catheterization.
- RVH and cavity size, contractility, morphology, and tricuspid valve function.
- ASD.

- Doppler flow studies:
  - Turbulent flow originating at the site of stenosis.
  - Pulsed and continuous wave Doppler measurement of the peak velocity across the point of stenosis.
- Estimated RVSp from tricuspid regurgitation jet.
- Note, for PPAS: the estimated pressure gradient across a branch PA stenosis does not necessarily reflect severity of stenosis. Rather, differential flow distributions are required to best assess this (see next section).

7.5 CT/MRI

- Axial imaging (CT/MRI) are useful to adequately evaluate the branch PAs for the presence and extent of associated PPAS. This is particularly important in the setting of genetic syndromes such as Alagille and Williams syndrome.
- MRI, as well as nuclear medicine perfusion scans, are useful to evaluate flow distributions between the branch PAs. This is the best way to assess relative stenosis and helps determine thresholds for intervention.

8 Indications for Intervention/Surgery and Timing

- Mild (peak-to-peak gradient < 40 mmHg, RVSp < 50% systemic).
  - Intervention not required.
- Moderate (peak-to-peak gradient 40–60 mmHg, RVSp 50 to < 75% systemic).
  - Elective intervention.
- Severe PS (gradient $\geq$ 60 mmHg, RVSp $\geq$ 75% systemic).
  - If asymptomatic, elective/semi-elective.
  - If symptomatic or RV dysfunction, more urgent.
- Critical PS (ductal dependency, use of prostaglandin E_1 (PGE1))—urgent, when post-natal stability achieved.
- Balloon pulmonary valvuloplasty—procedure of choice.
- PPAS:

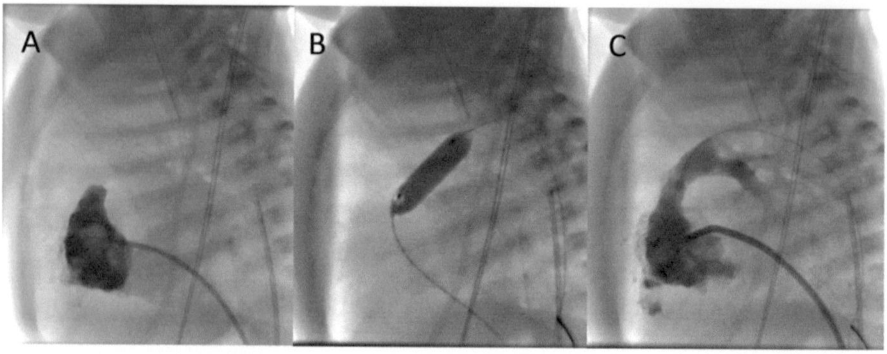

Fig. 1 Pulmonary balloon dilation in a newborn boy with critical stenosis. **a** lateral projection angiogram demonstrating hypoplastic right ventricle with minimal anterograde flow through a pinhole pulmonary orifice. **b** The child underwent a series of balloon dilations, culminating in a 7 × 20 mm Sterling balloon. **c** Repeat lateral projection angiogram demonstrating flow through the pulmonary valve

- Isolated branch PPAS: flow differential < 25% to the affected side typically warrants intervention.
- Bilateral or more complex PPAS disease, a rising RVSp (typically 50–75% systemic) should warrant intervention.
- Balloon angioplasty vs surgical pulmonary arterial reconstruction, depending on the anatomy (discrete vs diffuse stenosis), the presence of additional surgical requirements, and case-specific considerations.
- Note: patients with Williams syndrome often have a lower success rate (and higher complication rate) due in part to diffuse hypoplasia of the pulmonary vascular bed commonly found.

9 Interventional/Surgical Strategy

9.1 Balloon Dilation

- Procedure of choice (Fig. 1).
- Balloon diameter ~ 20–30% greater than the valve annulus.
- During inflation, observe for disappearance of the balloon waist.

9.2 Surgical Valvotomy

- For patients with dysplastic pulmonary valves (not amenable to balloon dilation) and/or a small valve annulus, or in those with multiple levels of obstruction.

- Open technique through the MPA.
- A trans-atrial infundibular resection may be required.
- Partial or often total removal of the valve may be required and a transannular patch if the annulus and MPA are hypoplastic.

10 Intensive Care Physiology and Management

10.1 Critical PS

- Persistent cyanosis after balloon dilation may occur, with resolution over weeks-to-months as RV compliance improves and right-left atrial shunting diminishes.
- A minority (~5–10%) are unable to maintain sufficient anterograde flow.
- If discontinuation of PGE_1 is not tolerated, continue PGE_1 with intermittent re-assessment of tolerance of ductal constriction, maintaining saturations $\geq$ 70%.
- Dynamic subvalvar obstruction may respond to beta-blockade.
- If ductal dependence persists, an alternative source of pulmonary blood flow is required, with ductal stenting the procedure of choice.
- If residual obstruction is valvar, surgery valvotomy indicated.
- Infective endocarditis prophylaxis typically not indicated.
- Treated patients or patients not meeting indications for intervention typically do not require activity restrictions.

11 Outcome

11.1 Balloon valvuloplasty

- Short and intermediate outcomes excellent.
  - With typical valve morphology—insignificant gradients (<20 mmHg) in > 85%.
  - Less optimal outcomes in those with dysplastic valves.
- Long-term outcomes (center-specific).
  - Freedom from re-intervention: > 80% at 10 years and ~ 75% at 15 years.
    - Surgical intervention after attempted balloon dilation in 12% (65% of which had dysplastic valves).
    - Repeat dilation performed in 8%.
- Overall a low incidence of complications but higher in neonates and infants, with pulmonary insufficiency (PI) the primary residual lesion, which can progress over time, but more often than not, well tolerated.

- Moderate PI is commonly encountered (~50% at 10–15 years post-intervention)
- Pulmonary valve replacement is rare (<5%)

11.2 Surgical Valvotomy

- 96% freedom from re-operation at 10 years with the majority (> 80%) in NYHA I.
- Post-operative PI rate is high.
- 25-year survival—97% with 97% of patients NYHA class I.
- Tend to have mildly decreased exercise tolerance.
- Higher incidence of ventricular ectopy.
- Re-intervention rate ~ 53% typically pulmonary valve replacement.

12 Alternative Strategies and Controversies

- Surgical and percutaneous approaches are equipoise for short and longer-term outcomes. The less invasive percutaneous approach as primary therapy is considered standard of care, with surgery indicated for more complicated lesions, including multi-level obstruction.

Bibliography

1. Earing MG, Connolly HM, Dearani JA, et al. Long-term follow-up of patients after surgical treatment for isolated pulmonary valve stenosis. Mayo Clin Proc. 2005;80(7):871.
2. Feltes TF, Bacha E, Beekman RH, et al. Indications for cardiac catheterization and intervention in pediatric cardiac disease: a scientific statement from the American Heart Association. Circulation. 2012;123:2607–52.
3. Garty Y, Veldtman G, Lee K, Benson L. Late outcomes after pulmonary valve balloon dilatation in neonates, infants and children. J Invasive Cardiol. 2005;17(6):318–22.
4. Hayes CJ, Gersony WM, Driscoll DJ et al (1993) Second natural history study of congenital heart defects. Results of treatment of patients with pulmonary valvar stenosis. Circulation. 87(2 Suppl):I28
5. Nugent EW, Freedom RM, Nora JJ, et al. Clinical course in pulmonary stenosis. Circulation. 1997;56(1 Suppl):I38-47.
6. Roos Hesselink JW, Meijboom FJ, Spitaels SE, et al. Long-term outcome after surgery for pulmonary stenosis (a longitudinal study of 22–33 years). Eur Heart J. 2006;27(4):482.

Tetralogy of Fallot (TOF)

Christoph Haller

Abstract Tetralogy of Fallot is the most common cyanotic cardiac defect. It is the result of malalignment of the ventricular septum with the infundibular septum, thereby resulting in a malalignment VSD, aortic override, hypoplastic or obstructed right ventricular outflow tract and right ventricular hypertrophy. Depending on the extent of right ventricular outflow obstruction, patients present with intermittent cyanosis (spells). If tolerated or adequately managed medically, patients are repaired electively between 3 to 6 months of age. Earlier repair (e.g. as a neonate) may be necessary in symptomatic patients. Primary repair is the preferred approach, consisting of VSD closure, right ventricular muscle bundle resection, pulmonary valvotomy or transannular patching and patching main/branch pulmonary arteries. Management of the right ventricular outflow tract is a key component of repair, aiming at adequate relief of obstruction and sparing the native pulmonary valve annulus when possible. Outcome is generally good with low surgical mortality and good long-term survival. However, reinterventions on the right ventricular outflow tract are common and most patients with transannular patch will come to need a pulmonary valve replacement later in life.

Keywords Tetralogy of fallot · TOF · VSD · Pulmonary stenosis · Right ventricular outflow tract obstruction · Valve sparing repair · Transannular patch · Infundibulotomy · Blalock-Taussig-Thomas shunt · PDA stent · RVOT stent · Pulmonary valve insufficiency · Valve replacement

Abbreviations

ASD	Atrial septal defect
AV	Atrioventricular
AVSD	Atrioventricular septal defect

C. Haller (✉)
Division of Cardiovascular Surgery, Labatt Family Heart Centre, Department of Surgery, The Hospital for Sick Children, University of Toronto, Toronto, ON, Canada
e-mail: christoph.haller@sickkids.ca

© The Author(s), under exclusive license to Springer Nature Switzerland AG 2024
A. I. Dipchand et al. (eds.), *Manual of Cardiac Care in Children*,
https://doi.org/10.1007/978-3-031-70973-9_12

BTT	Blalock Taussig Thomas
DORV	Double outlet right ventricle
JET	Junctional ectopic tachycardia
LAD	Left anterior descending
LPA	Left pulmonary artery
LV	Left ventricle
MAPCAs	Multiple aortopulmonary collaterals
MPA	Main pulmonary artery
OR	Operating room
PA	Pulmonary artery
PDA	Persistent ductus arteriosus
PI	Pulmonary insufficiency
RPA	Right pulmonary artery
RV	Right ventricle
RVH	Right ventricular hypertrophy
RVOT	Right ventricular outflow tract
TOF	Tetralogy of fallot
VSD	Ventricular septal defect

Key Points

- Most common cyanotic cardiac defect.
- Malalignment of ventricular and infundibular septum (anterior and superior deviation), resulting in:
  - Malalignment ventricular septal defect (VSD).
  - Aortic override.
  - Hypoplastic or obstructed right ventricular outflow tract (RVOT), usually at multiple levels.
  - Right ventricular hypertrophy.
- Presentation variable, depending on extent of RVOT obstruction.
- Cyanotic spells are the classic clinical presentation but can simply have progressive cyanosis.
- If tolerated, patients are repaired electively between 3 and 6 months of age.
- Earlier repair or palliation (e.g. as a neonate) may be necessary in symptomatic patients.
- Primary repair is the preferred approach, consisting of
  - Right ventricular muscle bundle resection and division.
  - Pulmonary valvotomy, infundibular patch or transannular patching, main and branch pulmonary artery (PA) patching as required.
  - VSD closure.

- Management of the RVOT is a key component of repair, aiming at adequate relief of obstruction but sparing the valve if possible.
- Restrictive physiology can complicate postoperative recovery.
- Outcome is generally good with low surgical mortality and good long-term survival.
- Small or high-risk symptomatic neonates/infants may need to be palliated with either RVOT stenting, persistent ductus arteriosus (PDA) stenting, or Blalock-Taussig-Thomas (BTT) shunt.

1 Nomenclature

- The defining feature of Tetralogy of Fallot (TOF) is antero-cephalad deviation of the infundibular septum. The resulting characteristics (VSD, aortic override, right ventricular outflow tract obstruction, right ventricular hypertrophy) are of variable extent.
- If aortic override is more than 50%, the lesion should be referred to as double outlet right ventricle. In severe cases, the aortic valve will no longer be in continuity with the mitral valve and this is unequivocal double outlet right ventricle (DORV).

2 Anatomy

- Antero-cephalad deviation of the infundibular septum. This single anatomic feature unifies the classic components of TOF (Fig. 1).
- Malalignment VSD.
- Overriding of the aorta.
- RVOT obstruction.
- Right ventricular hypertrophy.
- A patent foramen ovale or atrial septal defect (ASD) may also be present. This is also known as pentalogy of Fallot.

2.1 Interventricular Septum

- The VSD is subaortic, large, and perimembranous.
- Aortic override is variable and may be greater than 50%.
- More than 50% override is termed DORV.
- Rarely, the VSD can extend to become doubly committed such there is no true infundibular septum (higher incidence in central America).

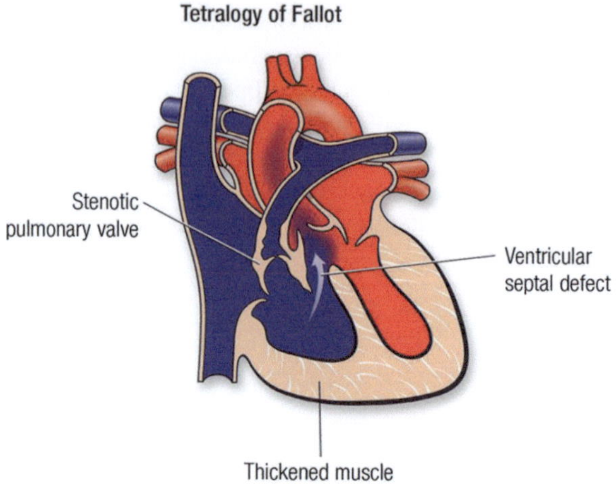

Fig. 1 Tetralogy of Fallot with its key characteristic features ventricular septal defect, overriding aortic valve, pulmonary valve stenosis with variable degree of right ventricular outflow tract obstruction, and right ventricular hypertrophy. Reprinted from AHA Website, Tetralogy of Fallot, https://www.heart.org/en/health-topics/congenitalheart-defects/about-congenital-heart-defects/tetralogy-of-fallot, with permission from American Heart Association, Inc

2.2 Right Ventricular Outflow Tract

- The RVOT obstruction is typically infundibular and valvar but may be only one or the other or affecting the central pulmonary arteries and branch origins as well. The pulmonary atresia variant of TOF is discussed in Chap. 14.
- The pulmonary valve is commonly thickened, dysplastic and may be bicuspid.
- Right ventricular hypertrophy (RVH) is mild in infancy and increases with age.

2.3 Pulmonary Artery

- The left PA (LPA) origin is typically more distant on the main PA (MPA) and takes off at an abnormal acute angle. LPA origin stenosis is common.
- Rarely the LPA can be disconnected from the MPA and arise exclusively from the PDA.
- Right PA (RPA) origin stenosis is less common.
- Bilateral small pulmonary arteries impacting surgical repair in 5–10%.

2.4 *Coronary Arteries*

- Anomalous coronary arteries crossing the RVOT include the left anterior descending artery arises from the right coronary artery in 2–4%, an accessory left anterior descending artery, or dominant conal branch. This may limit options to perform a trans-annular incision.

3 Embryology

- Concept of monology promoted by Van Praagh.
- Small infundibulum leads to
  - Outflow obstruction.
  - Malalignment of the infundibulum, which in turn causes.

    Malalignment VSD.
    Aortic override.
  - Right ventricular hypertrophy.
- Septoparietal trabecular malformation in addition to malalignment (Anderson).

4 Epidemiology

4.1 *Incidence/prevalence*

- The prevalence is approximately 1/4000 livebirths.
- Most common cyanotic congenital heart lesion.

4.2 *Population at Risk, Inheritance*

- 2.5–3% inheritance risk for children of patients with TOF.
- Equally distributed among male and female patients.
- Risk of congenital heart disease in future pregnancies.

5 Clinical Physiology and Presentation

- The predominant presenting feature is cyanosis and murmur (systolic ejection murmur heard over the upper left sternal border).

- Infants with severe obstruction may present with profound continuous cyanosis upon closure of the PDA.
- Hypercyanotic spells with arterial saturations transiently dropping below tolerable levels are known as “tetralogy spells”.
- Mild forms of TOF may present with signs of pulmonary congestion (heart failure) similar to patients with isolated VSDs.
- Infants with mild obstruction may be fully saturated and present with murmur on auscultation.
- Older children may have clubbing of the fingers and toes due to chronic cyanosis.

5.1 Natural History

- Depending on extent of right ventricular outflow tract obstruction.
- 25% of all untreated patients with TOF die within the first year.
- Milder, well-balanced forms may survive to adulthood with a late increase in mortality due to right ventricular (RV) failure and chronic cyanosis.

6 Associated Lesions

6.1 Common

- ASD.
- Anomalous origin of coronary artery crossing RVOT, including left anterior descending (LAD) from the right coronary artery (2–4%), dual LAD, large conal artery.
- Right aortic arch (15%).
- Left superior vena cava (10%).
- 22q11 microdeletion (Di George syndrome) (15%).

6.2 Less Common Associations

- Multiple VSDs.
- AVSD.
- Non-confluent pulmonary arteries or major collateral arteries (MAPCAs).
- VACTERL, CHARGE syndromes and many non-cardiac developmental abnormalities.

7 Diagnostic Studies

7.1 ECG

- Normal axis with right ventricular hypertrophy.
- In older children, the P waves may be peaked indicating right atrial enlargement.

7.2 CXR

- Classically shows a boot shaped heart with a paucity of shadow at the site of the MPA. The characteristic shape is due to the right ventricular hypertrophy and the relatively small main PA.

7.3 Echocardiography

- Echocardiography (Fig. 2) adequately delineates the anatomy in over 95% of cases and helps to define.
- VSD (size, position, alignment).
- RVOT i.e., infundibular chamber and pulmonary valve.
- Size and potential stenosis of branch pulmonary arteries.
- Aortic valve and its override over the VSD.
- Ventricular cavities.

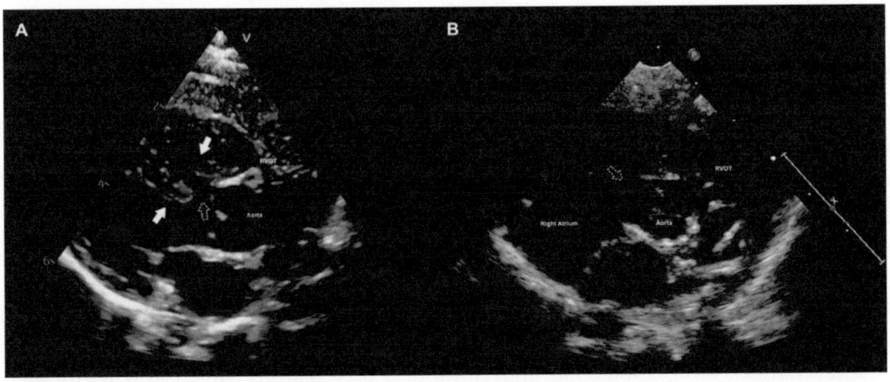

Fig. 2 Echocardiographic image of VSD and outflow tract delineating the antero-cephalad deviation of the outflow septum. ALong-axis view of LV outflow tract and aorta with VSD and aortic override. The bold arrows indicate the deviation of the septum that leads to RVOT obstruction and aortic override. The dashed arrow indicates the VSD. BShort-axis view at the level of the aortic valve showing the relation of VSD, aortic valve and RVOT

- Tricuspid and mitral valve (regurgitation, stenosis, potential straddling etc.).
- Coronaries arteries—CT or cath may be required if unable to clear by echo.

7.4 CT/MRI

- If the branch pulmonary arteries or coronary pattern are not well visualized, MRI or CT may be indicated.
- MRI preferred if flow and volume measurements are needed and CT if anatomical definition needed.

7.5 Cardiac Catheterization

- Rarely needed.
- Used, if suspicion of aortopulmonary collaterals.
- May be used to improve pulmonary blood flow with pulmonary valve dilation, or RVOT or PDA stenting.

8 Indications for Intervention/Surgery

- Presence of disease indicates repair. Best outcomes are achieved with repair between 3 and 9 months. There does not appear to be any benefit in delaying repair unless other major non-cardiac issue takes priority.

9 Timing of Intervention and Management Strategy

- $> 90\%$ are repaired electively.
- Elective repair at 3–6 months of age has best outcomes.
- Repair earlier if saturations are consistently $< 80\%$.
- Tet spells can be ameliorated with β-blocker therapy to delay surgery if necessary.
- 5–6% are repaired as neonates (increasing proportion in recent series).
- 5–10% require initial neonatal palliative procedure to improve pulmonary blood flow and/or promote pulmonary artery growth. BTT shunt is the classical surgical intervention, but catheter lab intervention is increasingly successful with either RVOT stenting or PDA stenting.
- On-going debate over neonatal repair vs palliation. Palliation preferred in high-risk cases, defined as prematurity, low birthweight (< 3 kg), small branch PAs (z-score < -2.5) or significant non-cardiac comorbidity. In cases of anomalous

LAD, repair will require an RV-PA conduit and palliation may help delay surgery until a larger conduit can be placed.

10 Surgical Strategy

- Surgical repair comprises.
  - Relief of RVOT obstruction.
  - VSD closure.
- Preservation of a functional pulmonary valve is ideal but may not be possible in some patients.
- Outflow tract procedures may range from simple valvotomies with infundibular muscle bundle resection to infundibular patch enlargement and transannular patching.
- Stepwise approach can prevent unnecessarily aggressive enlargement of the RVOT.
- RV/LV systolic pressure ratio of < 0.75 is usually acceptable but < 0.6 is preferred.
- 30–60% of patients will require a transannular patch in most studies. A monocusp can be created to reduce the amount of pulmonary regurgitation.
- Repair is usually performed with a transatrial, transpulmonary approach (see Fig. 3).
- Patients with moderate or less pulmonary annular hypoplasia (z-score > -3) are good candidates for valve-sparing approaches.
- Combined important residual PI and stenosis should be avoided.
- Anomalous LAD may require an RV-PA conduit unless a valve-sparing repair can be achieved.
- Common practice is to leave a small ASD to allow R-L shunting post-op in the setting of RV dysfunction, so improving systemic cardiac output at the cost of mild desaturation.

11 Intensive Care Physiology and Management

- Emergent preoperative management may be required for a severe or prolonged Tet spell. Medical management includes sedation/analgesia, volume expansion, systemic betablocker, increase systemic afterload (positioning or vasopressor), or unplanned intervention.
- Early postoperative or OR extubation for elective repairs done at 3–6 months of age.
- Those requiring continued ventilation should be ventilated with the lowest mean and positive end-expiratory airway pressures.

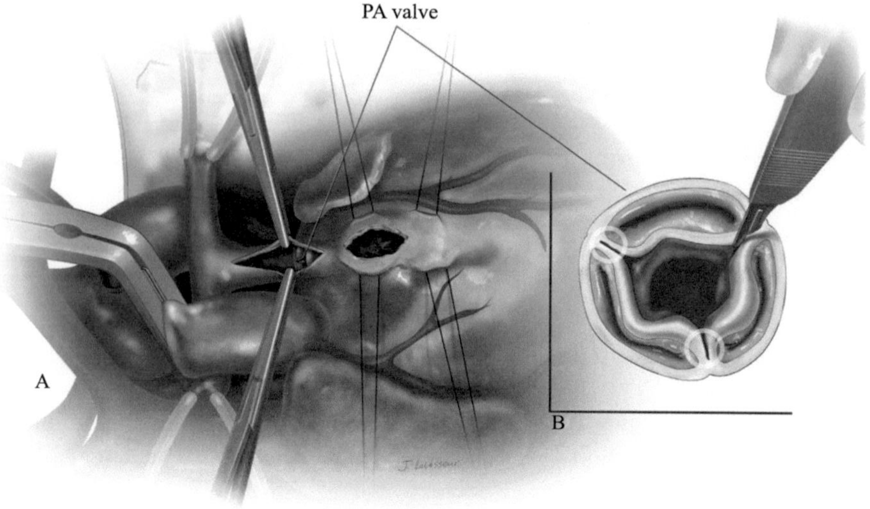

Fig. 3 Valve-sparing approach to Tetralogy of Fallot with incision on main pulmonary artery and subpulmonary infundibulum. The thickened and fused pulmonary valve is enlarged with commissurotomies (see inset B). Reprinted from Operative Techniques in Thoracic and Cardiovascular Surgery, Vol 18, Issue 4, Bacha E, Valve-sparing options in tetralogy of Fallot surgery, pp 316–327, 2013, with permission from Elsevier

- RV diastolic dysfunction and restrictive physiology is common since the procedure involves muscle resection in a hypertrophied ventricle and usually creates some degree of pulmonary incompetence. A stiff and restrictive RV may result in low cardiac output and require high right atrial and systemic venous pressures. This restrictive physiology is characterized by the atrial systolic contraction contributing to antegrade flow in the pulmonary arteries, reflecting the stiff nature of the RV (visible by echocardiography).
- Those with restrictive physiology are more likely to develop pleural effusions and experience prolonged chest tube drainage.
- The impact of restrictive physiology can be mitigated by intentionally leaving a small ASD to decompress the right atrium, decrease systemic venous pressures, and increase left ventricular preload at the expense of systemic desaturation.
- Neonates and cases at risk of restrictive physiology should have both pleural spaces drained with consideration given to a peritoneal drain).
- Milrinone load in the OR and infusion in the ICU. Aim to avoid epinephrine if possible as this can worsen diastolic dysfunction and promote tachyarrhythmias.
- Tachyarrythmias are a common complication. JET and then His bundle tachycardia are the commonest and may require topical cooling, sedation/muscle relaxation, atrial pacing (to maintain AV synchrony), or may need anti-arrhythmic therapy (e.g. amiodarone). They are temporary but can cause severe low cardiac output especially if in combination with restrictive RV physiology.

- Dysfunction of AV node may also present as transient heart block (may coexist with JET).
- Opening the sternum can be effective for relief of tissue tamponade associated with RV diastolic dysfunction.

12 Outcome

- Overall < 1% operative mortality. Neonatal repair has higher mortality in most series (3–5%) but lower if no risk factors (see above).
- Operative mortality has constantly decreased over the years.

13 Alternative Strategies and Controversies

- Palliative (staged) strategies as described above for high-risk symptomatic neonates and small infants.
- Increasing role for catheter-based palliation if necessary. Management is a balance between avoiding residual obstruction (risk of needing early reintervention) with the longer-term deleterious effects of severe PI and RV dilatation.
- Transannular patching remains the most common approach to TOF globally.
- Monocusp implantation is used to preserve some pulmonary valve function in patients with transannular patching but usually has only short-term benefit. The majority develop PI and RV dilatation.
- Intraoperative balloon dilatation of the pulmonary valve annulus does not preserve RV dimensions in the long-term despite initial positive effects.
- Complex pulmonary valve reconstructive strategies can achieve valvar competence despite aggressive annular enlargement, but long-term data is missing.

Acknowledgements The author would like to acknowledge Dr. Prisca Pondorfer and Dr. Sara Hussein for their contributions to this chapter.

Bibliography

1. Al Habib HF, Jacobs JP, Mavroudis C, et al. Contemporary patterns of management of tetralogy of fallot: data from the Society of Thoracic Surgeons Database. Ann Thorac Surg. 2010;90(3):813–9.
2. Hofferberth S, Nathan M, Marx G, et al. Valve-sparing repair with intraoperative balloon dilation in tetralogy of fallot: midterm results and therapeutic implications. J Thoracic Cardiovasc Surg. 2018;155(3):1163–73.

3. Kwon M, Bacha E. Pulmonary valve-sparing techniques for tetralogy of fallot: a systematic approach for maximizing success and minimizing risk. Semin Thorac Cardiovasc Surg Pediatr Card Surg Annu. 2020;23:24–8.
4. Romeo J, Takkenberg J, Cuypers J, et al. Timing of pulmonary valve replacement in patients with corrected fallot to prevent QRS prolongation. Eur J Cardiothorac Surg. 2020;58(3):559–66.
5. Samuel B, Marelli A, Vanasse A, et al. The 30-year outcomes of tetralogy of fallot according to native anatomy and genetic conditions. Can J Cardiol. 2020;37(6):877–86.
6. Smith C, McCracken C, Thomas A, et al. Long-term outcomes of tetralogy of fallot: a study from the Pediatric Cardiac Care Consortium. JAMA Cardiol. 2019;4(1):34–41.
7. Vonder Muhll IF. Timing and results of pulmonary valve replacement for pulmonary regurgitation in repaired tetralogy of fallot: a challenge for evidence-based medicine. Can J Cardiol. 2019;35(12):1620–2.

Tetralogy of Fallot with Absent Pulmonary Valve

Christoph Haller

Abstract Tetralogy of Fallot (TOF) with absent pulmonary valve is a relatively rare disease, characterized by absence of the pulmonary valve that results in a stenotic and regurgitant RVOT, leading to very enlarged and pulsatile proximal pulmonary arteries. TOF with absent pulmonary valve accounts for 3–6% of all TOF. The clinical presentation varies depending on extent of pulmonary artery enlargement, airway compression and respiratory compromise. Severely compromised neonates require immediate postnatal medical management to ensure adequate ventilation and oxygenation. If possible, symptomatic patients should be stabilized to promote somatic growth. Surgical repair focuses on reduction of the enlarged branch pulmonary arteries with or without implantation of a valved conduit. Early surgical mortality is low, but long-term survival can be significantly limited, and the reintervention rate is high. Reinterventions are primarily performed for recurrent airway disease, pulmonary valve, and pulmonary artery complications.

Keywords Tetralogy of fallot · Absent pulmonary valve · Tracheomalacia · Bronchomalacia · Pulmonary artery enlargement · Airway compression · Air trapping · Atelectasis · Hyperinflation

Abbreviations

ASD	Atrial septal defect
AVSD	Atrioventricular septal defect
LPA	Left pulmonary artery
MAPCAs	Multiple aortopulmonary collaterals
PA	Pulmonary artery
PDA	Persistent ductus arteriosus
PI	Pulmonary insufficiency

C. Haller (✉)
Division of Cardiovascular Surgery, Labatt Family Heart Centre, Department of Surgery, The Hospital for Sick Children, University of Toronto, Toronto, ON, Canada
e-mail: christoph.haller@sickkids.ca

© The Author(s), under exclusive license to Springer Nature Switzerland AG 2024

A. I. Dipchand et al. (eds.), *Manual of Cardiac Care in Children*,
https://doi.org/10.1007/978-3-031-70973-9_13

RPA	Right pulmonary artery
RV	Right ventricle
RVOT	Right ventricular outflow tract
SVC	Superior vena cava
TOF	Tetralogy of fallot
VSD	Ventricular septal defect

Key Points

- Form of Tetralogy of Fallot (TOF) characterized by absence of the pulmonary valve resulting in extensive enlargement of the pulmonary artery branches and airway compression.
- Variable clinical presentation, mainly depending on airway compromise.
- Elective repair (as in isolated TOF) if clinically stable or able to be supported with medical management. Severe cases have profound airway compression and need urgent intervention.
- Symptomatic patients should be stabilized, if possible, to allow for somatic growth.
- Surgical repair follows key concepts of TOF repair with reduction plasty of branch pulmonary arteries with or without placement of a valved right ventricle to pulmonary artery conduit and use of Lecompte maneuvre if necessary.
- Early postoperative mortality is low, but long-term mortality approaches 20%.
- High rate of reintervention for airway compromise, pulmonary valve, or pulmonary artery procedures.

1 Nomenclature

- As in isolated TOF (Chap. 12), antero-cephalad deviation of the infundibular septum is the hallmark for diagnosis.

1.1 Characteristics Determining the Subtype Absent Pulmonary Valve

- Absent pulmonary valve (i.e. patent RV outflow as opposed to pulmonary atresia) with pulmonary stenosis and severe insufficiency. The annulus is small but there is no true valvar tissue, only a fibrous ring of tissue within the annulus.
- Pulmonary artery dilatation can be extreme and is usually restricted to the main PA and the central LPA and RPA.
- Absent PDA

2 Anatomy

- The intracardiac features of TOF are described in detail in Chap. 12 and are similar in TOF absent pulmonary valve.

2.1 *Right Ventricular Outflow Tract and Pulmonary Valve*

- Pulmonary stenosis or right ventricular outflow tract obstruction is usually less dominant than in regular TOF, and patients are not usually severely cyanosed at birth.
- Remnants of valve leaflets are severely dysplastic and non-functional with resultant significant pulmonary regurgitation.
- Small pulmonary valve annulus.

2.2 *Pulmonary Trunk and Arteries*

- The pulmonary trunk, LPA and RPA are dilated (see Figs. 1 and 2).
- Varying degree of dilatation (asymptomatic to extreme forms with severely enlarged arteries reaching beyond the hilum).
- Airway compression and associated bronchomalacia at the level of the main bronchus or hilum caused by dilated arteries.

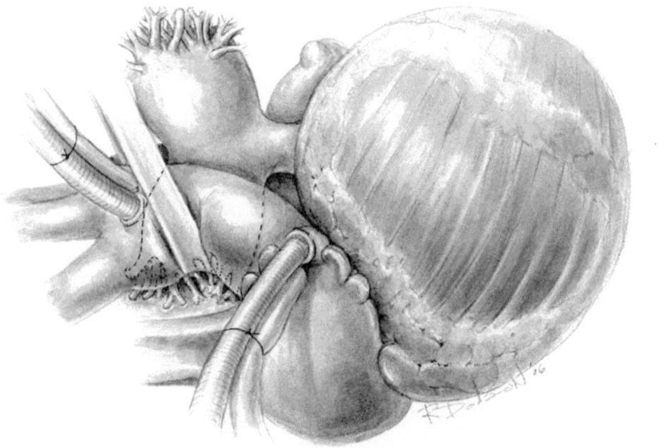

Fig. 1 Anatomic depiction of tetralogy of fallot with absent pulmonary valve. While the intracardiac features are similar to isolated Tetralogy of Fallot, the typical feature is the extensive dilatation of the branch pulmonary arteries. Reprinted from Operative Techniques in Thoracic and Cardiovascular Surgery, Vol 12, Issue 1, Welke FK, Ungerleider RM, Repair of Tetralogy of Fallot with absent pulmonary valve syndrome, pp. 25–35, 2007, with permission from Elsevier

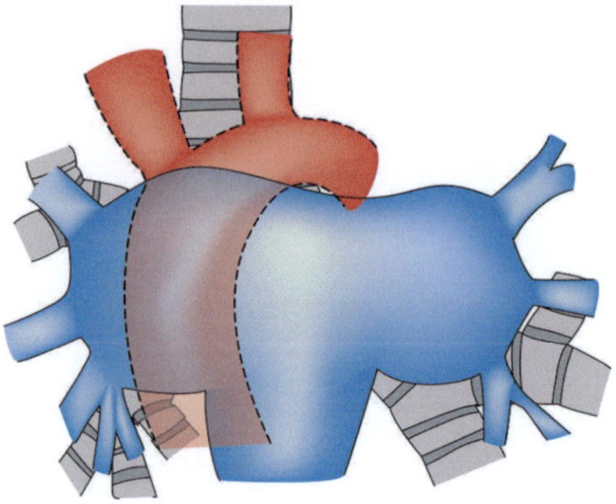

Fig. 2 Dilated pulmonary arteries in relation to trachea and bronchi

- Right pulmonary artery dilatation is more likely to affect airway.
- Airway compression can lead to air trapping and atelectasis.

2.3 Variations

- Aberrant origin of branch pulmonary artery from aorta.
- Dextrocardia.

3 Embryology

- Embryologic aspects regarding the antero-cephalad deviation of the infundibular septum are discussed in (Chap. 12.)
- Absence of the PDA is common as it leads to a more stable circulation, although cases with persistence are described.
- An aberrant ductal origin of a pulmonary artery may exist, with the duct not connected with the central pulmonary artery. The supplied pulmonary segment is not affected by dilatation.
- Increased compliance of artery wall. Dilatation is a hemodynamic effect, resulting from to-and-fro pulmonary blood flow and pressure.

4 Epidemiology

4.1 Incidence/Prevalence

- Approximately 3–6% of patients with TOF.

- TOF with absent pulmonary valve is seen in approximately 0.001% of all pregnancies.
- Isolated absent pulmonary valve syndrome with an intact ventricular septum is extremely rare.
- Incidence of absent pulmonary valve syndrome irrespective of associated TOF is 0.6% among all referrals to our institution.

4.2 Population at Risk, Inheritance

- Association with microdeletion 22q11.2 has been shown in 25%. These patients have a higher incidence of associated lesions.

5 Clinical Physiology and Presentation

- Patients typically show increased Q_p:Q_s, compared to that seen in classic TOF.
- Clinical presentation is variable and mostly dependent on the extent of airway compromise. Presentation ranges from asymptomatic with normal saturations, to congestive heart failure, to severe respiratory distress and cyanosis.
- Severe cases may present with immediate postnatal ventilation and oxygenation failure and require medical management, including intubation, positive pressure ventilation, prone positioning (offload pulmonary artery compression from airways).
- To-and-fro murmur heard along left sternal border.
- Size of pulmonary arteries does not necessarily correlate with clinical symptoms.
- Less symptomatic patients may present with recurrent upper respiratory tract infections and exercise intolerance.
- Cyanotic signs of TOF due to right-to-left shunting are uncommon. Cyanosis rather results from airway compromise.
- The greater the right ventricular outflow tract obstruction the more the presentation may resemble that of routine TOF.

5.1 Natural History

- 58–70% live births among those diagnosed prenatally.
- Severe airway impairment can lead to prompt deterioration and death after birth (up to 50% mortality in first year if left untreated) or are ventilator-dependent at birth.
- In less severe cases, the progression of enlargement of the pulmonary arteries can lead to further airway compression, progressive clinical deterioration, and eventually right ventricular failure.

- Rarely, asymptomatic patients may remain undiagnosed and can reach adulthood.

6 Associated Lesions

6.1 Common

- Right aortic arch.
- Absent PDA or ligamentum arteriosum.
- Bronchomalacia.

6.2 Less Common Associations

- ASD.
- Aberrant left subclavian artery.
- Aberrant origin of branch pulmonary artery from aorta or PDA.
- Absent left pulmonary artery.
- AVSD.
- MAPCAs.

7 Diagnostic Studies

7.1 ECG

- Right atrial enlargement.
- Right ventricular hypertrophy.

7.2 CXR

- Dilated pulmonary arteries, wide mediastinum, cardiomegaly.
- Atelectasis/collapse or hyperinflation.

7.3 Echocardiography

- Echocardiography is sufficient to make the diagnosis.
- Adequate assessment of

- ASD.
- VSDs.
- Pulmonary valve remnants.
- Degree of pulmonary insufficiency (PI) and stenosis.
- Proximal pulmonary artery dimensions (although limited peripherally).
- Right ventricular outflow tract anatomy and obstruction.
- Ventricular function.
- Aortic override.
- Atrioventricular valve function.
- Coronary arteries.
- Associated defects.

7.4 *CT-Angiography*

- Best imaging technique to assess airway (tracheal/bronchial compression) and pulmonary parenchyma (atelectasis, lobar collapse, air trapping, hyperinflation, lobar herniation).
- Allows for visualization of intraparenchymal pulmonary arterial tree.

7.5 *MRI*

- Rarely used in neonates.
- Diagnostic tool for right ventricular function/volume or PI during long-term follow-up after corrective surgery.

7.6 *Cardiac Catheterization*

- Not usually necessary. May be used to assess hemodynamics and/or to perform catheter-based intervention for residual lesions (e.g., balloon dilatation of branch pulmonary artery stenoses).

7.7 *Bronchoscopy*

- Indicated to determine site and mechanism of airway compression (pulmonary artery-mediated pulsatile compression on direct inspection versus tracheobronchomalacia).

8 Indications for Intervention/Surgery

- Presence of the disease.

9 Timing of Intervention and Management Strategy

- Timing is highly dependent on clinical symptoms (see Fig. 3).
- Conservative approach in neonates, if physiologically tolerated.
- In patients who are symptomatic because of airway compromise, conservative management (including noninvasive ventilation, intubation) to allow for growth if manageable, otherwise urgent repair.
- Prone positioning can have positive dramatic effects on respiratory symptoms and stability by allowing the pulmonary arteries to pull away from the airway.
- Intubation and use of muscle relaxants can be associated with cardiovascular collapse due to loss of contribution of chest wall effects on pulmonary arteries and airways that occur with spontaneous breathing.
- May need emergent sternotomy to relieve airway compression, or to initiate ECMO.
- For those who need urgent surgery, residual airway issues are common because the developmental component of bronchomalacia may be more important than actual airway compression.

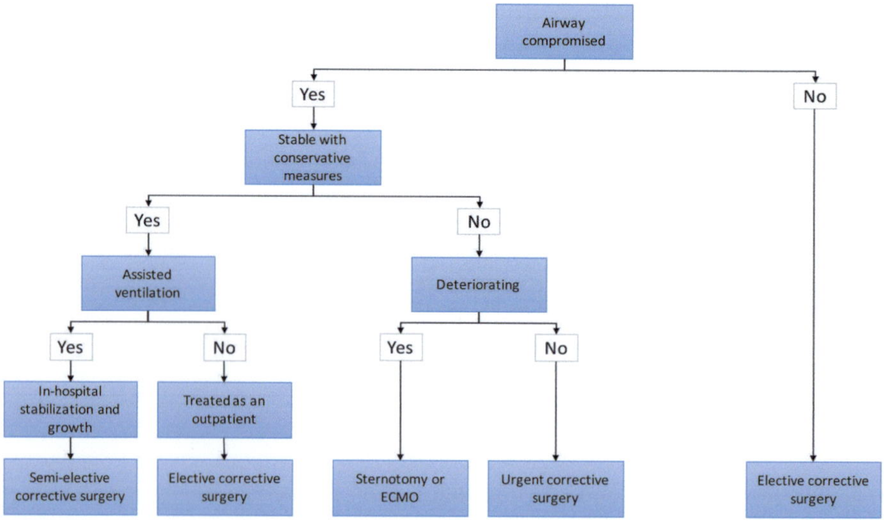

Fig. 3 Treatment algorithm for patients with Tetralogy of Fallot with absent pulmonary valve

10 Surgical Strategy

- Surgical Strategy aims at complete repair of the defect, including closure of the VSD, relief of the right ventricular outflow tract obstruction and reduction of the pulmonary arteries.
- The intracardiac component of the repair is similar to the technique used in regular TOF (Chap. 12).
- The right ventricular infundibulum may be relatively large and may not need extensive resection/enlargement.
- Pulmonary valve replacement is usually necessary to abolish the to-and-fro regurgitant flow that exacerbates the PA dilatation. This can be achieved with a valved RV to PA conduit (bovine jugular vein or a homograft). Patients with minimal airway compression may not require a valved conduit.
- Reduction in the size of the pulmonary arteries can be done by simple plication, resection of the anterior wall, or most effectively by combined resection of anterior and posterior pulmonary artery wall to ensure maximal relief of airway compression. The resection should be extended as far distally as possible (Fig. 4).

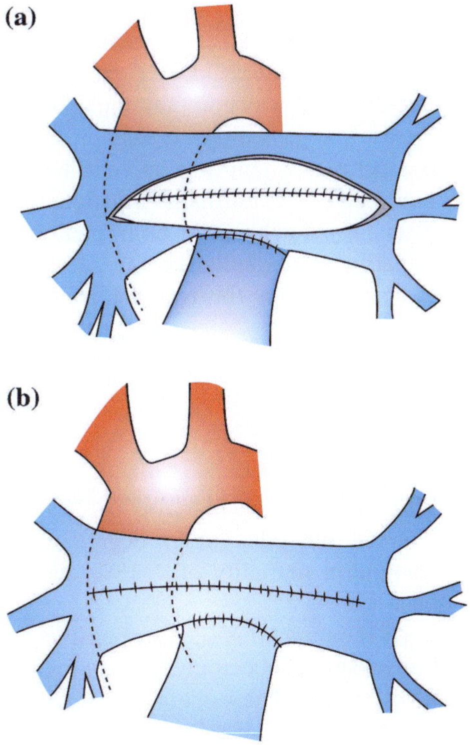

Fig. 4 Combined resection of anterior and posterior wall. **a** Resected and closed posterior wall seen through the open anterior pulmonary artery wall. **b** Completed repair, with reconstructed pulmonary artery and pulmonary valve/trunk replacement

- A Lecompte maneuver has been used in severe cases of airway obstruction to bring the PAs forward and away from the airways. This has been extremely effective in some small series.
- Intraoperative ventilation and bronchoscopic assessment of the airway can determine effectiveness of repair. If persistent compromise, placement of suspension sutures to aorta and/or pulmonary artery and temporarily leaving the chest open can be beneficial.

11 Intensive Care Physiology and Management

- Preoperative management highly dependent on severity of airway compromise.
- Postoperative extubation depends on severity of residual airway obstruction.
- Prolonged ventilation with high PEEP to overcome increased airway resistance from airway collapse may be necessary.
- Delayed sternal closure is common, especially in neonates.
- Persistent airway compression can be assessed by bronchoscopy.
- Suspension of thoracic vessels can improve ventilation and may be guided by bronchoscopy.
- Extensive lung reduction measures such as anterior translocation or lobectomy (often right middle lobe) if persistent ventilation or oxygenation failure from intolerable airway compression and air-trapping.
- Restrictive physiology is less pronounced than in regular TOF (depending on preoperative extent of right ventricular outflow tract obstruction and pulmonary blood flow) and milrinone infusion may help RV dysfunction.
- Neonates should have both pleural spaces drained to minimize additional impairment of ventilation.
- Echocardiogram for residual lesions and pericardial/pleural/abdominal fluid collection.

12 Outcome

- Early postoperative mortality 1–5% and almost entirely in neonates needing urgent intervention, reflecting the degree of airway compromise.
- Long-term mortality of 7–18%, mostly related to issues with chronic airway obstruction.
- Early reintervention (i.e., suspension suture of vessels, anterior pulmonary artery translocation, lobectomy) mainly for residual airway compromise in 13.5–14.8%.
- Most common late reoperations are related to the pulmonary valve (38.2%, median follow-up of 13 years).
- Freedom from reoperation approximates 80% at 5 years, 69% at 10 years, and 52% at 20 years (89% at 5 years, 59% at 10 years at our institution).

13 Alternative Strategies and Controversies

- Isolated resection of anterior or posterior pulmonary artery wall has been reported.
  - This is less efficient for relief of airway obstruction. Reduction of pulmonary artery dimensions significant only for combined approach.
- Lecompte-like anterior translocation (with or without transection of aorta).
  - Can be used for severe neonatal cases or for those not responding to pulmonary artery resection. Rate of reoperation in combined resection does not necessitate more extensive approach. Take care to avoid causing SVC compression from the translocated large RPA.
- Intrahilar reduction plasty.
  - Reduction should be performed as far distally as possible but may be limited for individual anatomic reasons.
- Bronchial stenting has been reported as an option for severe obstruction.
  - Last resort if other options fail. Lack of growth potential. Need for redilation/replacement.

Bibliography

1. Alsoufi B, Williams W, Hua Z, et al. Surgical outcomes in the treatment of patients with tetralogy of Fallot and absent pulmonary valve. Eur J Cardiothorac Surg. 2007;31(3):354–9.
2. Momma K, Kondo C, Matsuoka R. Tetralogy of Fallot with pulmonary atresia associated with chromosome 22q11 deletion. J Am Coll Cardiol. 1996;27(1):198–202.
3. Welke K, Ungerleider R. Repair of tetralogy of fallot with absent pulmonary valve syndrome. Op Tech Thorac Cardiovasc Surg. 2007;12(1):25–35.
4. Wertaschnigg D, Jaeggi M, Chitayat D, et al. Prenatal diagnosis and outcome of absent pulmonary valve syndrome: contemporary single-center experience and review of the literature. Ultrasound Obstet Gynecol. 2013;41(2):162–7.
5. Yong M, Yim D, Brizard C, et al. Long-term outcomes of patients with absent pulmonary valve syndrome: 38 years of experience. Ann Thorac Surg. 2014;97(5):1671–7.

Tetralogy of Fallot with Pulmonary Atresia

Osman O. Al-Radi

Abstract A subset of patients with Tetralogy of Fallot (TOF) have associated pulmonary atresia also referred to as 'Pulmonary Atresia with VSD'. The branch pulmonary arteries are usually confluent and normally developed, fed by the arterial duct, and the intracardiac anatomy is that of TOF with a well-developed right ventricle, large VSD and overriding aorta. By definition, these are duct dependent at birth and management is either primary repair or initial palliation with a ductal stent or a surgical systemic to pulmonary artery shunt (BTT most commonly). Definitive repair, whether as a primary or staged procedure, involves VSD closure with either an RV-PA conduit or a trans-annular patch if there is membranous atresia. Mortality is low and reoperation is usually for conduit replacement.

Keywords Tetralogy of fallot · Pulmonary atresia · Ventricular septal defect

Abbreviations

ASD	Atrial septal defect
BTT	Blalock Taussig Thomas
CVP	Central venous pressure
MAPCAs	Multiple aortopulmonary collaterals
MPA	Main pulmonary artery
PA	Pulmonary artery
PA/VSD	Pulmonary atresia/VSD
PDA	Persistent ductus arteriosus
PFO	Persistent foramen ovale
PS	Pulmonary stenosis
RV	Right ventricle
RVH	Right ventricular hypertrophy

O. O. Al-Radi (✉)
Cardiac Surgery, Department of Surgery, King Abdulaziz University, Jeddah, Saudi Arabia
e-mail: oradi@kau.edu.sa

© The Author(s), under exclusive license to Springer Nature Switzerland AG 2024

A. I. Dipchand et al. (eds.), *Manual of Cardiac Care in Children*,
https://doi.org/10.1007/978-3-031-70973-9_14

RVOT	Right ventricular outflow tract
TOF	Tetralogy of fallot
TOF/PA	Tetralogy of fallot/pulmonary atresia
VSD	Ventricular septal defect

Key Points

- Duct dependent circulation.
- Primary neonatal repair if weight > 2.5–3.0 kg and branch pulmonary arteries > 3–4 mm in diameter.
- In low-birth-weight neonates or small branch pulmonary arteries, consider a PDA stent, or a modified Blalock-Taussig-Thomas (BTT) shunt.
- Principles of repair: VSD closure and RV to PA conduit (or transannular patch if membranous atresia).
- Conduit of choice is bovine jugular vein (Contegra) or Pulmonary Homograft.

1 Nomenclature

- TOF/PA: A congenital cardiovascular malformation that is a variant of TOF in which there is no direct communication between the RV and the pulmonary arterial tree. Can be muscular or membranous atresia.
- By definition, the condition is duct dependent. The native PAs are supplied by the duct.
- In TOF/PA the native pulmonary arteries are the main source of pulmonary blood supply.
- Patients with associated Major Aorto-Pulmonary Collateral Arteries (MAPCAs) are dealt with in Chap. 15.

2 Anatomy

- The terms Pulmonary Atresia with Ventricular Septal Defect (PA/VSD) and Tetralogy of Fallot with pulmonary atresia (TOF/PA) are used interchangeably.
- The native PA system is usually well developed and supplied by a duct, which is often tortuous or S-shaped.
- The intracardiac anatomy is that of TOF.
  - TOF/PA shares the intra-cardiac anatomical features of other forms of TOF, namely:
  - Anterior deviation of outlet septum and aortic override.
  - Perimembranous VSD.

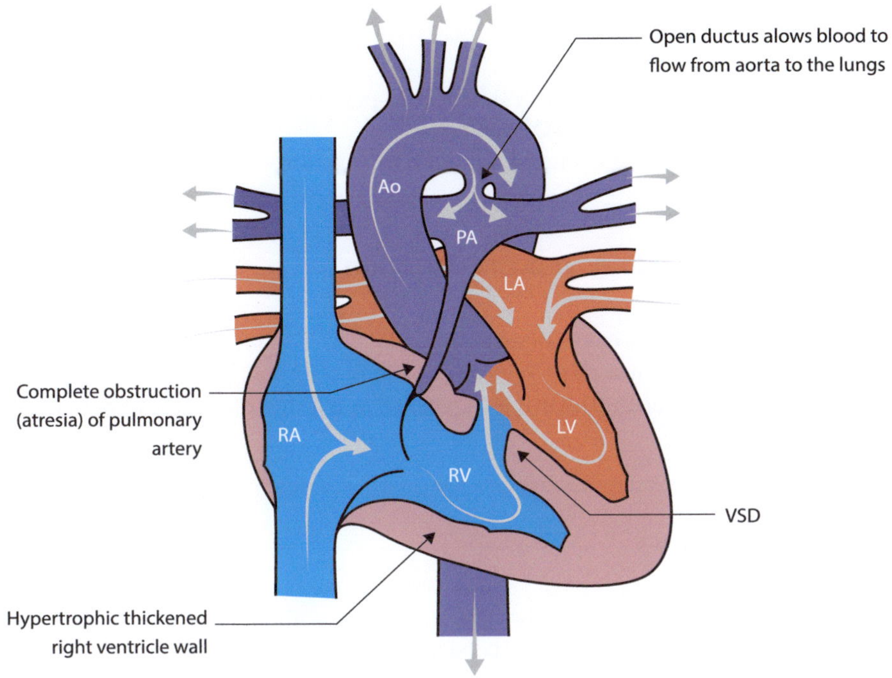

Fig. 1 Anatomy and physiology of tetralogy of fallot with pulmonary atresia. Reprinted from The Royal Children's Hospital website, Pulmonary Atresia with VSD, https://www.rch.org.au/cardiology/heart_defects/Pulmonary_Atresia_with_VSD/, with permission from Dr. Michael Cheung, Director of Cardiology, Royal Children's Hospital, Melbourne, Australia

- RVH (if long-standing).
- Counter-clockwise rotation of the aortic root.
- Instead of PS there is valvar or infundibular and valvar atresia (see Fig. 1).

3 Embryology

- The MPA originates from the process of septation of the common arterial trunk.
- The intra-pericardial pulmonary arteries originate from the 6th aortic arches.
- The intrapulmonary arteries originate from the vascular plexus of the lung buds.
- As is the case with TOF the main process that leads to TOF/PA is an imbalance in the process of septation of the common arterial truck in favor of the aorta.

4 Epidemiology

- The prevalence is approximately 0.013–0.07 per 1000 live births.
- It constitutes about 10% of TOF patients.
- Chromosome 22q11 deletion is a common association.

5 Clinical Physiology and Presentation

- The diagnosis is often made antenatally.
- Cyanosis in the first few days to weeks of life is common.
- The circulation is dependent on ductal patency as it is the sole source of pulmonary blood flow.

6 Natural History

- The disease is usually fatal in the neonatal period without intervention.
- Some cases survive longer due to persistent patency of the arterial duct.

7 Associated Lesions

7.1 Common

- ASD.
- Chromosome 22q11 deletion.
- Absent thymus and hypocalcemia, DiGeorge syndrome.

7.2 Less Common

- Multiple VSDs.
- Non-confluent PAs, bilateral PDA.

8 Diagnostic Studies

8.1 ECG

- Normal axis or right axis deviation with RVH.

8.2 CXR

- Classically shows a boot shaped heart due to paucity of shadow at the site of the main pulmonary artery.

8.3 Echocardiography

- Echocardiography adequately delineates the anatomy in over 95% of cases.
- Perimembranous VSD usually with outlet extension, rarely multiple VSDs.
- Absence of forward flow across the pulmonary valve.
- Branch pulmonary arteries of normal size and potential stenosis or non-confluence.
- Aortic valve that overrides the VSD.
- Two well developed ventricular cavities.
- If the branch pulmonary arteries are not well visualized, further study is indicated.

8.4 CT

- Limited chest CT can be done in neonates without sedation.
- Only needed if branch PAs not clearly seen on echo, or if concern over additional sources of pulmonary blood supply (MAPCAs). It may aid in planing of PDA stunting.

8.5 Cardiac Catheterization

- If there is a question of aortopulmonary collaterals or high pulmonary vascular resistance.
- PDA stenting if primary surgery is deemed risky (e.g. low weight or hypoplastic branch PAs).

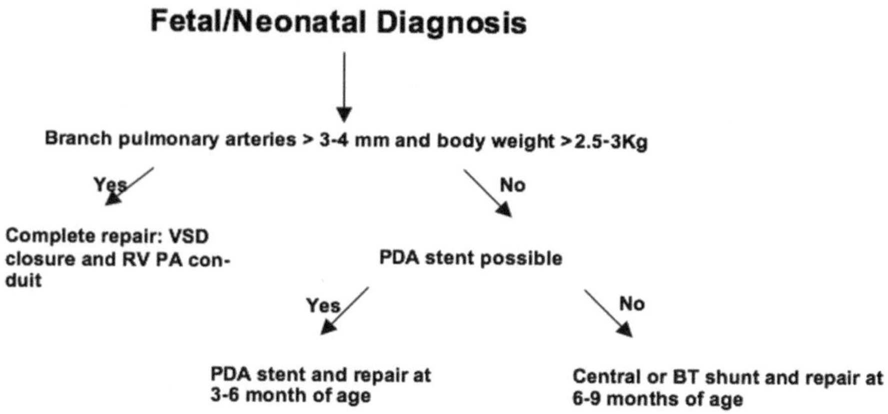

Fig. 2 Treatment algorithm for tetralogy of fallot with pulmonary atresia

9 Indications for Intervention/Surgery

- Presence of the disease.

10 Timing of Intervention and Management Strategy

- Complete repair with VSD closure and RV-PA conduit can be considered in neonatal period if the branch pulmonary arteries are > 3–4 mm in diameter and the body weight is ≥ 2.5–3.0 kg depending on the expertise of the surgical and intensive care teams.
- PDA stenting or BTT shunt, with complete repair at 3–6 month of age is a safe alternative especially in cases with small pulmonary arteries or low birthweight.
- If PDA stenting fails or is not suitable based on anatomy, a Right mBTT Shunt or central shunt is used.
- Treatment algorithm is shown in Fig. 2.

11 Surgical Strategy

- PDA ligation.
- Transatrial or transventricular closure of VSD.
- RV incision for proximal conduit anastomosis, most commonly a pulmonary homograft or Contegra (bovine jugular vein) conduit.
- Alternatively in membranous atresia a transannular incision with outflow tract patch. A tailored pulmonary valve creation with heterograft pericardium can be considered.

- Consider PA augmentation with autologous or heterograft pericardium.
- If the branch PAs are non-confluent, establish PA continuity and decide either primary repair or initial shunt based on branch PA size and body weight.

12 Intensive Care Physiology and Management

- In the absence of residual lesions, management is relatively routine and straightforward.
- Expected restrictive physiology consider leaving a PFO open.
- A peritoneal drain is sometimes needed.
- May need to leave the chest open for a few days. The chest can be closed when RV diastolic dysfunction resolves indicated by reduced fluid drainage from the peritoneal drain and lower CVP.
- Milrinone load in the OR and in the ICU (0.25–0.1 μg/kg/ml).
- Echocardiogram for residual lesions and pericardial fluid.

13 Outcome

- Mortality is < 3% using the outlined approach.
- Reinterventions are mainly for conduit replacement. Typically, 40–50% of conduits will need reintervention within 5 years.
- Risk of heart block should be <1%.

14 Alternative Strategies and Controversies

- Staged repair with initial palliation with PDA stenting or a systemic to pulmonary shunt is an acceptable approach and may be preferred depending on the surgical and perioperative experience and expertise.
- PDA stenting versus a systemic to pulmonary shunt (central or modified BTT) is an area of controversy. There is no clear difference in PA growth or need for reinterventions between the two palliative options. The choice depends on the level of expertise with PDA stenting and the surgical expertise in dealing with stent related distortion of the proximal pulmonary arteries at the time of complete repair.
- Perforation of membranous atresia in the cath lab with RVOT stent is an emerging alternative palliation. A surgical RV-PA conduit with a small goretex tube graft (4 or 5 mm) is the surgical equivalent of this if primary repair not felt to be feasible.
- Early stent extraction and systemic to PA shunt should be considered if the PDA stent placement is suboptimal. For example, if the stent is too deep into the one of the branch PAs crossing the upper lobe branch.

- In membranous atresia, in conjunction with a tranannular patch a tailored bicuspid or tricuspid pulmonary valve formation has been described with the use of equine pericardium which may improves perioperative outcomes and may delay RV dilatation and chronic dysfunction.
- Alternative conduit choices include femoral vein homografts or hand-sewn valved goretex conduits.

Bibliography

1. Goldstein BH, Petit CJ, Qureshi AM, et al. Comparison of management strategies for neonates with symptomatic tetralogy of fallot. J Am Coll Cardiol. 2021;77(8):1093–106. https://doi.org/10.1016/j.jacc.2020.12.048.
2. Hoffman JI, Kaplan S. The incidence of congenital heart disease. J Am Coll Cardiol. 2002;39(12):1890–900. https://doi.org/10.1016/s0735-1097(02)01886-7.
3. Jaobs JP, Franklin RCG, Béland MJ, et al. Nomenclature for pediatric and congenital cardiac care: unification of clinical and administrative nomenclature—the 2021 international paediatric and congenital cardiac code (IPCCC) and the eleventh revision of the international classification of diseases (ICD-11). World J Pediatr Congenit Heart Surg. 2021;12(5):E1–18. https://doi.org/10.1177/21501351211032919.
4. Mercer-Rosa L, Elci OU, DeCost G, et al. Predictors of length of hospital stay after complete repair for tetralogy of fallot: a prospective cohort study. J Am Heart Assoc. 2018;7(11): e008719. https://doi.org/10.1161/JAHA.118.008719.
5. Mitchell SC, Korones SB, Berendes HW. Congenital heart disease in 56,109 births incidence and natural history. Circulation. 1971;43(3):323–32.

Pulmonary Atresia with Ventricular Septal Defect and Major Aortopulmonary Collateral Arteries

Osami Honjo

Abstract Pulmonary atresia/ventricular septal defect with major aortopulmonary collateral arteries (PA/VSD/MAPCAs) is a rare, complex, and heterogeneous congenital heart diseases where pulmonary blood flow is supplied by multiple MAPCAs. Physiology varies greatly depending on the number, size, and presence or absence of stenosis of the MACPAs, as well as their relationship and extent of the native pulmonary artery system. Patients can be cyanotic, balanced, or have excessive pulmonary blood flow depending on the total amount of pulmonary blood flow from MAPCAs. The goal of surgical intervention is to unifocalize all important MAPCAs to recruit as many lung segments with concomitant or subsequent achievement of biventricular physiology by closing the VSD and establishing a right ventricle-to-pulmonary artery continuity. One stage unifocalization at 4–8 months of age is a preferred approach although a subgroup of patients with diminutive branch pulmonary arteries requires a staged approach with an initial central shunt (Mee shunt). Our treatment algorithm and intraoperative pulmonary flow study to determine the feasibility of VSD closure are included.

Keywords Pulmonary atresia · Major aortopulmonary collateral arteries · Unifocalization

Abbreviations

ASD	Atrial septal defect
AVSD	Atrioventricular septal defect
CHD	Congenital heart disease
CHF	Congestive heart failure
CPB	Cardiopulmonary bypass
DORV	Double outlet right ventricle

O. Honjo (✉)
Division of Cardiovascular Surgery, Department of Surgery, Labatt Family Heart Centre, The Hospital for Sick Children, University of Toronto, Toronto, ON, Canada
e-mail: Osami.honjo@sickkids.ca

© The Author(s), under exclusive license to Springer Nature Switzerland AG 2024

A. I. Dipchand et al. (eds.), *Manual of Cardiac Care in Children*,
https://doi.org/10.1007/978-3-031-70973-9_15

iNO	Inhaled nitric oxide
LA	Left atrium
LV	Left ventricle
MAPCAs	Major aortopulmonary collaterals
MPA	Main pulmonary artery
PA	Pulmonary artery
PA/VSD	Pulmonary atresia/ventricular septal defect
PA/VSD/MAPCAs	Pulmonary atresia/ventricular septal defect with major aortopulmonary collateral arteries
PDA	Persistent ductus arteriosus
PGE	Prostaglandin
Qp	Pulmonary blood flow
Qs	Systemic blood flow
RV	Right ventricle
RVSP	Right ventricular systolic pressure
TGA	Transposition of the great arteries
TOF	Tetralogy of fallot
TOF/PA	Tetralogy of fallot/pulmonary atresia
VSD	Ventricular septal defect

Key Points

- Pulmonary atresia/ventricular septal defect with major aortopulmonary collateral arteries (PA/VSD/MAPCAs) is a rare, complex, and heterogeneous congenital heart disease (CHD) where pulmonary blood flow is supplied by MAPCAs.
- Physiology depends on the number, size, and presence or absence of stenosis of the MAPCAs. Patients can be cyanotic, balanced, or overcirculated depending on the total amount of pulmonary blood flow from MAPCAs and relationship/extent of the native pulmonary artery (PA) system.
- Lung segments may have sole supply from a MAPCA, or may have dual supply from native PAs and MAPCAs.
- The goal of surgical intervention is to unifocalize all important MAPCAs to recruit as many lung segments as possible and to achieve biventricular physiology by closing the VSD and establishing a right ventricle (RV)-to-PA continuity.
- One stage unifocalization at 4–8 months of age is a preferred approach although a subgroup of patients with diminutive branch PAs requires a staged approach with an initial central shunt (Mee shunt).
- Feasibility of biventricular repair, i.e., VSD closure, is largely dependent on the quality and extent of the pulmonary vasculature and subsequent PA pressure after full unifocalization, for which intraoperative pulmonary flow study is a useful method.

1 Anatomy

- Intracardiac morphology is essentially that of Tetralogy of Fallot (TOF) with large VSD, anterior deviation of the outflow septum and aortic override but no patent connection from RV to main PA (MPA).
- PA/VSD can be classified into four types based on anatomy of native PAs, PDA, and MAPCAs (Fig. 1).
  - Type I: Intrapericardial PAs are present and fully developed. There are no MAPCAs and pulmonary blood flow is supplied by PDA (Chap. 14).
  - Type II: Absent MPA with confluent central PAs supplied by a PDA without MAPCAs.
  - Type III: Confluent central PAs with MAPCAs but no PDA.
  - Type IV: Non-confluent or absent central PAs with MAPCAs (10–15% of cases have absent intrapericardial PAs).
  - A fifth sub-group has also been described who have both a PDA and MAPCAs (see below).
- Congenital Heart Surgery Nomenclature and Database divides PA/VSD into 3 subtypes, which is further defined by whether the branch PAs are confluent, and by the presence of absence of the MPA trunk.
- MAPCAs typically originate from the descending aorta but they can originate from other vessels, including the subclavian artery, internal mammary artery, intercostal artery, and extremely rarely from the coronary artery.
- The PDA is usually absent. If present, then it usually supplies a relatively normal native PA system to one lung, with MAPCAs supplying the contralateral lung.

2 Epidemiology

- PA/VSD accounts for approximately 2.5% of all CHD with the incidence of 0.07 per 100 live births.
- Among patients with PA/VSD, approximately 30–65% of the patients have MAPCAs.
- Approximately 25% of patients with PA/VSD (not specifically with MAPCAs), have associated chromosomal abnormalities and syndromes.
  - Most common is DiGeorge syndrome (22q11 deletion syndrome) – especially associated with Type IV subtype.
  - Others include VACTRL association, Alagille syndrome, CHARGE syndrome.
- Maternal diabetes and maternal intake of benzodiazepines are associated with increased incidence.

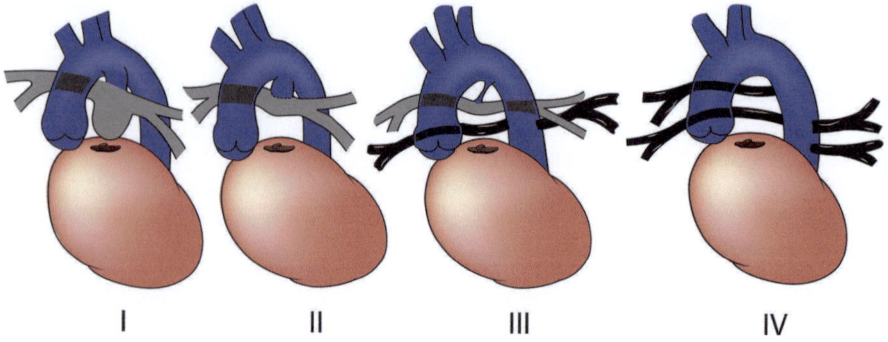

Fig. 1 One of the anatomical classifications of PA/VSD/MAPCAs based on the anatomical characteristics of native pulmonary arteries, PDA, and MAPCAs. Type I: Intrapericardial PAs are present and fully developed. There are no MAPCAs and pulmonary blood flow is supplied by PDA Type II: Absent MPA with confluent central PAs supplied by a PDA without MAPCAs. Type III: Confluent central PAs with MAPCAs but no PDA. Type IV: Non-confluent or absent central PAs with MAPCAs (10–15% of cases have absent intrapericardial PAs). Reprinted from Sabiston and Spencer Surgery of the Chest, 7th Edition, Emani SM (author), Sellke FW, del Nido PJ, Swanson SJ (eds), Pulmonary atresia with ventricular septal defect and right ventricle-to-pulmonary artery conduits, pp 2147–2161, 2016, with permission from Elsevier

3 Clinical Physiology and Presentation

- Clinical physiology and presentation mainly depend on the amount of pulmonary blood supply through MAPCAs.
- Patients with large unobstructed MAPCAs may have excessive pulmonary blood flow and pulmonary overcirculation resulting in early onset of congestive heart failure (CHF) and rarely systemic hypoperfusion.
- Some patients with moderate to large MAPCAs have a balanced circulation in which patients have minimal symptoms except mild cyanosis.
- Patients with small and/or stenotic MAPCAs may have reduced pulmonary blood flow resulting in moderate or severe cyanosis. Those patients are typically not responsive to Prostaglandin (PGE) administration as the PDA is usually absent.

4 Natural History

- The natural history of patients with PA/VSD/MAPCAs is mainly determined by the fate of MAPCAs.
- Some large MAPCAs remain unobstructed and provide a large amount of blood flow to the area of lungs, causing 'patchy' pulmonary hypertension in specific lung segments. These patients may be in high output cardiac failure initially but if untreated, may develop pulmonary hypertension.

- Many MAPCAs develop stenosis (and even occlude), typically at the origin from the descending aorta, resulting in progressive severe cyanosis.
- The worst spectrum of the disease has poorly developed pulmonary vasculature and profound cyanosis from an early age.
- Patients with progressive cyanosis may develop non-specific arterio-venous collateral circulations to compensate for low oxygen saturation.
- Approximately 60% of untreated infants with PA/VSD/MAPCAs survive more than 1 year.

5 Associated Lesions

- Double outlet right ventricle (DORV).
- Atrial septal defect (ASD)
- Right aortic arch.
- Transposition of the great arteries (TGA) and complete atrioventricular septal defects (AVSD) have very rarely been associated with MAPCAs.

6 Diagnostic Studies

6.1 Electrocardiogram

- Right axis deviation.
- Right ventricular hypertrophy.
- In older children, p waves may peak indicating right atrial enlargement.

6.2 Chest X Ray

- A boot shaped heart due to small or absent branch PAs.
- Pulmonary vascular markings can be increased, decreased or unremarkable depending on the size of MAPCAs and subsequent amount of pulmonary blood flow.
- Right aortic arch shadow (up to 50%).

6.3 Echocardiography

- Echocardiography is the most important modality to delineate intracardiac lesions but has a limited role delineating anatomy of MAPCAs.

- VSD: usually in the perimembranous portion with outlet extension and an anteriorly deviated infundibular septum (anteriorly malaligned VSD).
- Presence or absence of additional muscular VSDs.
- Degree of aortic override [> 50% override is defined as DORV (Chap. 5)].
- Nature of pulmonary atresia and pulmonary valve.
- Presence or absence of main and branch PAs. If present, confluency and size of the branch PAs.
- Ventricular function.
- Valvular regurgitation.
- Other associated lesions.
- Presence of MAPCAs or non-specific collaterals.

6.4 Chest CT

- Chest CT is the first-line non-invasive modality to delineate detailed MAPCA and native branch PA anatomy.
- MAPCA and native PA anatomy (if present).
  - Number of MAPCAs.
  - For each MAPCA: origin, size, the number of lung segment(s) supplied, and presence or absence of stenosis.
  - Communication between MAPCAs and central or peripheral branch PA (intra-parenchymal communication) can often be delineated with chest CT but it may not be as definitive as traditional angiogram.

6.5 Cardiac Magnetic Resonance (CMR)

- CMR may provide supplemental but important blood flow and physiology data, particularly on pulmonary circulation.
- Total pulmonary blood flow (Qp) and pulmonary blood flow to each lung (it is difficult to quantify blood flow through each MAPCA).
- Pulmonary to systemic flow (Qs) ratio (Qp:Qs).
- Blood flow pattern of each MAPCA by phase contrast flow velocity mapping.
- Ventricular volume and function.

6.6 Cardiac Catheterization (Fig. 2)

- Cardiac catheterization and angiogram are the gold standard to obtain complete delineation of MAPCA and native PA anatomy, thereby providing essential data for surgical planning.

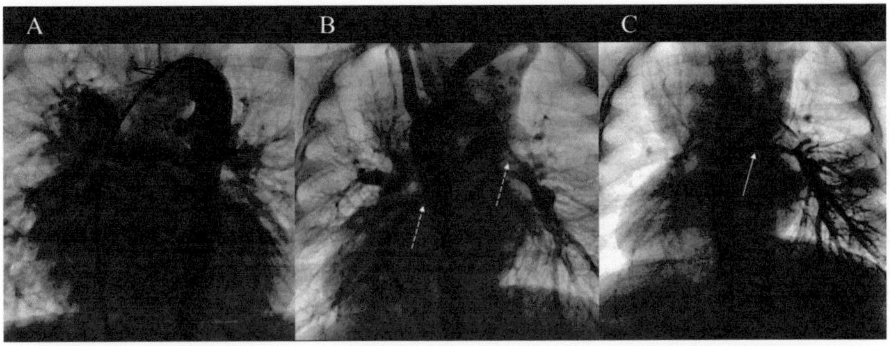

Fig. 2 Aortograms of 2 patients with PA/VSD/MAPCAs. A: Patient #1 has well-developed multiple MAPCAs arising from the descending aorta. Almost all lung segments are perfused by MAPCAs. NO central pulmonary arteries are visualized. B: Patient#2 has moderate-sized multiple MAPCAs with multiple stenosis (dotted arrows). C: Patient#2 has a confluent but diminutive central pulmonary arteries that are only visualized through an intra-parenchymal communication from one of the left MAPCAs

- Delineation of MAPCA and native PA anatomy.
- Angiography is better diagnosing or visualizing the following anatomic information compared to cardiac CT.
  - Presence or absence of intra-parenchymal communication or dual supply from both MAPCA and native PA to specific segments (Fig. 2c).
  - Presence or absence, and degree of arborization abnormalities of the peripheral branch PAs.
  - The number of lung segments supplied by each MAPCAs or native PAs.
  - Interventions during cardiac catheterization may optimize patient's operative candidacy.
  - Balloon angioplasty or occasionally stent placement to the stenotic MAPCAs.
  - Coil occlusion of non-specific collaterals or MAPCAs that have dual and competitive flow to native PAs.
  - Perforation and/or stenting of native right ventricular outflow tract, in the cases of membranous PA to promote antegrade pulmonary blood flow and PA growth.

7 Treatment

7.1 Indication for Surgical Treatment

- The diagnosis of this lesion is an indication for surgical intervention. Contraindications for surgical interventions include:
  - Poorly developed MAPCAs and native PAs that are not amenable to any interventions (usually some sort of palliative shunt is feasible in these cases).

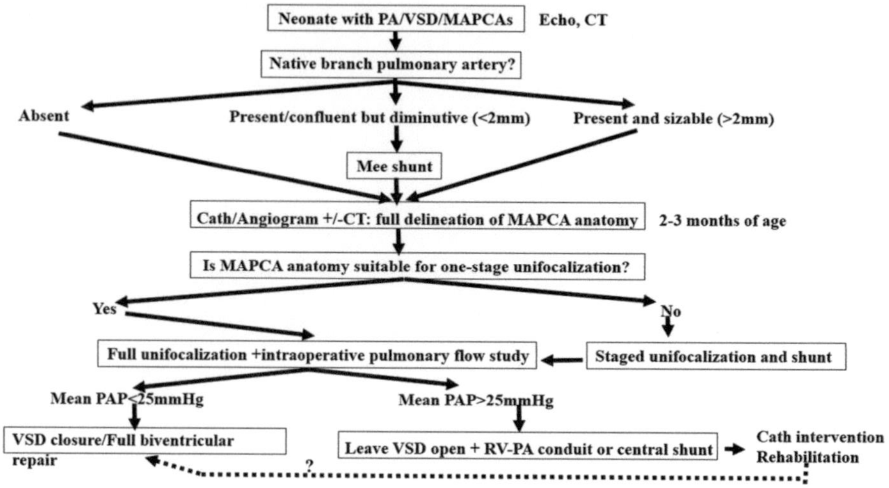

Fig. 3 Investigation and treatment algorithm for patients with PA/VSD/MAPCAs in The Hospital for Sick Children. PAP, pulmonary artery pressure

- Late diagnosis and (1) occluded major MAPCAs and lost substantial lung segments, (2) unobstructed large MAPCAs that caused irreversible pulmonary hypertension to the supplied segments.

7.2 *Treatment Algorithm (Fig. 3)*

- The aim is to perform complete unifocalization of all MAPCAs at 4–8 months of age before MAPCAs starts developing significant stenosis or occlusion, or before pulmonary hypertension develops in over-perfused segments.

7.3 *Management Strategy During Neonatal and Early Infantile Periods*

- No medical or surgical intervention is indicated when physiology is balanced. Patients can be managed as an outpatient. However, a clinically balanced physiology could consist of a combination of underperfused and overperfused areas of the lung, and therefore complete and early imaging assessment is essential.
- Diuretic therapy is indicated when patients have significant CHF and/or pulmonary edema from pulmonary overcirculation caused by unrestrictive large MAPCAs. Early unifocalization is considered when patients have persistent failure to thrive or poor growth.

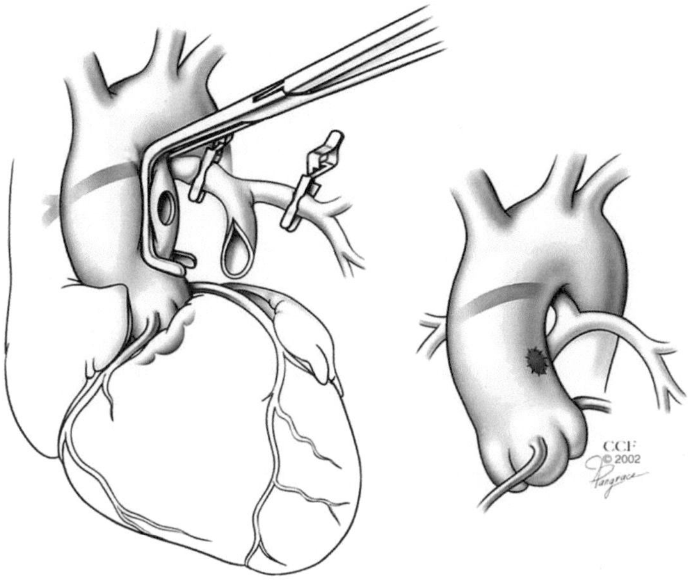

Fig. 4 Mee shunt (and end-to-side anastomosis between the origin of the main pulmonary artery and the ascending aorta) for the confluent but diminutive (< 2 mm) for the purpose of promoting pulmonary artery growth. This procedure can be done without cardiopulmonary bypass. Right pulmonary artery and/or anastomotic stenoses are relatively common complications. Reprinted from The Journal of Thoracic and Cardiovascular Surgery, Vol 126, Issue 3, Duncan BW, Mee RBB, Prieto LR et al., Staged repair of tetralogy of Fallot with pulmonary atresia and major aortopulmonary collateral arteries, pp 694–705, 2003 with permission from Elsevier

- Cyanotic neonates and young infants with this lesion are extremely difficult to treat. Supplemental oxygen may be indicated. A central shunt or Mee shunt (when there are native branch PAs) may be indicated although shunt procedure may not dramatically increase arterial saturation.
- Mee shunt (and end-to-side anastomosis between the origin of the MPA and the ascending aorta) is indicated with the central branch PAs are present and confluent but diminutive (< 2 mm) for the purpose of promoting PA growth (sometimes called native PA 'rehabilitation') (Fig. 4).

7.4 Unifocalization

- Optimal timing of complete unifocalization is 4–8 months of age and is sometimes up to 12 months of age as long as MAPCAs do not develop stenosis or when the native PA needs time to grow after Mee shunt placement.

- Complete unifocalization can typically be achieved via a median sternotomy approach, although a thoracotomy prior to sternotomy to control MAPCAs that are difficult to access via sternotomy is an option.
- Staged unifocalization strategy is uncommon but sometimes employed when some MAPCAs, particularly the ones that run posterior to the bronchus, are extremely difficult to access via one approach.
- All MAPCAs that provide blood flow to distinctive lung segments should be unfocalized to the central PAs to recruit as much lung segment and PA cross-sectional area as possible. General rule is to try and recruit as much vascular tissue as possible.
- Branch PAs, regardless of previous shunt procedure, require patch reconstruction in order to achieve biventricular repair.

7.5 *VSD Closure and Biventricular Repair*

- After complete unifocalization, biventricular circulation is achieved when VSD is closed and the continuity between the RV and PA is established by a valved conduit.
- VSD is safe to be completely closed when:
  - Reconstructed branch PAs with all MAPCAs unfocalized have sufficient lung segments and PA cross-sectional area (target > 15/20 lung segments).
  - PA pressure is low enough that does not cause significant RV hypertension.
- Intraoperative pulmonary flow study, which is performed right after complete unifocalization, is an effective method to estimate mean PA pressure and subsequent RV systolic pressure (RVSP) after VSD closure (see Fig. 5).
- VSD closure and biventricular repair can be achieved as one operation with unifocalization of MAPCAs or as a separate operation when peripheral PAs are rehabilitated and optimized.
- If not felt to be safe to close the VSD then it is left open and either a central shunt placed into the unifocalized confluence or place a deliberately restrictive RV-PA conduit.

7.6 *Operative Techniques of Unifocalization*

- After a median sternotomy, all MAPCAs are mobilized and controlled before cardiopulmonary bypass (CPB) is initiated. All native PA branches also mobilized. A thoractomy may be used first, to control posterior MAPCAs that are difficult to access via a sternotomy.

- Normothermic CPB is initiated and all MAPCAs are divided from the aorta at their origin. Unifocalization of all MAPCAs to the central PAs is achieved. Vessels are controlled with spring-loaded clips (Yasargil) or clamps.
- Patch reconstruction of the branch PAs is achieved, completing full unifocalization and PA reconstruction. Pulmonary homograft is the preferred material, or a treated autologous pericardium (if homograft not available).
- Cardioplegic cardiac arrest is achieved. When the heart is completely decompressed,intraoperative pulmonary flow study is performed.

7.7 *Intraoperative Pulmonary Flow Study (Fig. 5)*

- A physiologic test to estimate mean PA pressure and subsequent RVSP if the VSD is closed.
- Under full CPB and cardioplegic cardiac arrest, full ventilation is maintained, and LA and LV are completely emptied.
- An additional arterial cannula is placed into the reconstructed central PA.
- Using a separate arterial pump, blood is infused into the pulmonary circulation while continuously measuring mean PA pressure by a needle placed in the central PA.
- Pulmonary blood flow is incrementally increased to 3L/m2/min.
- If mean PA pressure is less than 25 mmHg, which generally results in < 2/3 systemic RVSP, the VSD is closed.
- Flow study is repeated at least twice to ensure the accuracy of the study.
- If mean PA pressure is consistently higher than 25 mmHg, the VSD is left open with establishment of pulmonary blood flow, either by a restrictive RV-PA conduit or a central shunt.

8 Intensive Care Physiology and Management

- Full unifocalization and/or VSD closure typically require many hours on CPB and therefore patients may have significant inflammatory response, vasoplegia, and sometimes hemolysis.
- RV can be exposed to variable degree of afterload, depending on the distal PA pressure. RV systolic dysfunction could occur when RVSP is high (> 70–75% of systemic pressure).
- RV may demonstrate variable degree of restrictive physiology, which is typically seen after TOF or its variants repair (Chap. 12).
- Unfocalized lung segments may experience reperfusion injury, particularly when the corresponding MAPCA was stenotic before unifocalization, which may result in pulmonary hemorrhage, hemoptysis and poor oxygenation.

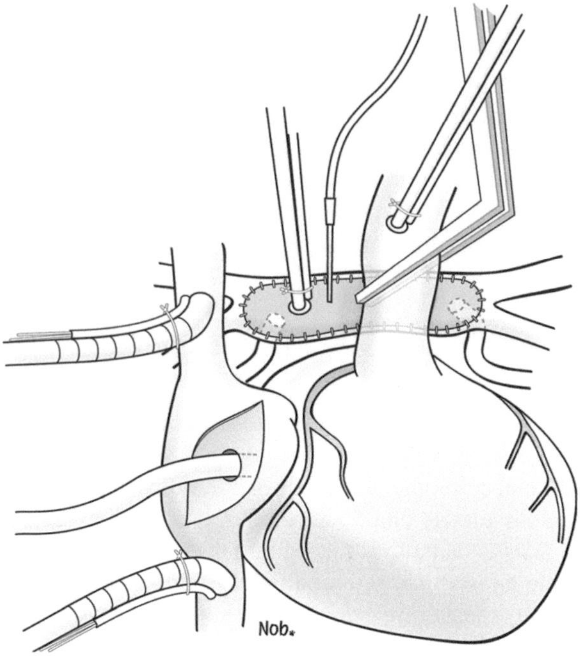

Fig. 5 Intraoperative pulmonary flow study. After complete unifocalization and patch reconstruction of the central pulmonary arteries, cardioplegic cardiac arrest is commenced and the left heart completely decompressed. Normal mechanical ventilation is maintained. An additional arterial cannula and a needle to measure mean pressure are placed into the reconstructed central pulmonary artery. Mean pulmonary artery is measured while 3L/m2/min of flow is perfused into the pulmonary circulation. Reprinted from Circulation, Vol 120, Issue 11_Suppl_1, Honjo O, Al-Radi, MacDonald C et al., The functional intraoperative pulmonary blood flow study is a more sensitive predictor that preoperative anatomy for right ventricular pressure and physiologic tolerance of ventricular septal defect closure after complete unifocalization in patients with pulmonary atresia, ventricular septal defect, and major aortopulmonary collaterals, pp S46–52, 2009, with permission from Wolters Kluwer Health, Inc

- Pulmonary vasodilation therapy (iNO, alkylanization, etc.) may be required if evidence of reactive pulmonary vasculature in high pulmonary blood flow lung segments and/or long CPB.
- Systemic oxygenation determined by degree of right-to-left intracardiac shunting (ASD or VSD) and co-existing lung disease (following CPB).
- If an atrial communication is left open, which is a common practice in many institutions, it may create a bidirectional or right-to-left shunt, resulting in various degree of desaturation. This desaturation is typically manageable with conservative management unless the communication and the amount of atrial-level shunt is too large.
- LV function is typically preserved although LV systolic and diastolic function can be compromised due to prolonged CPB.

- Patients can be weaned from ventilation and be extubated within 24–48 h after surgery unless exhibiting significant physiologic problems.
- Bronchial compression could occur after unifocalization and extensive PA reconstruction, which may result in difficulty weaning from mechanical ventilation.

9 Outcome

- Operative mortality of unifocalization and intracardiac repair in the experienced centres is 1–3% in the current era.
- Approximately 75–90% of the patients who undergo unifocalization procedures achieve VSD closure, although sometimes as a staged procedure.
- 1- and 5-year survival after unifocalization is 85–90% and 75–85%, respectively.
- More than 2/3 of patients require catheter-based interventions to the reconstructed PAs and/or unfocalized MAPCAs in the first 5 years.
- There is a small minority of patients with poor pulmonary vasculature who can never achieve VSD closure and remain palliated with shunts or stented vessels.

10 Alternative Strategies and Controversies

- Some centres focus on promoting growth of the native PAs ('rehabilitation') and prefer to ligate MAPCAs as opposed to unifocalization.
- Although one-stage complete unifocalization is a common practice, some centres still prefer staged unifocalization approach.
- There are various ways to establish a Mee shunt or a central shunt to promote native PA growth, including artificial graft use versus the direct connection between the MPA and the aorta.
- Some centres prefer early (2–3 months of age) unifocalization as opposed to 4–8 months of age.
- A central shunt or a RV-PA conduit can be applied as a pulmonary blood source after unifocalization when VSD cannot be closed and PA and MAPCAs need further growth and optimization. RV-PA conduit facilitates Cath-based rehabilitation.

Acknowledgements The authors would like to acknowledge Dr. Jiaquan Zhu, MD for his contribution to this chapter.

Bibliography

1. Balaguru D, Dilawar M. Pulmonary atresia with ventricular septal defect: systematic review. Heart Views. 2007;8(2):52–61.
2. Barron DJ, Kutty RS, Stickley J, et al. Unifocalization cannot reply exclusively on native pulmonary arteries: the importance of recruitment of major aortopulmonary collaterals in 249 cases. Eur J Cardiothorac Surg. 2019;56(4):679–87.
3. Brizard CP, Liava'a M, d'Udekem Y. Pulmonary atresia, VSD and Mapcas: repair without unifocalization. Semin Thorac Cardiovasc Surg Pediatr Card Surg Annu. 2009;139–144.
4. Duncan BW, Mee RB, Prieto LR, et al. Staged repair of tetralogy of Fallot with pulmonary atresia and major aortopulmonary collateral arteries. J Thorac Cardiovasc Surg. 2003;126(3):694–702.
5. Emani SM. Pulmonary atresia with ventricular septal defect and right ventricle-to-pulmonary artery conduit. In: Sellke FW, del Nido PJ, Swanson SJ, editors. Sabiston and Spencer surgery of the chest. 7th ed. Philadelphia: Elsevier Saunders; 2005. p. 2147–61.
6. Grosse-Wortmann L, Yoo SJ, van Arsdell G, et al. Preoperative total pulmonary blood flow predicts right ventricular pressure in patients early after complete repair of tetralogy of Fallot and pulmonary atresia with major aortopulmonary collateral arteries. J Thorac Cardiovasc Surg. 2013;146(5):1185–90.
7. Honjo O, Al-Radi OO, MacDonald C, et al. The functional intraoperative pulmonary blood flow study is a more sensitive predictor than preoperative anatomy for right ventricular pressure and physiologic tolerance of ventricular septal defect closure after complete unifocalization in patients with pulmonary atresia, ventricular septal defect, and major aortopulmonary collaterals. Circulation. 2009;120(11 Suppl):S46–52.
8. McElhinney DB, Asija R, Zhang Y, et al. 20-year experience with repair of pulmonary atresia or stenosis and major aortopulmonary collateral arteries. J Am Coll Cardiol. 2023;82(12):1206–22.
9. Tchervenkov CI, Roy N. Congenital heart surgery nomenclature and database project: pulmonary atresia–ventricular septal defect. Ann Thorac Surg. 2000;69(4 Suppl):S97–105.
10. Zhu J, Meza J, Kato A, et al. Pulmonary flow study predicts survival in pulmonary atresia with ventricular septal defect and major aortopulmonary collateral arteries. J Thorac Cardiovasc Surg. 2016;152(6):1494–1503.e1.

Pulmonary Atresia with Intact Ventricular Septum

Seth B. Gray

Abstract Pulmonary atresia with intact ventricular septum (PA/IVS) results from membranous or muscular atresia of the right ventricular (RV) outflow tract and obstruction to antegrade pulmonary blood flow. This results in right ventricular hypertrophy (RVH) with variable RV size and morphology (ranging from normal to diminutive), tricuspid valve abnormalites including hypoplasia/stenosis/regurgitation, an obligate right-to-left shunt across the atrial septum, and potential coronary artery anomalies that include extensive ventriculocoronary connections or RV dependent coronary circulation (RVDCC). Maintaining patency of the PDA is imperative as the source of pulmonary blood flow until cardiac catheterization or surgical interventions are performed. Prognosis and management are contingent on the degree of right ventricular hypertrophy, degree of right ventricle and tricuspid valve hypoplasia (z-score), and presence of RVDCC for myocardial perfusion. In the absence of RVDCC, establishing antegrade RV to PA circulation is the priority for patients with adequately sized right ventricle and tricuspid valve inflow. Supplemental pulmonary blood flow by PDA stenting or BTT shunt may be required while awaiting regression of RV hypertrophy (RVH) and establishing a biventricular circulation, or as initial single ventricle palliation. A one-and-a half ventricle repair with bidirectional cavopulmonary shunt as a second intervention may be required for those with borderline RV and/or TV size. RVDCC increases in frequency with degree of RV hypoplasia and is associated with high mortality that may benefit from primary cardiac transplantation and possible high-risk ventricular device support.

Keywords Pulmonary atresia with intact ventricular septum · Hypoplastic right heart syndrome · Right ventricle dependent coronary circulation · Coronary fistulae · Coronary sinusoids

S. B. Gray (✉)
Department of Critical Care Medicine, Division of Cardiac Critical Care, The Hospital for Sick Children, 555 University Avenue, Toronto, ON M5G 1X8, Canada
e-mail: seth.gray@sickkids.ca

© The Author(s), under exclusive license to Springer Nature Switzerland AG 2024

A. I. Dipchand et al. (eds.), *Manual of Cardiac Care in Children*,
https://doi.org/10.1007/978-3-031-70973-9_16

Abbreviations

ASD	Atrial septal defect
BCPS	Bidirectional cavopulmonary shunt
BTT	Blalock Taussig Thomas
ECMO	Extracorporeal membrane oxygenation
LA	Left atrium
LV	Left ventricle
LVOT	Left ventricular outflow tract
MPA	Main pulmonary artery
PA	Pulmonary artery
PA/IVS	Pulmonary atresia / intact ventricular septum
PDA	Persistent ductus arteriosus
PFO	Persistent foramen ovale
PGE	Prostaglandin
PI	Pulmonary insufficiency
PVR	Pulmonary vascular resistance
Qp	Pulmonary blood flow
Qs	Systemic blood flow
RA	Right atrium
RV	Right ventricle
RVDCC	Right ventricle dependent coronary circulation
RVH	Right ventricular hypertrophy
RVOT	Right ventricular outflow tract
TR	Tricuspid regurgitation
TV	Tricuspid valve

Key Points

- A heterogenous set of lesions with right ventricular outflow tract obstruction due to imperforate pulmonary valve and variable tricuspid valve and right ventricular size and function.
- May be membranous atresia (consisting of an imperforate pulmonary valve with well-formed semilunar cusps and complete commissural fusion) or muscular atresia (consisting of long segment muscular atresia of the right ventricular outflow tract).
- Extensive ventriculocoronary connections (fistulas) may exist; coronary circulation is considered RV dependent if associated with ostial or proximal stenosis or atresia.
- Prognosis and management is dependant on right ventricle chamber size and anatomy, tricuspid valve size (z-score), and presence of right ventricle dependent coronary circulation (RVDCC) for myocardial perfusion.

- A PDA is necessary to maintain pulmonary blood flow and an obligate right-to-left shunt across the atrial septum to maintain left ventricular preload and cardiac output.
- Patients present with cyanosis after PDA closure ± low cardiac output if atrial septal defect restrictive.
- Management ranges from establishment of right ventricular outflow tract patency and right ventricle decompression to achieve a biventricular circulation in those with favorable right ventricle anatomy and normal coronary circulation; initial palliation with PDA stenting to support pulmonary circulation toward a biventricular repair, one-and-a-half ventricle physiology, or single ventricle palliation in those with unfavorable right ventricle anatomy.
- RVDCC is a high risk lesion that may benefit from listing for primary cardiac transplantation.

1 Nomenclature

- Situs solitus, concordant atrio-ventricular and ventricular-arterial connections, and a left sided aortic arch. Atretic RV to PA connection; open ASD/PFO. Ebstein anomaly of the tricuspid valve is rare.

2 Anatomy

- Fig. 1 demonstrates native anatomy of PA/IVS.
- Pulmonary atresia.
  - May consist of membranous atresia (imperforate pulmonary valve with well-formed semilunar cusps and complete commissural fusion) or muscular atresia (long segment muscular atresia of the RVOT).
- RV anatomy.
  - Ranges from a tripartite ventricle with a well-formed inlet, apical trabecular, and outlet components, to a moderately hypoplastic bipartite ventricle with an inlet and outlet component, to a unipartite ventricle with a severely hypoplastic diminutive inlet chamber. The LV usually demonstrates normal size and anatomy.
- TV anatomy.
  - Variable anatomy, ranging from normal size to severe hypoplasia and stenosis, to severe regurgitation.
  - Size (z-score) correlates with RV size and morphology, with the smallest TV correlating with smaller RV cavities and attenuated apical trabecular and outlet portions.

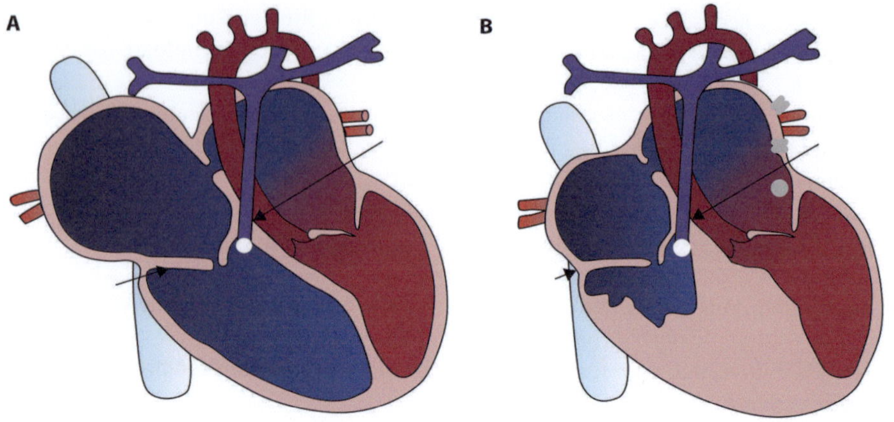

Fig. 1 **Anatomic** spectrum of PA/IVS. Panel A demonstrates a plate-like valve atresia with two well-formed ventricles, and a good size tricuspid valve that undergoes a biventricular repair. The diminutive right ventricle and tricuspid valve in Panel B are highly associated with coronary artery anomalies and require single ventricle palliation or primary transplantation depending on presence of RV dependent coronary circulation. Reprinted from ISUGO.org page, Pulmonary atresia with intact ventricular septumPatient information SeriesWhat you should know, what you should ask, 2022, with permission from Delgado, Raquel G

  - Also inversely correlated with the presence of significant coronary artery anomalies, with the smallest TVs more likely to be associated with coronary sinusoids and RVDCC.
- Atrial septal defect (ASD).
  - There is an obligate right-to-left shunt across either a PFO or ASD to volume load the left side of the heart for LV preload and cardiac output in the setting of restrictive RV physiology.
  - Rarely restricted to flow.
- Coronary artery anatomy.
  - Coronary artery anomalies are found in up to 75% of cases.
  - Three main types of abnormalities include (1) RV-to-coronary artery fistulas and sinusoids (RV to subepicardial coronaries); (2) coronary artery stenosis; (3) coronary artery occlusion or ostial atresia.
  - Fistula connections primarily to right coronary or left anterior descending arteries.
  - Can result in coronary myointimal hyperplasia in the presence of a rich background of glycosaminoglycans, ranging from mild intimal and medial thickening to loss of normal arterial wall morphology and severe stenoses or luminal occlusion.
  - Up to 35% of patients have at least one coronary artery interruption and up to 40% have RVDCC.

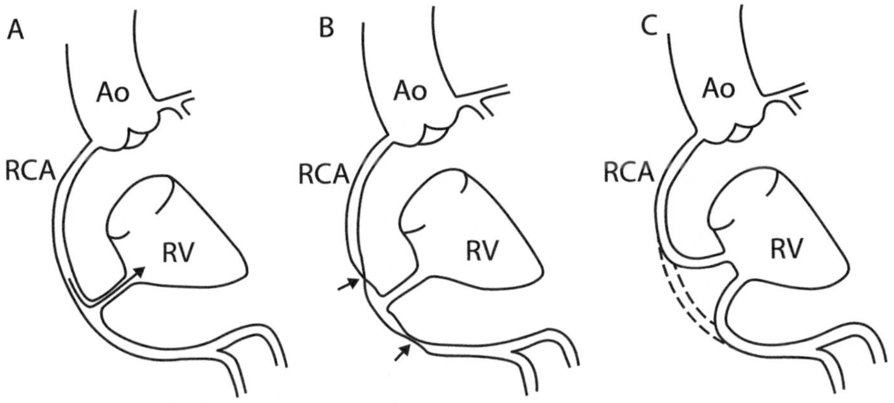

Fig. 2 Coronary-cameral fistulas. **a** Unobstructed fistula connection from RV to right coronary artery; **b** Proximal or distal stenosis to RV coronary fistula. Myocardium distal to stenosis at risk for coronary steal with RV decompression; **c** Coronary sinusoids with atresia of coronary. Distal myocardium at risk of isolation and/or myocardial infarction. Reproduced from Circulation, Vol 86, Issue 5, Giglia TM, Mandell VS, Connor AR, et al., Diagnosis and Management of Right Ventricle-Dependent Coronary Circulation in Pulmonary Atresia With Intact Ventricular Septum., pp 1516–1528, 1992, with permission from Wolters Kluwer Health Inc

  - RVDCC occurs when a significant portion of the ventricular myocardium relies on retrograde flow from the hypertensive RV to the coronaries for myocardial perfusion. Defined as severe proximal stenoses of two or more major coronary arteries or interruption of aortocoronary (ie coronary ostial atresia), or profound coronary-cameral steal through coronary fistula (Fig. 2).

- Left ventricular outflow tract (LVOT).
  - LVOT obstruction due to a leftward protrusion of the ventricular septum and crowding caused by the suprasystemic right ventricular pressures have been described.
- Pulmonary arteries.
  - Pulmonary arteries are well formed (or mildly hypoplastic) and supplied by a PDA. MAPCAs are rare and associated with poor outcomes.

3 Embryology

- A precise embryological cause has not been identified. Possibly due to failure of separation of the pulmonary valve after cardiac septation as evidenced by normal or mildly hypoplastic proximal MPA and branch PAs.

4 Epidemiology

4.1 Incidence/Prevalence

- Annual incidence of 0.6/10,000 live births.
- Fetal incidence may be underestimated due to high rates of spontaneous and elective abortions.

4.2 Population at Risk, Inheritance

- Insufficient evidence to establish a genetic association for PA/IVS.
- No predilection for female versus male sex.

5 Clinical Physiology and Presentation

- PDA dependent pulmonary ciruculation due to valve atresia and absence of antegrade flow.
- An obligate right-to-left shunt exists across an unrestrictive PFO or ASD in order to maintain LV preload and cardiac output; dilation of restrictive ASD may be necessary to avoid systemic venous hypertension and end-organ congestion/dysfunction.
- Oxygen saturation depends on the interplay between the obligate right-to-left shunt of systemic venous blood across the atrial septum mixing with pulmonary venous blood in the left atrium, and higher oxygenation saturations correlate with excessive pulmonary blood flow.
- Many patients are now identified through routine antenatal ultrasound screening, especially when marked RV hypoplasia is present.
- Postnatal diangnosis may be made during routine neonatal screening or worsening cyanosis and hypoxemia with PDA closure. Patients with restrictive atrial septum may demonstrate low cardiac output, poor perfusion, acidosis, and multisystem organ dysfunction.
- Arrhythmias and ECG abnormalities (ST-T wave changes) may occur due to coronary ischemia.
- Initial management includes maintaining PDA patency with PGE infusion. Dilation of ASD is rare and only required if low cardiac output. As the PVR decreases, close attention should be paid to ensuring adequate systemic blood flow in the setting of high pulmonary blood flow.

5.1 *Natural History*

- Untreated patients will develop progressive cyanosis, hypoxemia and cardiogenic shock as the PDA closes, ultimately resulting in death. Death occurs in 50% within 2 weeks of birth and in 85% by 6 months of age; rare cases of longer-term survival have been reported in the setting of a persistent PDA or systemic-to-pulmonary artery collateral blood flow.

6 Associated Lesions

- PA/IVS is associated with Ebstein anomaly of the tricuspid valve in up to 10% of patients.

7 Diagnostic Studies

7.1 *ECG*

- Frontal QRS vector + 30 to + 90.
- Paucity of right-sided forces, dominant left-sided forces.
- Frequently have ST-T wave abnormalities due to coronary anomalies and subendocardial ischemia

7.2 *CXR*

- Often will have normal cardiac silhouette with reduced pulmonary vascular markings until PDA is reopened.
- Worsening pulmonary edema as PVR falls in the setting of a patent PDA.
- Massive cardiomegaly may occur if Ebstein anomaly present.

7.3 *Echocardiogram*

Transthoracic echocardiography remains the mainstay of diagnostic imaging.

- Morphology of the pulmonary valve atresia (membranous versus muscular atresia).
- MPA and branch PA size.
- RV size and morphology (unipartite, bipartite, tripartite).

- TV size (z-score), anatomy, and function (Ebstenoid, dysplasia, stenosis or regurgitation).
- Presence of ventriculocoronary connections (sinusoids, fistulas).
- Presence of aorto-coronary continuity.
- Unrestrictive ASD.
- PDA presence and morphology.
- LV size and function and outflow tract obstruction.

7.4 Cardiac Catheterization and Angiography

- Coronary angiography by aortic root or selective coronary injections is necessary to evaluate for coronary artery stenoses, interruptions, and RVDCC prior to pulmonary valve intervention and RV decompression.
- RV ventriculogram to confirm RV anatomy, RVOT anatomy, and ventriculocoronary connections (fistulas, sinusoids).
- Hemodynamic assessment for RV systolic and end-diastolic pressures, ASD gradient.

8 Surgical and Cardiac Catheterization Management Strategy

- Management options guided primarily by size of RV and TV, and presence of RVDCC.
- Tripartite right ventricle, membranous atresia, TV z-score > -2.5, no RVDCC or major sinusoids.
  - Decompression of RV and establishment of antegrade pulmonary blood flow via percutaneous radiofrequency perforation of pulmonary valve and pulmonary valve balloon dilations.
  - ASD is left open to allow right-to-left shunt across atrial septum while the RV remodels. Percutaneous ASD device closure considered if defect does not close spontaneously in the future.
  - Surgical RVOT repair (reconstruction or patch augmentation), pulmonary valve repair or replacement, or TV repair may be required in the future.
- Bipartite right ventricle, membranous atresia, TV z-score −2.5 to −5, + major sinusoids, no RVDCC.
  - Decompression of RV and establishment of antegrade pulmonary blood flow with primary goal to allow for potential RV growth.
  - Systemic saturations determined by antegrade pulmonary blood flow and right-to-left atrial level shunt.
  - PGE infusion for PDA patency may be necessary to allow for PVR to fall.

  - If cyanosis persists will require additional pulmonary blood flow via stenting of PDA or surgical systemic-to-pulmonary artery shunt (ie BTT shunt).
  - Restrictive ASD may require dilation to avoid systemic venous hypertension while the RV remodels.
- Hypoplastic unipartite right ventricle, muscular atresia, TV z-score < -5, absence of RVDCC.
  - Staged single ventricle palliation with initial intervention to establish reliable pulmonary blood flow through PDA stent or BTT shunt.
  - Planned bidirectional cavopulmonary shunt (BCPS) at 4–6 months if favourable hemodynamics.
- Hypoplasic unipartite right ventricle, muscular atresia, TV z-score < -5, presence of RVDCC.
  - RVDCC dictates that RV-to-PA continuity is avoided due to high likelihood of myocardial ischemia once RV pressure and coronary perfusion pressures decrease.
  - Management options include pursuing a staged single ventricle palliation pathway and/or listing for primary cardiac transplantation.
  - Listing for primary cardiac transplantation is strongly considered with evidence of RVDCC, ± coronary ischemia or LV dysfunction.
    - Pulmonary blood flow supported with PGE infusion or PDA stent. BTT shunt possible but generally avoided.
    - Staged Single Ventricle pathway if transplantation not an option. Establish stable source of pulmonary blood flow via PDA stent or BTT shunt.

8.1 Considerations for Transcatheter Perforation of Pulmonary Valve

- Offers advantage of avoiding RV incision and cardiopulmonary bypass.
- Femoral vein used to access the RV and perform either wire or radiofrequency catheter perforation of the membranous pulmonary valve plate and balloon dilations of the right ventricular outflow tract.
- Additional source of pulmonary blood flow may be required to allow time for RV growth and remodeling; options include PDA stent, systemic-to-pulmonary artery shunt, or prolonged PGE infusion.
- Cardiac CT angiography may be useful for ductal stent pre-procedural planning.
- An alternative to the percutaneous approach is a hybrid per-ventricular approach via median sternotomy for RVOT access and balloon dilation of pulmonary valve and RVOT.

8.2 *Anesthesia and Bypass Considerations*

- In the presence of RV-coronary fistulas, adequate RV preload and systemic diastolic blood pressure are essential to maintain coronary perfusion pressure.
- Hemodynamic management of patients with PA/IVS and functional single ventricle physiology is focused on maintaining Qp:Qs balance and adequate systemic cardiac output.
- Inadequate RV pressurization on cardiopulmonary bypass or with full veno-arterial extracorporeal membrane oxygen (ECMO) support in patients with RVDCC can lead to myocardial infarction.
- Maintain RV filling pressures in the setting of restrictive RV physiology.
- Monitor closely for signs and symptoms of circular shunt in patients following pulmonary valve perforation with PI, TR, and systemic-to-pulmonary artery connection (PDA or BTT shunt).

9 Intensive Care Physiology and Management

- Post-operative and post-procedural management dictated by intervention or surgical pathway.
- Monitor closely for signs of coronary steal and coronary ischemia.
- Oxygen saturations are determined by total pulmonary blood flow (depends on residual RVOT obstruction, RV size, RV systolic and diastolic dysfunction, and right-to-left shunt across atrial communication). Oxygen saturations assess adequacy of pulmonary blood flow; low saturations ($< 70\%$) suggest inadequate pulmonary blood flow, pulmonary venous desaturation, or systemic venous desaturation. High oxygen saturations often signify excessive pulmonary blood flow.
- The presence of arrhythmias or new ECG ST-T wave changes raise suspicion for coronary insufficiency.
- Patients with systemic-to-pulmonary shunt (ie modified BTT shunt) are monitored closely for shunt thrombosis.
- Early extubation or early spontaneous breathing can decrease RV afterload and increase pulmonary blood flow post-procedure.
- Must confirm unrestrictive nature of the ASD in patients with evolving low cardiac output.
- Circular shunt physiology may develop in patients with re-established antegrade pulmonary blood flow, a systemic-to-pulmonary shunt or PDA to augment pulmonary blood flow, and significant TR; systemic blood flow transits from aorta to the pulmonary arteries, back into the RV (PI), into the RA (TR), and across ASD back into the LA. Leads to profound systemic hypoperfusion and shock. Management often includes surgical interventions to narrow the shunt or decrease TR.

- Extracorporeal membrane oxygenation (ECMO) presents additional challenges, as decompressing the right heart may lead to further coronary steal and myocardial ischemia.

10 Outcomes

- Overall survival rates are approaching 70–90%.
- Most common risks include coronary ischemia, myocardial infarction and arrhythmias related to coronary insufficiency.
- The highest mortality exists in those with PA/IVS palliated down the staged single ventricle pathway, with the presence of RVDCC and coronary sinusoids pertaining to higher risk.
- In patients with RVDCC, mortality is reported as high as 50–60%.
- Future surgical interventions depend on RV size and morphology and ability to support a biventricular circulation.
  - RV and TV size and function assessed by echocardiography or cardiac MRI.
  - Following PV perforation, adequate RV size may require device closure of PFO/ASD.
  - Further intervention may be necessary to ensure unobstructed outflow tract.
  - If inadequate RV size, one-and-a half ventricle repair considered, including superior BCPS to volume offload the RV, ± closure of PFO/ASD.

11 Alternative Strategies and Controversies

- Listing for primary cardiac transplantation as primary therapy remains controversial, with many surgical programs favoring routine listing only in the setting of RVDCC (consider de-listing if successfully achieve BCPS while waiting cardiac transplantation).
- Technique for perforation of pulmonary valve and RV decompression remains controversial, with options including radiofrequency perforation of pulmonary valve followed by balloon dilations of RVOT (local preference), surgical valvotomy and RVOT patch augmentation, or hybrid per-ventricular access of RVOT for transcatheter pulmonary valvuloplasty.
- Strategy to provide additional pulmonary blood flow remains controversial, including PDA stent or surgical BTT shunt. PGE infusion is preferred for transient therapy while awaiting for drop in PVR or awaiting heart transplantation.
- Emerging experience with Ventricular Assist Device (VAD) support of high risk transplant candidates (PA/IVS with RVDCC) with or without evidence of acute ischemia.

Bibliography

1. Cheung EW, Richmond ME, Turner ME, et al. Pulmonary atresia/intact ventricular septum: influence of coronary anatomy on single-ventricle outcome. Ann Thorac Surg. 2014;98(4):1371–7.
2. Gleich S, Latham GJ, Joffe D, et al. Perioperative and anesthetic considerations in pulmonary atresia with intact ventricular septum. Semin in Cardiothorac Vasc Anesth. 2018;22(3):256–64.
3. Hanley FL, Sade RM, Blackstone EH, et al. Outcomes in neonatal pulmonary atresia with intact ventricular septum. A multiinstitutional study. J Thorac Cardiovasc Surg. 1993;105(3):406–423,424–427
4. McArthur JD, Munsi SC, Sukumar IP, et al. Pulmonary valve atresia with intact ventricular septum. Report of a case with long survival and pulmonary blood supply from an anomalous coronary artery. Circulation. 1971;44(4):740–745.
5. Schneider AW, Blom NA, Bruggemans EF, et al. More than 25 years of experience in managing pulmonary atresia with intact ventricular septum. Ann Thorac Surg. 2014;98(5):1680–6.
6. Shaddy RE, Penny DJ, Feltes TF, Cetta F, Mital S. Moss and Adams' Heart disease in infants, children, and adolescents: including the fetus and young adult. 10th ed. Philadelphia: Wolters Kluwer Health; 2021.
7. Sukhavasi A, McHugh-Grant S, Glatz AC, et al. Pulmonary atresia with intact ventricular septum: intended strategies. J Thorac Cardiovasc Surg. 2022;164(5):1277–88.
8. Ungerleider RM, Nelson K, Meliones J, Quartermain M, Jacobs J, editors. Critical heart disease in infants and children. 3rd ed. Philadelphia: Elsevier; 2018.

Cor Triatriatum (Divided Atrium)

Devin Chetan and Christoph Haller

Abstract Divided left atrium or cor triatriatum sinister is a rare congenital anomaly characterized by a fibromuscular partition between a proximal left atrial compartment containing the pulmonary veins and a distal left atrial compartment in continuity with the left atrial appendage and the mitral valve. The clinical presentation is variable and based on the degree of restriction of the distal chamber and left ventricular inflow and the associated cardiac lesions (found in up to 80% of patients with this congenital malformation). Clinical features are similar to mitral stenosis and severe cases may require urgent neonatal repair for pulmonary congestion and low cardiac output. Echocardiography is the diagnostic test of choice. Surgical excision of the membrane is the definitive management and has excellent outcomes. A divided right atrium (cor triatriatum dexter) has been described as well and refers to a functional division by large remnants of embryonic valvar structures between the sinus venosus and the distal right atrium.

Keywords Divided atrium · Cor triatriatum

Abbreviations

ASD	Atrial septal defect
LA	Left atrium
LAA	Left atrial appendage
LSVC	Left SVC
LV	Left ventricle

D. Chetan
Division of Cardiology, Labatt Family Heart Centre, The Hospital for Sick Children, Toronto, ON, Canada
e-mail: devin.chetan@sickkids.ca

C. Haller (✉)
Division of Cardiovascular Surgery, Labatt Family Heart Centre, Department of Surgery, The Hospital for Sick Children, University of Toronto, Toronto, ON, Canada
e-mail: christoph.haller@sickkids.ca

© The Author(s), under exclusive license to Springer Nature Switzerland AG 2024

A. I. Dipchand et al. (eds.), *Manual of Cardiac Care in Children*,
https://doi.org/10.1007/978-3-031-70973-9_17

PAPVD	Partial anomalous pulmonary venous drainage
RA	Right atrium
RVH	Right ventricular hypertrophy
TAPVC	Total anomalous pulmonary venous connection

Key Points

- Rare congenital anomaly (0.4% of congenital heart disease).
- Partial division of the left atrium into two chambers, with one containing pulmonary veins and the other containing the left atrial appendage and mitral valve
- Variable clinical presentation (primarily depending on degree of obstruction between proximal and distal compartment).
- Surgical repair indicated for obstruction, timing variable.
- Frequently obstructed, 75% have some degree of restriction. If severe, may necessitate urgent repair.
- Primarily diagnosed by echocardiography.
- Results of surgical correction are excellent.

1 Nomenclature

- A divided leftatrium (cor triatriatum) is defined by a separating structure within the atrium separating a pulmonary venous component from a vestibular component containing mitral valve and left atrial appendage (LAA). A divided right atrium shows a separating structure within the atrium separating a systemic venous component from a vestibular component.

2 Anatomy

- Division of the morphologic left atrium (LA) into proximal and distal components by a fibromuscular shelf or diaphragm.
- Pulmonary venous drainage into the proximal part of the divided LA.
- Vestibule and atrial appendage forming parts of the distal atrial chamber.
- Distal atrial chamber communicates with the mitral valve and LAA.
- Fibromuscular partition dividing LA is different in structure and histology from lesions obstructing inflow to the LV (e.g. supramitral ring). Usually a double layer of myocardium.
- There is usually an atrial septal communication that can be to either chamber, usually the distal chamber.
- Pulmonary venous connection is usually normal

- Cor triatriatum dexter - Division of the morphologic right atrium (RA) is a consequence of persistent embryologic structures. If fenestrated, commonly referred to as a Chiari network.

3 Classification

I: Proximal chamber receives all pulmonary veins and communicates directly with distal chamber. This can be either with intact atrial septum (Fig. 1A), with an ASD (Fig. 1B) or with a decompressing levocardinal vein (Fig. 1C).

II: Proximal chamber receives all pulmonary veins but does not communicate directly with distal chamber. This falls into the spectrum of cardiac-type TAPVC (Fig. 1D and E).

III: Subtotal cor triatriatum (rare). A form of partial anomalous pulmonary venous connection in association with the cor triatriatum (Fig. 1F, G and H).

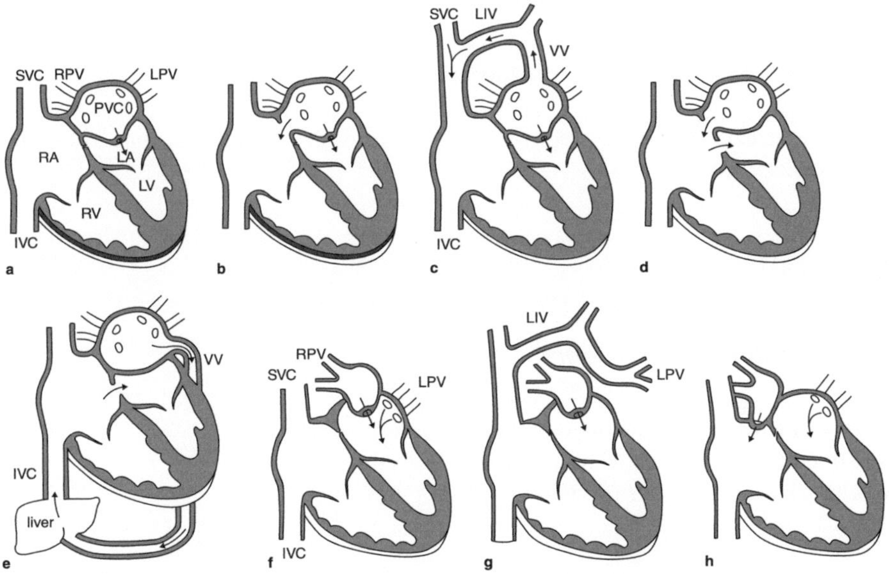

Fig. 1 Anatomic types of cor triatriatum sinister. A Classic cor triatriatum. B Direct communication between proximal and distal component with atrial septal defect. C Direct communication between proximal and distal component with decompressing levocardinal vein. D No direct communication between proximal and distal component with atrial septal defect. (Similar to cardiac-type TAPVC). E No direct communication between proximal and distal component (similar to infra-cardiac TAPVC). F Proximal chamber connected to left atrium. Partial pulmonary venous return to distal left atrial chamber. G Proximal chamber connected to left atrium. Partial pulmonary venous return to systemic venous component. H Proximal chamber connected to right atrium. Partial pulmonary venous return to distal left atrial chamber. *Reprinted from WK Health Book, 7th Edition, Shaddy RE, Penny DJ, Feltes TF* et al., *Moss and Adams Heart Disease in infants, children and adolescents, pp 788, 2021, with permission from Wolters Kluwer Health Inc*

4 Embryology

4.1 Cor Triatriatum Sinister

- Exact morphogenesis remains unclear.
- Different theories have been suggested:
  - Malincorporation (i.e., failed incorporation of common pulmonary vein into LA).
  - Entrapment (i.e., pulmonary veins prevented from incorporating into the LA by left sinus venosus; this could explain the higher occurrence of LSVC in patients with Cor triatriatum).
  - Malseptation (by abnormal growth of septum primum).

4.2 Cor Triatriatum Dexter

- Persistence of large valvar structures that guide oxygenated blood across the atrial septum.
- These structures usually regress and persist as the Eustachian and Thebesian valves.

5 Epidemiology

5.1 Incidence/Prevalence

- 0.4% of patients with congenital heart disease at autopsy.
- Found in less than 0.1% of congenital heart disease.
- Cor triatriatum dexter (division of RA) is very rare.

5.2 Population at Risk, Inheritance

- May be associated with other congenital cardiac lesions in up to 80% of pediatric cases.
- Roughly equivalent prevalence in males and females.

6 Clinical Physiology and Presentation

- Age and symptoms at diagnosis are highly variable and dependent on the degree of pulmonary venous obstruction as well as associated cardiac lesions.
  - Physiologic consequences directly related to degree of obstruction within the respective communicating pathways between proximal and distal chamber and atrial communication.
  - Significant obstruction can mimic mitral stenosis or TAPVC.
  - Obstruction leads to increased LA pressures and pulmonary congestion.
  - Dyspnea can range from mild to more severe.
- The most common presenting features in the pediatric population include pulmonary hypertension, respiratory complaints including tachypnea, congestive heart failure, failure to thrive, feeding intolerance, and cyanosis.
- Over 75% of patients are symptomatic, the remainder are referred because of incidental finding or after detection of a heart murmur.
- Adults are often asymptomatic because of an unrestrictive foramen with no pressure gradient between proximal and distal compartment.
  - Symptoms of exertional dyspnea, orthopnea, and hemoptysis can occur secondary to fibrosis or calcification of the accessory membrane.
  - Symptoms can also arise in high output states (i.e., pulmonary edema during labor).
- Patients may present with atrial arrhythmias or embolic events due to thrombus formation in an enlarged accessory chamber.

6.1 Natural History

- Highly dependent on the degree of obstruction in the pulmonary venous drainage pathway from proximal to distal chamber.
- If the communication between proximal and distal chamber is very small (< 3 mm) survival is limited to only few months without intervention. Survival remains severely limited for all restrictive lesions if not treated.

7 Associated Lesions

7.1 Common

- ASD
- PAPVC / TAPVC

- LSVC to LA
- Division of the RA is associated with pulmonary stenosis/atresia and tricuspid atresia.

8 Diagnostic Studies

8.1 *Auscultation*

- Diastolic murmur with a loud P2 when the patient has pulmonary hypertension.
- Murmur intensity varies with velocity of flow.
- The absence of an opening snap or loud S1 characterize the difference between a divided LA and mitral stenosis.

8.2 *ECG*

- Can often see features of RVH.
- Frontal mean QRS axis between $+120$ and $+140°$.
- May see broad P waves as a consequence of RA enlargement.

8.3 *CXR*

- Cardiomegaly, increased pulmonary vascularity, pulmonary edema.
- 'Staghorn' or 'butterfly wing' sign may be seen due to prominent venous engorgement of the upper pulmonary veins.
- Pulmonary artery hypertension may be reflected by a prominent pulmonary knob.

8.4 *Echocardiography*

- Delineate morphology of proximal and distal chamber and associated cardiac lesions
- Definition of communicating pathways between pulmonary veins, proximal and distal chamber, and right atrium.
- Assessment of trans-membrane pressure gradients via Doppler.
- Measurement of pulmonary artery pressures.
- Assessment of right ventricular function.

8.5 MRI

- Demonstrates detailed anatomy and abnormal pulmonary venous connections.
- Cine-MRI depicts fenestration within the membrane with associated flow turbulence.

8.6 CT

- May be helpful to delineate abnormal pulmonary venous drainage pathways.

8.7 Cardiac Catheterization

- Rarely used.
- Gradient between proximal and distal compartment estimated by elevated pulmonary artery wedge pressure and normal LV end-diastolic pressure.
- Angiography can show differential filling of the two distinct atrial chambers and respective connections.

9 Indications for Intervention/Surgery

- Primary treatment is surgical. Completely unrestrictive defects may not require any intervention.
- When patients with relatively unimpaired blood flow develop exertional dyspnea or signs of pulmonary congestion, diuretics and preload reduction are indicated.

10 Timing of Intervention and Management Strategy

- Patients who are symptomatic may need intervention on an urgent basis.
- Patients with insidious symptoms are operated electively.

11 Surgical Strategy

- In classic cor triatriatum sinister, resection of the dividing wall between proximal and distal compartment is performed on cardiopulmonary bypass with cardioplegic arrest. Having resected all the membrane, the atrial septum is reconstructed with a patch to ensure a widely open left atrium.

- Access is via the RA. Care has to be taken to identify landmarks as the anatomy can be deceiving.
- Surgical correction may include the ligation of a pulmonary-to-systemic venous pathway, correction of anomalous pulmonary venous drainage, or closure of an ASD.
- Surgical correction of cor triatriatum dexter aims at complete resection of the dividing membrane

12 Intensive Care Physiology and Management

- Postoperative course dependent on degree of preoperative obstruction.
- Most common immediate postoperative complications include prolonged ventilation, pulmonary hypertension, acute arrhythmia, and cardiac dysfunction.

13 Outcome

- Operative risk of death is < 5%. Death is uncommon after surgical repair and has been reported mostly in children who presented in critically ill condition, had complex associated anomalies, or after misdiagnosis.
- Life expectancy approximates that of the general population.
- Most patients are clinically asymptomatic at follow-up.
- Patients approach near-normal cardiac dimensions at follow-up.

14 Alternative Strategies and Controversies

- There are a few reports of balloon catheter dilation of the communication between proximal and distal compartment, but long-term outcomes have yet to be determined.

Bibliography

1. Alphonso N, Nørgaard M, Newcomb A, et al. Cor triatriatum: presentation, diagnosis and long-term surgical results. Ann Thorac Surg. 2005;80(5):1666–71.
2. Arrantz JE, Riopel DA, Catalano PW. Cor triatriatum: preoperative diagnosis and successful surgical correction in a ten-week old infant. Chest. 1973;63(6):1027–28.
3. Bharucha T, Spicer D, Mohun T, et al. Cor triatriatum or divided atriums: which approach provides the better understanding? Cardiol Young. 2015;25(2):193–207.

4. Jegier W, Gibbons JE, Wigglesworth FW. Cor triatriatum: Clinical, hemodynamic and pathological studies: surgical correction in early life. Pediatrics. 1963;31(2):255–267.
5. Rudienė V, Hjortshøj C, Glaveckaitė S, et al. Cor triatriatum sinistrum diagnosed in the adulthood: a systematic review. Heart. 2019;105(15):1197–202.

Total Anomalous Pulmonary Venous Connection

Rachel D. Vanderlaan and Andreea Dragulescu

Abstract Total anomalous pulmonary venous connection (TAPVC) encompasses a spectrum of lesions in which all the pulmonary veins are connected to the right atrium (RA) or its systemic venous tributaries. For survival a right-to-left shunt is required, and this is typically at the atrial level. Significant obstruction to pulmonary venous drainage results in pulmonary edema and cardiogenic shock which is lethal if untreated. Surgical results for the treatment of TAPVC have greatly improved over the last three decades, reducing operative mortality to less than 10%.

Keywords Total anomalous pulmonary venous connection (TAPVC) · Total anomalous pulmonary venous drainage (TAPVD) · Pulmonary veins · Vertical vein · Sutureless repair

Abbreviations

ASD	Atrial septal defect
AVSD	Atrioventricular septal defect
DORV	Double outlet right ventricle
ECMO	Extracorporeal membrane oxygenation
HLHS	Hypoplastic left heart syndrome
LA	Left atrium
LPA	Left pulmonary artery
LV	Left ventricle
PDA	Persistent ductus arteriosus

R. D. Vanderlaan (✉)
Division of Cardiovascular Surgery, Labatt Family Heart Centre, Hospital for Sick Children, Department of Surgery, University of Toronto, Toronto, ON, Canada
e-mail: Rachel.vanderlaan@sickkids.ca

A. Dragulescu
Division of Cardiology, Labatt Family Heart Centre, Hospital for Sick Children, Department of Paediatrics, University of Toronto, Toronto, ON, Canada
e-mail: Andreea.dragulescu@sickkids.ca

© The Author(s), under exclusive license to Springer Nature Switzerland AG 2024

A. I. Dipchand et al. (eds.), *Manual of Cardiac Care in Children*,
https://doi.org/10.1007/978-3-031-70973-9_18

PGE	Prostaglandin
PV	Pulmonary vein
RA	Right atrium
TAPVC	Total anomalous pulmonary venous connection
TGA	Transposition of the great arteries
TOF	Tetralogy of fallot
VSD	Ventricular septal defect

Key Points

- Total anomalous pulmonary venous connection (TAPVC) results in all pulmonary veins draining into the right side of the heart (RA or its venous tributaries)
- Right to left shunt is required—this is typically at the atrial level
- TAPVC can be an isolated lesion but can also occur with other complex congenital lesions such as AVSD, TGA, DORV and coarctation of the aorta. TAPVC can also occur in the setting of heterotaxy syndrome (see Chap. 35).
- Obstructed TAPVC requires urgent decompression - either emergent surgery, ECMO or vertical vein stenting
- Individual pulmonary veins may be hypoplastic or stenotic
- Post repair pulmonary vein stenosis occurs in 5–10% of all TAPVC and is associated with reinterventions and poor outcome

1 Nomenclature

- With isolated TAPVC the cardiac anatomy is Situs solitus, levocardia, atrioventricular connections and ventriculo-arterial connections are concordant, and the aortic arch is usually left sided. Systemic venous anatomy is normal.
- Description of pulmonary venous connection (location, size and presence of obstruction). Description of pulmonary veins.
- Associated cardiovascular anomalies can be present, so full segmental assessment is required.
- Anomalous pulmonary venous drainage is often present in isomeric lesions (Chap. 35)

2 Anatomy

- There are 4 main subgroups based on the level of connection of the anomalous veins (Fig. 1):

1. Supracardiac (50%)—The common vein connects to central venous structures above the heart, most commonly the innominate vein or superior vena cava
2. Infracardiac (20%)—The common vein connects to central venous structures below the heart, most commonly the inferior vena cava or the portal venous system. All TAPVC to portal vein are physiologically obstructed.
3. Cardiac (20%)—The common vein connects to cardiac structures (i.e., RA or coronary sinus)
4. Mixed (10%)—The veins connect in a combination of ways (example: 2 veins draining to RA, 2 veins draining to innominate vein).

- The presence or absence of obstruction should be noted with the nature and level of obstruction detailed.
- Common source of obstruction:
  - Supracardiac—Anatomic vice (level of left main bronchus, LPA, aorta), insertion into innominate vein
  - Infracardiac—crossing diaphragm, insertion into portal vein or hepatic vein
- A right to left shunt is required and this is typically an interatrial communication—restrictive ASDs and associated gradient should be noted

3 Embryology

- In the initial stages of developments, the primitive lung drains via the splanchnic venous plexus into the cardinal and umbilical veins.
- The connexion of a lumenized common pulmonary vein (PV) then connects to the LA and to the lung plexus, followed by a regression of the connections between the common PV and the systemic veins through a remodelling process.
- The persistence of these connections is the likely substrate of anomalous extracardiac PV drainage, probably related to the abnormal developments of the common PV, while cardiac anomalous PV drainage seem to result from absent or impaired mesenchymal contribution to atrial septation.

4 Epidemiology

- TAPVC accounts for 1–2% of all congenital heart disease
- There is a male preponderance for infracardiac TAPVC
- Familial inheritance has been documented and it is also associated with syndromes such as cat eye syndrome, heterotaxy and Holt-Oram.

5 Clinical Physiology and Presentation

- The clinical presentation of TAPVC depends on two critical elements:
  - Degree of obstruction to the pulmonary venous drainage
  - Degree of obstruction to the compensatory right-to-left shunt
- Obstructive TAPVC present with profound cyanosis, respiratory distress, and hemodynamic collapse requiring intubation with positive pressure ventilation and 100% oxygen immediately after birth.
- PGE may preserve cardiac output but pulmonary complications of obstructed venous return and can lead to worsening cyanosis.
- Severe obstruction with impaired cardiac output, or oxygenation/ventilation failure may require emergency ECMO prior to surgical repair.
- Unobstructed TAPVC with good atrial mixing can present hemodynamically stable with mild cyanosis and signs of heart failure in which case surgical repair may be deferred for several weeks.

6 Associated Lesions

- Smaller left sided cardiac chambers (LA and LV) are common but can usually support a biventricular circulation
- The majority of TAPVC have an adequate ASD, with a small proportion of patients have associated VSD or PDA as their shunt lesion
- More complex associated congenital heart disease have been described, such as heterotaxy (more commonly right atrial isomerism), HLHS, TOF, DORV.

7 Diagnostic Studies

7.1 CXR

- Obstructed TAPVC present with a reticular pattern and extensive pulmonary edema
- 'Snowman sign' (widened upper mediastinum) can be seen in older infants with supracardiac TAPVC

7.2 Echocardiography

- Echocardiography remains the main imaging modality for diagnosis
- Anatomical delineation of the individual veins, the confluence and vertical vein

- Presence, location, and degree of obstruction
- Atrial communication, size, flow
- Signs of pulmonary hypertension: septal position, tricuspid regurgitation jet for right ventricular systolic pressure, PDA shunt direction
- Ventricular function
- Associated lesions

7.3 MRA/CTA

- Delineate pulmonary vein anatomy and level of obstruction, especially with mixed TAPVC

8 Indications and Timing for Intervention/Surgery

- Surgical correction and timing are dictated by degree of obstruction

8.1 Obstructed TAPVC

- Requires urgent surgical correction or vertical vein stenting as a bridge to surgery
- May require stabilization on ECMO prior to surgical/interventional management
- Relief of obstruction by vertical vein stenting can be done as bridge to surgery if cardiopulmonary bypass contraindicated and optimizing end organ dysfunction is required.

8.2 Unobstructed TAPVC

- Elective surgical correction typically by 4–6 weeks of life
- May require medical management of heart failure symptoms due to high degree of left to right shunt

9 Management Strategy

9.1 Surgical Strategy

- Repair requires cardiopulmonary bypass with cooling to 28–32 degrees can be done if repair strategy requires low flow (cooled to 18 degrees if circulatory arrest is required)
- For supracardiac or infracardiac TAPVC, direct anastomosis of the confluence to LA (conventional technique) or using the 'sutureless technique' by creating a pericardial well and attaching the parietal pericardium to the opened-out LA.
- Sutureless technique may decrease rates of post repair pulmonary vein stenosis (Fig. 2)
- Cardiac TAPVC requires unroofing of the coronary sinus (incising into the anterior wall) and patch closure to septate the atrium.
- Vertical Vein ligation is recommended to encourage blood flow into the pulmonary vein confluence. Vertical vein can be left open resulting in a small left to right shunt that typically closes on it own or may require device closure if significant residual shunt.

9.2 Catheter-Based Interventions

- Balloon dilation with/without stenting of vertical vein stenosis can be considered in setting of extremis to allow for hemodynamic and lung recovery prior to corrective bypass surgery
- Common areas include anatomic vice or vertical vein insertion to innominate vein/SVC in supracardiac lesions or at level of diaphragm or insertion to hepatic vein/IVC in infracardiac lesions

10 Intensive Care Physiology and Management

- If unobstructed, patients are typically extubated within the first 24 h after surgery
- Obstructed TAPVC usually require prolonged intubation following repair
- Pulmonary hypertension can be seen in all types of TAPVC with increased incidence in those that were obstructed, and is treated with oxygen therapy and inhaled nitric oxide in the early postoperative period
- Low cardiac output due to small, non-compliant left sided structures may prolong stay in ICU but is self-resolving. LA pressure line can be used to help monitor and manage a non-compliant LV.
- Arrhythmia, particularly supraventricular arrhythmias, can occur in 5–10% of TAPVC

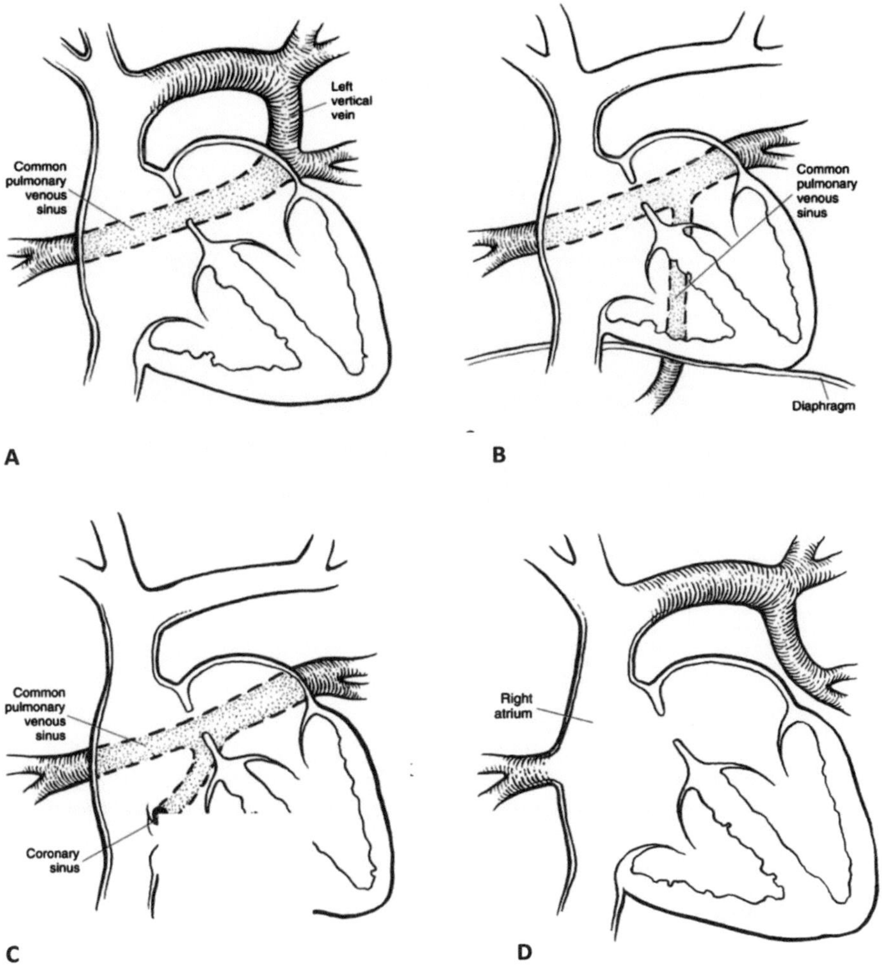

Fig. 1 Types of TAPVC. A) Supracardiac, B) Infracardiac, C) Cardiac, D) Mixed. *Reprinted from Kirklin-Barratt-Boyes-Cardiac-Surgery, 4th Edition, Morphology, diagnostic criteria, natural history, techniques, results and indications, Total anomalous pulmonary venous connection, Kirklin JW, Kouchoukos NT, 2013, with permission from Elsevier*

- Stenosis of anastomosis or individual veins can occur early and must be investigated if suspected

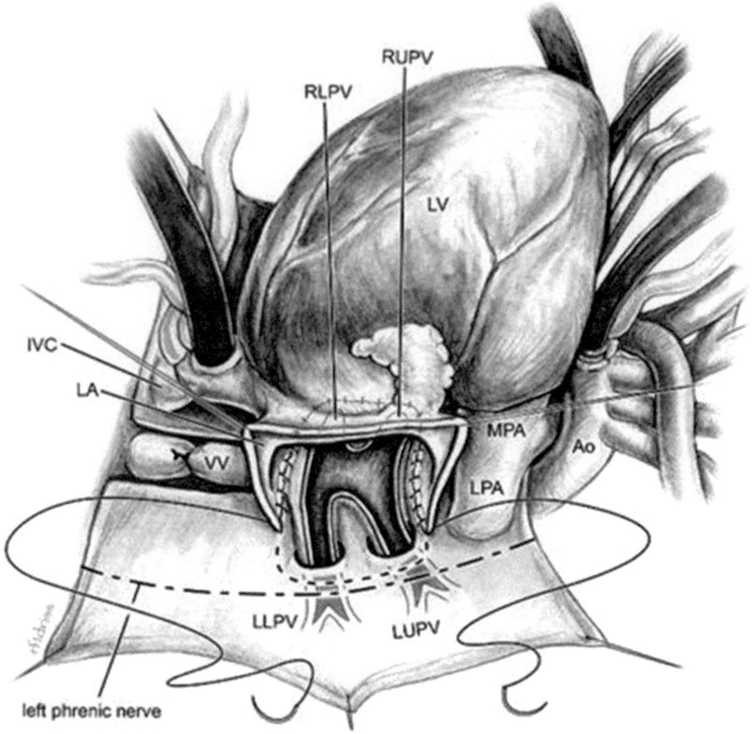

Fig. 2 Sutureless repair in infracardiac TAPVC. *Reprinted from* ***Pediatric Cardiac Surgery*** *5th Edition, Constantine* ***Mavroudis and Carl L Backer, pp 781, 2023, with permission from John Wiley and Sons***

11 Outcomes

11.1 Mortality

- Survival has improved with a 5-year survival of approximately 95%
- Obstructed TAPVC have a 5-year survival of approximately 86%
- Worse survival for high-risk groups with single ventricle physiology or heterotaxy.

11.2 Morbidity

- Major morbidity occurs in approximately 5–15% after TAPVC repair
- Reintervention due to stenosis at the anastomotic site or in the individual veins occurs in around 10% of cases. This can be addressed either surgically (typically sutureless technique) or with cath based procedures (angioplasty vs drug

eluting stent). In difficult cases, intraoperative stent deployment can be done. (See Chap. 19)

- Atrial arrhythmias and sinus node dysfunction can also contribute to morbidity.

Bibliography

1. Bleyl S, Ruttenberg HD, Carey JC, et al. Familial total anomalous pulmonary venous return: a large Utah-Idaho family. Am J Med Genet. 1994;52(4):462–6.
2. Chaturvedi K, Deshmukh A, Thakur P, et al (2022) Palliative vertical vein stenting in a critical neonate with obstructed infradiaphragmatic total anomalous pulmonary venous connection. Cardiol Young. 2:1–2. Epub ahead of print.
3. Douglas YL, Jongbloed MR, Deruiter MC, et al. Normal and abnormal development of pulmonary veins: state of the art and correlation with clinical entities. Int J Cardiol. 2011;147(1):13–24.
4. Karamlou T, Gurofsky R, Al Sukhni E, et al. Factors associated with mortality and reoperation in 377 children with total anomalous pulmonary venous connection. Circulation. 2007;115(12):1591–8.
5. Shi G, Zhu Z, Chen J, Ou Y, Hong H, Nie Z, Zhang H, Liu X, Zheng J, Sun Q, Liu J, Chen H, Zhuang J, et al. Total anomalous pulmonary venous connection: the current management strategies in a pediatric cohort of 768 patients. Circulation. 2017;135(1):48–58.
6. Spigel ZA, Edmunds EE, Caldarone CA, et al. Total anomalous pulmonary venous connection: influence of heterotaxy and venous obstruction on outcomes. J Thorac Cardiovasc Surg. 2022;163(2):387-395.e3.

Pulmonary Vein Stenosis

Rachel D. Vanderlaan and Andreea Dragulescu

Abstract Pulmonary vein stenosis (PVS) is a rare disease associated with high mortality. Clinically, it can be broadly categorized into primary PVS or post repair PVS. While children can present with variable involvement of pulmonary veins, children with 2 or more stenotic veins or bilateral PVS typically have a poor prognosis. Children with progressive disease develop secondary pulmonary hypertension and subsequent right heart failure. Prematurity is a non-modifiable risk factor associated with PVS. Multidisciplinary approach to treat disease includes surgery and catheter-based interventions (balloon angioplasty, stents). Experimental medications (Imatinib, sirolimus, losartan) have been used at some centers as adjuncts. 1 year survival is approximately 60% for children with progressive multivessel disease).

Keywords Pulmonary Vein Stenosis (PVS) · Right heart failure · Pulmonary hypertension · Primary PVS · Post-repair PVS

Abbreviations

ASD	Atrial septal defect
AVSD	Atrioventricular septal defect
LA	Left atrium
PDA	Persistent ductus arteriosus
PVS	Pulmonary vein stenosis
RVH	Right ventricular hypertrophy
RVSP	Right ventricular systolic pressure

R. D. Vanderlaan
Division of Cardiovascular Surgery, Labatt Family Heart Centre, Hospital for Sick Children, Department of Surgery, University of Toronto, Toronto, ON, Canada
e-mail: Rachel.vanderlaan@sickkids.ca

A. Dragulescu (✉)
Division of Cardiology, Labatt Family Heart Centre, Hospital for Sick Children, Department of Paediatrics, University of Toronto, Toronto, ON, Canada
e-mail: Andreea.dragulescu@sickkids.ca

© The Author(s), under exclusive license to Springer Nature Switzerland AG 2024

A. I. Dipchand et al. (eds.), *Manual of Cardiac Care in Children*,
https://doi.org/10.1007/978-3-031-70973-9_19

TAPVC	Total anomalous pulmonary venous connection
VSD	Ventricular septal defect

Key Points

- Progressive multivessel pulmonary vein stenosis (PVS) is associated with high mortality due to pulmonary hypertension and right heart failure
- Distinct subpopulations: primary (congenital) PVS and post repair PVS
- Clinical spectrum of disease: variable number of veins affected and location of stenosis
- Intrapulmonary flow redistribution transfers flow from obstructed pulmonary segments to segments with less obstruction. Consequently, echocardiography-derived indices of obstruction (flow gradients) may underestimate progression of disease in obstructed pulmonary veins.
- Multi-disciplinary approach to treatment involving cardiac surgery, interventional cardiology, Imaging and echocardiography specialists, lung transplant and palliative care teams

1 Nomenclature

- Cardiac anatomy in primary (congenital) PVS is typically situs solitus, levocardia, atrioventricular and ventriculoarterial concordance.
- Pulmonary veins have normal connection to the LA with focal stenosis, diffuse stenosis or atretic pulmonary vein(s).
- In post repair PVS, anomalous drainage of the pulmonary veins has been corrected and the pulmonary vein confluence drains into the LA. Patients can also have associated congenital heart disease (left to right shunts or complex congenital lesions).

2 Anatomy

- PVS is diagnosed when there is a narrowing or blockage in one or more pulmonary veins (Fig. 1).

- The stenosis impedes returning blood flow from the affected lung segment.
- The intraluminal stenosis is caused by hypercellular neointimal lesions made up of myofibroblast-like cells and deposition of extracellular matrix.

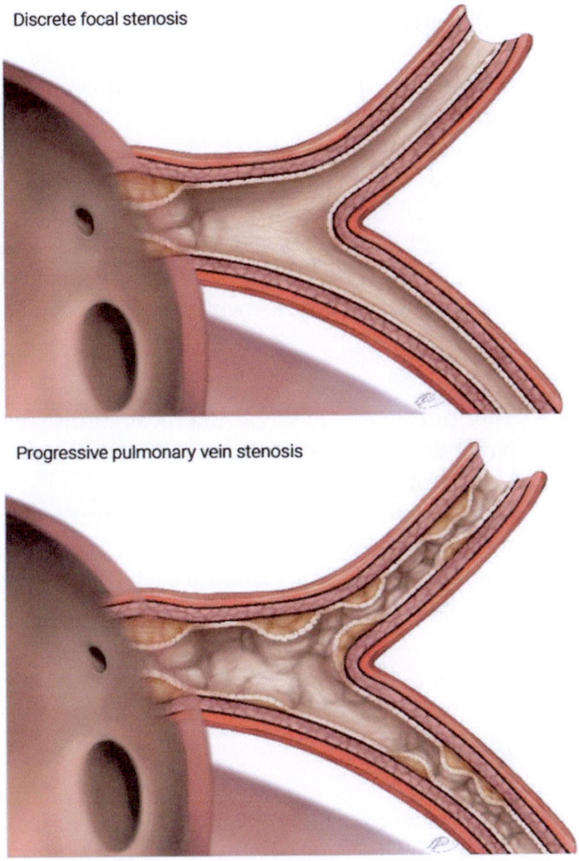

Fig. 1 Progressive pulmonary vein stenosis

2.1 *Classification of Pulmonary Vein Stenosis*

2.1.1 *Primary (Congenital) PVS*

- Disease occurs in pulmonary veins that are normally connected to the LA and occurs without any previous intervention on the veins themselves.
- It can be associated with simple (left to right shunts) or complex congenital heart disease
- Ex-premature infants are increasingly recognized as an important sub-category with important lung pathology such as bronchopulmonary dysplasia and pulmonary arterial hypertension

2.1.2 *Post-Repair PVS*

- Disease occurs in pulmonary veins following repair of anomalous pulmonary venous return.
- This occurs in approximately 5–15% of total anomalous pulmonary venous connection (TAPVC) repairs with the highest risk being within 6 months of repair.
- Risk factors for post-repair PVS include preoperative pulmonary vein obstruction, a small pulmonary venous confluence, younger age, mixed type TAPVC, infracardiac TAPVC, and intraoperative residual stenosis after initial repair
- Disease presentation varies with:
  - Location of stenosis: Veno-atrial junction, intraparenchymal distal pulmonary veins
  - Type of stenosis: Discrete and focal, diffuse hypoplasia, atretic or occluded
  - Number of pulmonary veins involved: Single to multiple vein involvement, Unilateral vs bilateral
  - Age at presentation: Neonatal or younger age infants have worse prognosis
  - Associated congenital heart disease or anomalous pulmonary vein anatomy
  - Associated pulmonary disease such as lymphangiectasis, scimitar syndrome, bronchopulmonary dysplasia.

3 Epidemiology

- Occurs in approximately 1.7/100,000 live births and constitutes ~ 0.5% of all congenital cardiac defects.
- The incidence of post repair PVS is approximately 5–15% following primary repair of TAPVC.
- To date there is no genetic predisposition associated with PVS
- Approximately 20–30% of children with PVS have a genetic syndrome, such as trisomy 21, CHARGE syndrome, VACTERL and others.

4 Clinical Physiology and Presentation

- Progression can be silent
- Narrowing of one or more of the pulmonary veins leads to flow redistribution away from the segment of high pressure. Persistent pulmonary venous hypertension can lead to elevated pulmonary vascular resistance and subsequent right heart failure.
- Infants can present with failure to thrive, tachypnea and signs of right heart failure.
- Recurrent infections and hemoptysis can lead to frequent hospital admissions and complications.

- Children with progressive disease present with secondary pulmonary hypertension and right heart failure.

5 Natural History

- The natural history of PVS is dictated by the number of veins involved and associated comorbidities in the heart or lungs.
  - Children with one vein involvement can typically compensate and will be asymptomatic.
  - PVS limited to involvement of a single pulmonary vein can progress to involvement of ipsilateral and/or contralateral pulmonary veins.
  - Bilateral disease involvement is associated with poor outcome. Unilateral involvement can lead to a functional single lung physiology.
  - If left untreated, children with involvement of most or all veins will die within 1–2 years following diagnosis due to right heart failure.
- Morbidity associated with PVS include infections, pleural effusions, and hemoptysis.

6 Associated Lesions

- Simple cardiac lesions associated with PVS include ASD, VSD or PDA
- Complex cardiac lesions associated with PVS include AVSD, TAPVC, heterotaxy, and univentricular circulations.
- Children born premature can have associated bronchopulmonary dysplasia and pulmonary arterial hypertension.
- Children can have extracardiac defects associated with underlying genetic syndromes

7 Diagnostic Studies

7.1 ECG

- Evidence of RVH.

7.2 CXR

- May show cardiomegaly, enlarged main pulmonary artery, increased pulmonary vascular markings and pulmonary edema in severe cases.

7.3 Echocardiography

- Size of proximal pulmonary veins and doppler gradients of proximal pulmonary veins
  - Flow redistribution to unaffected lung segments may lead to underestimation of the pulmonary vein gradients
- Important to assess for signs of pulmonary hypertension and right heart failure: RVSP, flow in the pulmonary arteries, RV function and size, and septal motion.
- Presence of anomalous pulmonary venous drainage or aorto-pulmonary collaterals
- Presence of shunts (PDA, ASD, VSD)
- Presence of associated congenital heart lesions

7.4 Computed Tomography Angiography (CTA)

- Excellent anatomical resolution of the pulmonary veins
- First choice for cross-sectional imaging
- Can be done without sedation (an important consideration in high-risk patients)

7.5 Magnetic Resonance Angiography (MRA)

- Good resolution of anatomy of the pulmonary veins
- Important functional measurements, such as blood flow and pattern in pulmonary veins and arteries
- Estimates of RV fibrosis with extracellular volume measurements
- Requires sedation which can be associated with increased risk

7.6 Cardiac Catheterization

- Typically used for intervention but can be diagnostic modality of choice if potential for balloon angioplasty or stenting
- Higher risk invasive procedure which requires sedation

- Determination of pulmonary artery pressures

8 Indications for Intervention/Surgery

- No consensus guidelines/indications exist amongst institutions

8.1 *Clinically Significant PVS*

- Moderate to severe echocardiography doppler gradients (mean gradient > 6 mmHg, in the absence of flow redistribution)
- Elevated right sided pressures (RVSP $\geq$ 1/2 systemic)
- CTA or MRA demonstrating anatomically significant narrowing with MRA also demonstrating decreased and abnormal flow patterns

8.2 *General Surgical Indications for PVS*

- Stenosis involving $\geq$ 2 pulmonary veins (or functional equivalent common pulmonary vein)
  - Proximal disease that is located near the veno-atrial junction
  - Presence of moderate to severe stenosis with good size upstream pulmonary vein diameter
- Stenosis involving 1 pulmonary vein
  - Undergoing cardiac surgery for other reasons

8.3 *General Catheter-Based Intervention Indications for PVS*

- Clinically significant pulmonary vein stenosis
- It can be a stand-alone therapy or adjunct to surgery by reaching peripheral lesions not amenable to surgery
- Consider when important comorbidities limit candidacy for surgical interventions

8.4 *Lung Transplantation*

- Disease not responsive to medical and surgical/intervention management.

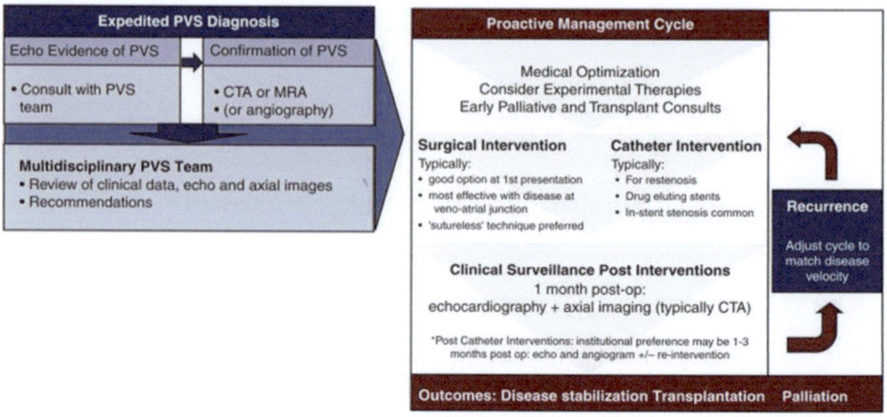

Fig. 2 SickKids algorithm for multidisciplinary team decision making for pulmonary vein stenosis patients

- Patients typically have diffuse disease with small intraparenchymal pulmonary veins

9 Timing of Intervention and Management Strategy

- If single pulmonary vein stenosis usually they are asymptomatic and can be managed expectantly.
- Infants and young children with suprasystemic or systemic right sided pressures with decreased RV function require urgent interventions and may require temporizing measures such as catheter-based interventions or mechanical pulmonary support (ECMO or PA-LA oxygenator (e.g. Novalung) to stabilize.
- Infants with new diagnosis of PVS are reviewed by the PVS Multidisciplinary team to ensure best intervention based on anatomy and clinical presentation (Fig. 2)

10 Surgical Strategy

10.1 Sutureless Repair Technique (Fig. 3)

- Preferred surgical technique for post repair and primary PVS.
- Minimizes intimal injury and anatomical distortion at the venoatrial junction therefore decreased turbulence which may be stimulus to drive further PVS
- Anatomical approach may be indicated in some cases involving extensive resection and patching of the pulmonary veins

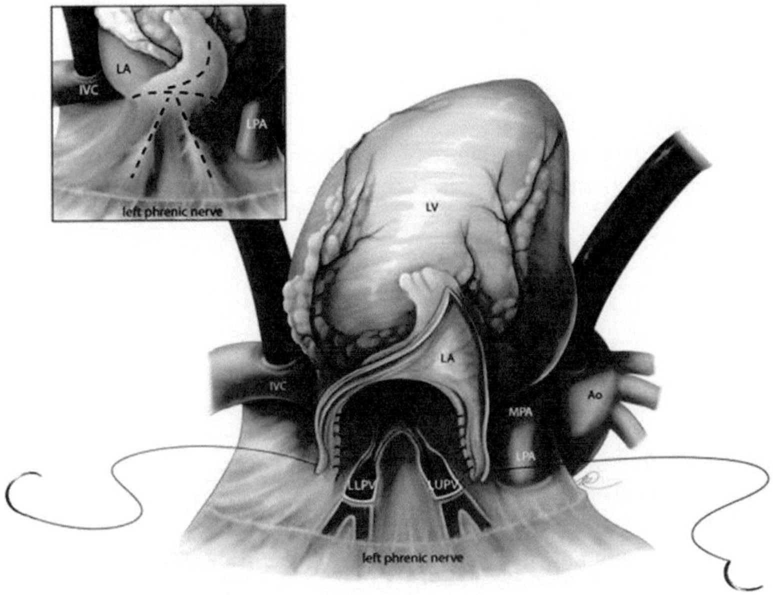

Fig. 3 Sutureless technique for pulmonary vein stenosis

- Rare complications of the sutureless repair include extra pleural hemorrhage, embolism, bronchopulmonary fistula

10.2 Interventional Strategy

- Choice of balloon angioplasty vs stent placement is driven by anatomy of the pulmonary veins and the need for future interventions.
- Balloon angioplasty is useful in small diameter pulmonary veins and veins with multiple branches.
- Drug eluting stents have a small increased freedom from reintervention compared to bare metal stents.
- In-stent restenosis is a significant problem and is a separate disease process than native pulmonary vein stenosis. In-stent restenosis may require subsequent balloon dilations
- Intra-op stenting in combination with surgical approach can be effective in management of multivessel disease

11 Intensive Care Physiology and Management

- Supporting RV function and sequelae of RV failure is goal of preoperative management
- Postoperative management focuses on pulmonary vascular reactivity with risk of pulmonary hypertension crisis (ventilation, sedation, pulmonary vasodilator therapy)
- Lung pathology can be a significant comorbidity in the ex-premature infant or post-repair PVS patients who initially presented as obstructed TAPVC.

12 Outcome

- Current operative mortality 1% for primary and post repair PVS.
- For multivessel progressive PVS, 1 year survival is approximately 60%.
- Re-stenosis and reintervention is common in progressive PVS.
- Contemporary outcomes in North America through the PVS Network Registry will help overcome limitations of single center reports (www.PVSNetwork.org)

13 Alternative Strategies and Controversies

13.1 Experimental Therapies

- Currently there is no randomized control trial that addresses the efficacy of experimental and antiproliferative therapies in PVS (Sirolimus, Imatinib, losartan). Single center reports report some improvement in outcomes, but larger studies are needed to truly evaluate efficacy.
- Use of pulmonary hypertension medications is controversial due to potential pulmonary edema, particularly in pulmonary-veno occlusive disease. Many centers in North America report using pulmonary hypertension medications such as sildenafil; however, benefit of these agents in pulmonary vein stenosis remains undetermined.

Bibliography

1. Aras MA, Psotka MA, De Marco T. Pulmonary hypertension due to left heart disease: an update. Curr Cardiol Rep. 2019;21(7):62. https://doi.org/10.1007/s11886-019-1149-1.
2. Frank DB, Levy PT, Stiver CA, et al. Primary pulmonary vein stenosis during infancy: state of the art review. J Perinatol. 2021;41(7):1528–39. https://doi.org/10.1038/s41372-021-01008-7.

3. Quinonez LG, Gauvreau K, Borisuk M, et al. Outcomes of surgery for young children with multivessel pulmonary vein stenosis. J Thorac Cardiovasc Surg. 2015;150(4):911–7. https://doi.org/10.1016/j.jtcvs.2015.06.050.
4. Vanderlaan RD, Rome J, Hirsch R, et al. Pulmonary vein stenosis: treatment and challenges. J Thorac Cardiovasc Surg. 2021;161(6):2169–76. https://doi.org/10.1016/j.jtcvs.2020.05.117.

Transposition of the Great Arteries (TGA)

Colm Breatnach and Alejandro A. Floh

Abstract Transposition of the great arteries (TGA) is the most common *neonatal* cyanotic congenital cardiac lesion. The parallel and separate circulations require the presence of an intracardiac lesion to ensure mixing and adequate systemic oxygenation, which is promoted by PDA flow to increase left atrial pressure. Associated lesions may include different coronary artery patterns, ventricular septal defect, pulmonary tract obstruction, and arch obstruction. Fetal diagnosis allows for co-ordination of delivery at or in close proximity to a cardiac intensive care unit with access to interventional cardiology. Severe postnatal hypoxemia necessitates immediate evaluation for a balloon atrial septostomy. Surgical correction of TGA with intact ventricular septum with an arterial switch operation (ASO) typically occurs within the first 10 days of life. Timing of repair of TGA with VSD depends on size and number of VSD and associated lesions; simple VSD is managed similar to TGA/IVS but complex TGA may need a staged approach. The ASO for TGA with intact ventricular septum has > 98% survival and excellent long-term outcomes; excellent outcomes are also seen for TGA with isolated VSD surgery. Increased risk is encountered with coronary artery anomalies. Treatment of TGA/VSD with additional lesions are contingent on underlying anatomy and residual lesions. TGA/VSD with obstruction to systemic outflow requires early corrective surgery or palliation. Repair of TGA/VSD with pulmonary stenosis are generally deferred for several months to decrease risk for a Rastelli or Nakaidoh operation.

Keywords Transposition of the great arteries · Arterial switch procedure · Left ventricular outflow tract obstruction · Lecompte procedure · Rastelli · REV · Nikaidoh

C. Breatnach
Children's Health Ireland at Crumlin, Dublin, Ireland
e-mail: Colm.breatnach@olchc.ie

A. A. Floh (✉)
Department of Critical Care Medicine, Division of Cardiac Critical Care Unit, Labatt Family Heart Centre, The Hospital for Sick Children, Toronto, ON, Canada
e-mail: alejandro.floh@sickkids.ca

© The Author(s), under exclusive license to Springer Nature Switzerland AG 2024
A. I. Dipchand et al. (eds.), *Manual of Cardiac Care in Children*,
https://doi.org/10.1007/978-3-031-70973-9_20

Abbreviations

ASD	Atrial septal defect
ASO	Arterial switch operation
AV	Atrioventricular
BAS	Balloon atrial septostomy
Cx	Circumflex
iNO	Inhaled nitric oxide
LV	Left ventricle
LVOT	Left ventricular outflow tract
LVOTO	Left ventricular outflow tract obstruction
MPA	Main pulmonary artery
PA	Pulmonary artery
PDA	Persistent ductus arteriosus
PFO	Persistent foramen ovale
PS	Pulmonary stenosis
REV	Reparation à l'étage ventriculaire
RV	Right ventricle
RVH	Right ventricular hypertrophy
RVOT	Right ventricular outflow tract
TGA	Transposition of the great arteries
TGA/IVS	Transposition of the great arteries/intact ventricular septum
TGA/VSD	Transposition of the great arteries/ventricular septal defect
VA	Ventriculo-arterial
VSD	Ventricular septal defect

Key Points

- Transposition of the great arteries (TGA) refers to a lesion in which there is atrioventricular (AV) concordance and ventricular-arterial (VA) discordance, such that the aorta originates from the right ventricle (RV) and the pulmonary artery connects to the left ventricle (LV) creating a non-mixing circulation in parallel.
- This lesion is often referred to d-TGA (Van Praagh) as it results from dextro looping of the great vessels during fetal development that result in the aorta being anterior and rightward to the pulmonary artery.
- Without the presence of an intracardiac shunt at birth (an unrestrictive ASD or VSD) extreme cyanosis occurs and cerebral ischemia rapidly evolves.
- The most common co-existing lesions include VSD with or without outflow tract stenosis. This has a major influence on presenting physiology, surgical planning, and outcomes.

- Coronary artery anatomy is carefully evaluated with pre-operative echocardiography as certain variations make surgical repair technically challenging and are associated with worse outcomes.
- Repair is typically performed with an ASO in the neonatal period although it may be delayed in the presence of an VSD and associated lesions.
- For complex forms of TGA may require alternative procedures as initial palliation or definitve repair.

1 Nomenclature

- Generally, situs solitus, levocardia, AV concordance and VA discordance, left aortic arch

2 Anatomy

- Isolated VA discordance occurs in 60% of patients with TGA.
- The aorta most commonly arises anterior and rightward of the pulmonary artery, although other orientations of the great vessels may occur (eg anterior–posterior, side by side).
- Several variations of coronary artery branching patterns exist (Fig. 1) with most common configuration of left anterior descending and circumflex originating in leftward sinus (1L,Cx) and right coronary artery from posterior rightward sinus (2R)
- VSDs are present in the other 40% of patients with TGA
- In patients with VSD, septal malalignment and outflow tract obstruction can occur; deviation of outflow septum typically occurs posteriorly into the LV resulting in pulmonary valve stenosis.

3 Embryology

- The cause of abnormal looping of the great vessels are not incompletely understood
- Normal heart: the cono-truncal region spirals and the right conal tissue is absorbed leaving VA concordance
- In TGA: there is absence of spiraling of the primitive truncus arteriosus leading to maldevelopment of the conus either with abnormal resorption or differential rates of conal growth (Van Praagh).
- Deviation of outlet septum may interfere with antegrade flow leading to underdevelopment of corresponding outflow tract and vessels (e.g., anterior-cranial deviation leads to hypoplastic ascending aorta, arch, and coarctation)

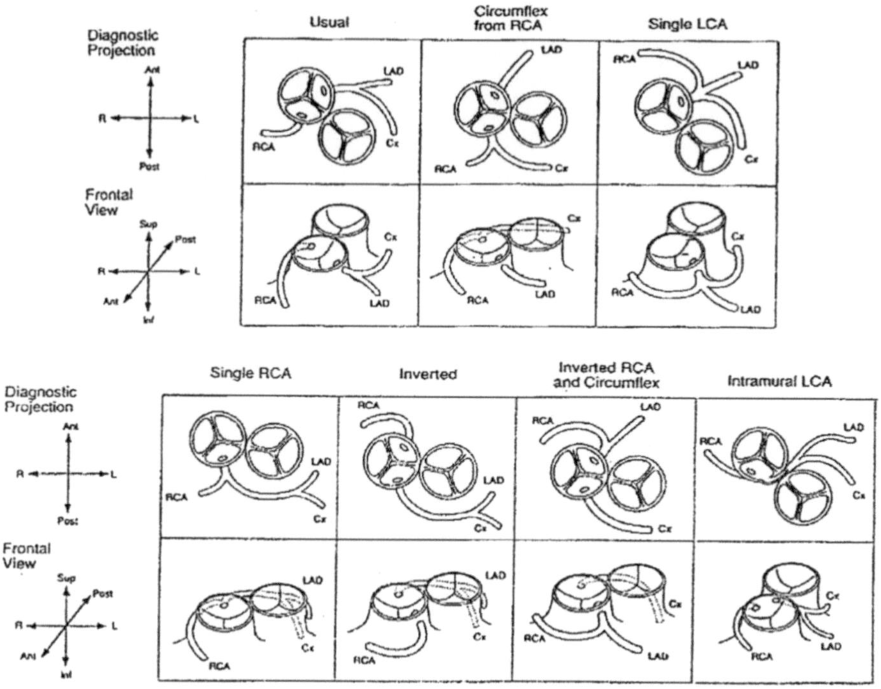

Fig. 1 Variations of coronary arteries in TGA. 1L/Cx2R is most common (top, left panel), followed by 1L2R, Cx (top, middle panel). *Reprinted from Coronary Artery Disease, Vol 4, Issue 2, Wernovsky G, Sanders S, Coronary artery anatomy and transposition of the great arteries, pp 148–151, 1993, with permission from Wolters Kluwer Health, Inc*

4 Epidemiology

- Most common cyanotic heart disease presenting in the newborn period, affecting 1 in 4000 live births
- 5–7% of congenital cardiac defects
- Male to female ratio of 2:1
- Extra cardiac abnormalities present in up to 10% of patients–risk factors include poorly controlled maternal diabetes, and alcohol, smoking, and maternal use of anti-convulsants in pregnancy.

5 Clinical Physiology and Presentation

- **Non-mixing lesion**: Rather than a normal "in series" circulation, oxygenated blood returns to lungs and desaturated blood pumped to systemic circulation.

- Oxygenation of systemic circulation only by “mixing” through septal defects across atria (ASD/PFO) and/or ventricles (VSD).
- Degree of mixing and systemic oxygenation is proportionate to size of septal defects
- PDA will promote mixing by raising left atrial pressure
- TGA/IVS is a high pulmonary blood flow lesion
- Reverse differential oxygen saturations (lower preductal versus postductal systemic saturations) are seen in presence of pulmonary hypertension or, less likely, coarctation of the aorta.

6 Natural History

- Cerebral hypoxemia occurs due to desaturated venous blood streaming from the superior vena cava into the RV which then ejects into the aorta and cerebral vessels.
- Fetal MRI has demonstrated a reduced forebrain volume
- Without surgical repair, mortality from TGA is 90% within the first year of life, often early after birth.
- Early stabilization achieved with a balloon atrial septostomy to improve atrial mixing
- The ASO that reconnects the PA to the RV and the aorta and coronary buttons to the LV is completed within the first week of life.
- Delay of ASO beyond 4–6 weeks of age associate with LV deconditioning and increased postoperative morbidity

7 Associated Lesions

- TGA with intact ventricular septum (TGA/IVS; simple TGA) account for 60% of cases
- Different coronary artery patterns (not 1 LCx/2R) occur in up to 40%—increased risk with side-by-side arrangement of great vessels
- Intramural coronary arteries seen in 2–5% of cases
- VSD is present in 40% which may occur with systemic (ascending aorta/arch/ coarctation) or pulmonary outflow tract obstruction – 15–25% pulmonary stenosis
- Coarctation of the aorta has been described in up to 5–10%

7.1 Taussig-Bing

- See Chap. 5 (Double outlet right ventricle)
- Refers to TGA, subpulmonic VSD, often with side-by-side arrangement of vessels and associated obstruction to aorta and arch

8 Diagnostic Studies

8.1 ECG

- Often normal but may show signs of right axis deviation and RVH.

8.2 CXR

- Typical description of an egg on a string may be seen due to a narrowed mediastinum.

8.3 ECHO

- Diagnostic modality of choice
- Confirms diagnosis with sequential anatomy and demonstrating parallel great vessel origins with ductal flow into the LVOT
- Aorta usually anterior and rightward to pulmonary valve but great vessels arrangements may vary
- Evaluates coronary artery anatomy—The presence of a single coronary ostium or intramural coronary artery is associated with worse prognosis
- Identifies additional lesions

8.4 CT

- Rarely employed to clarify coronary artery anatomy or other vascular concerns

9 Preoperative Management

- Antenatal diagnosis is optimal from a care perspective to ensure that delivery occurs at an appropriate institution with rapid access to interventional cardiology.
- Neonatal team should be prepared for severe hypoxemic if ventricular septum intact.
- Fetal determination of the degree of atrial septum restriction is challenging and not always reliable.
- Early IV access should be obtained after birth and PGE infusion instituted
- Balloon atrial septostomy (BAS) is indicated if severe (< 70%) systemic desaturation

- BAS is vital if atrial septum intact/restrictive—through umbilical or femoral access and care taken to avoid injury or stroke
- BAS indicated for delayed repair, even with adequate saturations, to lower left atrial pressure
- Fluid boluses, systemic vasoconstriction, and treating anemia can be trialed if desaturated despite open PDA (while mobilizing for BAS)
- Severe pulmonary hypertension may also occur (reverse cyanosis) and treated with adequate ventilation and vasodilation (iNO).

10 Indications for Intervention/Surgery

- Surgical repair is performed in all patients with TGA/IVS without contraindications.
- Late presentation may require 2-stage correction: first to retrain the LV prior to a definitive ASO.

11 Timing of Intervention and Management Strategy

- TGA/IVS is generally corrected within the first week of life
- Prior to surgery circulation may be unstable if open PDA with a rare risk systemic hypoperfusion
- If surgical repair is performed beyond 5–6 weeks, the LV may become deconditioned and become dysfunctional following ASO with the increased afterload of the systemic circulation.
- In the presence of an unrestricted VSD, the LV will remain pressure-loaded and surgery may be delayed but at risk for increase pulmonary blood flow and congestive heart failure
- Earlier surgery, if possible, is indicated to optimize neurodevelopmental outcomes
- Taussig-Bing (TGA/subpulmonic VSD/arch obstruction) requires early surgery to avoid systemic hypoperfusion
- For TGA with LVOTO (i.e. sub-pulmonary obstruction), securing adequate pulmonary blood flow by PDA stent or systemic-to-pulmonary shunt may be required. Timing of correct surgery typically performed within the first year of life (Rastelli, Nikaidoh, or REV)

12 Surgical Strategy

12.1 Simple TGA

- The ASO is the standard treatment
- A median sternotomy is preformed, and an autologous pericardial patch is harvested for the PA reconstruction
- The aorta and pulmonary artery are separated, and branch pulmonary arteries are mobilized, and coronary anatomy confirmed with visual inspection
- The PDA is ligated and divided after going on cardiopulmonary bypass
- Initial cardioplegia is delivered anterograde directly into the aortic root. Subsequent doses of cardioplegia are through direct coronary artery administration
- The aorta is transected distal to the sino-tubular junction and coronary buttons are harvested.
- Intramural coronary arteries may be addressed by unroofing with/without the creation of a sinus pouch (saddle bag) anastomosis to neo-aorta
- The MPA is then transected, and the coronary arteries are re-implanted. Reimplantation can occur using the open technique (prior to reconstruction of neo-aorta) or using the closed technique (after reconstruction of the neo-aorta)
- Care must be taken to minimize coronary artery rotation and kinking using techniques such as medially hinged trapdoor verses direct anastomosis to sinuses. The height of coronary reimplantation must also be considered.
- The Lecompte maneuver (anterior translocation of the pulmonary arteries relative to the aorta) is performed with care to further mobilize the branch PAs to avoid tension after reconstruction. If the great vessels are side by side, the Lecompte maneuver may not be possible.
- Once the neo-aorta is reconstructed, the ASD is closed, and the cross clamp can be removed and the heart re-perfused.
- The defects from coronary button harvest in the neo-PA root (original aortic root) are then reconstructed using autologous pericardium and the neo-PA anastomosis is completed while the heart is reperfusion and rewarming on bypass.
- Late presentation is rare in developed countries, but LV deconditions (thinning of myocardium due to lower resistance pulmonary circulation) beyond 6–8 weeks. Echo and hemodynamic criteria can be used to assess indication of a staged ASO.
- Rapid retraining of LV myocardium to allow for staged ASO is typically achieved by increasing afterload using PA band prior to switch procedure. The strategy of increased pressure overload can be done in combination with volume loading strategy (typically PDA or systemic to pulmonary shunt).

12.2 Complex TGA (VSD/PS)

- If the mechanism of LVOTO is amenable to relief, ASO with LVOTO relief and VSD closure remains an option.
- Procedural selection depends on multiple anatomic factors including the size and location of the VSD and the coronary distribution. Options include:
  - Rastelli operation—baffling of the ventricular septum to incorporate the aortic outflow tract into the left ventricular and placement of a right ventricular to pulmonary artery conduit.
  - Réparation à l'étage ventriculaire (REV)—baffling of the ventricular septum as above but through an RV incision. The sub-pulmonary infundibulum is resected to prevent later evolution of subaortic stenosis. Using a Lecompte maneuver, the main pulmonary artery is resected and re-implanted into the RV incision avoiding a conduit.
  - Nikaidoh procedures—the pulmonary valve is excised, and the aortic root is posteriorly translocated RV over the LV. The VSD is closed, and an RV-PA conduit is sited. A Lecompte maneuver is also employed here.
- Taussig-Bing—The ASO with VSD closure via median sternotomy is the standard treatment for patients with TGA
  - Ascending aorta and arch reconstruction are necessary in about 50% of cases. In these cases, staged repair with initial arch repair and PA band is an alternative to complete primary repair

13 Postoperative Intensive Care Management

- Transesophageal or epicardial echocardiogram is used to evaluate the anatomic repair and coronary artery patency
- Early extubation for uncomplicated repairs that remain hemodynamically stable
- Early postoperative course may be complicated by systemic inflammatory response, bleeding, or ventricular dysfunction—support for LV with inotropy and afterload reduction vital if ASO delayed
- Concern sometimes raised for coronary impingement from subpulmonary artery dilation (secondary to pulmonary hypertension or rapid volume expansion)
- Pulmonary artery hypertension is rare and can be treated with pulmonary vasodilators once anatomic stenosis excluded
- LA lines inserted intraoperatively if increased concern of LV deconditioning or dysfunction.
- Concern for coronary stenosis if ventricular dysfunction with regional wall motion abnormalities, low cardiac output exceeds expectations, or ventricular ectopy/arrhythmias

- Early coronary imaging (within 1–2 months) for high-risk cases (e.g., Intramural, inter-arterial coronaries or single coronary origin)

14 Outcome

- Excellent postoperative outcomes: Simple TGA < 2% surgical mortality, and 2–3% for isolated TGA/VSD. Overall mortality for TGA/VSD approximately 5% due to increased complexity, largely due to anomalies to coronary arteries and associated arch problems or LVOTO.
- Increased mortality associated with coronary arteries arising from single osteum or with intramural course
- Healthcare burden after infancy is extremely low
- Reinterventions are uncommon (7–10%) and can be divided into 3 periods:
  - First year –often coronary reinterventions and almost all related to intramural or single coronary origins
  - 2–8 years—commonest reinterventions are on the branch pulmonary arteries or RVOT (>50% successfully resolved by catheterization)
  - 20–40 years—aortic root dilatation and AR which is rare but is an emerging concern
- Coronary artery stenosis rare but concern for stenosis primarily in patients with challenging coronary artery patterns
- Repeat operations often required for TGA/VSD with PS to upsize RV-PA conduit
- Excellent long-term outcomes for simple transposition with normal functional health status

15 Emerging Controversies

- Immediate corrective ASO to avoid BAS in cyanotic patients with restrictive atrial septum and/or poor mixing.

Bibliography

1. Jatene AD, Fnontes VF, Paulista PP, et al. Successful anatomic correction of transposition of the great vessels. A preliminary report Arg Bras Cardiol. 1975;128(4):461–64.
2. Martins P, Castela E. Transposition of the great arteries. Orphanet J Rare Dis. 2008;3:27.
3. Pasquali SK, Hasselblad V, Li JS, et al. Coronary artery pattern and outcome of arterial switch operation for transposition of the great arteries: a meta-analysis. Circulation. 2002;106(20):2575–80.

4. Rashkind WJ, Miller WW. Creation of an atrial septal defect without thoracotomy. A palliative approach to complete transposition of the great arteries. JAMA. 1966;196(11):991–92.
5. Wernovsky G. Transposition of the great arteries and common variants. Pediatr Crit Care Med. 2016;17(8 Suppl 1):S337–43.

Congenitally Corrected Transposition of the Great Arteries (ccTGA)

David J. Barron

Abstract Rare condition characterized by atrio-ventricular and ventriculo-arterial discordance—this creates a physiologically 'corrected' circulation but leaves the morphologic right ventricle (mRV) in the systemic position. Very heterogenous condition—majority of cases have associated lesions, most commonly a VSD and the presence or absence of pulmonary or sub-pulmonary obstruction. Management depends on the associated lesions but has to take into account the unpredictable function of both the mRV and the tricuspid valve (TV) in the systemic position. This makes for complex management strategies that can either focus on 'physiological correction' of the associated lesions (leaving the mRV as the systemic ventricle) or 'anatomical correction' that also restores the morphologic left ventricle (mLV) to the systemic position. The latter are referred to as the 'double switch' procedures that involve both an atrial switch and correction of the outflow tracts—either arterial switch or Rastelli-type procedure. Anatomical repair is generally reserved for the younger age-groups and may require re-training of the mLV with pulmonary artery banding (PAB) if it has become deconditioned. Management is controversial and has to be individualized since occasional cases never require any intervention yet the majority require surgery and anatomical repair if possible is preferred when suitable.

Keywords Congenitally corrected transposition · Levo-transposition · l-TGA double switch · Rastelli-senning · Pulmonary artery banding · Left ventricle re-training

Abbreviations

AV	Atrioventricular
AVV	Atrioventricular valve
BCPS	Bidirectional cavopulmonary shunt

D. J. Barron (✉)
Division of Cardiovascular Surgery, Labatt Family Heart Centre, The Hospital for Sick Children, Department of Surgery, University of Toronto, Toronto, ON, Canada
e-mail: David.barron@sickkids.ca

© The Author(s), under exclusive license to Springer Nature Switzerland AG 2024

A. I. Dipchand et al. (eds.), *Manual of Cardiac Care in Children*,
https://doi.org/10.1007/978-3-031-70973-9_21

ccTGA	Congenitally corrected transposition of the great arteries
CHB	Complete heart block
CoA	Coarctation of the aorta
CRT	Cardiac resynchronization therapy
DORV	Double outlet right ventricle
IVC	Inferior vena cava
LA	Left atrium
LCA	Left coronary artery
LVOTO	Left ventricular outflow tract obstruction
mLV	Morphologic left ventricle
mRV	Morphologic rightventricle
PA	Pulmonary artery
RCA	Right coronary artery
RA	Right atrium
RV	Right ventricle
SVC	Superior vena cava
TGA	Transposition of the great arteries
TR	Tricuspid regurgitation
TV	Tricuspid valve
VA	Ventriculo-arterial
VSD	Ventricular septal defect

Key Points

- mRV and TV are in the systemic position and have unpredictable behaviour with tendency to fail
- Management is dictated by the associated lesions: VSD in 70% and between 30 and 60% have pulmonary/subpulmonary obstruction with VSD (commoner in the Eastern Hemisphere)
- Physiological repair corrects associated lesions but leaves mRV in systemic position
- Anatomical repair requires atrial together with arterial switch or Rastelli
- Pulmonary artery banding may be needed to re-train mLV prior to Double Switch—rarely possible after 10 y of age
- Anatomical repair has most reliable long-term survival but at the cost of high-reintervention

1 Nomenclature

- Also called l-TGA or 'double-discordance'.

- Associated with situs inversus in 10%, dextrocardia in 15% and mesocardia in 30%.
- Rare subtypes include ccTGA with DORV and left isomerism with l-TGA.

2 Anatomy

- VSD in 70% Usually perimembranous. Can be remote inlet VSD.
- Great vessels transposed with the aorta anterior and to the left
- LVOTO is common (30–70%) and usually multilevel. Pulmonary atresia in extreme cases.
- Tricuspid valve can be displaced apically and described as 'ebsteinoid', where it is more likely to be regurgitant.
- AV node is displaced superiorly and the bundle runs antero-superiorly under the pulmonary valve
- Coronary anatomy is reversed with RCA posterior and LCA anterior. Single or intramural patterns are very rare

3 Embryology

- Levo-rotation of the primitive heart tube in early development. Leads to AV and VA discordance and left-handed topology
- No strong genetic or chromosomal links identified

4 Epidemiology

- 0.5% of all congenital heart disease
- Associated LVOTO (pulmonary or sub-pulmonary obstruction) has geographical variation, being commoner in the Eastern Hemisphere—up to 60% or all cases compared to 30–35% in the west.

5 Clinical Physiology and Presentation

- Depends entirely on associated lesions. If none ('isolated ccTGA') then can remain symptom free indefinitely (although most will develop TR and RV dysfunction—see below)
- Cases with VSD present as for any infant with large left-to-right shunt and pulmonary over-circulation

- Cases with LVOTO will have variable degrees of cyanosis depending on degree of obstruction, severe cases are duct dependent and may require neonatal intervention
- Congenital complete heart block may be presenting feature in isolation or together with other lesions
- Regardless of associated lesions, the systemic mRV and TV may show deteriorating function at any age, with TR being common and usually progressive.
- Age at presentation and mRV function is key to decision-making with preference for anatomical repair if < 10 years and any mRV dysfunction

6 Natural History

- In isolated ccTGA (5–10% of all ccTGA) this is dictated by mRV function and TR. 50% of cases will be in heart failure by the age of 20 y. Occasional patients may remain well into old age but if there is moderate mRV dysfunction in childhood then survival is only 50% at 20 y.
- Associated lesions dictate outcome for the remainder. Excluding duct-dependent lesions, survival is 50% at the age of 15 y without intervention
- Congenital CHB can be present at birth and there is a 2% per year risk of developing block

7 Associated Lesions

- VSD in 70%
- LVOTO (pulmonary/sub-pulmonary obstruction) in 30–70% Pulmonary Atresia 3–8%
- CCHB in 5–10%
- Ebsteinoid TV 10–20%
- Arch hypoplasia/CoA 10%

8 Diagnostic Studies

- ECG can show variable degrees of block. CXR will reflect associated lesions. Situs inversus in 10%
- Echocardiography provides diagnosis to demonstrate AV- and VA-discordance and especially to define mRV and TV function. Position and size of VSD and any degree of LVOTO.
- MRI or CT may be necessary to demonstrate arch anatomy and to define relationship of VSD to the aorta in cases for potential Rastelli or Nikaidoh repair.
- Coronary anatomy can usually be defined on CT but may require cardiac catheterization if not clear.

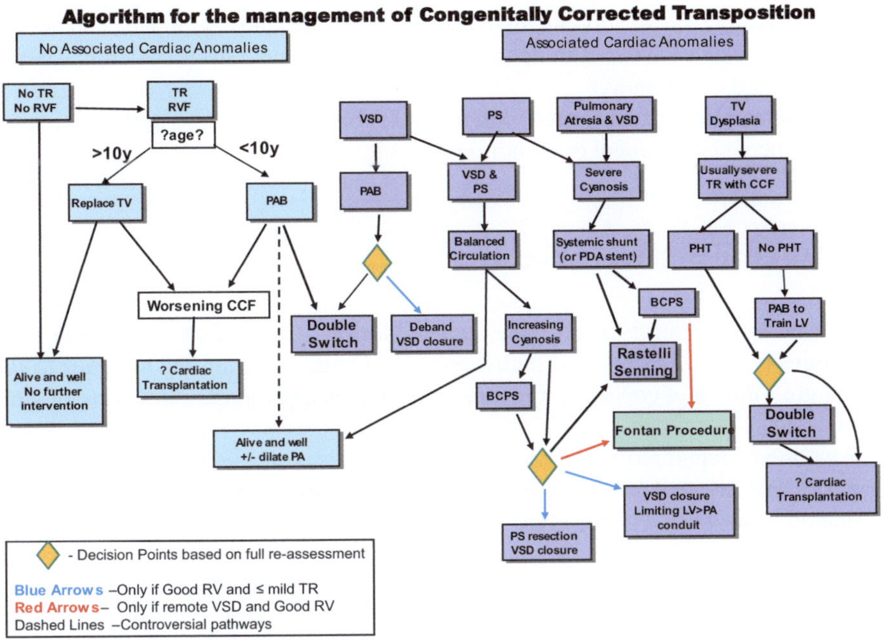

Fig. 1 Algorithm for management of ccTGA. *Adapted from Barron DJ, Brawn WJ. Surgery for corrected transposition of the great arteries. Sabiston & Spencer Surgery of the Chest, Eds. FW Sellke, PJ Del Nido and SJ Swanson 9th Edition, Elsevier 2016*

- Cases that have undergone PA banding to re-train the mLV require careful assessment with cardiac catheter, stress testing and MRI to show preparedness for anatomical repair.

9 Indications for Surgery/Intervention (Fig. 1)

- Dictated by associated lesions. Cases with isolated ccTGA and ≥ mod TR or progressive mRV dysfunction should be considered for PA band with a view to double switch—even if symptom-free.
- Older patients with ≥ mod TR should be considered for TV replacement even if symptom free.

10 Timing of Intervention

- Mainly dictated by the associated lesions.
- Neonatal interventions are required for duct-dependent lesions, arch hypoplasia/CoA or congenital CHB.

- Best outcomes for the double-switch are if performed at < 3y of age. The double switch is usually avoided in neonates and small infants (atrial switch has better outcomes if > 3 months)
- Significant VSDs often treated with initial PA band as this keeps options open for subsequent conventional or anatomical repair.

11 Surgical Strategy (Fig. 2)

- Conventional repair is as per the associated lesions. Care should be taken in VSD closure to avoid the unusual pathway of the bundle anterior and superior to the margin. (note that conduction reverts to normal orientation in the setting of situs inversus)
- Anatomical repair requires arterial switch, which is performed as in d-TGA. Coronaries are inverted but arise from the facing sinuses and variants in coronary anatomy are rare. The atrial switch can be either Mustard or Senning, but the majority of reports favour Senning.
- If there is LVOTO or atresia, then anatomical repair is with Rastelli or Nikaidoh. Usually, the VSD is large, but it may require enlargement—avoiding the outlet septum beneath the pulmonary valve due to the conduction tissue. Some centres offer a BCPS as an interim stage prior to anatomical repair as this also simplifies the atrial switch at time of repair.
- PAB is usually required prior to double switch: either to protect from overcirculation in the setting of a VSD, or to re-train the mLV if intact septum. In the latter the band should increase mLV to 60–70% pressure initially with no sign of dysfunction.
- Re-training typically takes 9–12 months and mLV should have reached 85–90% systemic pressure (up to 100% with Dobutamine stress) with LV mass index of $\geq 50\ gm^{-2}$. Re-training is rarely attempted at > 10 y of age.
- Remote VSD in the setting of LVOTO may be better managed with Fontan circulation so long as TV function is good.
- Patients with CHB require epicardial pacing (avoids leads in the atrial pathways) and biventricular leads allow for CRT pacing, which has evidence for better synchronization in ccTGA patients.
- The TR usually improves after anatomical repair and so interventions on the TV are rarely necessary in this setting. However, in conventional repair then TV replacement is more reliable than repair if the valve is incompetent.

12 Intensive Care Physiology and Management

- Anatomical repairs are complex procedures with long bypass and cross-clamp times. Moderate inotropic support often needed. Chest may be left open.

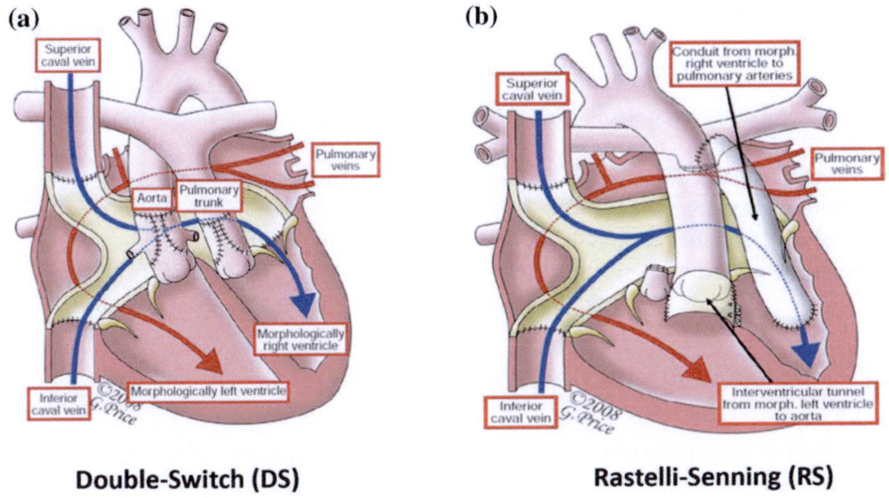

Fig. 2 Two most common types of anatomical repair for ccTGA. An atrial switch (Mustard or Senning) has been performed to divert the pulmonary venous blood to the left ventricle and the systemic venous blood to the right ventricle. A) If the LVOT is normally developed then an arterial switch is performed to overcome the transposition of the great arteries. This is the Double Switch (DS) procedure. B) If the LVOT is stenotic or atretic, then the transposition is overcome with a Rastelli procedure to commit the LV though the VSD to the aorta, and an RV-PA conduit is placed to provide pulmonary blood flow. This is the Rastelli-Senning (RS). *Reproduced from Anderson's Pediatric Cardiology, Vol 4, Barron D, Stumper O,* et al. *Congenitally corrected transposition, pp 712, 2019, with permission from Elsevier*

- LA pressure line helps to monitor systemic ventricle preload and function.
- Thorough echo to assess atrial switch pathways, AVV function and ventricular function. Neo-aortic regurgitation is common and should be monitored
- SVC pathway is long in atrial switch and pressures can initially be high, but do not reflect RV filling. Direct RA line or IVC line may be necessary to give accurate value.
- Patients banded to re-train the mLV can develop LV dysfunction and failure in the first 48 h (especially older children) and should be monitored closely. A line can be left in the mLV (similar to a swan-ganz) to monitor pressure.

13 Outcomes

- Conventional repair has overall disappointing outcomes with 10–15% operative mortality and 50% risk of significant TR and mRV failure within 10 years
- Anatomical repair has 5–10% operative mortality (less in the elective group) and 80% freedom from heart failure at 20 years. Reintervention rates are 30% at 10 years for most anatomical repairs and include conduit changes in the

Rastelli group but also 10–15% needing neo -Aortic Valve repair or replacement at 20 years.
- Around 15% of anatomical repairs develop late mLV failure by 20y post-op. This appears to be related to older age at double-switch and is very rare in those repaired at < 2 years.
- Post-operative CHB risk is 5–10% in addition to the natural history for heart block in these patients.
- PAB itself can be therapeutic in isolated ccTGA by splinting the inter-ventricular septum and reducing the amount of TR.

14 Controversies and Alternative Strategies

- ccTGA management remains very controversial. A small minority of patients with sustained good mRV function and no TR do extremely well with conventional repair but the majority develop mRV failure.
- Anatomical repair is generally regarded as gold standard if there is any RV dysfunction or TR—but is only achievable in younger children (around 10 y). Attempting to re-train the mLV in older agegroups is controversial with unreliable results.
- Prophylactic PAB in isolated ccTGA is controversial but is being offered by some centres. Also, PAB as definitive treatment may have a role in some cases, preventing progression of TR.
- The one-and-a-half repair simplifies the atrial switch and is favoured by some centres.
- Fontan in the setting of remote VSD and LVOTO has good outcomes. Small subgroup with balanced VSD and PS may be very stable.
- CRT has an important role in preserving function in patients with heart block.

Acknowledgements The author would like to acknowledge Dr. Maryam Alomair for her contributions to this chapter.

Bibliography

1. Cui H, Hage A, Piekarski BL, et al. Management of congenitally corrected transposition of the great arteries with intact ventricular septum: anatomic repair or palliative treatment? Circ Cardiovasc Interv. 2021;14(7): e010154.
2. Hraska V, Vergnat M, Zartner P, et al. Promising outcome of anatomic correction of corrected transposition of the great arteries. Ann Thorac Surg. 2017;104(2):650–6.
3. Lundstrom U, Bull C, Wyse RK, et al. The natural and "unnatural" history of congenitally corrected transposition. Am J Cardiol. 1990;65(18):1222–9.
4. Metton O, Gaudin R, Ou P, et al. Early prophylactic pulmonary artery banding in isolated congenitally corrected transposition of the great arteries. Eur J Cardiothorac Surg. 2010;38(6):728–34.

5. Murtuza B, Barron DJ, Stumper O, et al. Anatomic repair for congenitally corrected transposition of the great arteries: a single-institution 19-year experience. J Thorac Cardiovasc Surg. 2011;142(6):1348–57.

Truncus Arteriosus

Daniel E. Ehrmann and Alejandro A. Floh

Abstract Truncus arteriosus (TA) occurs when a common artery arises from the heart giving rise to the aorta and pulmonary arteries. This lesion results from failure of septation of the embryologic truncus and may occur as an isolated defect or associated with DiGeorge syndrome. It is classified primarily by the origins and configuration of the pulmonary arteries. TA is associated with VSD, variable truncal valve override into the RV, right aortic arch, and interruption of the aortic arch. The truncal valve is most commonly tricuspid but may have one to four cusps; valvar regurgitation and/or stenosis portend poor prognosis. Surgical correction consists of septating the heart by closing VSD and directing the LV to the truncal valve, establishing the RV to PA continuity, and arch reconstruction if required. Surgical repair is associated with good outcome, with increased morbidity associated with prematurity, low birth weight, aortic arch interruption, and valvar dysplasia and regurgitation.

Keywords Truncus arteriosus · Neonatal cardiovascular surgery

Abbreviations

ASD	Atrial septal defect
CoA	Coarctation of the aorta
CPB	Cardiopulmonary bypass
IAA	Interrupted aortic arch
iNO	Inhaled nitric oxide
LAD	Left anterior descending
LCA	Left coronary artery

D. E. Ehrmann
Department of Pediatrics, University of Michigan Medical School, Ann Arbor, MI, USA
e-mail: Dehrmann@med.umich.edu

A. A. Floh (✉)
Department of Critical Care Medicine, Division of Cardiac Critical Care Unit, Labatt Family Heart Centre, The Hospital for Sick Children, University of Toronto, Toronto, Canada
e-mail: Alejandro.floh@sickkids.ca

© The Author(s), under exclusive license to Springer Nature Switzerland AG 2024

A. I. Dipchand et al. (eds.), *Manual of Cardiac Care in Children*,
https://doi.org/10.1007/978-3-031-70973-9_22

LPA	Left pulmonary artery
LV	Left ventricle
PA	Pulmonary artery
PAB	Pulmonary artery band
PDA	Persistent ductus arteriosus
PI	Pulmonary insufficiency
RCA	Right coronary artery
RAA	Right aortic arch
RV	Right ventricle
RVOT	Right ventricular outflow tract
Qp	Pulmonary blood flow
Qs	Systemic blood flow
TA	Truncus arteriosus
VSD	Ventricular septal defect

Key Points

- Truncus arteriosus refers to a common arterial vessel arising from the base of the heart that gives rise to the systemic arteries, pulmonary arteries, and coronary arteries
- Usually occurs as an isolated defect but can be associated with DiGeorge syndrome
- Right aortic arch (RAA), interrupted aortic arch (IAA), and coronary anomalies are relatively common associations
- Clinical presentation relates to extent of pulmonary blood flow and the severity of truncal valve disease
- Surgical correction is performed typically during the first week of life to avoid development of heart failure and subsequent pulmonary hypertension
- Right and left ventricular systolic and diastolic dysfunction, and arrhythmias are common post-operative concerns
- Good short and long-term outcomes, with re-intervention required on the RV-PA conduit eventually and patients with ongoing significant truncal valve disease.

1 Nomenclature

- Three different nomenclatures exist: Collet & Edwards, Van Praagh, and Anderson. All are based on how the pulmonary arteries arise from a common arterial trunk ± associated defects
- Only Van Praagh classification incorporates isolated PA and IAA.

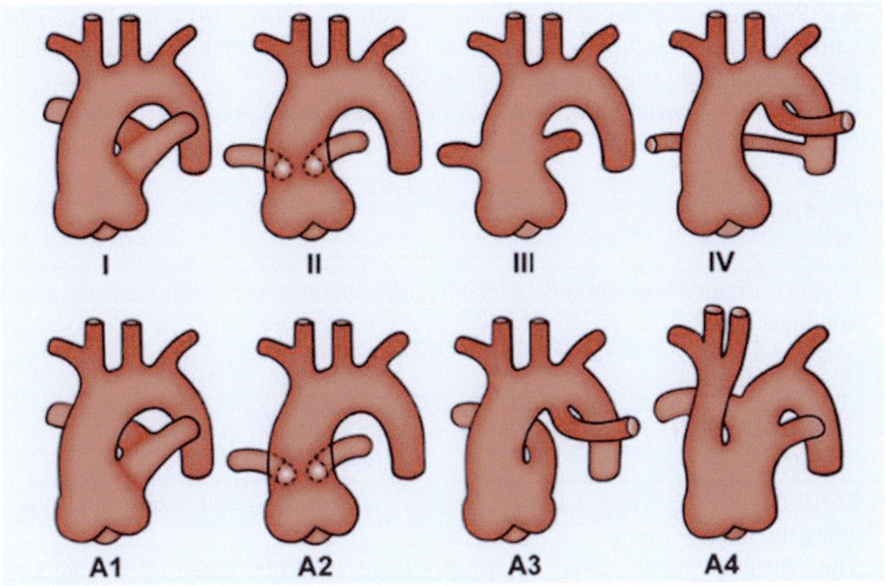

Fig. 1 Collet and Edwards and Van Praagh classification systems for truncus arteriosus. Reprinted from Operative Techniques in Thoracic and Cardiovascular Surgery, Vol 12, Issue 1, Moss & Adams Fig. 2 in Chap. 42, Welke KF, Ungerleider RM, Repair of tetralogy of Fallot with absent pulmonary valve syndrome, Classification systems for persistent truncus arteriosus, pp 25–35, 2007, with permission from Elsevier

1.1 Collet and Edwards (Fig. 1)

- I: Pulmonary arteries arise from a single pulmonary trunk off the common arterial trunk
- II: Pulmonary arteries arise separately but adjacent to each other off the common arterial trunk
- III: Pulmonary arteries arise separately but on opposite sides of the common arterial trunk
- IV: Pulmonary arteries arise separately, not from the common arterial trunk and outside the pericardium (e.g., from the descending aorta)

1.2 Van Praagh and Van Praagh

- A1: Same as Collet & Edwards type I
- A2: The branch pulmonary arteries arise directly from the common arterial trunk (does not distinguish between close together or far apart, therefore includes all Collet & Edwards type II and III phenotypes)

- A3: Pulmonary arteries arise separately, with one arising from inside the pericardium (e.g., from the common arterial trunk) and one arising from outside the pericardium (e.g., from the descending aorta)
- A4: Common arterial trunk with IAA or coarctation (CoA)

1.3 Anderson

- Lesion is divided into common arterial trunk with pulmonary dominance or aortic dominance

2 Anatomy

- Collet & Edwards Types I and II truncus comprise nearly all cases, with Type I being the most common
- The ventricular septal defect is typically large, muscular outlet (60%), adjacent to the truncal valve, and situated between the limbs of the septal band
  - The conduction system is typically remote from the VSD but pass closely along the leftward aspect of the posterior-inferior in cases with a perimembranous VSD (40%)
- The truncal valve can be unicuspid, bicuspid, tricuspid, or quadricuspid, with tricuspid being the most common (approximately 66% of patients)
- Truncal valve regurgitation not uncommon but true stenosis is rare (increased velocity often seen across valve due to high flow)
- The truncal valve is overriding the ventricular septal defect, and very rarely emerges entirely from the right ventricle
- Coronary artery variations and malformations are seen in over 33% of patients
  - RCA typically arises from the right anterolateral aorta and LCA from the left posterolateral aorta
  - Anterior/posterior position on the aorta as well as proximity to the pulmonary arteries can vary and may be of surgical importance
  - The LAD is frequently small and displaced leftward thereby leading to prominent conal branches of the RCA which may supply the RVOT.

3 Embryology

- Failure of division of embryonic truncus arteriosus into aorta and pulmonary trunks by fusion of truncal swellings proximally and distally by invagination of the roof of the aortic sac.

4 Epidemiology

- Usually occurs as an isolated defect with 30% associated with DiGeorge syndrome (increases to 60% with IAA)
- Increased incidence of disease in relatives of patients with truncus arteriosus suggest possible genetic component
- Maternal diabetes is a risk factor.

5 Clinical Physiology and Presentation

- Clinical presentation pre-operatively relates to extent of pulmonary blood flow and the severity of truncal valve disease
- Considered cyanotic heart disease but cyanosis is usually mild perinatally and often disappears completely due to excessive pulmonary blood
- Degree of pulmonary blood flow dependent on pulmonary artery (PA) size and pulmonary vascular resistance
- Excessive pulmonary blood flow may manifest as progressive respiratory symptoms and rarely signs of marginal systemic cardiac output (e.g., poor feeding) if severe and/or associated with severe truncal valve insufficiency
  - Gentle diuresis may be beneficial in patients with evidence of significant pulmonary congestion/symptomatology
- Increased Qp:Qs volume loads the heart thereby increasing metabolic demand
  - May be exacerbated by liberal use of supplemental oxygen
- Myocardial supply/demand mismatch and myocardial ischemia, especially in the setting of low diastolic blood pressure and coronary steal due to diastolic runoff into pulmonary arteries and and/or truncal valve insufficiency.

6 Natural History

- Left untreated, nearly all infants develop heart failure in infancy and are unable to survive past 1 year of life
- Hypertensive pulmonary vascular disease develops quickly after birth and may become irreversible in early infancy.

7 Associated Lesions

- Arch anomalies are relatively common

  - RAA occurs in approximately 33% of patients
  - IAA in approximately 15% of patients
  - CoA not seen

- PDA is absent and seen only with IAA or isolated LPA
- One PA is absent in up to 15%, typically missing on the same side as the aortic arch (e.g. truncus arteriosus with left aortic arch missing the LPA)
- Secundum ASD is present in 10–20% of cases
- Extracardiac anomalies (i.e., skeletal, renal, GI) are present in up to 1/4 of patients

8 Diagnostic Studies

8.1 CXR

- Typically shows cardiomegaly and increased pulmonary vascular markings

8.2 Echocardiography

- Typically, the only study needed to delineate intracardiac anatomy (connections, size and position of pulmonary arteries, coronary artery pattern), truncal valve function, arch sidedness and patency, ventricular function, and presence of other associated defects
- Diagnosis often made prenatally using fetal echocardiography

8.3 CT Angiography

- Occasionally required to delineate aortic arch and branching when interrupted

8.4 Cardiac Catheterization

- Not usually needed except in cases of delayed diagnosis to calculate indexed pulmonary arteriolar resistance and determine surgical candidacy

9 Indication for Surgery

- The diagnosis is universally surgically corrected.

10 Timing of Intervention

- Due to the natural history of disease, surgical correction is performed in early infancy, typically during the first week of life
- Patients monitored for systemic perfusion and evidence of end-organ dysfunction from pulmonary run-off, including coronary ischemia

11 Surgical Strategy

- Via median sternotomy, standard aortic and bicaval cannulation, cardiopulmonary bypass and mild to moderate hypothermia, the pulmonary arteries are separated from the truncus, RV-PA continuity is established, the VSD is closed, and associated defects are repaired
- Since the repair is typically performed in the first week of life, RV-PA continuity is achieved most often using pulmonary homografts and Contegra valved grafts
- Direct connection of the RV to PAs can be achieved with a transannular patch (increased incidence of PI but fewer outflow tract reinterventions)
- Truncal valve intervened upon at original surgery usually when more than moderate truncal valve regurgitation
- Multiple techniques exist for repair of the truncal valve with significant pathology, including suturing leaflets together at the commissure, extension of leaflets with pericardium, or other creative approaches to valve reconstruction
- Exclusion of a cusp in quadricuspid valves or bicuspidisation also done
- Surgical risk highest with more than moderate truncal regurgitation or IAA.
- Risk factors also include prematurity, low birth weight, preoperative instability
- Bilateral pulmonary artery banding (PAB) can be considered as temporizing measure if cardiopulmonary bypass contraindicated, or risk is prohibitive. Balances pulmonary and systemic circulations and allows for end-organ recovery. Surgical correction is completed as soon as safe to reduce long-term risk of PA stenosis.

12 Intensive Care Physiology and Management

- Full repair decreases LV volume loading and coronary steal from diastolic run-off
- Early focus on key elements of repair and residual lesions including RV and LV dysfunction, residual truncal valve disease, evidence of elevated RV systolic and/or diastolic pressures, and confirmation of unobstructed ventricular outflows and coronary arteries. A residual atrial level shunt may be purposely left if the concern for RV dysfunction or pulmonary hypertension is high
- RV systolic dysfunction is common due to elevated pulmonary pressures present pre-operatively, RV ventriculotomy, and neonatal CPB

  - Hemodynamic support with epinephrine to support systolic function, and/or iNO to decrease pulmonary vascular resistance is common
- RV diastolic dysfunction is relatively common due to hypertrophy exacerbated by preoperative pressure loading
  - Patients may present with an element of restrictive RV physiology and attention must be paid to volume status and central venous pressure to optimize RV filling
- Ventilation strategies should focus on minimizing mean airway pressure and pulmonary vascular resistance by achieving normal pH/CO_2 and functional residual capacity
  - Negative pressure ventilation (i.e., extubation) should be achieved as soon as safe
- LV dysfunction may arise from injury to coronary arteries during surgery and/or the inflammatory effects of neonatal surgery with CPB
  - Reduction of systemic vascular resistance with milrinone or other agents may reduce low cardiac output and be beneficial if there is significant residual truncal valve stenosis/insufficiency and unobstructed arch
  - Reduction to systemic vascular resistance may challenge management if RV dysfunction is present by promoting suboptimal ventricular-ventricular interactions and interfering with LV filling
- Tachyarrhythmias are commonly seen after repair of truncus arteriosus, and these patients are considered at high risk for junctional ectopic tachycardia
  - Complete heart block can also occur, albeit relatively rarely
  - Ventricular arrhythmias are relatively rare and should prompt investigation for coronary injury or compression (e.g., from the RV-PA conduit)
- Management of comorbidities from DiGeorge syndrome may be relevant post-operatively, including airway issues or significant hypocalcemia, which is specifically important for neonatal myocardial function.

13 Outcome

- In the modern era, in-hospital mortality is less than 5% for most patients with truncus arteriosus and intact aortic arch, with patients having IAA, complex comorbidities or truncal valve dysfunction experiencing higher rates of mortality
- Long term survival among those who make it to hospital discharge approaches 90% at 10 years following surgery
- Development should be closely followed as has become the standard of care for all neonatal cardiac surgeries

- Short- and long-term cardiac follow-up is focused on monitoring for truncal valve dysfunction, function of the RV-PA homograft/conduit, development of branch PA stenosis, and systolic and diastolic RV and LV function
- Moderate or worse truncal valve insufficiency before repair has been independently associated with decreased long-term survival at 20 years
- Need for re-intervention on the RV-PA conduit is universal, with median time to conduit re-intervention of approximately 5 years
  - Size of conduit used at initial repair is an important risk factor for earlier conduit re-intervention

14 Alternative Strategies and Controversies

- Management of early, persistent severe truncal valve dysfunction is challenging and the optimal strategy for repair or replacement has not been identified
- Techniques for replacement of obstructed RV-PA conduits vary between centers, with some using a "peel" technique in which the old conduit is removed and a prosthetic roof (usually pericardium) is reapplied with concomitant insertion of a bioprosthetic valve.

Bibliography

1. Bibevski S, Friedland-Little J, Ohye R, Thor T, Gaies M. Truncus arteriosus. In: Pediatric and congenital cardiology, cardiac surgery and intensive care, London: Springer; 2014, pp. 1983–2001.
2. Cabalka A, Edwards W, Dearani J. Truncus arteriosus. In: Moss and Adams heart disease in infants, children, and adolescents: including the fetus and young adult. Philadelphia: Lippincott Williams & Wilkins; 2015. p. 1053–64.
3. Ezon D, Goldberg J, Kyle W. Truncus arteriosus communis. In: Atlas of congenital heart disease nomenclature: an illustrated guide to the Van Praagh and Anderson approaches to describing congenital cardiac pathology. Houston: CreateSpace Independent Publishing Platform; 2015. p. 74–7.

Congenital Mitral Valve Disease

Christoph Haller

Abstract Mitral valve disease usually occurs in association with other congenital lesions. Regurgitation or stenosis may occur isolated or in combination. Defects resulting in a dysfunctional mitral valve can be related to any structure of the valve, including supravalvular obstruction, annular and leaflet abnormalities, or pathologies of the subvalvar apparatus (i.e., papillary muscles and chordae). Mitral valve pathologies typically present with variable signs of heart failure and pulmonary venous hypertension. Limited by the options for valve prostheses, valve repair is favored, even though higher than usual residual dysfunction must be accepted. A multitude of surgical techniques have been described to specifically address the various underlying pathologies. Valve replacement has been shown to impair outcome and is limited by annular size and early need for re-replacement. Catheter valves implanted in a hybrid procedure may offer new options as they allow replacement in small patients and offer stepwise dilation to accommodate growth.

Keywords Mitral valve · Mitral regurgitation · Mitral stenosis · Mitral valve replacement · Mitral valve repair · Supramitral ring · Parachute mitral valve

Abbreviations

ASD	Atrial septal defect
AVSD	Atrioventricular septal defect
CoA	Coarctation of the aorta
HLHS	Hypoplastic left heart syndrome
LV	Left ventricle
MR	Mitral regurgitation
MS	Mitral stenosis
PDA	Persistent ductus arteriosus

C. Haller (✉)
Division of Cardiovascular Surgery, Labatt Family Heart Centre, Department of Surgery, The Hospital for Sick Children, University of Toronto, Toronto, ON, Canada
e-mail: christoph.haller@sickkids.ca

© The Author(s), under exclusive license to Springer Nature Switzerland AG 2024

A. I. Dipchand et al. (eds.), *Manual of Cardiac Care in Children*,
https://doi.org/10.1007/978-3-031-70973-9_23

VSD Ventricular septal defect

Key Points

- Mitral valve disease may occur as an isolated entity (less common) or with associated lesions (more common).
- Mitral regurgitation (MR) or stenosis (MS) may occur as isolated lesions or combined.
- All parts of the valvar apparatus can be affected (supravalvar, valvar [annulus, leaflets], subvalvar [chordae, papillary muscles]), either isolated or combined.
- Typically presents with variable signs of heart failure and pulmonary venous hypertension.
- Valve sparing repair should be attempted in most patients (especially the very young), even if higher than usual residual regurgitation (or stenosis) is accepted.
- Valve replacement options are limited due to annular size and early need for re-replacement.
- Catheter valve prostheses may offer new options that allow interventional valve dilation postoperatively.

This chapter covers isolated mitral valve pathologies only. Mitral valve lesions that are part of other anomalies (e.g. AVSD, MS in the setting of HLHS, endocarditis, rheumatic valve disease etc.) are addressed in the respective chapters.

1 Nomenclature

- Mitral valve dysplasia may be seen, varies based on underlying pathology (i.e., supramitral ring, valve prolapse, cleft, elongated chordae, chordal rupture, papillary muscle anomalies), and is described as such.
- Congenital mitral valve disease may occur in association with any other congenital cardiac anomalies.

2 Anatomy

- The normal mitral valve consists of a fibrous annulus, an anterior and a posterior leaflet (which significantly differ from each other in size and shape), chordae tendineae and papillary muscles (Fig. 1). The size of the leaflets is supposed to be much larger than the valve orifice (about twice its size) leading to a large area of coaptation (area where both leaflets abut during systole).

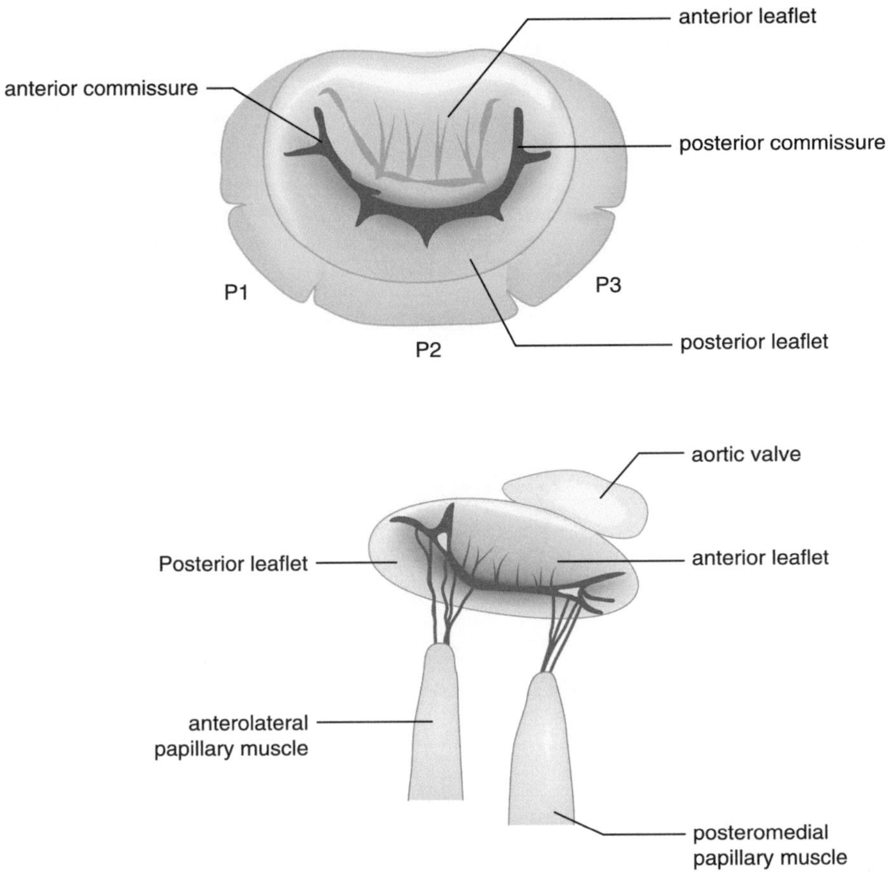

Fig. 1 Normal mitral valve anatomy

- Valve disease can be separated in regurgitant or stenotic lesions. A combination of regurgitation and stenosis may occur. Although some of the anatomical lesions may predominantly cause regurgitation or stenosis respectively, valve lesions may impair both closure and opening of the valve.
- Regurgitation may be caused by one or a combination of the following
  - Annular dilation
  - Cleft in anterior or posterior leaflet.
  - Leaflet prolapse
  - Leaflet tethering
  - Elongated chordae
  - Ruptured chordae.
- Regurgitation can be classified according to Carpentier to describe its mechanism (Fig. 2).

Fig. 2 Carpentier classification of mitral valve regurgitation

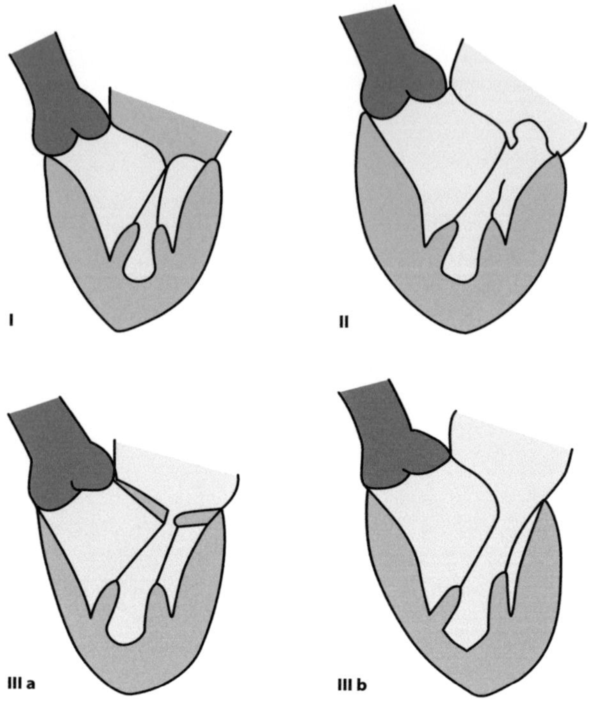

I Normal leaflet motion
II Excessive leaflet motion (i.e., prolapse)
III Restricted leaflet motion

a. Restriction affects opening
b. Restriction affects closure.

- Stenosis may be caused by one or a combination of the following:
  - Supramitral ring
  - Commissural fusion
  - Mitral arcade, hammock mitral valve
  - Shortened chordae
  - Enlarged or fused papillary muscles (e.g., parachute mitral valve).
- Anatomical lesions should be differentiated from functional lesions in the setting of reduced myocardial function and a structurally normal valve apparatus.

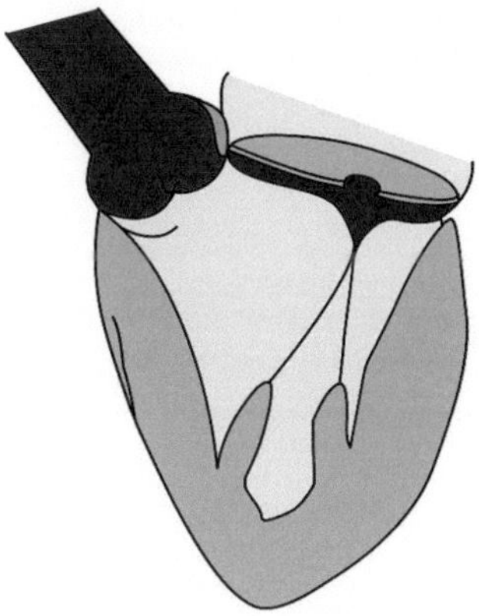

Fig. 3 Supramitral ring

2.1 *Supramitral Ring*

- Supramitral ring is a fibrous structure proximal to the mitral valve leaflets and orifice (Fig. 3). As opposed to Cor triatriatum, the ring is distal to both atrial appendage and pulmonary veins.

2.2 *Hammock Mitral Valve*

- Also called anomalous mitral arcade. It is regarded as an arrest of chordal development. Chordae are shortened leading to a "hammock"-like appearance when viewed from the atrium. It leads to decreased mobility of the leaflets, regurgitation and/or stenosis.
- Normal sized orifice
- Short, thickened chordae
- Little space between chordae
- Chordae to posterior leaflet usually better developed.

2.3 *Parachute Mitral Valve*

- Parachute mitral valve is defined by a single papillary muscle from which all chordae originate (Fig. 4). This leads to restrictive opening of the valve and valve stenosis.

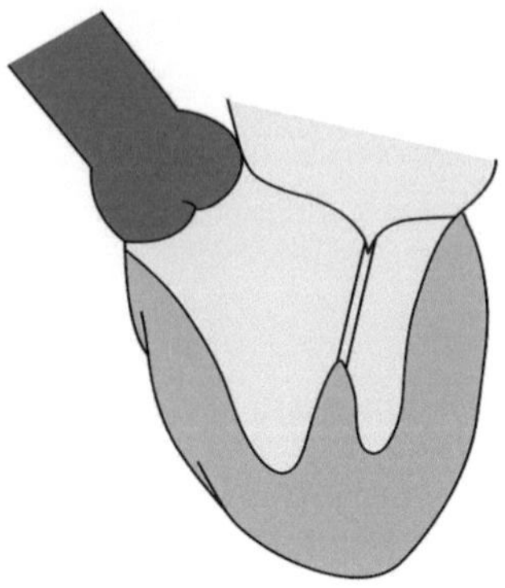

Fig. 4 Parachute mitral valve

3 Embryology

- Atrioventricular valve development is closely associated with both atrioventricular septation (i.e., separation of left and right AV valves) and ventricular delamination (formation of leaflets and papillary muscles).
- A muscular ridge in the ventricle undergoes delamination and its anterior and posterior part form the papillary muscles. Failure of this delamination process leads to either asymmetric papillary muscles or true parachute mitral valve.
- Failure of delamination of cushion tissue can lead to tethering of leaflets, shortened or absent chordae (as in Hammock mitral valve) or the very rarely reported Ebstein's malformation of the mitral valve. The latter usually affects the posterior leaflet only, which remains tethered.

4 Epidemiology

4.1 Incidence/Prevalence

- Commonly occurs in combination with other malformations.
- Exact numbers are not well reported.
- 65 in 13,400 (0.004%) of echocardiographically examined patients $\leq$ 18 years have been reported.

4.2 Population at Risk, Inheritance

- Familial clustering shown in both primary and secondary MR.
- MS is often part of a wide spectrum of associated lesions and resulting LV hypoplasia with complex inheritance pattern.

5 Clinical Physiology and Presentation

- Presentation is highly variable, ranging from asymptomatic or mildly symptomatic patients to patients in heart failure.
- Symptoms are based on severity of the mitral valve dysfunction
  - Failure to thrive
  - Difficulty feeding
  - Dyspnea
  - Recurrent infection
  - Signs of heart failure

6 Natural History

- Widely variable and commonly related to the individual severity of the mitral valve dysfunction and associated lesions.
- MR or MS (if mild) may be tolerated well for years. Severe dysfunction causing symptoms or ventricular failure may indicate early intervention.

7 Associated Lesions

- ASD
- VSD
- PDA
- CoA
- Most notably is the association of MS with LV hypoplasia and Shone complex, which consists of:
  - Supramitral ring
  - Parachute mitral valve
  - Subaortic membrane
  - Coarctation of the aorta
  - Shone's Syndrome: MS in association with one or more other obstructive left sided lesions (left outflow tract stenosis, aortic stenosis, coarctation).

8 Diagnostic Studies

- As associated lesions are common, diagnostic findings of mitral valve disease may be obscured. It is therefore even more important to direct attention on mitral valve pathologies to rule out any defect, that needs to be addressed when correcting associated lesions.

8.1 ECG

- Signs of LA enlargement.
- Longstanding pulmonary venous hypertension can lead to RV hypertrophy.
- LV dilation may be seen if ongoing regurgitation is present.

8.2 CXR

- Enlarged cardiac silhouette.
- Signs of pulmonary venous congestion.
- Pulmonary edema may be seen in more severe cases.

8.3 Echocardiography

- Echocardiography is the mainstay of diagnostic imaging.
- Anatomical valve dysfunction needs to be differentiated from functional problems caused by ventricular dysfunction.
- All aspects of the mitral valve apparatus can be described
  - Supramitral ring (and its relation to pulmonary veins and left atrial appendage)
  - Annular size
  - Valve leaflets (size, mobility, cleft, prolapse)
  - Valve orifice (size, commissural fusion)
  - Chordal attachments (length, relation to leaflet edge and papillary muscles, structure etc.)
  - Papillary muscles (size, position, separation)
  - Mechanism of valve dysfunction
  - Functional aspects (severity, regurgitant jet size/direction/number, vena contracta, inflow gradient, etc.)
- Coexisting lesions (especially obstructive lesions in case of MS) can be diagnosed simultaneously.

Table 1 Echocardiographic criteria for severity of MR

Mild	Severe
Small jet < 20% of LA	Large jet > 40% LA
Small vena contracta	Large vena contracta
No or little flow convergence	Flow reversal in pulm. Veins
A-wave dominance	E-wave dominance
Normal chamber dimensions	Enlarged LA / LV
Regurgitant fraction < 30%	Regurgitant fraction > 50%

- Echocardiographic criteria for severity of mitral regurgitation can be found in Table 1.
- Echocardiographic criteria for severity of MS needs to take into consideration the presence of associated lesions. A large left-to-right ventricular shunt or PDA can result in a mild gradient across a normal mitral valve based on flow alone and can lead to an overestimate of the actual degree of mitral stenosis in the setting of an abnormal valve. Conversely, a shunt at atrial level, downstream obstruction and/or an elevated end diastolic pressure can lead to a lower gradient and an underestimate of the degree of MS. In general, a mean gradient greater than 10–12 mmHg is considered severe. Secondary information including markers of right-sided pressures are also important in assessing the degree of MS.

8.4 MRI

- Rarely necessary for isolated valve disease.
- Quantification of regurgitation fraction and cardiac output.
- Important role in decision-making in borderline LV dimensions.

8.5 CT

- Uncommon for isolated valve disease unless coexisting lesions mandate further investigation.

8.6 Cardiac Catheterization

- May be helpful in assessment of gradients and pulmonary pressures if echocardiographic results are ambiguous.
- Usually not indicated.

9 Indications for Intervention/Surgery

- Indications for surgical intervention in children are less precisely defined than in adult patients. Especially in low bodyweight patients, the lack of a suitable valve prosthesis, the proven better outcome of valve repair and the technical challenges of surgery usually favor a conservative management if tolerated.
- Severe MS/MR.
- Symptomatic.
- Pulmonary hypertension
- Likelihood of ability to repair the valve.
- Mitral valve repair is preferred, especially if the patient's size does not allow implantation of an adult size valve prosthesis.
- Mitral balloon valvuloplasty can be used in the setting of MS but should be chosen with regard to the obstructing pathology.

10 Timing of Intervention and Management Strategy

- If clinically tolerated, valve intervention is delayed to increase likelihood of durable repair or implantation of a large valve prosthesis.
- However, some structural defects may be easier to repair at early stages as persistent stress on the valve may cause further damage (e.g., chordal rupture).
- Acute valve dysfunction is usually not tolerated well and may require early intervention.
- Conservative stabilization does not improve the underlying defect but instead the hemodynamics and symptoms. It mainly addresses heart failure caused by the valve pathology and can defer surgical intervention significantly.
- Mitral regurgitation
  - Volume restriction
  - Diuresis
  - Afterload reduction
  - Inotropic medication
  - Anticoagulation
- Medical management of severe MS can be difficult and is less effective than that of MR.
  - Diuresis (if signs of congestive heart failure)
  - Reduction in heart rate (to increase time of diastolic filling)
  - Anticoagulation
- Positive pressure ventilation (invasive or non-invasive) may be required in severe cases.

11 Surgical Strategy

- Mainstay of surgical treatment is valve repair, addressing the specific structural problem leading to valve dysfunction. A wide variety of techniques are described. Valve sparing repair should be attempted especially in the very young, even if higher than usual residual lesion (MR or MS) must be accepted. Mild MS is well tolerated if needed to achieve lesser grades of MR.
- Each part of the valvular apparatus can be addressed. Valve repair usually consists of a combination of these techniques:
- Annuloplasty (usually partial in children to preserve growth potential) (Fig. 5a).
- Reduction of the annular diameter by placing and tying a suture at the annular level.
  - This increases the zone of coaptation of anterior and posterior leaflet.
- Leaflet plication.
  - Folding and suturing of excess leaflet tissue allows for reversion of the repair.
  - Plication may reduce pliability and leaflet motion.

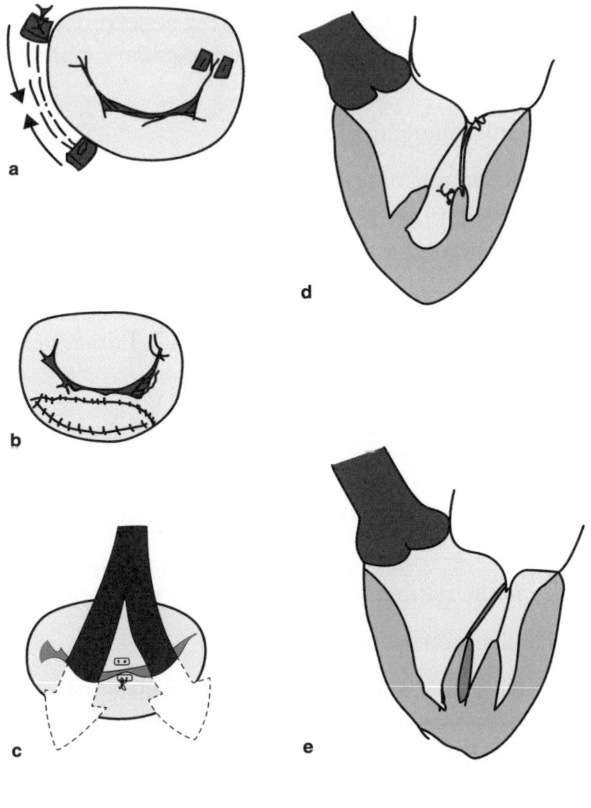

Fig. 5 Concepts of mitral valve repair. A Partial annuloplasty. B Patch augmentation of posterior mitral leaflet. C Alfieri stitch to create a double orifice. D Neochord insertion to posterior leaflet. E Longitudinal division to separate single papillary muscle

- Leaflet resection.
  - Triangular or quadrangular resections can reduce excess leaflet tissue in areas of prolapse.
- Leaflet extension (Fig. 5b).
  - Increase of area of coaptation by patch insertion (usually at the base of the leaflet). Treated Pericardium is commonly used.
- Commissurotomy.
  - Separation of fused commissures.
- Commissuroplasty (Fig. 5a).
  - Fusion of a commissure to reduce leakage or increase leaflet coaptation.
- Alfieri stitch (Fig. 5c).
  - Creation of a double orifice by adaptation of opposing parts of anterior and posterior leaflet edges.
- Chordal reinsertion.
  - Reinsertion of ruptured native chord.
  - Chordal replacement (GoreTex neochordae) (Fig. 5d).
  - Implantation of sutures from papillary muscle tip to leaflet edge (mimicking chordae tendineae).
- Chordal shortening/plication.
  - Reduction of chordal length by plication/folding of chordae. Usually includes the tip of the papillary muscle.
- Chordal division/relief of tethering.
  - Increases mobility of leaflets by reducing tethering while maintaining the level and heights of the coaptation zone. Primary chords are usually kept intact.
- Papillary muscle division (Fig. 5e).
  - Division (longitudinal) of papillary muscles to increase mobility and ventricular inflow, e.g., in parachute mitral valve.
- Papillary muscle shortening.
  - Similar to chordal shortening. Can be used to reduce prolapse of valve tissue in the setting of abnormally long papillary muscles
- Papillary muscle repositioning.
  - May be used to improve ventricular inflow and leaflet coaptation. Can be necessary in straddeling or LV outflow tract obstruction.
  - Resection of supravalvar/valvar/subvalvar fibrous tissue (i.e., supramitral ring)

11.1 Supramitral Ring

- Resection of the fibrous ring can be sufficient.
- The structure is usually located in close proximity to the mitral valve leaflets and care must be taken not to damage leaflets and adjacent structures (i.e., circumflex coronary artery).

11.2 Parachute and Hammock Mitral Valve

- To increase mobility of the valve leaflets in parachute mitral valve splitting of the single or fused papillary muscle can be used.
- Usually this aims at separate papillary muscles, supporting each commissure.
- In hammock mitral valves or mitral arcade, longitudinal division of the shortened chordae may increase mobility.
- Commissurotomy can be necessary.
- Detachment of the leading edge from papillary muscle and patch plasty with reinsertion to the muscle has been described.

11.3 Valve Replacement

- Options for valve replacement in the pediatric patient group are discussed in the respective chapter. In the mitral position, mechanical valve prostheses are favored due to the longer durability and lesser height.
- The use of mechanical valve prostheses is limited due to patient-prothesis mismatch and patient growth. Therefore, valve replacement should be regarded as a bailout if adequate valve repair cannot be achieved rather than a primary option.
- Valve implantation in small patients is usually performed in a supraannular position. Care must be taken to avoid damage to the circumflex artery and to ensure unimpaired leaflet opening.
- Surgical implantation of catheter valves (i.e., Medtronic Melody) have been used as alternatives, as partial expansion allows implantation in very small annuli and as these valves are dilatable once the patient grows. The valve cage is minimized and a sewing ring added to the valve by the surgeon. The collapsed valve is implanted into the mitral position and the valve then opened to the desired size with a balloon under direct vision.

12 Intensive Care Physiology and Management

- Postoperative management is to minimize afterload on the repaired valve and will be also dependent on degree of any residual MR or MS (unless associated defects exist). Therefore, medical management is similar to the therapeutic steps taken preoperatively.
- Anticoagulation is important and recommended for 3 months after repair or life-long after mechanical valve replacement. Unless a high risk of bleeding is suspected, anticoagulation should be initiated early postoperatively (after 6 h). Heparin is used and switched to warfarin, once chest tubes and pacing wires are removed.
- INR range 2.5–3.5 is targeted after mechanical valve replacement. The addition of low-dose ASA is recommended. INR of 2.5 is sufficient after valve repair.

13 Outcome

- Outcome is highly influenced by both mechanism of mitral valve disease and associated lesions. Intervention required in infancy carries much higher risk that in older children.

13.1 Valve Repair

- 3–4% in-hospital mortality
- 94% 5y survival
- 76% 5y freedom from reintervention

13.2 Valve Replacement

- 12–15% 30 day mortality
- 70% 5 year survival
- 62% 15 year survival
- Bleeding (6%)
- Thrombosis, thromboembolism (5%)
- Heart block, necessitating pacemaker (6%)
- Late arrhythmias (14%)
- (Prosthetic valve) endocarditis (6%)

14 Alternative Strategies and Controversies

- Although the experience with catheter mitral valve implantation in the pediatric population is limited, the strategy offers an interesting bailout option in very small patients with unrepairable valves, and has the additional possibility to dilate the valve, once a patient outgrows the implanted valve size.

Bibliography

1. Carpentier A, Adams D, Filsoufi F. Carpentier's reconstructive valve surgery. London: Elsevier Health Sciences; 2011.
2. Hetzer R, Delmo Walter E. Repair of congenital mitral valve insufficiency. Operative Tech Thorac Cardiovasc Surg. 2010;15(4):260–72.
3. Honjo, O., Chetan, D., Fan, C. P. S., Kadowaki, S., Marshall, A. C., Chaturvedi, R. R., ... & Barron, D. J. (2024). Surgical Melody mitral valve: a paradigm shift for infants with unrepairable mitral valve disease. The Annals of Thoracic Surgery, 118(3), 623–632. https://doi.org/10.1016/j.athoracsur.2024.04.037
4. Isaacson E, Lucjak C, Johnson W, et al. Mitral valve surgery in neonates, infants, and children: surgical approach, outcomes, and predictors. Semin Thorac Cardiovasc Surg. 2020;32(3):541–50.
5. Oppido G, Davies B, McMullan DM, et al. Surgical treatment of congenital mitral valve disease: midterm results of a repair-oriented policy. J Thorac Cardiovasc Surg. 2008;135(6):1313–21.
6. Pluchinotta F, Piekarski B, Milani V, et al. Surgical atrioventricular valve replacement with melody valve in infants and children: a multicenter study. Circ Cardiovasc Interv. 2018;11(11): e007145.

Aortic Stenosis

Conall Morgan and Lee Benson

Abstract Valvar aortic stenosis in infants and children is due to a congenital abnormality of the aortic valve complex, commonly associated with bicuspid or unicuspid valve morphology. This results in a reduction in the effective valve orifice leading to obstruction to outflow, and of varying degrees of severity. The severity of aortic valve stenosis is assessed using echocardiography and can be underestimated in the presence of left ventricular dysfunction. Critical or severe aortic valve stenosis in the newborn can present with cardiovascular collapse and shock. Older children are often asymptomatic. In many institutions balloon valvuloplasty is the preferred treatment modality of choice, however surgical valvotomy is an acceptable alternative strategy. Long term outcomes are good, however repeat interventions are not uncommon, with aortic valve replacement surgery often required in the long term.

Keywords Aortic stenosis · Bicuspid aortic valve · Balloon valvuloplasty · Aortic valvotomy

Abbreviations

AI	Aortic insufficiency
AS	Aortic stenosis
EFE	Endocardial fibroelastosis
HLHS	Hypoplastic left heart syndrome
LV	Left ventricle
MR	Mitral regurgitation

C. Morgan (✉) · L. Benson
Division of Cardiology, Department of Paediatrics, Labatt Family Heart Centre, The Hospital for Sick Children, University of Toronto, Toronto, ON, Canada
e-mail: Conallthomas.morgan@sickkids.ca

L. Benson
e-mail: Lee.benson@sickkids.ca

© The Author(s), under exclusive license to Springer Nature Switzerland AG 2024

A. I. Dipchand et al. (eds.), *Manual of Cardiac Care in Children*,
https://doi.org/10.1007/978-3-031-70973-9_24

PDA Persistent ductus arteriosus
VSD Ventricular septal defect

Key Points

- Bicuspid aortic valve (BAV) most common morphology (often the substrate for congenital or acquired stenosis, frequently seen with coarctation of the aorta).
- Critical aortic stenosis (ductal dependent systemic blood flow) in the neonate results from severely restricted forward flow and presents with poor peripheral perfusion and cyanosis when the arterial duct restricts or closes.
- Infants with severe, but not critical, stenosis may present with heart failure.
- Older children are rarely symptomatic and are generally identified by the presence of the characteristic murmur, and an ejection click.
- Obstruction in congenital valvar stenosis is often progressive, even if at presentation the gradients are low.
- Urgent treatment is indicated with severe obstruction, especially in the critically ill neonate and infant with heart failure.
- The decision to treat the asymptomatic older children is based on the systolic gradient, in the absence of left ventricular dysfunction *(see below assessment of severity).*
- Commonly, the initial treatment of choice is balloon valvuloplasty, regardless of the age and weight, however surgical valvotomy can also be considered
- Endocarditis prophylaxis is no longer recommended except in those with a prior history of endocarditis or who require prosthetic heart valves.

1 Nomenclature

Most Common Anatomical Setting

- Situs solitus
- Levocardia
- Atrioventricular concordance
- Ventriculoarterial concordance
- Left aortic arch.

2 Anatomy

- The aortic valve is positioned between the left ventricular outflow tract and the ascending aorta (see Fig. 1).
- The normal aortic valve consists of:

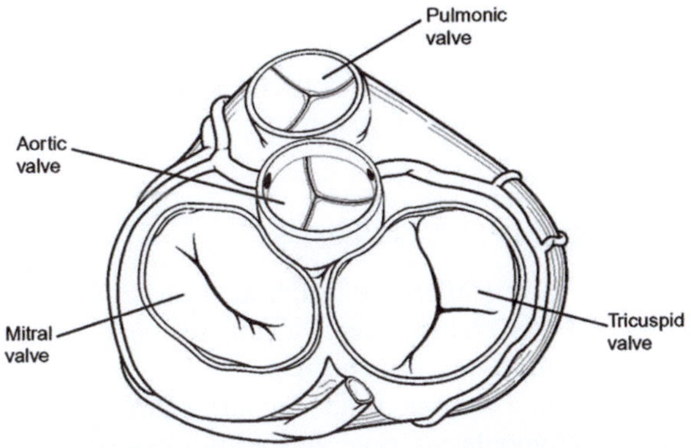

Fig. 1 Base of the heart delineating anatomic relations of the aortic valve and other heart valves

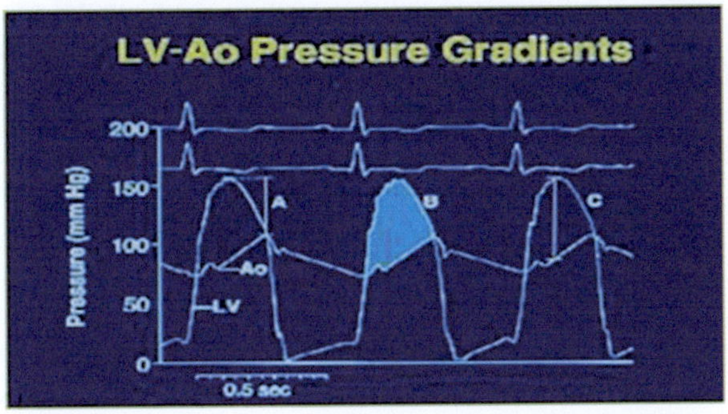

Fig. 2 Left ventricle versus aortic pressure gradients. A) peak-to-peak gradient, B) mean gradient, C) peak instantaneous gradient. LV—left ventricle; Ao—aorta

- Annulus

  Level of the junction of the aortic valve and the ventricular septum.
  Provides structural support to the aortic valve complex.
  Extends to the level of the aortic sinuses attached to the aortic wall media distally and the membranous and muscular ventricular septum proximally and anteriorly.

- Cusps

  Three valve cusps.
  Half-moon or semilunar in shape and each associated with an aortic sinus (sinus of Valsalva).
  The respective coronary ostia identify them as left, right, and posterior (or noncoronary).
  Each cusp has 1 free edge, shared with the adjacent cusp.

- Commissures

  The small spaces between each cusp's attachments and are equally spaced around the aortic root.

- Stenosis can be:
  - Valvar (~ 75% of cases)

    Valve leaflets are dysplastic (thickened).
    Often bicuspid: representing fusion of 2 of the leaflets with a resulting raphe, and an eccentric orifice.
    Can be unicuspid (acommissural/unicommisural), bicuspid, tricuspid (hypoplastic ring, dysplastic, cuspal inequality), quadracuspid; or six-cuspid.
    A unicuspid valve is seen in the neonatal expression of the disease.
    Secondary calcification in childhood is extremely rare.
    Valve annulus may in itself be hypoplastic, often associated with mitral or left ventricular hypoplasia.

3 Embryology

- The aortic valve is formed from cavitation of the conotruncal tissue ridge forming the 3 triangular valve leaflets; the right and left cusps form at the junction of the ventricular and arterial ends of the conotruncal canal, while the posterior cusp forms from additional conotruncal canal tissue.
- Abnormalities in this area lead to the development of incomplete separation (or fusion) of valve tissue, resulting in stenosis of the valve (most commonly the right and left) resulting in a smaller hemodynamic aortic orifice.
- Abnormal fetal hemodynamics likely contribute to the development of valve stenosis.

4 Epidemiology

- Incidence of congenital heart disease is ~ 8 per 1000 live births; aortic valve stenosis accounts for ~ 3–5%.
- A bicuspid but functionally normal aortic valve is estimated to occur in ~ 1% of the general population.
- There may be a higher prevalence in white than in black or Hispanic children.
- Male-to-female ratio is ~ 4:1.
- Recurrence risk in offspring of an affected father is ~ 3% and ~ 15% from an affected mother.

- A genetic defect has not been identified, but a bicuspid aortic valve can be identified in multiple family members and is a common defect in children with Turner syndrome.
- Isolated aortic valve stenosis is usually nonsyndromic; known associations with Turners, Jacobsen and Williams syndrome (mainly supravalvar disease) are common.

5 Clinical Physiology and Presentation

- Valvar aortic stenosis (AS) results in left ventricular hypertrophy, which is commensurate with the degree of obstruction.
- Mild-to-moderate degrees of obstruction are usually well tolerated, with minimal hypertrophy and normal LV function. If the hemodynamic orifice enlarges with growth, the degree of obstruction tends not to worsen. However, this is often not the case in valvar AS, with the obstruction worsening with somatic growth (increased stroke volume and oxygen demands with age).
- With severe hypertrophy and valvar obstruction, myocardial ischemia can result from a fixed cardiac output, reduced coronary perfusion and increased myocardial oxygen demand.
- A small, fixed, hemodynamic orifice will limit cardiac output increases with exercise and may result in exercise-induced syncope or sudden death.
- In utero, severe obstruction may lead to degrees of left heart hypoplasia (e.g., the forerunner of HLHS), endomyocardial fibroelastosis (EFE), decreased ventricular function, and important mitral valve regurgitation (MR).
- Neonates (~ 10% of affected individuals present in the neonatal period) are typically symptomatic and present with signs of congestive heart failure, poor feeding, tachypnea, decreased urine output, and irritability. When the arterial duct closes in the first days of life, systemic blood flow decreases, and the child may present with circulatory failure and cardiogenic shock.
- Older children are generally asymptomatic, the lesion often detected during a routine physical, school or pre-athletic examination. Symptoms that can occur include effort angina, syncope, dyspnea on exertion and fatigability. However, symptoms are rare until the disease is severe.
- The differential diagnosis of valvar AS includes hypertrophic cardiomyopathy, supra- and subvalvar AS.

6 Natural History

- The outcomes of children with congenital AS are dependent on valve morphology and the response to intervention. As noted above, the severity of obstruction varies widely, ranging from asymptomatic in those with a bicuspid but functionally normal valve with no stenosis to the critically ill neonate.
- Mortality is higher in neonates and infants who present with severe or critical disease, although this has decreased significantly over the past 2 decades.
- Mortality is often influenced by associated cardiac anomalies, which occur in 20% of children.
- Undetected, severe AS is a known cause of sudden death and accounts for ~ 1% of all cause sudden death in the young.
- Re-interventions (either surgical or percutaneous) are more often required in children diagnosed at a younger age (< 1 years) or more severe disease.

7 Associated Lesions

7.1 Common

- VSD
- Aortic coarctation
- Mitral valve abnormalities
- Left heart hypoplasia.

8 Diagnostic Studies

8.1 ECG

- Left ventricular hypertrophy with possible LV strain. The presence of a strain pattern indicates a degree of subendocardial ischemia and a greater severity of the obstruction. Its absence, particularly in the newborn, is reassuring. Infants without LV strain is at a low risk of sudden cardiac death.

8.2 CXR

- May note pulmonary venous congestion, and cardiomegaly.

8.3 Echocardiography

- Diagnostic imaging modality of choice.
- The following should be assessed:
  - Aortic valve morphology
  - Aortic valve annular diameter
  - Severity assessment
- Severity can be graded by measurement of the maximum instantaneous peak Doppler velocity and mean aortic transvalvular pressure gradient (Fig. 2). Importantly, severity can be underestimated in the presence of decreased LV function. In older children, an assessment of the valve area by the continuity equation can also be used.
  - Trivial stenosis Vmax < 2 m/s
  - Mild stenosis Vmax 2.0–2.9 m/s or mean gradient < 20 mmHg
  - Moderate stenosis Vmax 3.0–3.9 m/s or mean gradient 20–39 mmHg
  - Severe stenosis Vmax ≥ 4.0 m/s or mean gradient ≥ 40 mmHg
- Presence of aortic insufficiency (AI; moderate or severe AI may lead to overestimation of the degree of stenosis).
- Aortic root, arch and thoracic aorta dimensions.
- LV hypertrophy and function.
- MV morphology and function.
- Presence of associated lesions (VSD, PDA, arch coarctation).

8.4 Cardiac MRI

- If there is a question regarding the adequacy of the LV to support biventricular circulation, a cardiac MRI is useful to estimate ventricular volumes, flows and further details of ventricular and arch anatomy.

8.5 Cardiac CT

- CT can be used in older children to assess the aortic root and ascending aorta for presence of associated aortopathy

8.6 Cardiac Catheterization

- Not used routinely for diagnosis. Reserved for intervention.

8.7 Exercise Testing

- May be useful to assess symptomology if unclear from history.
- Useful for risk stratification in borderline cases where heart rate, blood pressure response, exercise duration and potential arrhythmias or ECG changes (signs of ischemia) can be evaluated.
- Helpful in assessing safety of exercise in mild to moderate cases, where no intervention is indicated by gradient alone. Often the child will report no limitations or symptoms on history, but objective findings on formal testing.

9 Indications for Intervention/Surgery

- Indications for intervention are based on the clinical status of the patient and transvalvar gradient, determined from echo-Doppler imaging.
- Indications for intervention:
  - In the newborn or child with decreased LV function the echo-Doppler-derived gradients may be low, and the clinical picture and morphology of the valve has to be considered.
  - Beyond infancy, in the asymptomatic child, intervention is based on mean transvalvar gradients, generally > 45 to 50 mmHg.
  - In adolescents and young adults, adult criteria can be applied based upon symptoms, gradient and calculated valve area (cm^2).

10 Timing of Intervention and Management Strategy

- Both surgical valvotomy and balloon valvuloplasty have similar outcomes. In experienced centers, a balloon approach is often considered as primary therapy, at any age in the absence of significant AI. In some centers particularly with a tricommisurate valve, surgery has been shown to have better outcomes. The more dysplastic the valve, the less the difference between balloon valvuloplasty and surgery.
- Surgical valvotomy is considered if there are hemodynamically significant additional lesions that warrant repair. However, often neonates with associated arch coarctation will undergo surgical arch repair followed by balloon valvuloplasty.
- In the case of acquired (post interventional) or primary severe AI, surgical intervention is required, either in the form of an aortic valve replacement, a Ross or Osaki procedure.
- Neonatal intervention is a choice between balloon valvuloplasty and surgical valvotomy/repair. Balloon valvuloplasty is more widely used but depends on institutional preference. Outcomes are very similar but freedom from AI is better in

the surgical group. Oversizing the balloon should be avoided as this can cause more AI.

- Balloon valvuloplasty continues to be effective in older age children, and is generally used as first choice, with surgical repair reserved for those with resistant stenosis or with co-existing AI.
- Surgical repair can be limited to valvotomy but also can include thinning of the leaflets, resection of nodules, false raphe and rebuilding commissures with a single patch.
- Unrepairable valves require replacement. First choice for replacement is the Ross procedure (pulmonary autograft, Fig. 3) as this is a living valve replacement that will grow with the child. Has the added advantage that it can be combined with root enlargement (Ross-Konno) to enlarge the LVOT where the annulus or subaortic area is small. Can be used in all age groups including neonates and for endocarditis.
- Contraindications to the Ross are abnormal/regurgitant pulmonary valve or dilated aortic annulus (> 20% larger than pulmonary annulus)
- Prosthetic aortic valve replacement is usually reserved for older children or when Ross is not possible. Annulus has to be large enough to accept the smallest manufactured valves (17 mm or in exceptional cases, 15 mm). Mechanical valves have lower profile and better hemodynamics in general—but require full anticoagulation using warfarin to a target INR of 2.5–3.5). Rarely, a homograft root can be used if no other options are available.
- An alternative to replacement in older children is the Osaki Procedure—three cusp aortic valve reconstruction, usually with treated pericardium as the leaflet material. This has mostly been used in adults and experience is very limited in children, as a minimum annulus size of 15 mm is needed.

11 Outcome

- Mortality associated with interventional procedures is low whether surgical or interventional—and mainly related to underlying LV function/EFE or associated MV disease.
- Balloon valvuloplasty or surgical valvotomy should be thought of as palliative procedures only as recurrence of the stenosis or development of regurgitation is common.
- Freedom from re-intervention is reported as 86% at 1 year, 67% at 5 years and 46% at 12 years.
- Ross procedure has operative mortality of 1–2% in most age-groups (10% in neonates, reflecting that it is only used in salvage situations) and freedom from autograft failure is 90% at 15 years.

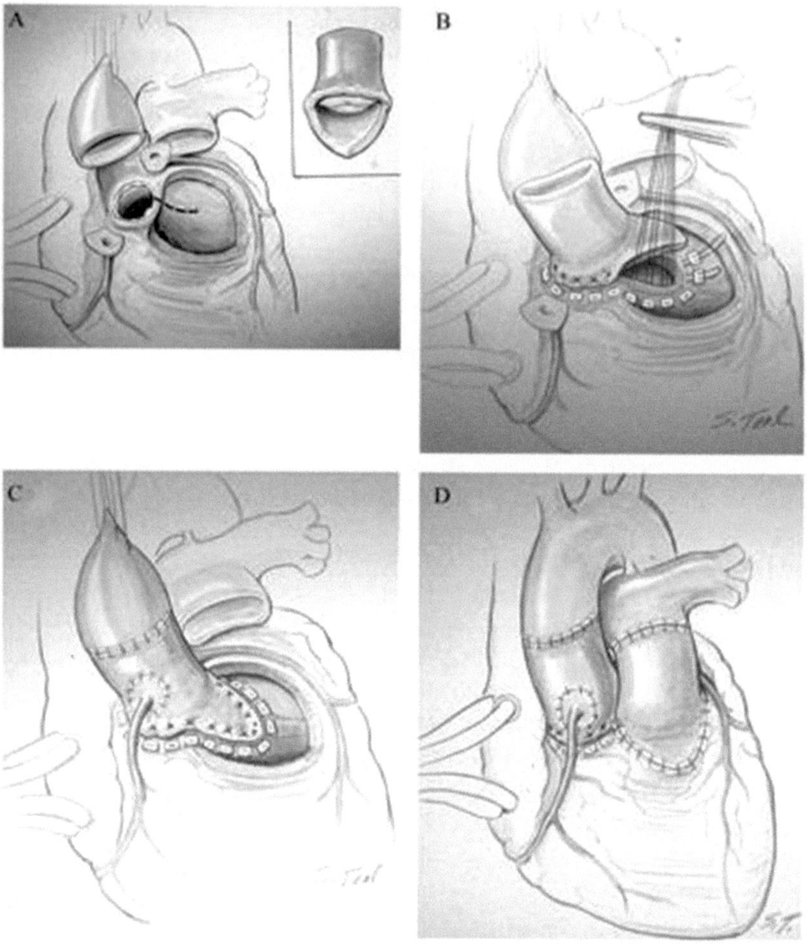

Fig. 3 The Ross-Konno Procedure. Reprinted from The Annals of Thoracic Surgery Vol 82, Issue 4, Brown JW, Ruzmetov M, Vijay P, et al., The Ross-Konno procedure in children: Outcomes, autograft and allograft function and reoperations, Pages 1301–1306, 2006, with permission from Elsevier

12 Alternative Strategies and Controversies

- Historically, the initial approach to management was primarily surgical. However, over the last 3 decades, percutaneous techniques have evolved, which in terms of therapeutic goals have equipoise with surgery. As such, a less non-invasive approach is attempted initially in most centres, but this does depend on institutional preference. Recurrent obstruction is treated with repeat balloon valvuloplasty, reserving surgical management to those with acquired severe regurgitation or annular hypoplasia.

Bibliography

1. Brown DW, Fulton DR, Armsby C. Valvar aortic stenosis in children. In: UpToDate Wolters Kluwer (2019). http://www.uptodate.com/contents/valvar-aortic-stenosis-in-children#H13529287. Accessed 21 Aug 2023
2. Feltes TF, Bacha E, Beekman RH 3rd, et al. Indications for cardiac catheterization and intervention in pediatric cardiac disease: a scientific statement from the American Heart Association. Circulation. 2011;123(22):2607–52.
3. Pedra CA, Sidhu R, McCrindle BW, et al. Outcomes after balloon dilation of congenital aortic stenosis in children and adolescents. Cardiol Young. 2004;14(3):315–21.

Supravalvar Aortic Stenosis

Christoph Haller

Abstract Supravalvar aortic stenosis is a rare type of left ventricular outflow tract stenosis and is most commonly localized at the sinotubular junction. It can be diffuse and extend into the distal aorta and supraaortic vessels. It can be part of more complex multilevel outflow obstructions. The disease is associated with Williams syndrome, an elastin gene mutation in 60–70% of cases. There is also an association with multiple branch pulmonary artery stenoses. Intervention is indicated if significant stenosis is present or symptomatic. Surgical risk is low and indication for surgery should consider potentially quick progression of the stenosis. Various patch techniques have been reported to address different aspects of the disease. Survival is good, but reintervention may be necessary.

Keywords Supravalvar aortic stenosis · Williams syndrome · Patch repair · Diffuse obstruction · Coronary artery stenosis · Left ventricular outflow tract obstruction

Abbreviations

LVOTO	Left ventricular outflow tract obstruction
PA	Pulmonary artery

C. Haller (✉)
Division of Cardiovascular Surgery, Labatt Family Heart Centre, Department of Surgery, The Hospital for Sick Children, University of Toronto, Toronto, ON, Canada
e-mail: christoph.haller@sickkids.ca

© The Author(s), under exclusive license to Springer Nature Switzerland AG 2024
A. I. Dipchand et al. (eds.), *Manual of Cardiac Care in Children*,
https://doi.org/10.1007/978-3-031-70973-9_25

Key Points

- Rare type of left ventricular outflow tract stenosis, usually localized at the sinotubular junction.
- Can be diffuse and extend into the distal aorta and supraaortic vessels and may involve the coronary ostia.
- Can be part of more complex multilevel outflow obstruction.
- Associated with elastin gene mutations (Williams syndrome).
- Treated if significant stenosis or symptomatic.
- Low threshold to operate as it can progress quickly, and risk of surgery is low.
- Surgery comprises resection of stenosis and patch plasty with various techniques.
- Outcome is good, with low surgical mortality, 90% long-term survival and 86% freedom from reintervention.

1 Nomenclature

- Supravalvar aortic stenosis commonly located at the sinotubular junction (if localized) or diffusely extending into ascending aorta and beyond.
- Aortic valve and sinus can be affected.
- Coronary artery ostial stenosis may be present and progress.

2 Anatomy

- Stenosis can vary in extent and there is thickening of the aortic wall as well as a characteristic hour-glass deformity. Usually localized but rarely is diffuse.
- Supravalvar stenosis usually starts at the level of the sinotubular junction (Fig. 1).
- This leads to enlargement of coronary arteries and the aortic root.
- Although often localized, the disease affects the aortic root and the aorta as well and can be very extensive into the arch and descending thoracic aorta in severe cases.
- Aortic valve leaflets can be thickened; coronary ostia and coronary artery flow can be impaired. Usually, the aortic valve is trileaflet with normal function—but bicuspid valves and leaflet dysplasia have been described.
- Multiple branch PA stenoses of variable severity may co-exist (particularly with William Syndrome)

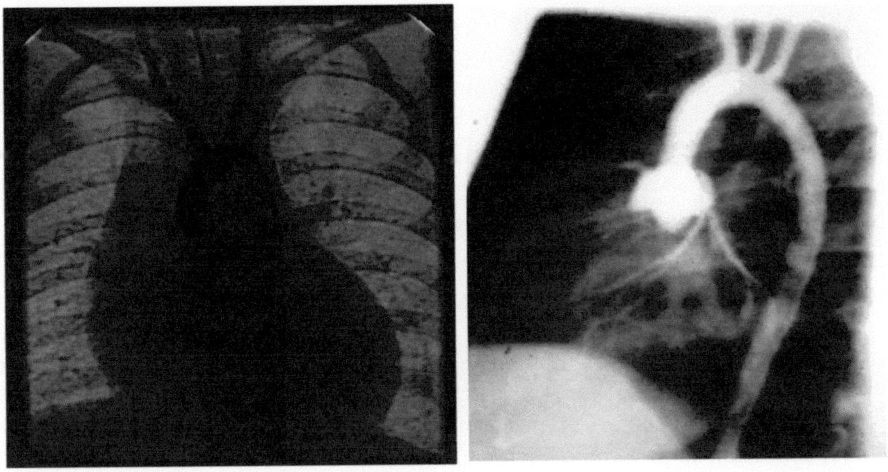

Fig. 1 Supraaortic stenosis on angiography

3 Epidemiology

3.1 Incidence/Prevalence

- Least common form of congenital aortic stenosis.
- 1/20,000 live births.
- Important isolated supravalvar aortic stenosis constitutes about 3% of patients with congenital left ventricular outflow tract obstruction.

3.2 Population at Risk, Inheritance

- High association with Williams syndrome (7q11.23 elastin gene mutation).
- Other familial associations have been reported but sporadic cases that are non-Williams still account for 30–40% of cases.

4 Clinical Physiology and Presentation

- Highly dependent on extent of narrowing and associated obstruction at other levels of the left ventricular outflow tract.
- Obstruction leads to left ventricular hypertrophy.
- Rarely symptomatic early in life.
- Symptoms are similar to other obstructions of the left ventricular outflow tract.

- Although stenosis is commonly located distally to the coronary artery origin, myocardial ischemia and angina may still occur due to ostial stenosis, impaired flow (supply–demand mismatch) into the coronaries, or early onset arteriosclerosis.

4.1 Natural History

- Risk of sudden death (as seen in other types of left ventricular outflow tract obstruction, LVOTO).
- Rapid progression more commonly seen than in other forms of outflow tract stenosis.
- Milder degrees of stenosis may not require intervention and remain stable.
- Freedom from surgical intervention 46% ± 6% at 10 years.

5 Associated Lesions

5.1 Common

- LVOTO at other levels
- PA stenoses
- Williams syndrome (7q11.23 elastin gene mutation)

5.2 Less Common Associations

- Bicuspid aortic valve
- Involvement of peripheral arteries

6 Diagnostic Studies

- Patients may have a murmur on auscultation.
- Elfin facies (short and upturned nose, wide set eyes, wide mouth) is a typical clinical appearance in patients with Williams syndrome.

6.1 ECG

- Normal early in life.

- Signs of left ventricular hypertrophy.
- Signs of ischemia if impaired coronary blood flow or with exercise (leading to supply–demand mismatch).

6.2 CXR

- Cardiomegaly
- Pulmonary congestion if severe stenosis and associated heart failure.

6.3 Echocardiography

- Echocardiography adequately delineates the anatomy in most cases.
- Location, extent, and severity of supravalvar aortic stenosis.
- Multilevel left ventricular outflow tract obstruction
- Aortic valve involvement (thickened or tethered leaflets)
- Coronary artery flow
- Ventricular hypertrophy and function.
- PA stenosis.

6.4 CT

- It is important to assess aorta and all branches as well as to define the extent of each lesion. Also assesses pulmonary vascular tree.
- CT preferred over MRI to image aortic anatomy.

6.5 MRI

- Rarely used unless assessment of ventricular function necessary.

6.6 Cardiac Catheterization

- Not regularly performed.
- Invasive measurement of gradients across the stenosis.
- Assessment of coronary artery anatomy and obstruction if concern of ostial involvement.
- Rarely used for intervention (more common in restenosis post repair).

7 Indications for Intervention/Surgery

- Not well defined in the literature.
- Significant stenosis can be considered if echocardiographic peak gradient > 50 mmHg, mean > 30–35 mmHg, or if the patient is symptomatic.
- Threshold to proceed with surgery lower than in valvular stenosis as surgical risk lower and higher rate of progression.
- If non-symptomatic and gradient less than moderate, managed expectantly. Gradual reduction in stenosis without treatment has been observed.
- If part of complex LVOTO, indication may be triggered by higher grade obstruction at another level.
- PA stenoses may be an indication for surgical intervention if RV pressure is close to systemic, especially if planning surgery for co-existing supraaortic stenosis. Stenoses tend to regress with age.

8 Timing of Intervention and Management Strategy

- Timing is determined based on severity of stenosis and symptoms (see section "Indications for Intervention/Surgery").
- Need for surgical intervention is highest within three years of diagnosis.

9 Surgical Strategy

- Surgical repair consists of resection of stenosis and patch augmentation of the respective aortic segment. In diffuse disease, extensive patch reconstruction of the ascending aorta, arch and descending aorta may be necessary.
- The aorta is incised longitudinally from the ascending aorta proximally into one or multiple aortic sinus.
- Fibrous stenosis can be resected or peeled off.
- Different patching techniques have been described (see Fig. 2)
  - Simple 1-patch: patch enlargement into the non-coronary sinus
  - Y-shaped patch (Doty): patch enlargement into both right- and non-coronary sinus (inverted Y-shape of the patch). This is most widely used technique and splits the supra-aortic ridge at two points.
  - 3-patch (Brom): separate enlargement of all three sinuses and end-to-end anastomosis of aorta
  - No patch: enlargement of all three sinuses with interdigitating incisions in the distal ascending aorta to avoid artificial material
  - If coronary ostia are involved, causing ostial narrowing then these need to be opened out and patched as part of the repair.

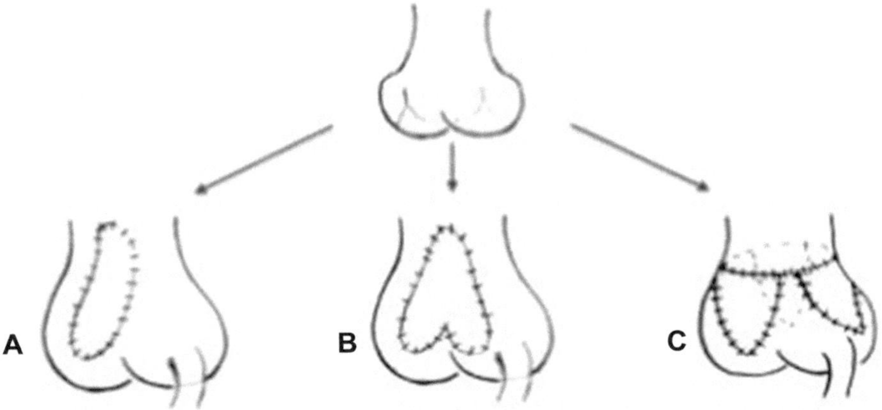

Fig. 2 Surgical repair techniques for supravalvar aortic stenosis. A Single patch technique. B Doty repair. C Brom technique

- Risk of coronary artery distortion with patching of sinuses.
  - H-repair is a two-patch technique that can avoid geometric distortion/dislocation of coronary artery origins.
- Risk of aortic valve distortion and resulting aortic insufficiency.
- Complex reconstructions of diffuse disease may necessitate hypothermic cardiac arrest, selective cerebral perfusion and/or alternative cannulation strategies (e.g., femoral cannulation).

10 Intensive Care Physiology and Management

- Postoperative care is usually the same as for all major cardiac procedures.
- Ventricular diastolic function can be impaired postoperatively and may need adequate preload.
- Coronary artery distortion is usually diagnosed intraoperatively and corrected, but residual aortic or coronary stenosis can occur.

11 Outcome

- Early postoperative mortality is low (3–4%) in the patient group with mixed types of supravalvar aortic stenosis.
- 10-year survival > 90%
- 20-year survival approaches 90%
- 10-year freedom from reintervention for recurrent stenosis is 73–86%.

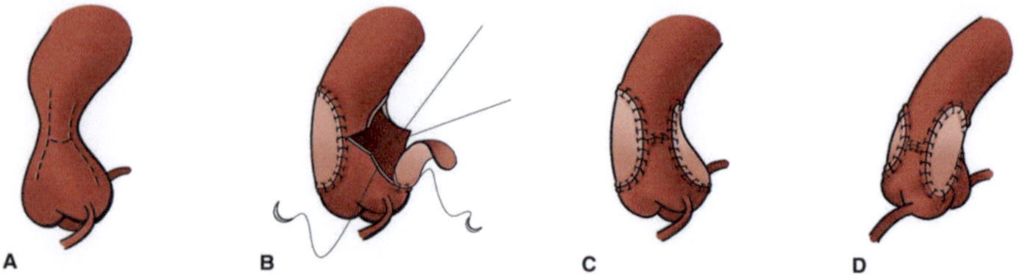

Fig. 3 H-technique for supravalvar aortic stenosis. Reprinted from JTCVS Techniques, Vol 6, Issue 4, Luo S, Haller C, Deng MX, Honjo O, H-repair in supravalvular aortic stenosis, pp. 114–117, 2021, with permission from Elsevier

12 Alternative Strategies and Controversies

12.1 Patch-Technique

- Patching may change the aortic root geometry significantly.
- Y-patch repair most commonly used.
- This increases the anterior length of the sinotubular junction and the ascending aorta with the risk of right coronary artery kinking.
- 3-patch technique is favored by some institutions to preserve a symmetric geometry of the aortic root.
- The H-repair aims to limit the longitudinal enlargement of the aorta by the patch, thereby reducing the risk of coronary artery kinking (see Fig. 3).

Bibliography

1. Doty DB, Polansky DB, Jenson CB. Supravalvular aortic stenosis. Repair by extended aortoplasty. J Thorac Cardiovasc Surg. 1977;74(3):362–71.
2. Luo S, Haller C, Deng MX, et al. H-Repair in supravalvular aortic stenosis. JTCVS Tech. 2021;6:114–7.
3. Hickey E, Jung G, Williams W, et al. Congenital supravalvular aortic stenosis: defining surgical and nonsurgical outcomes. Ann Thorac Surg. 2008;86(6):1919–27.
4. Fricke T, d'Udekem Y, Brizard C, et al. Surgical repair of supravalvular aortic stenosis in children with williams syndrome: a 30-year experience. Ann Thorac Surg. 2015;99(4):1335–41.

Subaortic Stenosis

Mimi Xiaoming Deng and Osami Honjo

Abstract Subaortic stenosis (SAS) is a rare congenital heart defect affecting 8 in 10,000 live births. SAS refers to a group of diverse defects with obstruction to systemic blood flow originating below the aortic valve, including subaortic membrane, fibromuscular ridge, accessory mitral valve tissue, septal hypertrophy, acute aortoventricular angle, and funnel-shaped left ventricular outflow tract (LVOT). Patients with SAS present similarly to aortic stenosis, with symptoms of exertional angina, syncope/presyncope, or even heart failure if diagnosed late. SAS can also be an incidental finding in asymptomatic patients. SAS is associated with other left-sided stenotic lesions, including congenital mitral stenosis, bicuspid aortic valve, aortic arch hypoplasia, or coarctation. Diagnosis is generally made by doppler echocardiography and can also be identified by computed tomography angiography or cardiac magnetic resonance imaging. Definitive surgical intervention to relieve the obstructing lesion is indicated if symptomatic, mean pressure gradient is $\geq$ 50 mmHg, or presence of left ventricular hypertrophy. Iatrogenic ventricular septal defect, mitral or aortic valve injury, complete heart block, residual stenosis due to incomplete resection, and left ventricular diastolic dysfunction are postoperative complications that must be monitored closely.

Keywords Subaortic stenosis · Fibromuscular ridge · Septal hypertrophy · Konno procedure

Abbreviations

AI	Aortic insufficiency
AS	Aortic stenosis

M. X. Deng · O. Honjo (✉)
Department of Cardiovascular Surgery, Labatt Family Heart Centre, Hospital for Sick Children, University of Toronto, Toronto, ON, Canada
e-mail: Osami.honjo@sickkids.ca

M. X. Deng
e-mail: Mimixiaoming.deng@sickkids.ca

© The Author(s), under exclusive license to Springer Nature Switzerland AG 2024

A. I. Dipchand et al. (eds.), *Manual of Cardiac Care in Children*,
https://doi.org/10.1007/978-3-031-70973-9_26

AVSD	Atrioventricular septal defect
CMRI	Cardiac magnetic resonance imaging
CoA	Coarctation
CT	Computed tomography
ECG	Electrocardiogram
HLHS	Hypoplastic left heart syndrome
HOCM	Hypertrophic obstructive cardiomyopathy
LV	Left ventricle
LVH	Left ventricular hypertrophy
LVOT	Left ventricular outflow tract
LVOTO	Left ventricular outflow tract obstruction
OR	Operating room
RV	Right ventricle
SAS	Subaortic stenosis
VSD	Ventricular septal defect

Key Points

- Subaortic stenosis (SAS) is a rare congenital heart defect that encompasses a spectrum of lesions originating below the aortic valve that obstruct to systemic blood flow
- Presentation can be asymptomatic to severe hemodynamic compromise from critical obstruction
- Associated with other left-heart obstructive lesions
- Definitive management, when indicated, is surgical and involves relieving source of obstruction
- Postoperative complications include congenital heart block, residual or recurrent stenosis, and/or iatrogenic injury to the aortic valve, mitral valve, or interventricular septum.

1 Anatomy

- The left ventricular outflow tract (LVOT) is the passage from the left ventricle (LV) to the ascending aorta, comprising of 3 components:
  1. Subaortic component formed by
     a. Anterior mitral valve leaflet—beneath left and non-coronary commissure
     b. Membranous septum—beneath right and non-coronary commissure
     c. Muscular septum—beneath left and right commissure
  2. Aortic valve and aortic root
  3. Supravalvular component above the sinotubular junction

- Subaortic stenosis (SAS) describes a group of obstructive lesions below the aortic valve (Fig. 1)
  - Subaortic membrane
  - Subaortic fibromuscular ridge
  - Septal hypertrophy [e.g., hypertrophic obstructive cardiomyopathy (HOCM)]
  - Accessory mitral valve tissue—accessory chordae or fibrous nodules/cysts
  - Abnormal aortoventricular angle
    - Systolic anterior motion of the mitral valve
    - Posterior deviation of the outlet interventricular septum in the setting of perimembranous or subaortic ventricular septal defect (VSD)
- Funnel-shaped LVOT (e.g., after atrioventricular septal defect [AVSD] repair)
- Bulging/intrusion of intraventricular septum (e.g., with right ventricular [RV] hypertension of any etiology)

2 Epidemiology

- SAS accounts for 1% of pediatric congenital heart defects (8 in 10,000 births) and 6.5% of adult congenital heart diseases
  - Greater male predilection, with 2:1 male:female prevalence ratio
  - 10–14% of SAS is observed in children with congenital aortic stenosis
- One theory suggests that SAS is caused by abnormal flow during embryonic development
  - A narrow LVOT, exaggerated aortic override, increased mitral-aortic septation, subaortic VSD, and steep atrioventricular septal angle may result in a chronic flow disturbance
  - Shear stress on interventricular septum induces endothelial and muscle proliferation, resulting in formation of fibromuscular ridge

3 Associated Lesions

- SAS is associated with other cardiac anomalies in 50–65% of cases
  - Aortic valve—aortic stenosis (AS), aortic insufficiency (AI)
  - Aortic coarctation, hypoplasia of ascending aorta and arch, interrupted aortic arch
  - Mitral valve lesions (e.g. supravalvular mitral membrane, parachute mitral valve)
  - AVSD
  - VSD

- Diffuse left-sided obstructions
    - Hypoplastic left heart syndrome (HLHS)
    - Shone complex—constellation of mitral valve abnormality with LVOT obstruction (LVOTO), ± aortic arch abnormality

4 Clinical Physiology and Presentation

- SAS, regardless of severity, has little impact during fetal circulation due to maintenance of systemic circulation through the RV via the patent ductus arteriosus
- Isolated SAS rarely presents in infancy and most cases present in older children
- Mild and moderate SAS
    - Usually asymptomatic, systolic ejection murmur over aortic area radiating to the suprasternal notch, that decreases with Valsalva maneuver
    - Failure to thrive and effort intolerance in some cases
    - Dynamic cardiac impulse, symmetrically diminished femoral pulses, palpable carotid or left parasternal thrill, cool pallid skin with mottling, hepatomegaly with subcostal recession
- Severe SAS
    - May have effort intolerance, failure to thrive, tachypnea, and subcostal recession
    - Episode of syncope or pre-syncope in severe cases and can present with sudden death
    - Critical cases have signs of low cardiac output state manifesting as hypotension, decreased urine output, lactic acidosis, decreased level of consciousness, or even death
- Neonatal SAS is usually seen as part of a constellation of left sided obstructive lesions including arch obstruction and interrupted arch

5 Natural History

- SAS can often be asymptomatic and diagnosed as an incidental finding
- Neonatal presentation of isolated SAS is rare, in which case it is usually associated with multiple left sided obstructive lesions
- Most cases of isolated SAS present in later childhood and are often asymptomatic
- Similar to aortic stenosis, LVOTO can lead to left ventricular hypertrophy (LVH) and heart failure, as well as risk of sudden cardiac death from lethal ventricular arrhythmias and myocardial ischemia

- Symptoms of severe SAS include increasing dyspnea on exercise, fatigue, exertional angina, syncope/pre-syncope with exercise

6 Diagnostic Studies

6.1 Electrocardiogram (ECG)

- LVH
  - Deep S-waves in V1, V2 and Tall R in V4-6
  - Strain indicated by T-wave inversion in II, III, AVF, V5, V6
- Q-wave in left precordial leads suggest septal hypertrophy

6.2 Chest X-ray

- Cardiomegaly if LVH
- Plethoric lung fields if RV dysfunction

6.3 Echocardiography (Fig. 2)

- Primary diagnostic modality
- LVOTO should be comprehensively interrogated for:

- Mechanism
  - Mode of obstruction—membrane, LVOT fibrosis, septal deviation, etc.
  - Anatomy of aortic and mitral valves—number of leaflets, thickness, mobility
  - Lesions—nodules or vegetation
- Severity—continuous wave and pulse wave doppler
- Presence and severity of associated left sided lesions (mitral stenosis, coarctation, AS)
- Assessment of LV function and hypertrophy

6.4 CT and MRI

- Computed tomography (CT) and cardiac magnetic resonance imaging (CMRI) are only necessary if needed to evaluate complex LVOTO and extent of LVH

Table 1 Indications and management of SAS

Doppler mean gradient (mmHg)	Management
< 30	Medical management if no LVH
30–50	Operative management if symptomatic, or if asymptomatic but demonstrates exertional ECG changes
> 50	Operative management

6.5 Cardiac Catheterization

- Predominantly replaced by CMRI and cardiac CT in the assessment of coronaries
- Catheterization can be used for both diagnostic and therapeutic purpose in children treated with primary balloon valvuloplasty in concomitant critical/severe AS

6.6 Cardiopulmonary Exercise Testing

- Provide objective evidence of functional limitation if baseline symptoms are vague

7 Indications for Intervention/Surgery

- Surgical repair is definitive treatment
- Indication and timing of surgery vary depending on severity of LVOTO and associated lesions
- In isolated SAS, surgical intervention is indicated if
  - Symptomatic
  - Mean doppler gradient > 50 mmHg
  - Signs of LVH
  - Worsening AI
- Threshold for intervention in LVOTO associated with VSD is lower due to increased VSD left-to-right shunting from outlet obstruction
- General principles of management are shown in Table 1

8 Surgical Strategy

- Isolated SAS
  - Hockey-stick aortotomy into the non-coronary sinus or transverse aortotomy at sino-tubular junction
  - Subaortic lesions are primarily treated working through the aortic valve
    - Membranes peel off myocardium easily with blunt and sharp dissection

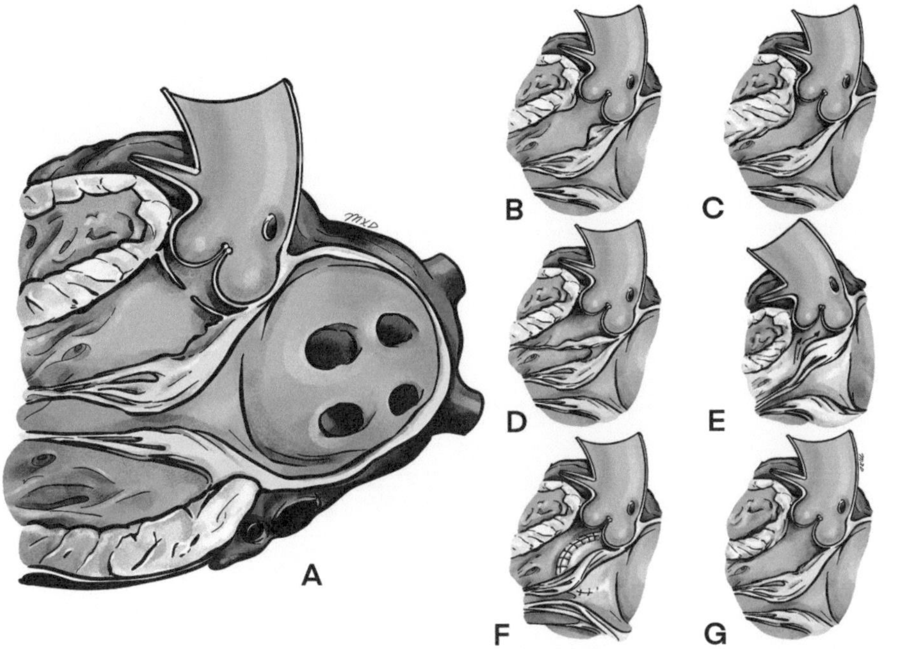

Fig. 1 Mechanisms of SubAortic Obstruction: A) Sub-aortic membrane, B) Sub-aortic fibrous ridge, C) Septal hypertrophy, D) Mitral valve accessory chordae, E) Abnormal atrioventricular angle causing systolic anterior motion of the mitral valve, F) Funnel-shaped LVOT after AVSD repair, G) Bulging of intraventricular septum from RV hypertension

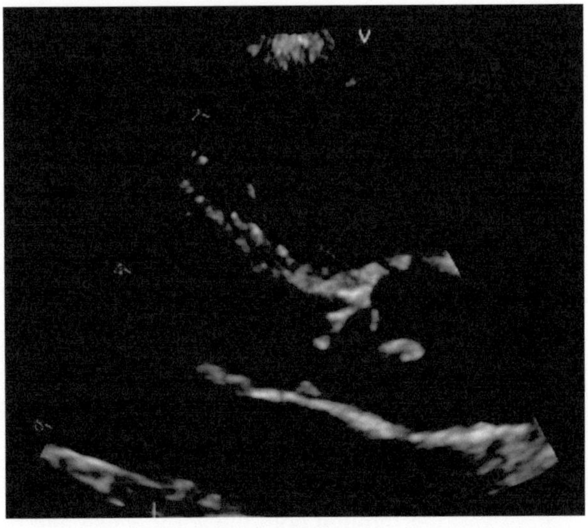

Fig. 2 Fibromuscular ridge on echocardiogram (parasternal long axis view). Reprinted from Circulation, Vol 114, Issue 22, Aboulhosn J, Child JS, Left ventricular outflow obstruction, pp 2414, 2006, with permission from Wolters Kluwer Health Inc

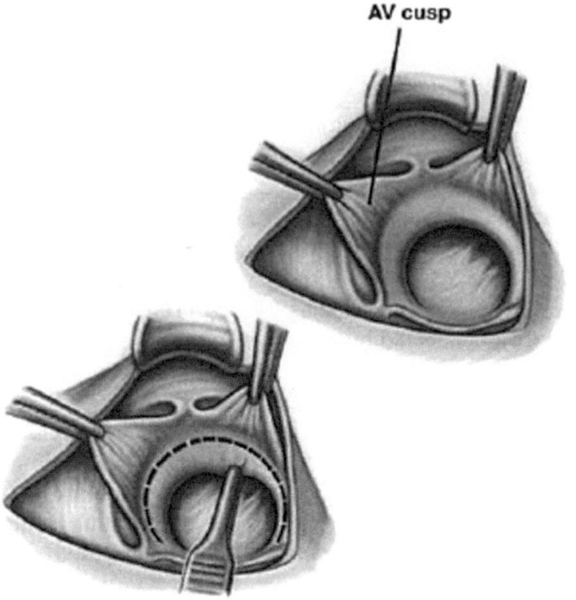

Fig. 3 Fibromuscular ridge resection. Surgery of the left ventricular outflow tract. Reprinted from Surgery for Congenital Heart Defects, 3rd edition, Stark JF, de Leval MR, Courtney M, Tsang VT, pp 503, 2006, with permission from John Wiley and Sons

- Fibromusuclar ridges are circumferentially excised completely into its mitral or aortic valve extension (Fig. 3)
- LVOT myectomy may be needed if significant septal LVH; many centres recommend routine resection of septal muscle wedge to minimise risk of recurrence
- Removal of accessory mitral valve chords, while maintaining mitral valve competence
- Remove mitral valve cysts and accessory tissue tags

- SAS with septal defect
  - In VSD repair, SAS lesion can be accessed through the tricuspid valve
  - In AVSD repair, SAS lesion can be accessed through the common AV valve
- SAS with functionally univentricular circulation – manage with single ventricle palliation
  - Norwood procedure if HLHS
  - Damus-Kaye-Stansel procedure if double-inlet left ventricle with normal arch
- Tunnel-type LVOTO
  - Normal aortic valve and annulus treated with a Modified Konno Procedure – working through both the aortic valve and the RV, muscle is resected and a VSD created to enlarge the subaortic region, followed by VSD patch repair placed on the RV side of the septum
  - More commonly, hypoplastic aortic valve and annulus treated with:

    - Ross-Konno procedure (aortoventriculoplasty) – preferred in infant and children; the autograft is harvested with larger muscle skirt than usual, and this is laid into the septal incision to augment the LVOT
    - Bentall procedure or Konno-Rastan is an alternative in adolescents and adults, using a prosthetic aortic valve

- Surgical complications of LVOT surgery
  - Iatrogenic VSD
  - Heart block from damage to bundle of His
  - Residual stenosis or recurrent stenosis
  - Anterior mitral valve injury
  - AR due to iatrogenic leaflet or commissural injury
  - Postoperative low cardiac output due to left ventricular diastolic dysfunction

9 Intensive Care Physiology and Management

- Elective cases undergo extubation in the operating room (OR) and require standard postoperative care of avoiding systemic hypertension in view of aortic suture lines
- LVH - rate control targeting low-normal heart rate, maintain sinus rhythm, avoid hypovolemia; volume resuscitation and pressors to treat hypotension
- Evaluate rhythm
  - Complications of complete heart block are generally identified in OR
  - Repair of neonatal SAS with VSD can be associated with junctional ectopic tachycardia.

10 Surgical Outcomes

- Isolated SAS repair
  - Operative mortality of < 2%
  - Reoperation in 10–15% of cases
  - 10-year survival > 95%.
  - Late AI in 20% of cases
- Tunnel LVOTO carry greater operative risk and decreased freedom from late death and reoperation than discrete SAS
- Independent predictors for reoperation are:
  - Female gender
  - Increasing LVOT gradient progression over time
  - Preoperative peak instantaneous LVOT gradient ≥ 80 mmHg
  - Age > 30 y at time of diagnosis.

11 Alternative Strategies and Controversies

- Alternative to myectomy is radio-frequency muscle ablation and/or selective alcohol septal ablation in cases of asymmetric muscular hypertrophy (see Chap. 40).
- Concomitant endocardial fibroelastosis resection can also be performed at time of index surgery to improve left ventricular compliance

Bibliography

1. Choi JY, Sullivan ID. Fixed subaortic stenosis: anatomical spectrum and nature of progression. Br Heart J. 1991;65(5):280–6.
2. Erentug V, Bozbuga N, Kirali K, et al. Surgical treatment of subaortic obstruction in adolescents and adults: long-term follow-up. J Card Surg. 2005;20(1):16–21.
3. Ezon DS. Fixed subaortic stenosis: a clinical dilemma for clinicians and patients. Congenit Heart Dis. 2013;8(5):450–6.
4. Karamlou T, Gurofsky R, Bojcevski A, et al (2007) Prevalence and associated risk factors for intervention in 313 children with subaortic stenosis. Ann Thorac Surg 84(3), 900–6; discussion 906.
5. Kitchiner D, Jackson M, Malaiya N, et al. Incidence and prognosis of obstruction of the left ventricular outflow tract in Liverpool (1960–91): a study of 313 patients. Br Heart J. 1994;71(6):588–95.
6. Liu CW, Hwang B, Lee BC, et al. Aortic stenosis in children: 19-year experience. Zhonghua Yi Xue Za Zhi (Taipei). 1997;59(2):107–13.
7. Oliver JM, González A, Gallego P, et al. Discrete subaortic stenosis in adults: increased prevalence and slow rate of progression of the obstruction and aortic regurgitation. J Am Coll Cardiol. 2001;38(3):835–42.
8. Said SM. The Ross-Konno procedure for congenital aortic stenosis. Ann Cardiothorac Surg. 2021;10(4):527–37.
9. Schlein J, Wollmann F, Kaider A, et al. Long-term outcomes after surgical repair of subvalvular aortic stenosis in pediatric patients. Front Cardiovasc Med. 2022;9:1033312.

Coarctation of the Aorta

Rachel D. Vanderlaan

Abstract Coarctation of the aorta, aortic arch hypoplasia and interrupted aortic arch are congenital lesions whereby the aortic arch is either atretic, discontinuous or small for body surface area. Coarctation of the aorta can present in the neonate, infant, child or rarely in the adult. The timing of presentation is dependent on the severity of the coarctation, the presence of a PDA, and any associated arch hypoplasia. In neonates with severe coarctation and duct dependant systemic circulation, early institution of PGEs is critical in initial management. For simple coarctation without significant proximal arch hypoplasia, an extended end to end anastomosis via a left thoracotomy is preferred with low rates of reintervention and low mortality. Associate transverse arch hypoplasia may require more extensive surgery. Older children are increasingly managed with interventional approaches including balloon dilatation and stenting.

Keywords Coarctation of the aorta (CoA) · End-to-end repair · Extended end-to-end repair · Subclavian flap repair · Aortic arch hypoplasia · Thoracotomy

Abbreviations

ASD	Atrial septal defect
AVSD	Atrioventricular septal defect
CoA	Coarctation of the aorta
DORV	Double outlet right ventricle
LSCA	Left subclavian artery
LV	Left ventricle
PDA	Persistent ductus arteriosus
PGE	Prostaglandin
TGA	Transposition of the great arteries
THAA	Tubular hypoplasia of the aortic arch

R. D. Vanderlaan (✉)
Division of Cardiovascular Surgery, Department of Surgery, Labatt Family Heart Centre, Hospital for Sick Children, University of Toronto, Toronto, ON, Canada
e-mail: Rachel.vanderlaan@sickkids.ca

© The Author(s), under exclusive license to Springer Nature Switzerland AG 2024

A. I. Dipchand et al. (eds.), *Manual of Cardiac Care in Children*,
https://doi.org/10.1007/978-3-031-70973-9_27

VSD Ventricular septal defect

Key Points

- 2 subgroups: symptomatic neonate/infant and asymptomatic older children
- Critically ill neonates with duct dependant systemic circulation can present with hemodynamic compromise and typically present within the first 2 weeks of life after ductal closure.
- Resection with end-to-end anastomosis via a left thoracotomy is surgical approach of choice for a simple coarctation without arch involvement.
- Extended end-to-end anastomosis via left thoracotomy is indicated for simple CoA with distal hypoplastic aortic arch.
- Arch reconstruction through a sternotomy should be considered if there is proximal arch hypoplasia.
- Important role of interventional techniques in older infants/children

1 Nomenclature

- Left aortic arch, coarctation of the aorta (location and severity), associated defects such as ventricular septal defect and left ventricular outflow tract obstruction (subvalvular, valvular, supravalvular).

2 Anatomy

- The aortic arch is divided into 3 main segments
  - Proximal arch: innominate artery to left common carotid artery
  - Distal arch: left common carotid to left subclavian artery
  - Isthmus: left subclavian artery to ductus arteriosus (or ligamentum arteriosus)
- Narrowing of the distal aorta typically at the isthmus just distal to the left subclavian artery
- Can present with tubular hypoplasia of the aortic arch (THAA)
- Clinically significant arm-leg blood pressure (BP) gradient of greater than 20 mmHg or anatomical narrowing of > 50% compared to the supradiaphragmatic descending aorta.

3 Embryology

3.1 Three Main Theories

1. Abnormal embryogenesis of the vessels in the arch
2. Abnormal ductal tissue in the wall of the aorta at the site of arterial duct insertion leads to posterior aortic shelf
3. Flow related lesion whereby high flow in the ductal arch (left-to-right shunts) can lead to underdevelopment of the transverse arch and isthmus during fetal life

4 Epidemiology

- Accounts for 4–7% of all congenital heart defects
- Prevalence of approximately 4 per 10,000 births
- Male predominance
- Associated with Turner's Syndrome (30%).

5 Clinical Physiology and Presentation

5.1 Neonates

- Clinical presentation will vary with severity of the coarctation
- With closure of ductus arteriosus, neonates with significant CoA will present with poor femoral pulses and differential BP gradient between the upper and lower extremities
- Severe CoA leads to hemodynamic decompensation with metabolic acidosis, impaired ventricular function and end-organ dysfunction.

5.2 Infants and Young Children

- Typically, those presenting with CoA in later infancy or childhood initially had less severe lesions and collateral arteries have developed to augment blood flow distal to the narrowing.
- Those with moderate lesions may present in early infancy with gradual decline and heart failure (may be biventricular) can manifest with tachypnea and failure to thrive
- Children usually asymptomatic and most commonly diagnosed as a chance finding due to identification of a murmur, hypertension, abnormal ECG or CXR.

6 Natural History

- Severe obstruction can result in neonatal demise if not surgically corrected.
- If the PDA closes slowly or there is less severe narrowing, collateralization to the distal aorta can occur. Clinically significant upper extremity hypertension can also develop.
- The hypertension can lead to extensive changes in the vasculature proximal to the CoA, with accelerated atherosclerosis, aortic dilatation (risk of dissection and rupture) and cerebral aneurysms.

7 Associated Lesions

7.1 Common

- Bicuspid aortic valve (up to 60%)
- VSD (30–40%).

7.2 Association with Other Congenital Heart Defects

- Shone's Complex (supravalvar mitral ring, parachute mitral valve, subaortic stenosis, and coarctation of aorta)
- Transposition of the great arteries with VSD and Taussig-Bing Anomaly (DORV of TGA-type)
- AVSD
- Small left-sided structures.

8 Diagnostic Studies

8.1 ECG

- Right ventricular hypertrophy in the first few months of life.
- In older children, predominant left ventricular hypertrophy.
- ECG is normal in about one third of children.

8.2 *CXR*

- Rib notching may be present in children with significant aortopulmonary collaterals

8.3 *Echocardiography*

- Echocardiography is a reliable tool and remains the gold standard in neonates and infants
- Side of aortic arch (note that CoA in a right sided arch is exceedingly rare)
- Location of narrowed arch segment
- Aortic arch anatomy and size
- Size, flow pattern and doppler velocity across the coarctation
- Flow pattern in the descending aorta
- Coexisting intracardiac anomalies, such as VSD and ASD
- Can be diagnosed or suspected antenatally by fetal echocardiography.

8.4 *CTA/MRA*

- Can provide detailed anatomy of aortic arch, descending aorta and collateral arteries in older children
- Essential in all older children/adults.

9 Indications for Intervention/Surgery

9.1 *Neonates and Infants*

- Clinically significant arm-leg BP gradient (greater than 20 mmHg) across the CoA and anatomical narrowing (> 50%) seen on echocardiography. The gradient can be lower in the setting of LV dysfunction.
- Hemodynamic compromise and/or signs of end organ compromise (left ventricular dysfunction, renal insufficiency, necrotizing enterocolitis)
- If diagnosis is unclear due to a large PDA, trial of PGEs discontinuation with close clinical and echocardiography follow up may be warranted.

9.2 Asymptomatic Child

- Hypertension > two standard deviations above normal in the upper extremity BP.
- BP gradient > 20 mmHg between upper and lower extremity.
- LV hypertrophy.

10 Timing of Intervention and Management Strategy

10.1 Neonates

- Administration of PGEs empirically or as soon as diagnosis is made.
- Surgery is preferred once hemodynamically stable and left ventricular function has stabilized and/or improved but may be performed urgently.
- Patients who present with significant dysfunction/heart failure and the PDA does not open or remains restrictive need immediate surgery.
- Proximal tubular hypoplasia of the aortic arch (THAA) is an important discriminator if surgery should be performed through median sternotomy and the need for cardiopulmonary bypass.
- Mild proximal THAA can be managed by extended end-to-end anastomosis via thoracotomy when proximal aortic arch diameter > body weight in kilograms. In borderline cases, THAA is variably defined as arch diameter $\leq$ the body weight in kilograms + 1, a z-score of < -2 or when the transverse arch is smaller than the dimension of the innominate artery.
- More extensive THAA requires CoA resection with end-to-end reconstruction of posterior wall with additional patch augmentation of the inner curvature of the aortic arch.

10.2 Infants

- Referral for elective surgical correction once clinically significant coarctation is identified.
- For infants greater than 3 months with clinically significant gradients without hemodynamic compromise, catheter-based intervention can be offered (see alternative strategies section).
- Patients who present with LV dysfunction/heart failure need timely surgery.

10.3 CoA with VSD

- Arch reconstruction with closure of VSD through the median sternotomy.

- If contraindications to cardiopulmonary bypass and simple coarctation, can consider thoracotomy for CoA repair and pulmonary artery banding
- If VSD is restrictive, repair of CoA is performed through thoracotomy and the VSD is reassessed during follow-up.

10.4 Older Children

- Catheter based interventions are often the first approach for both discrete coarctation and / or shorter segment arch hypoplasia amenable to balloon dilatation or stenting
- Surgical approach by thoracotomy and extended end-to-end anastomosis can be considered if catheter-based intervention not technically possible or does not relieve the obstruction adequately
- Long segment coarctation with diminutive arch and descending aorta may require resection with interposition graft or extra-anatomical bypass.

11 Surgical Strategy

- The surgical approach should be tailored to the anatomy of the patient.
- The main stay for coarctation repair is the extended end to end anastomosis.
- Simple end-to-end anastomosis, use of left subclavian flap or patch aortoplasty can also be used if needed.
- The subclavian flap has good results, but the LSCA has to be sacrificed and it has become less popular given the excellent results with extended end-to-end repair.
- If significant proximal arch hypoplasia, arch reconstruction via sternotomy is required.

11.1 Extended End-to-End Anastomosis (Fig. 1)

- Serratus sparing left posterolateral thoracotomy through the 3rd or 4th intercostal space.
- Dissection and mobilization of the transverse arch and descending aorta as much as possible.
- Care taken to avoid injury to the recurrent laryngeal and vagus nerve.
- Proximal aortic cross-clamp just distal to the innominate artery to achieve augmentation of proximal aortic arch.
- Complete resection of the CoA tissue and distal isthmus.
- Transverse arch is incised proximally along the inner curvature and extended anastomosis is performed with an end-to-end type of connection of the distal aorta to the transverse arch typically to the level of the left common carotid artery.

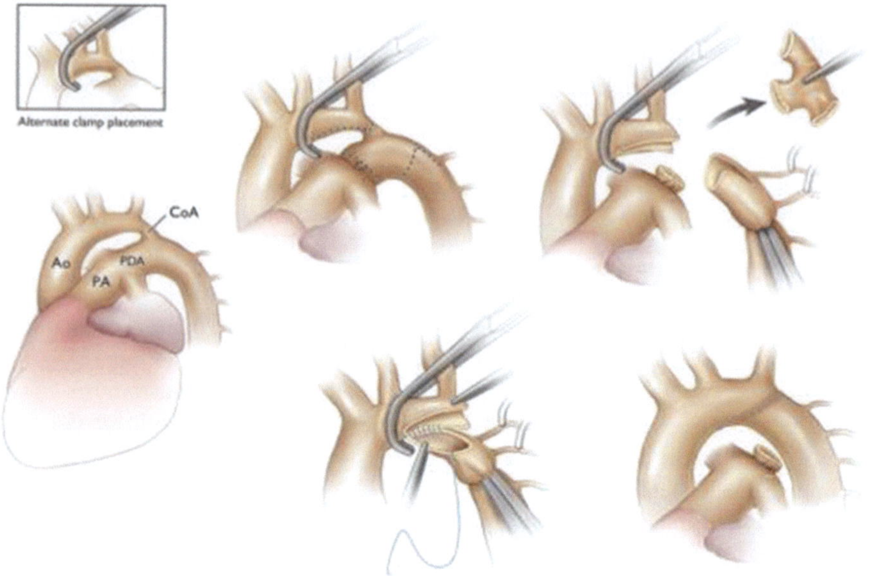

Fig. 1 Extend end to end anastomosis repair of coarctation of the aorta. The aortic arch, neck vessels and descending aortal are fully mobilized. The PDA is tied, and then proximal and distal clamps are applied. The coarctation tissue is resected and the proximal incision is extended into the undersurface of the arch. The extended end to end anastomosis is then completed. After completion, the clamps are removed, and BP gradient is preformed to confirm a satisfactory repair. *Reprinted from Annals of Thoracic Surgery, Vol 100, Mery CM, Guzmán-Pruneda FA, Trost JG Jr,* et al. *Contemporary results of aortic coarctation repair through left thoracotomy, pp 1039–1049, 2015, with permission from Elsevier Science & Technology Journals*

- In older children, surgical steps are the same, but the tissue is more friable, less elastic and more collaterals can be found. Usually only performed if the CoA lesion is very discrete.

11.2 Arch Reconstruction via Median Sternotomy

- Median sternotomy and initiation of cardiopulmonary bypass with hypothermia (18°–28°).
- Antegrade cerebral perfusion via Gore-Tex graft to the innominate artery is utilized in the majority of cases (or advance arterial cannula into the innominate artery).
- Dissection of entire aorta, PDA and proximal control of the head vessels.
- Cross clamp and cardioplegia delivery after reaching goal temperature.
- Resection of CoA tissue with subsequent reconstruction of the posterior aortic wall and patch augmentation of the arch typically using glutaraldehyde fixed

autologous pericardium or bovine pericardial patch (or pulmonary homograft in neonates).

12 Intensive Care Physiology and Management

- PGE infusion to open or maintain PDA
- Inotropic support may be required preoperatively in setting of ventricular dysfunction
- Extubation early if hemodynamically stable
- 4-limb BP for surveillance of CoA repair
- Management of hypertension post operatively.

12.1 Paradoxical Hypertension

- Hypertension can be persistent even after release of stenosis.

12.2 Postcoarctectomy Syndrome

- Mainly occurs in older children.
- Pulsatile flow to mesenteric arteries can cause vessel injury or reflex vasoconstriction, leading to abdominal pain and distention. Ischemic bowel can occur.

12.3 Left Recurrent Laryngeal Nerve Palsy

- Stridor, hoarseness, swallowing difficulties

12.4 Chylothorax

- Rare. Caused by injury of lymphatic vessels crossing the left subclavian artery.

12.5 *Paraplegia*

- Extremely rare (< 0.2%) but has been recorded due to spinal cord ischemia during clamping (most recorded cases were in older children and with prolonged clamp-times).

13 Outcome

13.1 *Mortality*

- < 1% mortality is achieved in simple CoA
- Mortality risk is increased in infants weighing < 2.5 kg.

13.2 *Morbidity*

Recurrent CoA

- Defined as resting arm-leg BP gradient of greater than 20 mmHg or a diameter loss of 50% or greater by image
- Balloon angioplasty is a reliable technique for re-CoA with 70% in reduction in BP gradient.

Aneurysm Formation

- More common in patients having patch augmentation of the aorta.

Recurrent Hypertension

- Increased risk with older age at initial repair. Important to ensure regular surveillance of BP.

14 Alternative Strategies and Controversies

- The threshold for thoracotomy vs sternotomy approach is not well defined. The arch anatomy, size of the proximal arch and risks of bypass all must be considered when deciding on thoracotomy vs sternotomy. A rule of thumb is that the proximal arch is at greater than or equal to the weight of the patient in kilograms. Growth of the proximal arch has been demonstrated.
- Native CoA that is mild that presents in infancy (> 3 months) can be treated with balloon angioplasty as an alternative to surgical correction with reintervention rates are approximately 11%. Anatomical considerations, parental preferences and multidisciplinary discussions are important for decision making.

- Older children can be successfully managed with CoA stenting as definitive treatment and this is becoming more widely used. Most regard 20 kg as minimum bodyweight and stents need to have the capability to be sequentially dilated to adult size. Associated THAA or proximity of the CoA to the LSCA origin are contraindications.
- Extra-anatomic bypass performed from the midline with a graft from the ascending to the descending thoracic aorta is an option in older children where the CoA segment is very long, tortuous or difficult to access—especially if concurrent intracardiac or aortic lesions require repair at the same time.

Bibliography

1. Dias MQ, Barros A, Leite-Moreira A, et al. Risk factors for recoarctation and mortality in infants submitted to aortic coarctation repair: a systematic review. Pediatr Cardiol. 2020;41(3):561–75.
2. Farag ES, Kluin J, de Heer F, et al. Aortic coarctation repair through left thoracotomy: results in the modern era. Eur J Cardiothorac Surg. 2019;55(2):331–7.
3. Karamlou T, Bernasconi A, Jaeggi E, et al. Factors associated with arch reintervention and growth of the aortic arch after coarctation repair in neonates weighing less than 2.5 kg. J Thorac Cardiovasc Surg. 2009;137(5):1163–7.
4. Mery CM, Guzmán-Pruneda FA, Trost JG Jr, et al. Contemporary results of aortic coarctation repair through left thoracotomy. Ann Thorac Surg. 2015;100:1039–46.
5. Sandoval JP, Kang SL, Lee KJ, et al. Balloon angioplasty for native aortic coarctation in 3- to 12-month-old infants. Circ Cardiovasc Interv. 2020;13(11): e008938.

Interrupted Aortic Arch

Rachel D. Vanderlaan

Abstract Interrupted aortic arch is a rare congenital defect whereby the aortic arch is discontinuous resulting in a duct dependant systemic circulation. Classification is based the anatomical location of interruption. Type B is most common, whereby there is an interruption between the left common carotid artery and the left subclavian artery. Primary surgical repair is required in the first few days after diagnosis unless contraindications to cardiopulmonary bypass exist. Almost all cases will have a significant intracardiac shunt or AP window. Common associated anomalies include a posterior malaligned ventricular septal defect which can be associated with left ventricular outflow tract obstruction and, rarely, hypoplastic left ventricle. Up to 50% of patients with interrupted aortic arch have DiGeorge syndrome. Surgical outcomes have improved in contemporary cohorts.

Keywords Interrupted aortic arch · Duct dependant circulation · Left ventricular outflow tract obstruction · Truncus-interruption · Aorto-pulmonary window

Abbreviations

AP	Aortopulmonary
AV	Atrioventricular
BP	Blood pressure
CoA	Coarctation of the aorta
IAA	Interrupted aortic arch
LA	Left atrium
LV	Left ventricle
LVOT	Left ventricular outflow tract
LVOTO	Left ventricular outflow tract obstruction
PA	Pulmonary artery

R. D. Vanderlaan (✉)
Division of Cardiovascular Surgery, Department of Surgery, Labatt Family Heart Centre, Hospital for Sick Children, University of Toronto, Toronto, ON, Canada
e-mail: Rachel.vanderlaan@sickkids.ca

© The Author(s), under exclusive license to Springer Nature Switzerland AG 2024

A. I. Dipchand et al. (eds.), *Manual of Cardiac Care in Children*,
https://doi.org/10.1007/978-3-031-70973-9_28

PGE	Prostaglandin
RV	Right ventricle
TGA	Transposition of the great arteries
VSD	Ventricular septal defect

Key Points

- Aortic arch is discontinuous resulting in a duct dependant systemic circulation. Closure of duct results in cardiovascular collapse and end-organ injury
- Primary total repair at time of diagnosis is preferred, unless contraindication for surgery/cardiopulmonary bypass
- Hybrid palliation if unable to do primary repair consisting of temporary bilateral pulmonary artery bands (to reduce pulmonary overcirculation and PGE), or initial Norwood procedure
- A Yasui procedure can be considered for those with severe left ventricular outflow tract obstruction. Alternatives include neonatal Ross Konno procedure depending on the individual anatomy.

1 Nomenclature

- Aortic arch sidedness.
- Left ventricular outlet tract obstruction (LVOTO; subvalvular, valvular, and supra valvular).
- Interruption of the aortic arch (IAA; classification based on location of interruption).
- Presence of intracardiac defects such as ventricular septal defect

2 Anatomy

- Absence of luminal continuity between the ascending and the descending aorta
- Duct dependent systemic circulation
- Proximal component may be relatively small (Aorta < 4 mm may require patch augentation).

The segments of the aortic arch are defined as

- Proximal aortic arch (derived from conotruncus): section of the aorta between the innominate artery and the left carotid artery
- Distal aortic arch (derived from 4th embryonic arch): section of the aorta between the left carotid artery and the left subclavian artery

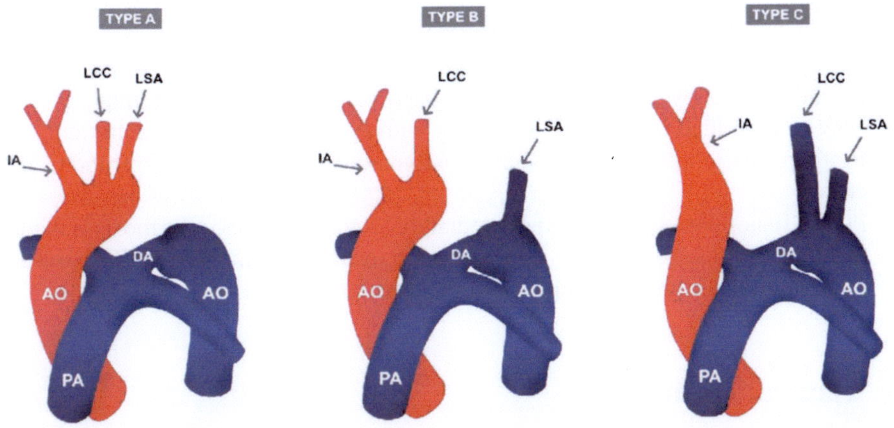

Fig. 1 Classification of interrupted aortic arch. Type A) interruption distal to the Left subclavian artery, Type B) interruption between left common carotid artery and left subclavian artery, Type C) interruption between the innominate artery and the left common carotid artery. Reprinted from Indian Heart Journal, Vol 70, Issue 1, Bravo-Valenzuela, N, Borges Peixoto, A, Araujo Júnior E, Prenatal diagnosis of congenital heart disease: A review of current knowledge. pp 150–164, 2018, with permission from Elsevier

- The isthmus region (derived from 6th embryonic arch): section of the aorta between the left subclavian artery and the area of the ductus arteriosus.

3 Classification (Celoria and Patton, Fig. 1)

- Type A: Interruption occurs at the isthmus, distal to the left subclavian artery. May be an extreme form of coarctation of the aorta (CoA)
- Type B: Interruption occurs between the left carotid and the left subclavian artery. Most common type. Associated with DiGeorge syndrome. Also commonly associated with having aberrant right subclavian artery.
- Type C: Interruption occurs between the innominate and the left carotid artery. Very rare.

4 Epidemiology

- Rare defect: 1% of all congenital heart defects.
- Prevalence of about 0.6 per 10,000 live births.
- Male predominance.
- Di George syndrome (22q11 del) may be present in 50% of patients with IAA Type B.

5 Clinical Physiology and Presentation

- Fetal diagnosis by echocardiography is becoming increasingly common.
- May be identified in postnatal screening with differential oxygen saturation.
- Profound metabolic acidosis and hemodynamic instability develop upon duct closure.
- PGE infusion should be started immediately after birth or once diagnosis is made.
- Severe heart failure develops due to volume overload from left-to-right intracardiac shunt and high afterload imposed by the closing duct.

6 Natural History

- IAA is lethal unless surgically corrected.
- 75% of all patients die within 1 month without treatment.
- Less than 10% survive to 1 year of age, in the setting of ductal patency.

7 Associated Lesions

7.1 Common

- Posterior malalignment VSD
  - Often seen in Type B
  - The posterior deviation of the conal septum towards the LV can result in LVOTO or hypoplastic aortic annulus
- Bicuspid aortic valve (BAV)
- Truncus arteriosus
- Single ventricle type lesions.

7.2 Rare

- TGA: Associated with Type A.
- Aortopulmonary window
- Double outlet right ventricle

8 Diagnostic Studies

8.1 ECG

- Can show right ventricular hypertrophy.

8.2 CXR

- Can show cardiomegaly with increased pulmonary vascularity. Absence of thymus could be indicated by narrow mediastinum.

8.3 Pulse Oximetry

- May show differential saturations (higher SaO2 levels in the arms compared to legs).

8.4 Echocardiography

- Echocardiography is a reliable tool and remains the gold standard
- Fetal diagnosis is increasingly common
- Arch sidedness
- Location of interrupted arch segment
- Aortic arch anatomy and size
- LV size, function, and presence of endocardial fibroelastosis
- Coexisting intracardiac anomalies, such as VSD, LVOTO, aortic annulus size.

8.5 CT/Magnetic Resonance Imaging

- Can provide anatomy of arch and descending aorta when echo images are unclear
- Physiological parameters for those with hypoplastic left-sided structures.

9 Indications for Repair

- Fig. 2
- Primary one-stage surgical repair is preferred
- Usually within first few days to 1st week of life

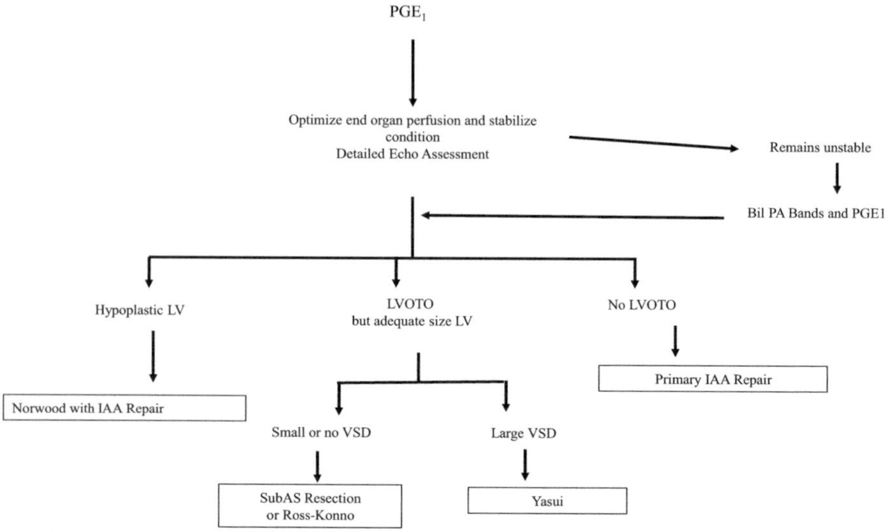

Fig. 2 Management Algorithm for Interrupted Aortic Arch

- Allow for recovery of end organ dysfunction if cardiovascular collapse due to duct closure at time of presentation
- Palliation with bilateral PA banding and PGE may be indicated if there are contraindications to primary repair (i.e. interventricular hemorrhage, persistent end organ dysfunction)
- Staged repair with arch repair and PA band can be considered in setting of a VSD, especially if complex intracardiac anatomy such as multiple VSDs or straddling AV valve.

10 Surgical Strategy

10.1 Repair of IAA

- Aortic arch reconstruction with selective antegrade cerebral perfusion via a median sternotomy
- Mild (28°) to deep (18°) hypothermia
- Two arterial in-flows are required for CPB: Aortic cannulation is typically with gortex side graft to the innominate to allow for selective cerebral perfusion and cannulation of the PDA to provide distal perfusion. The PDA is snared proximally to prevent flow to the pulmonary circulation once on bypass
- Direct back wall anastomosis is usually feasible, patch augmentation to the lesser curvature of the arch (with glutaraldehyde treated autologous pericardium or pulmonary homograft) is recommended, to avoid undue tension on the arch and

augment arch size. Incising up into the origins of the head-and-neck vessels can help increase the perimeter of native tissue-to-tissue anastomosis.

10.2 Repair of Co-existing Anomalies

- Subpulmonary VSD—Trans-pulmonary or trans-atrial approach. Care should be taken not to compromise the pulmonary valve and the right ventricular outflow tract.
- Perimembraneous VSD—right atrial approach.
- AP window is repaired by separating the aorta and main PA and patch repair of both defects.
- Truncus repair is completed as described in Chap. 22. The patch used to reconstruct the lesser curve of the aorta can also be used to repair the defect created by excision of the branch PAs from the common trunk.

10.3 Repair of IAA with VSD and LVOTO

- Yasui procedure (Fig. 3) is considered for those with hypoplasia of the LVOT.
- Usually less than 4 mm in diameter and tunnel-like LVOT is an indication.
- Consists of Damus-Kaye-Stansel anastomosis, VSD closure, IAA repair, and RV-PA conduit.
- If the aortic annulus is an adequate size, then careful resection of the subaortc knuckle of outflow septum with VSD closure may be possible.
- Alternative procedures could include Ross Konno procedure, depending on the individual anatomy. Outcomes with Yasui have been superior to Ross-Konno.

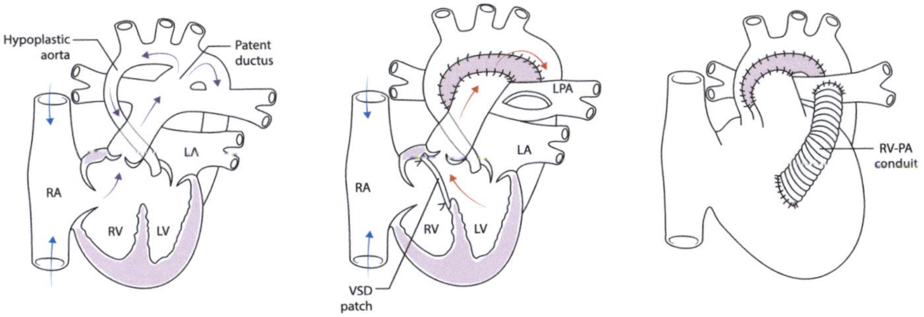

Fig. 3 Yasui Procedure. Reprinted from The Annals of Thoracic Surgery, Vol 84, Issue 1, Moorthy PSK, McGuirk SP, Jones TJ, Brawn WJ, Barron DJ, Damus-Rastelli Procedure for Biventricular Repair of Aortic Atresia and Hypoplasia, pp 142–146, 2007, with permission from Elsevier

11 Intensive Care Physiology and Management

11.1 Preop

- Administration of PGE should be started as soon as diagnosis is made. As lower body perfusion is maintained through the duct, the pulmonary resistance should be maximized.
- Vasodilator, such as milrinone is also useful to reduce systemic vascular resistance.
- Target pCO2 level of 40–50 mmHg with paralysis and ventilation if difficulty to control with above management.

11.2 Postop

- Chest may be left open if necessary, especially if a conduit has been used (truncus or Yasui).
- Consider LA pressure line if concern over LV size.
- DiGeorge patients may require management of hypocalcemia.
- Tracheobronchial compression by the reconstructed arch is rare but should be considered if persistent left lung atelectasis post-operatively.
- Recurrent laryngeal nerve palsy can occur with any arch reconstruction and should be monitored for following surgery.

12 Outcomes

12.1 Mortality

- Improved outcomes in contemporary cohorts
- Multicenter study shows 4-year survival is 63% in heterogeneous population
- Operative mortality is 7–10%. Higher in single ventricle group or in truncus group
- Recent cohorts demonstrate improved survival of ~ 90% at 15 years for isolated IAA repair.

12.2 Morbidity

Aortic Arch Obstruction/Restenosis

- Arm-Leg BP gradient of greater than 20 mmHg or a diameter loss of 50% or greater by imaging modality requires intervention—typically balloon angioplasty.

- Freedom from reintervention for aortic arch obstruction is ~ 85% at 3-years.
- Risk factors include presence of residual ductal tissue, anastomotic tension and type of repair. Patch augmentation techniques have lowest risk of recurrence.

Left Ventricular Outflow Tract Obstruction

- Risk factors for reintervention on the LVOT include patients with a smaller aortic annulus or elevated LVOT gradient at time of primary repair
- Reintervention for LVOTO is reported between from 5–25% from various centers.

Bibliography

1. Flint JD, Gentles TL, MacCormick J, et al. Outcomes using predominantly single-stage approach to interrupted aortic arch and associated defects. Ann Thorac Surg. 2010;89(2):564–9.
2. Hirata Y, Quaegebeur JM, Mosca RS, et al. Impact of aortic annular size on rate of reoperation for left ventricular outflow tract obstruction after repair of interrupted aortic arch and ventricular septal defect. Ann Thorac Surg. 2010;90(2):588–92.
3. Jonas RA. Management of interrupted aortic arch. Semin Thorac Cardiovasc Surg. 2015;27(2):177–88. https://doi.org/10.1053/j.semtcvs.2015.04.003.
4. Jonas RA, Quaegebeur JM, Kirklin JW, et al. Outcomes in patients with interrupted aortic arch and ventricular septal defect. A multiinstitutional study. Congenital heart surgeons society. J Thorac Cardiovasc Surg. 1994;107(4), 1099–1109; discussion 1109–13.
5. LaPar DJ, Baird CW. Surgical considerations in interrupted aortic arch. Semin Cardiothorac Vasc Anesth. 2018;22(3):278–84. https://doi.org/10.1177/1089253218776664.
6. Mery CM, Khan MS, Guzmán-Pruneda FA, et al. Contemporary results of surgical repair of recurrent aortic arch obstruction. Ann Thorac Surg. 2014;98(1):133–40; discussion 140–1. https://doi.org/10.1016/j.athoracsur.2014.01.065.
7. Salem MM, Starnes SV, Wells WJ, et al. Predictors of left ventricular outflow obstruction following single-stage repair of interrupted aortic arch and ventricular septal defect. Am J Cardiol. 2000;86(9):1044–7.

Vascular Rings, Slings, and Related Disorders

Lars Grosse-Wortmann, Evan J. Propst, and Osami Honjo

Abstract The three predominant forms of vascular ring/sling are: Double aortic arch (40–50%), Right arch with left duct (usually with diverticulum of Kommerell) 25–30%, and Pulmonary artery sling 15–20%. Surgical decision-making is guided by respiratory and dysphagia symptoms. Cross-sectional imaging is essential for surgical planning. Complete tracheal rings are associated in 50–67% of pulmonary artery sling patients. Need for surgical correction by slide tracheoplasty determined by symptomatology and natural history of growth. The prognosis of left pulmonary artery sling syndrome is variable and determined primarily by the associated airway abnormalities.

Keywords Vascular ring · Pulmonary artery sling · Tracheal rings · Airway compression · Diverticulum of Kommerell

Abbreviations

BIPAP	Bilevel positive airway pressure
CPAP	Continuous positive airway pressure
DAA	Double aortic arch
ECMO	Extracorporeal membrane oxygenation

L. Grosse-Wortmann (✉)
Division of Cardiology, Department of Pediatrics, Oregon Health and Science University, CDRC, 707 SW Gaines, St. Portland, OR 97239, USA
e-mail: grossewo@ohsu.edu

E. J. Propst
Department of Otolaryngology, The Hospital for Sick Children, Otolaryngology, University of Toronto, Toronto, ON, Canada
e-mail: evan.propst@utoronto.ca

O. Honjo
Division of Cardiovascular Surgery, Department of Surgery, Labatt Family Heart Centre, The Hospital for Sick Children, University of Toronto, Toronto, ON, Canada
e-mail: osami.honjo@sickkids.ca

© The Author(s), under exclusive license to Springer Nature Switzerland AG 2024

A. I. Dipchand et al. (eds.), *Manual of Cardiac Care in Children*,
https://doi.org/10.1007/978-3-031-70973-9_29

ETT	Endotracheal tube
LAA	Left aortic arch
LPA	Left pulmonary artery
MPA	Main pulmonary artery
PDA	Persistent ductus arteriosus
RAA	Right aortic arch
RPA	Right pulmonary artery

Key Points

- Edwards' hypothetical pluripotent double aortic arch (DAA) model allows the understanding of the pathogenesis of all branching anomalies of the aortic arch.
- With the exception of a DAA, a complete vascular ring is extremely rare in the setting of a left aortic arch (LAA).
- The most common types of vascular mediated airway compromise are DAA, right aortic arch (RAA) with aberrant left subclavian artery and diverticulum of Kommerell, as well as retroesophageal circumflex RAA.
- Surgical decision-making is guided by respiratory and dysphagia symptoms.
- Cross-sectional imaging is essential for surgical planning.
- Pulmonary artery sling syndrome is commonly associated with complex tracheobronchial malformations.
- Flexible or rigid bronchoscopy is required to diagnose complete tracheal rings.
- Need for surgical correction by slide tracheoplasty determined by symptomatology and natural history of growth.
- The prognosis of left pulmonary artery (LPA) sling syndrome is variable and determined primarily by the associated airway abnormalities.

1 Anatomy

- The variations of arch and branching abnormalities are considerable. A review of the embryology of human thoracic artery development is helpful in understanding the presenting anatomy (Fig. 1).
- During human embryological development, six paired vessels ('arches') connect the truncoaortic sac of the embryonic heart tube with the paired dorsal aortae.
- A complex system of growth and sequential involution of these arches leads to the normal LAA with the usual sequence of origins of the head and neck vessels.
- Aortic arch anomalies are explained by variations on the involution of the sixth arches.
- Based on this theory, Edwards' hypothetical DAA model serves to explain the vast majority of arch anomalies.

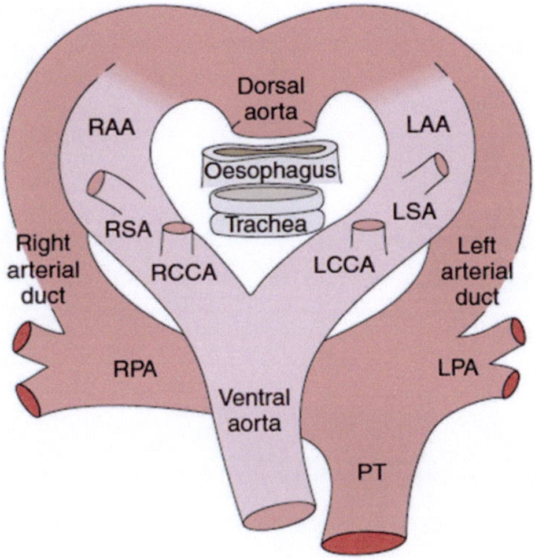

Fig. 1 Edwards' hypothetical double aortic arch model with an aortic arch and a ductus arteriosus on each side during embryological development, as well as the descending aorta in the midline. Modified from Edwards JE: Anomalies of the derivatives of the aortic arch system. Med Clin N Am 1948; 32:925–948

- Vascular rings may encircle the trachea and the esophagus, whereas non-circular lesions compress the trachea from anterior or posterior without primarily compromising the esophagus.

1.1 Double Aortic Arch (DAA)

- Most common symptomatic vascular ring (Fig. 2).
- The right arch is typically dominant, and one side (most often the left) may be atretic or stenosed.
- Atresia can occur anywhere along the arch: proximal to the head-and-neck arteries, distal to the branches, or between the common carotid and subclavian arteries.

1.2 Right Aortic Arch with Aberrant Left Subclavian Artery Arising from a Diverticulum of Kommerell

- Second most common vascular ring.
- Components of the complete ring around the trachea and esophagus:
  - Heart and main pulmonary artery anteriorly.
  - Aortic arch on the right.
  - Diverticulum of Kommerell and aberrant subclavian artery posteriorly.
  - Patent ductus arteriosus (PDA) or ductal ligament and LPA on the left.
- Very rarely, a LAA with right sided duct ligament can exist as a rare type of vascular ring but mirror image of this arch anomaly (LAA and an aberrant right

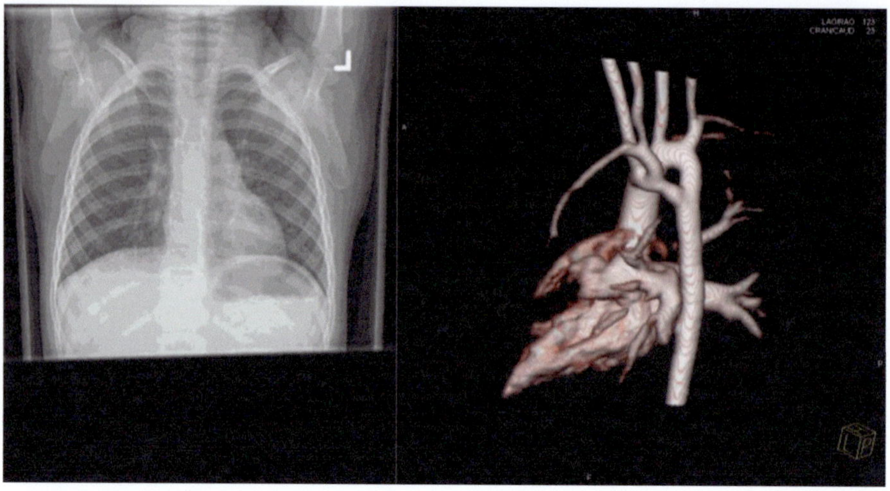

Fig. 2 Double aortic arch. A) The chest X-ray shows compression and mild deviation of the trachea to the left. B) The volume rendered reconstruction of a contrast-enhanced magnetic resonance angiogram in a two-year-old shows a double aortic arch with hypoplastic left arch

subclavian artery), typically does not have a right-sided duct or ductal ligament and, therefore, does not form a vascular ring. Feeding difficulties can still occur because of the retroesophageal course of the aberrant right subclavian artery ('dysphagia lusoria').

- Rarely, a small outpouching, or dimple, on the left-sided aspect of a distal RAA in the presence of mirror image (i.e., normal) branching of the head and neck vessels is an indicator of a left-sided duct, also completing a vascular ring.

1.3 Right Aortic Arch with Retroesophageal Circumflex Aortic Arch

- In patients with a RAA, the descending aorta often reaches the left side at the level of the diaphragm. In contrast, a retroesophageal circumflex aortic arch courses to the left high in the mediastinum. Left-sided ductal ligament is typically present and completes the vascular ring.
- The mirror image of this lesion, i.e., a LAA and a right-sided descending aorta, is exceedingly rare.

1.4 Compression of the Trachea by the Innominate Artery

- The innominate artery crosses the trachea.

- In individuals with a reduced anteroposterior thoracic diameter and/or a lateralized origin of the innominate artery, this vessel can cause tracheal compression without forming a ring.

1.5 Pulmonary Artery Sling

- The LPA arises more distally than normal, effectively arising as a branch from the RPA, and courses between the trachea and esophagus to reach the left lung (Fig. 3).
- Commonly associated with malformations of the trachea and bronchi, most often in the form of complete cartilaginous rings and tracheal stenosis, as well as complex bronchial branching abnormalities (Fig. 4).
- Vascular and airway pathologies together are known as 'pulmonary artery sling syndrome' or 'ring and sling complex'.

2 Epidemiology

- Uncommon; < 1% of all congenital cardiac defects.
- Males and females are affected equally.
- DAA and RAA with left ligamentum arteriosum account for 85–95% of all cases.
- Pulmonary artery sling syndrome is very rare and has been estimated to occur in 59 out of 1,000,000 school children.
- Vascular compression of the trachea is also common following mediastinal surgery, whereby the suspensory ligaments of the heart and trachea are disrupted. Intrusion of the trachealis muscle into the airway is common in children before and after tracheoesophageal fistula repair.

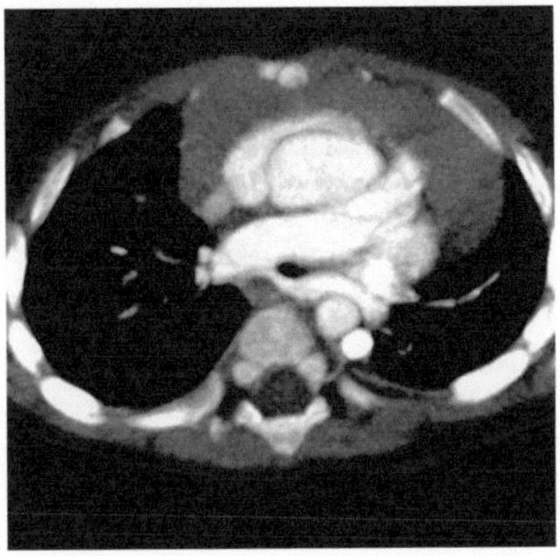

Fig. 3 Artery sling syndrome. Computed tomography angiogram in a patient with Tetralogy of Fallot and left pulmonary artery (LPA) sling syndrome shows the LPA arising more distally than normal and encircling the trachea.

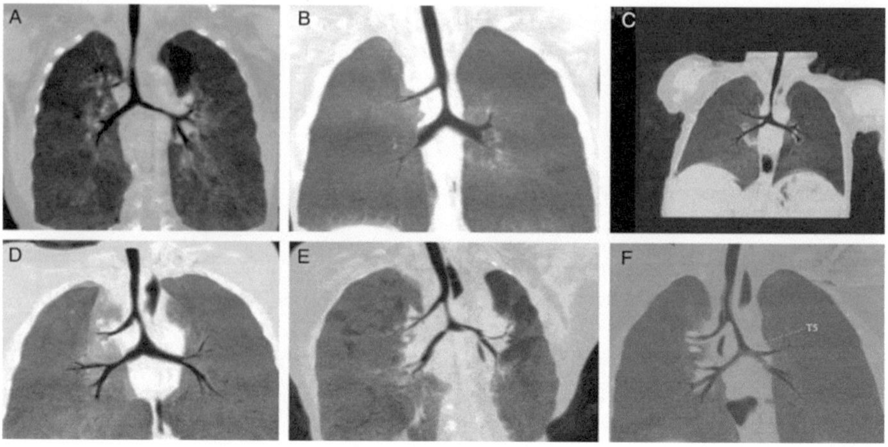

Fig. 4 CT examples of complex and variable airway malformations in patients with left pulmonary artery (LPA) sling syndrome, consisting of long segment tracheal stenosis and a separate right upper lobar bronchus

3 Clinical Physiology and Presentation

- Presentation is variable. Vascular rings and other forms of vessel-related airway compromise are not uncommonly detected incidentally in asymptomatic patients.
- When they are not associated with airway and/or esophageal compromise, the prognosis of these lesions is favorable. This is less common in DAAs and especially with pulmonary artery slings.
- DAA vascular rings are usually tight and associated with symptoms.
- Most rings involving Kommerell's diverticulum are mild or asymptomatic.
- Dysphagia is a frequent presenting symptom, with onset in an infant commonly presenting shortly after the introduction of solid foods.
- Respiratory symptoms are common.
  - Inspiratory stridor and expiratory wheezing.
  - Often misdiagnosed as asthma/reactive airways.
  - Dyspnea occurs on exertion or occasionally at rest and is often positional depending on the degree of tracheomalacia and airway malformations.
  - Frequent chest infections, especially with pulmonary artery sling syndrome.
- Unilaterally diminished brachial pulses can be a sign of a stenotic or isolated subclavian artery.
- Cervical aortic arch often presents with a pulsatile mass in the supraclavicular fossa or in the neck.

4 Associated Lesions

- A high percentage of patients with arch anomalies, especially with anomalous origin of the subclavian artery, have 22q11 microdeletion.
- Significant intracardiac malformations are rare in vascular rings, except for in LAA with aberrant right subclavian artery.
- Associated other congenital heart disease occurs in 50–71% of patients with pulmonary artery sling syndrome, most often septal defects and PDA. Extracardiac defects of other organ systems are also not infrequent.
- Cervical aortic arch (transverse arch above the level of the clavicles) is not infrequently associated with a vascular ring, and coarctation of the aorta.

5 Diagnostic Studies

- The following anatomical features need to be identified:
  - Arch-sidedness, i.e., the course of the transverse arch, relative to the spine.
  - Location of the descending aorta relative to the spine.
  - Branching of the head and neck vessels, i.e., the sequence in which the subclavian and common carotid arteries leave the thoracic aorta.
  - Presence, location, course of a patent duct or ductal ligament.
  - Arch dominance in the presence of a DAA.
  - Location, degree and severity of tracheal and/or esophageal compression.
  - Associated airway anomalies (e.g. tracheal rings, see below).
  - Associated extracardiac or intracardiac lesions.

5.1 Chest X-Ray

- On plain films, the relationship of the arch to the trachea can be determined by direct visualization and tracheal compression can be visualized.

5.2 Echocardiography

- Often suggests the diagnosis of a vascular ring or related lesion.
- Arch-sidedness is determined by the branching pattern off the aortic arch and, with less certainty, the course of the aortic arch. Nearly always the first branch (either the innominate or common carotid artery) arises as the first branch contralateral to the side of the arch. Rare exceptions to this rule are a) a retroesophageal innominate artery, b) an isolated innominate artery, or c) congenital absence of the carotid artery contralateral to the arch.

5.3 CT/MRI

- Routinely used to confirm the diagnosis, evaluate the airways, and for surgical planning.
- The choice of modality co-depends on local expertise, anaesthesia support and availability.
- A DAA with unilateral atresia can be difficult to differentiate by non-invasive imaging from a RAA with aberrant left subclavian artery and a diverticulum of Kommerell.
- The appearance of the take-off of the left subclavian artery and the orientation of the ligamentous structure (cranially in an atretic LAA and caudally in a ligamentum arteriosum) are important clues to the underlying anatomy.
- CT with contrast and axial, coronal and 3D reconstruction of the trachea and vasculature are essential.
- Compared with bronchoscopy findings to identify which vessels are causing any pulsatile compression.

5.4 Bronchoscopy

- Typically reserved for lesions with known or suspected airway compromise.
- Identifies pulsatile external compression of the airway and confirms complete tracheal cartilaginous rings (see below) and aberrant bronchial branching patterns seen in LPA sling syndrome.
- Institutionally used routinely only in patients in whom the LPA courses between the trachea and esophagus and who are considered for surgical repair.

5.5 Other Investigations

- Cardiac catheterization is not routinely needed.
- Sometimes suspected by a posterior indentation of the esophagus on a barium-swallow esophagogram for dysphagia. Once the anatomy has been established by CT or MRI, a barium-swallow study is rarely necessary, as the indication for surgery hinges on symptoms.

6 Indications for Interventions/Surgery

- The indication for surgical repair is based on symptoms. Most centers do not divide a ring or repair a compressing vascular lesion in an asymptomatic patient.

- An exception may be significant tracheal compression without definite related symptoms, in order to prevent progressive compression of the trachea.
- Other factors that impact the indication and timing for repair include:
  - Size and age of the patient.
  - Severity and course of symptoms.
  - Expected outcome and complications of the repair.
  - Associated cardiac and extracardiac malformations.

7 Timing of Intervention and Management Strategy

7.1 Double Aortic Arch

- Approach is via a left thoracotomy in the majority of cases and may be suitable for minimally invasive thoracoscopic approach.
- The smaller arch, which is almost always the left, is divided either between the common carotid artery and the subclavian artery, or more usually distal to the subclavian artery, depending on accessibility and length of the segment to be divided.
- A ductal ligament is usually also present in addition to the double arch and *must* be divided as well at the time of surgery.

7.2 Vascular Ring Other Than Double Aortic Arch

- Treatment consists of division of the ductal ligament or PDA.
- Some cases are amenable to thoracoscopic techniques.
- On occasion, older patients require more extensive arch reconstruction for complete relief of tracheal compression.

7.3 Compression of the Trachea by the Innominate Artery

- Treatment options include expectant management, waiting for the tracheomalacia to resolve, more proximal reimplantation of the innominate artery, or suspension of the innominate artery and/or the arch to the sternum

7.4 Pulmonary Artery Sling Syndrome

- Management is focused on avoiding and reducing inflammation of the airway: use of steroids, nebulized epinephrine, and non-invasive positive pressure ventilation with longer expiratory time than usual (if needed) for respiratory distress.
- Laryngeal mask airway may bypass concomitant upper airway obstruction.
- When mechanical ventilation is necessary, proper positioning of endotracheal tube above complete tracheal rings is paramount (see below). Do not try to intubate past the complete tracheal rings.
- Reimplantation of the LPA more proximally into the MPA, creating a course anterior to the trachea. Any arterial stenosis is relieved at that time.
- The tracheobronchial malformations are addressed through a collaboration across Cardiovascular Surgery or Thoracic Surgery and Otolaryngology—Head & Neck Surgery, (as indicated) during the same setting, and pose a much greater surgical challenge with various strategies, options, and outcomes.
- Cardiovascular anomalies are repaired first during the same operation, and the trachea is repaired second.

8 Intensive Care Physiology and Management

- Dependent on residual lesions, primarily airway narrowing and/or tracheomalacia.
- If concurrent slide tracheoplasty for tracheal rings, see strategies below.

9 Outcome

- The prognosis after vascular ring repair is generally favorable.
- An innominate artery that compresses the trachea can be more challenging to relocate and relief of symptoms may be incomplete.
- Existing tracheo- or bronchomalacia typically improves over the course of months and sometimes years.
- Overall survival is approximately 88% in patients undergoing slide tracheoplasty.
- The long-term outcome after surgery for LPA sling syndrome depends nearly entirely on the airway reconstruction, and residual symptoms are not uncommon, although most patients improve with somatic growth.

10 Tracheal Rings

- Complete cartilaginous tracheal ring(s) with absence of membranous trachea—leads to luminal narrowing by varying degrees (average width 2.5 mm). Most distal rings are usually the most narrow.
- Approximately 1 in 64,500 live births.
- Length of narrowing can be short or long and can extend down one or both main bronchi. Extension of narrowing to hilum is much more difficult to repair surgically.
- Can be classified according to morphology or symptoms (Supplementary Table 1).
- Common Associations
  - LPA sling at site of tracheal narrowing (48%) (Fig. 4)
  - 1/3 of children with complete tracheal rings have an LPA sling, whereas 2/3 of children with an LPA sling have complete tracheal rings
  - Congenital intracardiac anomalies (47%)
  - Tracheal "pig" bronchus of right upper lobe (13%)
  - Main bronchi have more acute takeoff forming upside down "T" shape on coronal imaging.
  - Rare: single lung (9%), Trisomy 21 (8%), anorectal malformation, duodenal atresia (7%), VACTERL/VATER association (6%), 22q11 microdeletion, Opitz G/BBB, and absent lung.
- Presentation
  - Asymptomatic or minimally symptomatic (10–50%) children may have mild biphasic stridor (often confused with well-controlled asthma) for whom tracheal rings grow over time (averaging 0.35% growth per month), attaining normal tracheal dimensions around 9 years of age.
  - Early symptomatic (50%) infants develop respiratory distress and biphasic stridor and may demonstrate air trapping and desaturations in first hours to weeks of life. Often due to a viral illness or discovered during intubation for another procedure.
  - Late symptomatic children present with exercise intolerance and biphasic stridor after first year of life. Presentation in adulthood is rare.
  - Air trapping possible as rings may act as one-way ball-valve obstruction with application of positive airway pressure ventilation (CPAP or BIPAP)—frequent pauses in ventilation with/without manual chest decompression may be required to prevent lung hyperinflation and pneumothorax.

10.1 CXR

- Classically shows narrowing of the trachea but does not confirm the diagnosis.

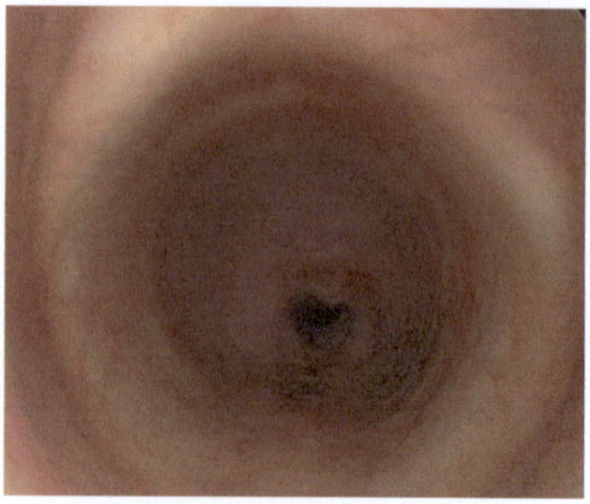

Fig. 5 Visualization of a complete ring of cartilage with absent posterior membranous trachea

10.2 Bronchoscopy

- Flexible or rigid—remains the gold standard for diagnosis complete tracheal rings. Visualization of a complete ring of cartilage with absent posterior membranous trachea is confirmatory (Fig. 5).
- Narrowing of the trachea alone may be due to vascular compression or the trachealis muscle intruding into the trachea from posteriorly.

10.3 Computed Tomography (CT) Imaging

- Assessment of the length of tracheal narrowing, presence or absence of a tracheal bronchus, involvement of the carina or main bronchi, presence of both lungs, and compression by a vascular ring or sling.

10.4 Echocardiography

- Delineate intracardiac or vascular anomalies (71%).

10.5 Repair

- Early for symptomatic infant on ECMO or bypass, cannot extubate, has repeated infections requiring steroids and admission to the intensive care unit.
- Late if causing exercise intolerance or baseline respiratory distress.
- May consider repair of trachea in an asymptomatic patient if opening chest for cardiovascular surgery.

10.6 Medical Management

- Early steroids (0.5 mg/kg) and nebulized epinephrine for respiratory distress.
- CPAP or BIPAP therapy may be required.
- Intubation (not deep and without force) is often necessary. Use an ETT that is small enough to fit through the vocal cords, but large enough that it will not get displaced inferiorly and traumatize the most proximal complete tracheal ring.

10.7 Surgical Management

- Slide tracheoplasty is the surgery of choice for repair of complete tracheal rings (Fig. 6).
- Tracheal and cardiovascular anomalies are repaired during the same surgery.
- Guided by bronchoscopy.
- Surgery should be performed immediately if on ECMO or bypass. However, surgery can be delayed in more stable patients until viral infections have cleared.
- Tracheostomy for complete tracheal rings is difficult and uncommon—ventilation challenges are unchanged or worsened (inflammation) if placed proximal to the rings, and placing it through the rings is not suggested/feasible (because they are usually lower than the neck).

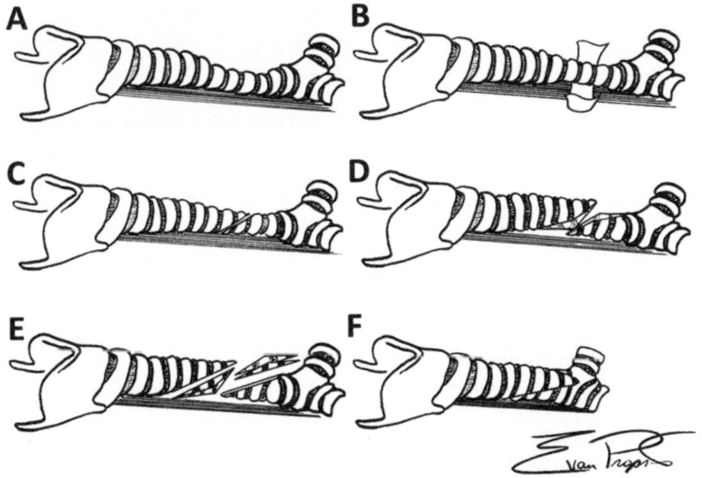

Fig. 6 Steps to perform slide tracheoplasty: A) Area of complete tracheal rings depicted above carina; B) Area of complete tracheal rings is isolated circumferentially and separated from the esophagus; C) The trachea is divided on a bevel; D) The proximal trachea is divided vertically in the midline posteriorly and the distal trachea is divided vertically in the midline anteriorly; E) The triangular edges are removed; F) The proximal trachea is slid overtop of the distal trachea and the two are sutured together

10.8 Intensive Care Physiology and Management

- Patients are usually extubated 2–7 days postoperatively.
- Repeat bronchoscopy per surgeons' preference.
- The tip of the endotracheal tube remains midway between the proximal and distal ends of the oblique anastomosis (between the horizontal clips on the chest x-ray) for mid-tracheal repairs, and above the anastomosis for repairs near the carina.
- Gentle suctioning to only 1–2 mm beyond the tip of ETT to maintain airway patency while preventing granulation formation.
- Maintain adequate humidity and nebulized steroids (Budesonide or Ciprodex) after several days of healing, as required for granulation tissue.
- Parenteral or oral steroids should be used only when absolutely essential.
- Flexible bronchoscopy to suction mucous plugs and reposition the ETT.
- Nasal intubation may decrease ETT movement in smaller children.

11 Outcomes

- Best in those who outgrow respiratory issues with minimal therapy.
- Overall survival is approximately 88%.

Bibliography

1. Butler CR, Speggiorin S, Rijnberg FM, et al. Outcomes of slide tracheoplasty in 101 children: a 17-year single-center experience. J Thorac Cardiovasc Surg. 2014;147:1783–90.
2. Cina CS, Althani H, Pasenau J, Abouzahr L. Kommerell's diverticulum and right-sided aortic arch: a cohort study and review of the literature. J Vasc Surg. 2004;39(1):131–9. Epub 2004/01/14
3. Dodge-Khatami A, Tulevski, II, Hitchcock JF, de Mol BA, Bennink GB. Vascular rings and pulmonary arterial sling: from respiratory collapse to surgical cure, with emphasis on judicious imaging in the hi-tech era. Cardiol Young 2002;12(2):96–104. Epub 2002/05/23.
4. Edwards JE. Anomalies of the derivatives of the aortic arch system. Med. Clin. North Am. 1948;32:925–49. Epub 1948/07/01.
5. Humphrey C, Duncan K, Fletcher S. Decade of experience with vascular rings at a single institution. Pediatrics 2006;117(5): e903–8. Epub 2006/04/06.
6. Manning PB, Rutter MJ, Lisec A, Gupta R, Marino BS. One slide fits all: the versatility of slide tracheoplasty with cardiopulmonary bypass support for airway reconstruction in children. J Thorac Cardiovasc Surg. 2011;141:155–61.
7. Yu JM, Liao CP, Ge S, Weng ZC, Hsiung MC, Chang JK, et al. The prevalence and clinical impact of pulmonary artery sling on school-aged children: a large-scale screening study. Pediatric Pulmonol. 2008;43(7):656–61. Epub 2008/05/20

Anomalous Left Coronary Artery from Pulmonary Artery (ALCAPA)

Conall Morgan and Jennifer L. Russell

Abstract ALCAPA is a rare congenital heart lesion. It occurs when the left coronary artery arises from the pulmonary trunk instead of the aorta. Patients usually present in infancy with acute heart failure or circulatory collapse due to poor left ventricular function and the lesion is often fatal if not promptly recognised and treated. Occasionally patients present in adulthood with sudden cardiac death or myocardial ischemia. ALCAPA usually occurs in isolation. Diagnosis can be made easily by echocardiography and should be excluded in any pediatric patient presenting with left ventricular dysfunction. Colour Doppler can demonstrate flow from the left coronary artery into the main pulmonary artery in diastole. Mitral regurgitation due to ischemia of the papillary muscle and annular dilation can be severe and may also provide a clue to the diagnosis. Surgical repair to establish an aortic connection to the left coronary should be undertaken as soon as possible. Long term survival is excellent, however survival is dependent on recovery of ventricular function and the degree of mitral regurgitation. Rarely, a ventricular assist device may be needed as a bridge to ventricular remodelling. Occasionally mitral valve repair or replacement may be warranted depending on the degree of secondary regurgitation.

Keywords Coronary artery · Ischemia · Cardiomyopathy · Heart failure · Mitral regurgitation · Ventricular assist device

Abbreviations

ALCAPA	Anomalous left coronary artery from the pulmonary artery
ARCAPA	Anomalous right coronary from the pulmonary artery
CoA	Coarctation of the aorta

C. Morgan · J. L. Russell (✉)
Division of Cardiology, Department of Paediatrics, Labatt Family Heart Centre, The Hospital for Sick Children, University of Toronto, Toronto, ON, Canada
e-mail: Jennifer.russell@sickkkids.ca

C. Morgan
e-mail: Conallthomas.morgan@sickkids.ca

© The Author(s), under exclusive license to Springer Nature Switzerland AG 2024

A. I. Dipchand et al. (eds.), *Manual of Cardiac Care in Children*,
https://doi.org/10.1007/978-3-031-70973-9_30

ECMO	Extracorporeal membrane oxygenation
EFE	Endocardial fibroelastosis
HLHS	Hypoplastic left heart syndrome
LA	Left atrium
LAD	Left anterior descending
LCA	Left coronary artery
LMCA	Left main coronary artery
LV	Left ventricle
MPA	Main pulmonary artery
MR	Mitral regurgitation
MV	Mitral valve
RCA	Right coronary artery
RVOT	Right ventricular outflow tract
TOF	Tetralogy of Fallot

Key Points

- Anomalous origin of the left coronary artery (LCA) from the pulmonary artery (ALCAPA).
- Usually presents with heart failure and possible circulatory collapse due to poor left ventricular (LV) function in infancy but can be asymptomatic.
- Urgent surgical reimplantation of the LCA is indicated upon diagnosis.
- Recovery of LV function is expected in the majority of patients, however this may be slow, rarely requiring ventricular assist device as a bridge to recovery.
- Mitral regurgitation (MR) can be severe and require surgical repair/replacement.

1 Nomenclature

- Situs solitus, levocardia, concordant atrioventricular and ventriculoarterial connections.
- Anomalous origin of the left coronary artery (LCA) from the pulmonary trunk.

2 Anatomy (Fig. 1)

- Origin of the left coronary arterial system from the pulmonary arterial trunk.
- Usually from the main pulmonary artery (MPA), arising from the left pulmonary valve sinus; rarely may arise from a branch pulmonary artery.

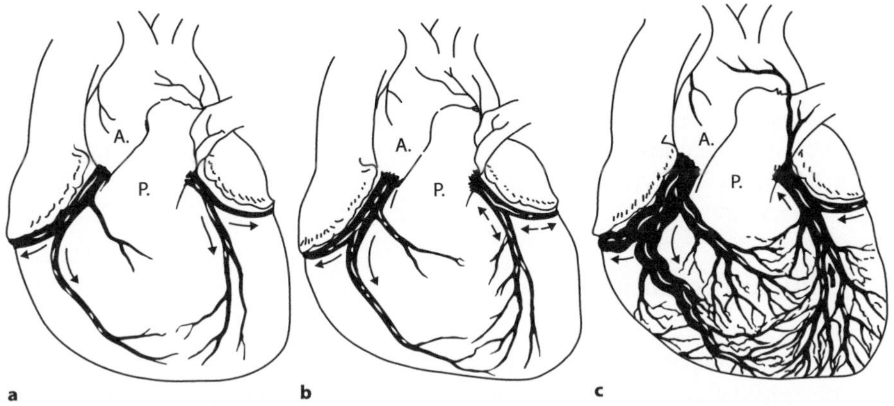

Fig. 1 Functional states in anomalous origin of the left coronary artery from pulmonary trunk

- The right coronary artery (RCA) is usually dilated with large collateral vessels evident on the epicardial surface of the heart. These collateral vessels may not be evident if the lesion is identified early.
- The LV and LA are dilated. Typically, there is moderate to severely reduced LV function. The LV wall may be thin.
- Endocardial fibroelastosis (EFE) may be evident in the LV/LA and mitral valve (MV) apparatus.

3 Epidemiology

- Overall incidence of 1 in 300,000 increasing to 1 in 250 to 400 in patients with congenitally malformed hearts.
- Males more commonly affected than females 2.3 to 1.

4 Pathophysiology

- As a fetus, no clinical effect is seen as the pressure and oxygen saturation are almost identical in the pulmonary artery and the aorta.
- After birth as the pulmonary vascular resistance falls and the arterial duct begins to close, the pulmonary artery pressure begins to decrease.
- LV coronary perfusion becomes compromised as collateral flow is initially insufficient, resulting in myocardial ischemia. Decreased function and increased end diastolic pressure subsequently follows.
- MR secondary to annular dilation or infarction and dysfunction of the anterolateral papillary muscle can worsen heart failure symptoms.

- As collateral vessels develop from the RCA system, coronary steal into the pulmonary artery can occur via the low pressure LCA instead of flow passing into the higher pressure vessels supplying the myocardium.
- Some patients develop effective collaterals and are apparently asymptomatic into adulthood. There may be no myocardial dysfunction or infarction in this subset. There is a net left to right shunt.

5 Clinical Presentation

- The majority of patients present after 4–6 weeks postnatally. Neonatal presentation is rare given elevated right heart pressures in the neonatal period.
- Usually present with symptoms and signs of heart failure. Rarely can present with cardiac arrest.
- Can also present with episodes of acute discomfort that are often mistaken for colic or reflux with pallor, grunting, diaphoresis, or shock. These episodes are angina pectoris.
- Associated lesions which result in ongoing elevation in pulmonary artery pressures may delay presentation.
- In any new presentation of ventricular dysfunction, a diagnosis of ALCAPA must be considered and excluded with certainty.
- Some patients present relatively asymptomatically as children or adults if effective coronary collaterization occurs and/or in the presence of pulmonary hypertension

6 Natural History

- In most cases if left untreated, the lesion is fatal.
- In those patients surviving past childhood, up to 90% will die from sudden cardiac death, acute heart failure or myocardial ischemia at a mean age of 35 years.
- Survival (unrepaired) over the age of 50 years is very rare.

7 Associated Lesions

- Usually occurs in isolation
- VSD
- TOF
- CoA
- HLHS

8 Diagnostic Studies

8.1 Electrocardiogram

- Abnormal Q waves in leads I, aVL and V 4–6

8.2 Echocardiography

- Diagnostic imaging modality of choice.
- Determine segmental anatomy.
- Origin of the LCA from the MPA is easily identified by echocardiography.
- Clue to the diagnosis:
  - Abnormal direction of flow by colour Doppler in the LAD and LMCA (retrograde).
  - Collaterals in interventricular septum by colour Doppler
  - Dilated RCA
- Colour Doppler will demonstrate flow from the LCA into the pulmonary artery in diastole.
- An echo bright myocardium and papillary muscle with an enlarged RCA should raise suspicion.
- Function and degree of MR should be assessed.
- Associated lesions should be ruled out.

8.3 CT/MR

- Cross-sectional imaging is used for older children or when there is diagnostic doubt.

8.4 Catheterization

- Not routinely used to diagnose ALCAPA.

9 Indications for Repair

- Presence of the disease.

10 Timing of Intervention and Management Strategy

- Surgery should generally be carried out as soon as possible after diagnosis in the setting of reduced heart function.
- Those presenting in severe heart failure (ventilation and inotrope dependent) require urgent repair.
- Those with mild symptoms and minimal heart failure can be repaired semi-electively.

11 Surgical Strategy

- Mobilisation and direct re-implantation of the LCA into the facing side of the aorta is usually possible.
- Myocardial protection is important and extra doses of cardioplegia can be given directly into the coronary ostium once exposed.
- If the coronary arises from the leftward side of the MPA (rare) then direct reimplantation is more difficult. A trap-door flap can be created from the aorta and then an additional patch placed anteriorly if necessary to complete the connection. Alternative is the Takeuchi technique of creating a tunnel within the pulmonary root, that is connected to the neighboring aorta by creating a small AP window. This is rarely used as it risks causing obstruction to the RVOT.
- MV repair is recommended if more than moderate MR is present. If due to ischemia and retraction of the papillary muscles then there is a high likelihood of recurrent MR and future MV replacement may be necessary.
- Ligation of the LCA to prevent the retrograde run-off was used historically, but the preference now is to re-establish antegrade flow in a two-coronary system.
- For those whose only pathology is the finding of ALCAPA (i.e., late presenting adults) some advocate interventional catheter occlusion.
- Transplantation may become indicated if there is refractory heart failure due to lack of improvement in myocardial function. Ventricular assist devices can be used as a bridge to recovery or transplantation should LV function not recover.

12 Intensive Care Physiology and Management

- Acute heart failure management including possible bridging with ECMO in the perioperative period.
- Often need to transition from acute to chronic heart failure management either with guideline-directed medical therapy or even ventricular assist device as a bridge to recovery of function over the weeks to months needed for ventricular remodeling.

13 Outcomes

- Excellent long-term outcomes are expected dependent on the extent of LV dysfunction and ischemic injury to the MV support apparatus.
- 10 year transplant free survival is 95%.

14 Alternative Strategies and Controversies

- Ligation of the LCA rather than reimplantation could be considered in older children and adults with evidence of adequate collateralization and preserved LV function.
- Occlusion of the LCA may be considered via percutaneous plug/coil.

15 Anomalous Right Coronary from the Pulmonary Artery (ARCAPA)

- Extremely rare anomaly with a prevalence of 0.002%.
- Rarely reported in the paediatric population. Most are diagnosed incidentally later in life.
- Considered more benign with ongoing controversy around indications for and timing of surgical intervention.
- A commonly accepted approach is to follow expectantly with a low threshold for surgical repair should cardiac function decrease or signs and symptoms of ischemia develop with age and time.

Bibliography

1. Edwards JE. The direction of blood flow in coronary arteries arising from the pulmonary trunk. Circulation. 1964;29:163–6.
2. Fierens CW, Budts B, Denef et al. A 72 year old woman with ALCAPA. Heart (Br. Card. Soc.) 2000;83(1).
3. Li RJ, Sun Z, Yang J, et al. Diagnostic value of transthoracic echocardiography in patients with anomalous origin of the left coronary artery from the pulmonary artery. Medicine (Baltimore). 2016;95(15): e3401.
4. Naimo PS, Fricke TA, D'Udekem Y, et al. Surgical intervention for anomalous origin of left coronary artery from the pulmonary artery in children. A long-term follow-up. Ann Thorac Surg. 2016;101(5):1842–8.
5. Singh TP, Di Carli MF, Sullivan NM, et al. Myocardial flow reserve in long-term survivors of repair of anomalous left coronary artery from pulmonary artery. J Am Coll Cardiol. 1998;31(2):437–43.

6. Thomas AS, Chan A, Alsoufi B, et al. Long-term outcomes of children operated on for anomalous left coronary artery from the pulmonary artery. Ann Thorac Surg. 2022;113(4):1223–30.
7. Tran A, Kochilas L, Thomas AS, et al. Long-term outcomes after repair for anomalous right coronary artery from the pulmonary artery. Cardiol Young. 2022;18:1–5.
8. Yamanaka O, Hobbs RE. Coronary artery anomalies in 126,595 patients undergoing coronary arteriography. Cathet Cardiovasc Diagn. 1990;21(1):28–40.

Anomalous Aortic Origin of a Coronary Artery

Anusha Jegatheeswaran

Abstract Anomalous aortic origin of a coronary artery (AAOCA), is a rare lesion whereby one or both coronary arteries does not arise from the usual location on the aorta. It is the second leading cause of sudden cardiac death in otherwise healthy young individuals. However, AAOCA remains a lesion with many unknowns. These relate to the true prevalence of this lesion, as most patients are incidentally diagnosed without any clinical consequences, and a lack of understanding regarding which anatomical variants are at high risk for ischemia and sudden cardiac events. This leads to an unclear picture regarding the optimal management for patients, whether surgical or medical. In addition, while repair of AAOCA can be achieved using many techniques, the long-term outcomes of each strategy remains unknown, and recently the higher-than-expected complications of repair were outlined in a multi-institutional Congenital Heart Surgeons' Society study. This chapter sheds light on these unknowns and provides clinicians with the current understandings regarding how to best manage this complex lesion.

Keywords AAOCA · Anomalous aortic origin of a coronary artery · Coronary artery anomaly · Ischemia · Sudden cardiac arrest · Sudden cardiac death · Sudden cardiac event

Abbreviations

AAOCA	Aanomalous aortic origin of acoronary artery
ACC	American college of cardiology
AHA	American heart association
CHSS	Congenital heart surgeons' society
CTA	Computed tomography angiography
ECG	Electrocardiogram

A. Jegatheeswaran (✉)
Great Ormond Street Hospital for Children, Great Ormond Street, London WC1N 3JH, UK
e-mail: anusha.jegatheeswaran@utoronto.ca

© The Author(s), under exclusive license to Springer Nature Switzerland AG 2024

A. I. Dipchand et al. (eds.), *Manual of Cardiac Care in Children*,
https://doi.org/10.1007/978-3-031-70973-9_31

MRI Magnetic resonance imaging

Key Points

- Anomalous aortic origin of a coronary artery (AAOCA), is a rare lesion whereby one or both coronary arteries does not arise from its normal location.
- It is the second leading cause of sudden cardiac death in otherwise healthy young individuals (after hypertrophic cardiomyopathy).
- AAOCA remains a lesion with many unknowns due to lack of understanding of the true prevalence and of which features predict high risk.
- Most patients are incidentally diagnosed without any clinical consequences.
- Indications for surgery are most clear when patients have had a sudden cardiac event or have inducible ischemia.
- Surgical repair can occur via multiple techniques based on the anatomical features present, however it can result in complications and adverse events.

1 Nomenclature

- Anomalous aortic origin of the coronary artery (AAOCA).
- Description of this lesion should include the detailed variations listed under Anatomy (see below).

2 Anatomy

- Multiple anatomic variations based on (see Fig. 1):
  - Which coronary artery is anomalous [left, right (most common), both] with a description of the sinus of origin, or whether the coronary artery has a high take-off.
  - The course of the coronary artery is variable and has to be defined for each case: interarterial (i.e., running between the two great vessels), intramural (i.e., running for a distance within the wall of the aorta), intraconal (i.e., running intramyocardial within the conal septum), and whether it is prepulmonic, retroaortic, or retrocardiac (i.e., pathway after leaving the aorta).
  - The morphology of the ostium (high orifice, slit-like orifice, acute take-off angle, proximal narrowing, and/or elliptical).

3 Epidemiology

- The true proportion of patients with AAOCA is unknown as individuals are not routinely screened for this lesion, and the majority of patients with AAOCA are diagnosed incidentally.
- Estimates vary widely between 0.1 and 1% of the general population (rarely as high as 2%).
- Currently, there is no data to suggest a genetic basis for AAOCA.

4 Clinical Physiology and Presentation

4.1 Clinical Physiology

- Theories regarding how ischemia can occur:
  - Vigorous physical exercise results in increased cardiac output leading to coronary ostial obstruction from vessel expansion. This can also cause aortic root dilation which can cause lateral compression of the interarterial or intramural region of the vessel.
  - Flow reserve may be limited in cases with small ostium, a narrowed proximal course, or a retrocommissural course (intramural vessel running behind the commissure which causes compression) which only becomes significant in times of increased cardiac output.

4.2 Presentation

- The majority of AAOCA patients are diagnosed incidentally and are asymptomatic.
- In the subset of patients with high risk lesions (see below), where the anatomy can result in ischemia, the first presentation may be a sudden cardiac event (arrest or death). In the majority of these cases however, high risk lesions present with the signs and symptoms of ischemia (e.g. chest pain with concomitant ECG or biomarker evidence, or syncope on exercise).

4.3 Natural History

- It remains unclear because there may be many undiagnosed patients who do not have any clinical consequences.

5 Associated Lesions

- There are no known associated lesions.

6 Diagnostic Studies

- Echocardiogrpahy is essential to assess regional wall motion and may identify coronary origins.
- Anatomical definition with ECG-gated CTA is essential to understanding the specific anatomy of the patient and preoperative planning.
- MRI with gadolinium gives additional functional and perfusion imaging.
- Assess ischemia using cardiac enzymes and ECGs in the acute setting.
- Provocative ischemia testing options include cardiopulmonary exercise testing, stress echocardiography, and stress cardiac MRI.
- Angiography with intravascular ultrasound and fractional flow reserve assessment using dobutamine can be used as adjuncts at sites with these capabilities, especially in patients with suspected intraseptal or myocardial bridges.
- Ensure that the territory of ischemia is supplied by the anomalous coronary artery.

7 Indications for Intervention/Surgery

- Surgery is clearly indicated for any patients with proven signs or symptoms of ischemia including aborted cardiac arrest, syncope following exertion which is not vasovagal in nature, or chest pain with corroborating evidence. Activity should be restricted and patients should proceed to surgery urgently.
- Patients with left AAOCA are generally felt to be higher risk, but surgery is only indicated if there is proven ischemia on provocative testing, or if there are several high risk features present (see below).
- Patients with right AAOCA are generally not offered surgery unless ischemia can be demonstrated.
- From the Congenital Heart Surgeons' Society study, the high risk features found to be associated with ischemia include:
  - Left AAOCA.
  - In patients with left AAOCA: an intramural course, a high take-off, and/or a slit-like orifice.
  - In patients with right AAOCA: a longer intramural course.

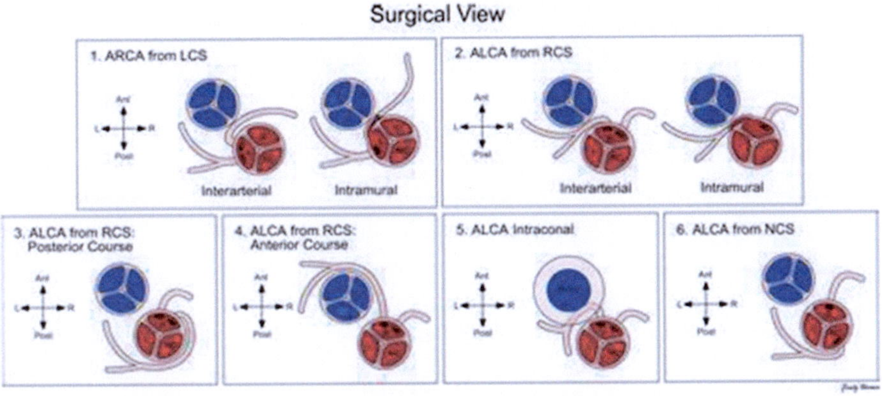

Fig. 1 Common variants of AAOCA. From, Sem Thorac Cardiovasc Surg, Fabozzo A et al., pp 791–800, 2016, with permission from Elevier

8 Timing of Intervention and Management Strategy

- Unless patients present with ischemia, patients generally do not undergo surgery until approximately 10 years of age when it is felt they are able to exert themselves adequately with exercise. There is significant center variation related to this.
- However, it should be noted that there have been patients younger than this who have presented with a sudden cardiac event.
- The AAOCA section from the 2018 AHA/ACC Guidelines for the Management of Adults with Congenital Heart Disease are summarised in Fig. 2.

9 Surgical Strategy

- Multiple strategies are available, depending on the specific anatomical features present. The principle is to move the orifice to the appropriate sinus with resolution of high-risk features.
- Unroofing of the intramural segment is the commonest technique. However, if the intramural course runs behind the commissural pillar, then this repair strategy may be associated with aortic insufficiency if commissural takedown and resuspension are required. Alternatives such as creation of an aortocoronary window, neo-ostial window creation, or reimplantation (with a button or following transection without a button) may be employed.
- Patch ostioplasty may be used in select cases with a narrowed orifice or proximal hypoplasia.
- Pulmonary artery translocation has been relegated to use primarily as an adjunct procedure (never alone), as it is now believed that it is generally an intramural course and not an interarterial course which is the substrate for ischemia.

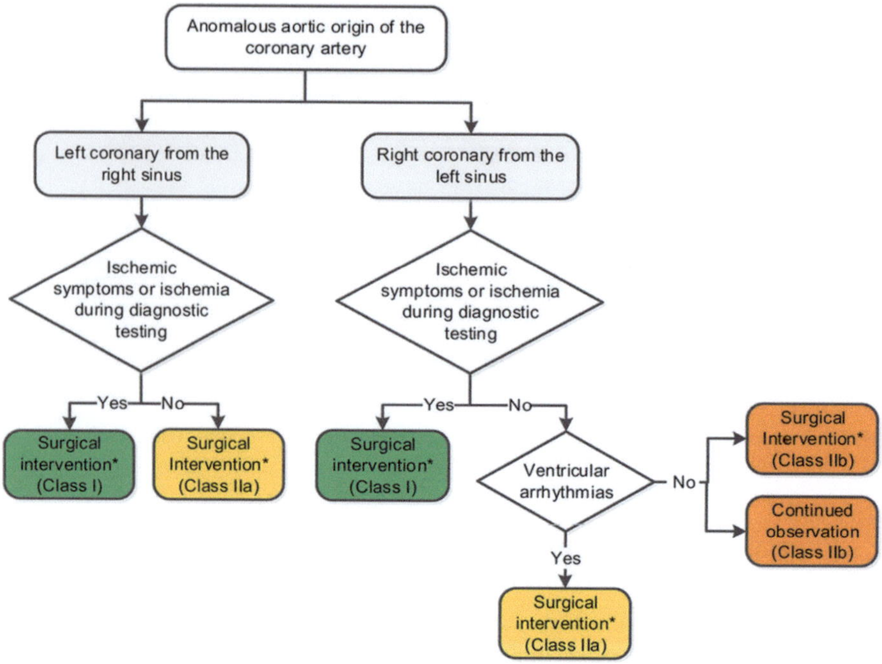

Fig. 2 Surgical intervention to involve unroofing or coronary revascularization for patients with concomitant fixed obstruction. Reprinted from Circulation Vol 139, The 2018 AHA/ACC Guideline for the Management of Adults with Congenital Heart Disease: A Report of the American College of Cardiology/American Heart Association Task Force on Clinical Practice Guidelines (Fig. 5), pp e698–e800, 2019, with permission from © 2018 American Heart Association, Inc.

10 Intensive Care Physiology and Management

- Monitor for acute ischemia following surgery. This can manifest as ECG abnormalities, arrhythmias, elevation of cardiac enzymes, and cardiac dysfunction.

11 Longer Term Follow Up

- Post-operative follow up should include an ECG and echocardiogram at 7–10 days and 4–6 weeks, with exercise stress testing with imaging at 3 months (only after this should patients resume competitive athletics, however if the patient presented with a sudden event this should be done at 12 months), and ecg and cardiac MRI at 6 months. These are used to obtain the baseline status of the patient.
- Annual follow-up should include an ECG and echocardiogram.

- Exercise stress testing should occur every 1–3 years based on degree of activity. If the patient is an athlete this should be performed annually, and if new symptoms occur nuclear perfusion or stress echocardiogram/MRI should be considered.
- If patients remain asymptomatic and do not undergo surgery, they should have annual ECG with echocardiogram every 1–2 years, and exercise stress testing as described above.
- Exercise restriction is no longer advocated unless a patient is awaiting surgery or cannot undergo repair.
- Indefinite treatment with low-dose aspirin has been recommended following surgery, and this is especially important depending on the type of repair performed and whether it involves the coronary ostia.

12 Outcome

- Surgery specific complications (from the CHSS study) are summarized in Fig. 3.
- Operative mortality (0.8%) and reoperation (3%) were higher than expected.

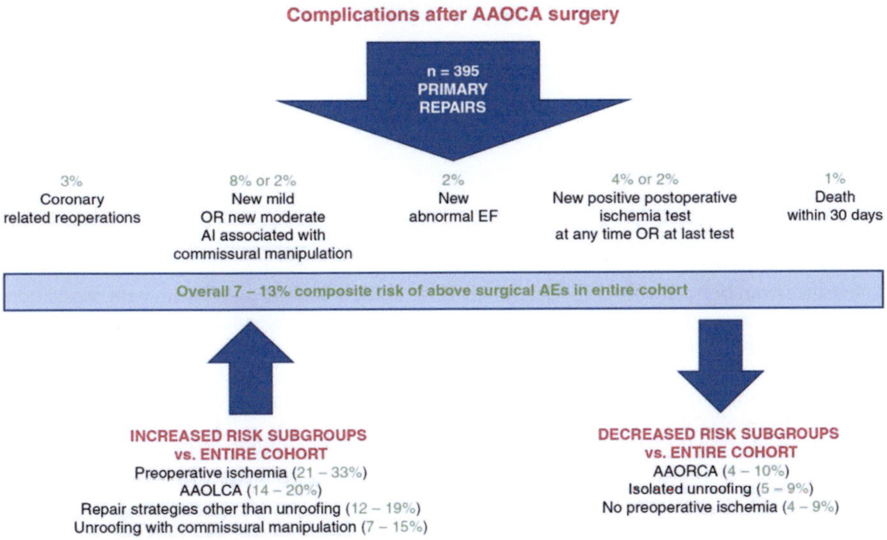

Fig. 3 Primary findings related to the surgical risks of AAOCA repair. Ranges for surgical adverse events based on calculations using occurrence of new mild or new moderate AI associated with commissural manipulation and new postoperative ischemia based on any or last postoperative ischemia test. AAOCA—Anomalous aortic origin of a coronary artery; AI—aortic insufficiency; EF—ejection fraction; AE—adverse event; AAOLCA—anomalous aortic origin of a left coronary artery; AAORCA—anomalous aortic origin of a right coronary artery. Reprinted from the Journal of Thoracic and Cardiovascular Surgery, Vol 160, Issue 3, Jegatheeswaran A, Devlin PJ, Williams WG et al., Outcomes after anomalous aortic origin of a coronary artery repair: A Congenital Heart Surgeons' Society Study, pp 757–771.e5, 2020, with permission from Elsevier

- In patients with proven ischemia pre-op, 80% had resolution, while 20% had persistent ischemia. In those without preoperative ischemia, 4% developed new ischemia.
- Higher risk subgroups: those with preoperative ischemia, those with left AAOCA, those undergoing repair strategies other than unroofing, and those undergoing unroofing with commissural manipulation.
- Lower risk subgroups: those with right AAOCA, those undergoing isolated unroofing without commissural manipulation, and those without preoperative ischemia.

13 Controversies/Unanswered Questions

- The true epidemiology of the lesion is unclear due to potentially undiagnosed cases without symptoms.
- Optimal protocols are required for preoperative provocative testing and postoperative clearance assessment.
- We need to determine which patients require surgery vs. medical management.
- We need to determine optimal surgical strategies based on the given anatomical features.

Bibliography

1. Brothers JA, Frommelt MA, Jaquiss RDB, et al. Expert consensus guidelines: anomalous aortic origin of a coronary artery. J Thorac Cardiovasc Surg. 2017;153(6):1440–57.
2. Jegatheeswaran A, Devlin PJ, McCrindle BW, et al. Features associated with myocardial ischemia in anomalous aortic origin of a coronary artery: a congenital heart surgeons' society study. J Thorac Cardiovasc Surg. 2019;158(3):822-834.e3.
3. Jegatheeswaran A, Devlin PJ, Williams WG, et al. Outcomes after anomalous aortic origin of a coronary artery repair: a congenital heart surgeons' society study. J Thorac Cardiovasc Surg. 2020;160(3):757-771.e5.
4. Molossi S, Agrawal H, Mery CM, et al. Outcomes in anomalous aortic origin of a coronary artery following a prospective standardized approach. Circ Cardiovasc Interv. 2020;13(2): e008445.
5. Padalino MA, Jegatheeswaran A, Blitzer D, et al. Surgery for anomalous aortic origin of coronary arteries: technical safeguards and pitfalls. Front Cardiovasc Med. 2021;8: 626108.
6. Stout KK, Daniels CJ, Aboulhosn JA, et al. 2018 AHA/ACC Guideline for the management of adults with congenital heart disease: a report of the American College of Cardiology/American Heart Association Task Force on Clinical Practice Guidelines. Circulation 2019;139(14):e698–800.

Hypoplastic Left Heart Syndrome and Variants

Bhavikkumar D. Langanecha

Abstract Hypoplastic left heart syndrome (HLHS) is a rare congenital heart disease in which the left ventricle and supporting structures are underdeveloped and unable to support the systemic circulation. The condition is universally fatal if untreated. Many patients are now identified prenatally but undiagnosed patients may present postnatally on routine neonatal screening or with respiratory distress and hemodynamic shock following PDA closure. Peri-operative management is dependent on maintaining unobstructed systemic outflow, optimizing cardiac output, and balancing of systemic and pulmonary circulations. Surgical correction is not possible, and most patients undergo staged surgical single ventricle palliation toward a Fontan physiology. The Norwood procedure is the first stage surgery and pulmonary blood flow can be achieved with RV-PA conduit or modified BTT shunt with similar long-term outcomes; the RV-PA conduit being most common. A hybrid procedure or primary transplantation are reserved for high-risk subgroups. Restrictive atrial septum may lead to arterialization of pulmonary veins and pulmonary lymphangiectasia and portends poor prognosis. Fetal interventions considered to improve patient outcomes include balloon dilation or stenting of intact or severely restrictive atrial communication and aortic valvuloplasty.

Keywords Hypoplastic left heart syndrome · Hypoplasia of left heart · Norwood with RV-PA conduit · Norwood with BTT shunt · Hybrid procedure · Restrictive atrial communication · Levoatrial cardinal vein · Endocardial fibroelastosis

Abbreviations

AA	Aortic atresia
AKI	Acute kidney injury
AS	Aortic stenosis

B. D. Langanecha (✉)
Division of Cardiac Critical Care, Department of Critical Care Medicine, Labatt Family Heart Centre, The Hospital for Sick Children, University of Toronto, Toronto, ON, Canada
e-mail: Bhavikkumar.langanecha@sickkids.ca

© The Author(s), under exclusive license to Springer Nature Switzerland AG 2024

A. I. Dipchand et al. (eds.), *Manual of Cardiac Care in Children*,
https://doi.org/10.1007/978-3-031-70973-9_32

ΔAVO2	Arterial-venous oxygen saturation difference
BCPS	Bidirectional cavopulmonary shunt
BTT	Blalock Taussig Thomas
CHD	Congenital heart disease
CoA	Coarctation of the aorta
CPB	Cardiopulmonary bypass
CPR	Cardiopulmonary resuscitation
ECMO	Extracorporeal membrane oxygenation
EFE	Endocardial fibroelastosis
HLHC	Hypoplastic left heart complex
HLHS	Hypoplastic left heart syndrome
ICH	Intracranial hemorrhage
LA	Left atrium
LV	Left ventricle
MA	Mitral atresia
MS	Mitral stenosis
MV	Mitral valve
MVO2	Mixed venous oxygen saturation
NEC	Necrotizing enterocolitis
NIRS	Near infrared spectroscopy
PA	Pulmonary artery
PDA	Persistent ductus arteriosus
PFO	Persistent foramen ovale
PGE	Prostaglandin
PVR	Pulmonary vascular resistance
Qp	Pulmonary blood flow
Qs	Systemic blood flow
RA	Right atrium
RV	Right ventricle
SV	Single ventricle
SVR	Systemic vascular resistance
TAPVC	Total anomalous pulmonary venous connection
TR	Tricuspid regurgitation
TV	Tricuspid valve
VSD	Ventricular septal defect

Key Points

- Hypoplastic Left Heart Syndrome (HLHS) is a rare (2–3%) CHD with a small or diminutive left ventricle (LV), mitral valve (MV) and systemic outflow.
- Universally fatal if untreated, not repairable, and palliated through a series of three operations.

- Increased risk associated with prematurity, small size, presence of genetic syndrome, MS/AA variant with coronary fistulas, intact/restrictive atrial septum, or right ventricle (RV) and tricuspid valve (TV) dysfunction.
- Norwood with RV-PA conduit is our institution's preference for the first stage single ventricle (SV) surgical palliation with BTT used in those with a dominant LV or severely hypoplastic pulmonary arteries.
- The hybrid procedure and primary transplantation reserved for high-risk patients.

1 Nomenclature

- Term HLHS was originally used by Noonan and Nadas.
- Defines a spectrum of cardiac malformations, characterized by underdevelopment of the left heart, including significant hypoplasia of the LV in setting of atresia/stenosis/hypoplasia of the aortic and/or mitral valves and hypoplasia of the ascending aorta and aortic arch.
- HLHS without intrinsic valvar stenosis or atresia is synonymous with the term hypoplastic left heart complex (HLHC)
- HLHS variants include anomalies with underdeveloped LV – including mitral atresia with VSD, double outlet RV variants, critical LV outflow obstruction with/without VSD, and unbalanced atriventricular septal defects (AVSD)

2 Anatomy

- Classical HLHS has situs solitus, levocardia, atrioventricular and ventricular-arterial concordance, mitral stenosis/atresia (MS/MA) and aortic stenosis/atresia (AS/AA), hypoplastic left aortic arch, possible coarctation (CoA)
- Situs abnormality can be present in HLHS variants, commonly in unbalanced AVSD
- Interventricular septum is intact in classical HLHS and include three major anatomic variants (Fig. 1):

  1. Mitral Atresia/Aortic Atresia (MA/AA)
     a. A slit like LV with no inflow or outflow
     b. LV within the left posterior aspect of the ventricular mass
     c. No valve tissue or endocardial fibroelastosis (EFE) is detected.
  2. Mitral Stenosis/Aortic Atresia (MS/AA)
     a. LV has inflow but no outflow leading to significant LV hypertrophy and hypoplastic LV cavity. The thick interventricular septum can distort the RV, TV, and RV outflow.
     b. Can be complicated by coronary-cameral connections
     c. EFE is more prominent in this subgroup
  3. Mitral Stenosis/Aortic Stenosis (MS/AS)

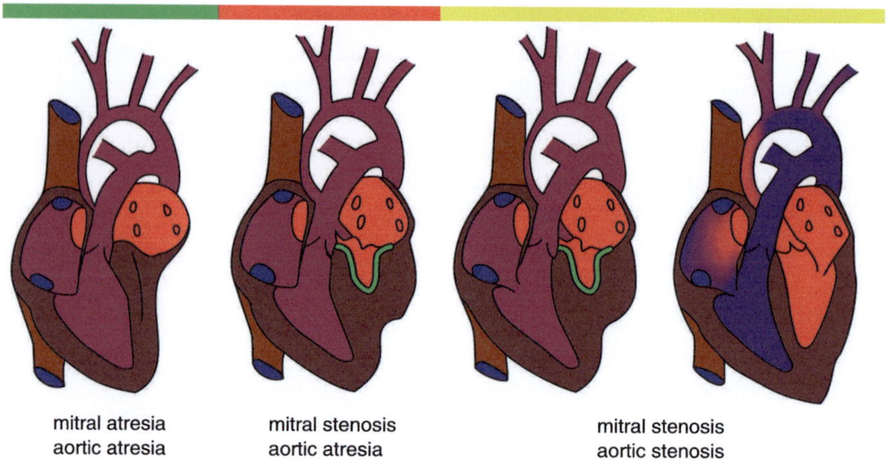

Fig. 1 The morphological spectrum of hypoplastic left heart syndrome

  a. Hypoplastic LV may approximate normal size and parietal thickness, but not apex-forming.
  b. A spectrum of critical AS
  c. Severe AS will present similar to MS and AA

- The right sided cardiac structures are larger than normal. The RV is enlarged and may also be hypertrophied.
- One third of patients have moderate to severely dysplastic TV.
- Atrial communication is restrictive in 25% of case and 1% have intact interatrial septum.
- LA can sometimes decompresses into innominate vein through a levoatrial cardinal vein with a severely restrictive or intact atrial septum
- Other associated lesions are TAPVC, coronary arterial origin anomalies and coronary sinusoid/fistula. Rarely dysplastic pulmonary valve with stenosis and/or regurgitation.

3 Embryology

- Most cases of HLHS are thought to arise secondarily because of decreased flow into the developing embryonic left ventricle (obstruction to LV inflow or outflow, or restriction at PFO). In some cases, abnormal LV growth could be the primary defect.

4 Epidemiology

- HLHS phenotype occurs in 0.016 to 0.036% of live births in Canada and the US.
- HLHS represents 2–3 of CHD cases but accounts for 23% of neonatal death from congenital malformations.
- No specific gene abnormality is identified for HLHS, even with strong supporting evidence of a genetic etiology. Nineteen percent of 1st degree relatives of infants with HLHS have CHD.
- Common syndromes associated with HLHS are Kabuki syndrome, Noonan syndrome, Smith-Lemli-Opitz syndrome, CHARGE syndrome and Holt-Oral syndrome
- Trisomies and monosomies associated with HLHS are Turner syndrome, trisomy 13, trisomy 18 and trisomy 21.

5 Fetal Diagnosis and Risk Factors

- Classical forms with severely hypoplastic LV can be detected at 11–14 weeks, but more commonly around 18–22 weeks of gestation
- Risk factors for poor outcome in fetal echocardiogram: restrictive or intact inter-atrial septum, obstructed TAPVC, RV dysfunction, moderate-to-severe TR, and coronary sinusoids
- Significant restriction at atrial communication (LA to RA flow) leads to LA and pulmonary venous hypertension (arterialization of the pulmonary venous vasculature) and pulmonary lymphangiectasia
- Fetal atrial septostomy or stent implantation can be done for restrictive atrial communication

6 Clinical Physiology and Presentation

- Most patients diagnosed prenatally or identified postnatally due to failed universal pulse oximetry testing or due to clinical concern.
- Most undiagnosed patients present in the first week of life in shock and respiratory distress due to PDA closure and drop in pulmonary vascular resistance (PVR).
- Patients with severely restrictive or intact atrial septum (or obstructed TAPVC) will have shock, oxygenation and ventilation failure from birth.
- Patients with excessive pulmonary blood flow will have tachypnea, high systemic oxygenation (SPO2 > 90 s) and impaired systemic blood flow.

7 Diagnostic Studies

7.1 CXR

- Pulmonary venous congestion and possible pleural effusion in patients with severely restricted atrial communication or obstructed levoatrial cardinal vein

7.2 Echocardiogram

- Primary mode of diagnosis of specific cardiac anatomy, atrial communication, ascending aorta and arch size, PDA size and flow, presence of coronary-cameral fistula and EFE, severity of valvar and ventricular dysfunction.

7.3 Cardiac CT/Cardiac MR

- Routine cross-sectional imaging is not required.
- Useful in difficult cases for delineation of TAPVC, levoatrial cardinal vein or difficult coronary imaging.

8 Management Options

- Single ventricle palliation (ultimate goal is Fontan physiology)
- Primary heart Ttransplantation or Hybrid procedure for high-risk subgroups
- Comfort care.

9 Pre-operative Management (Fig. 2)

10 Indications of Cardiac Catheterization Before Stage 1 Palliation

- Restrictive atrial communication or obstructed levoatrial cardinal vein required immediate decompression of LA by balloon dilatation or/and stenting of atrial communication or stenting of obstructed vein.

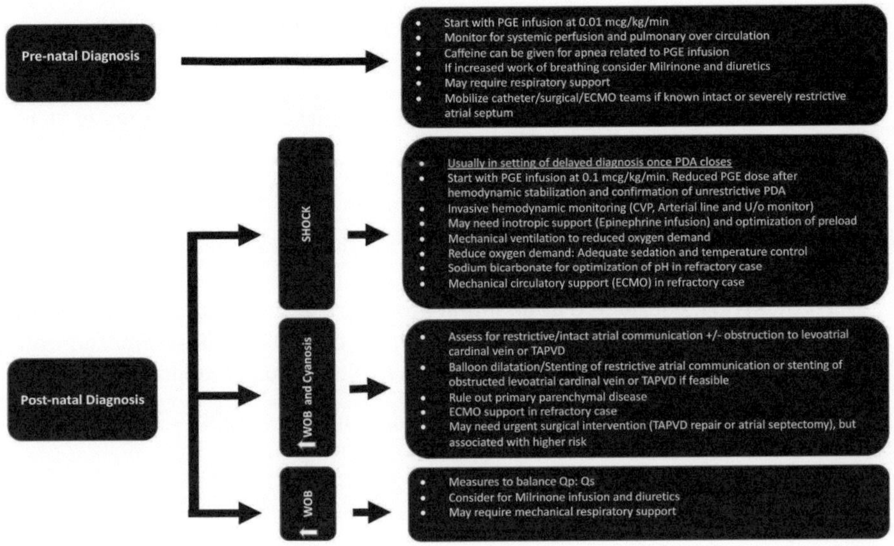

Fig. 2 Pre-Operative management of hypoplastic left heart complex according to clinical presentation. From Crucean A, Alqahtani, A., Barron, D. J. et al. Orphanet Journal of Rase Diseases, 2017; 12(1): 138, licensed under the Creative Commons Attribution 4.0 International License (http://creativecommons.org/licenses/by/4.0/)

11 Surgical Intervention

- Stage 1 palliation includes Norwoord with RV-PA conduit or BTT shunt, or hybrid procedure. The RV-PA conduit is most common and preferred option at SickKids for routine risk patients (>2.5 kg)
- Goals of Stage 1 Palliation
  - Unobstructed systemic outflow
  - Regulated source of pulmonary blood flow
  - Unobstructed pulmonary venous inflow (and inter-atrial communication)
  - Minimal AV valve regurgitation
- Surgical intervention performed in first week of life between 2 to 7 days of life
- Norwood procedures includes:
  - Damus-Kaye-Stansel (division of main PA and anastomosis with proximal ascending aorta)
  - Aortic arch reconstruction
  - Atrial septectomy
  - Source of pulmonary blood flow: RV-PA conduit or BTT shunt
    - BTT shunt with HLHS varients with a dominant LV, and considered to promote growth of severely hypoplastic PAs

    - RV-PA conduit may be modified to BTT if inadequate PA growth
- Hybrid Procedure
  - Bilateral PA bands, maintain PDA (PGE or stent), atrial septostomy or stent
    - Further Atrial septal intervention 7–10 days post PA band placement if needed
  - May be used as a Norwood alternative in routine-risk patients (institutional preference)
  - At SickKids, considered as an initial procedure in premature, small for gestation (<2 kg), hemodynamic instability, or patients with severe end-organ dysfunction (NEC, AKI, ICH) as bridge to Norwood procedure.
    - Conversion to RV-PA conduit at predetermined weight (~3 kg) and/or 4–6 weeks post hybrid
    - Possible bridge to transplantation
- Primary Transplantation
  - For high-risk subgroups (e.g. moderate-to-severe ventricular or valvar dysfunction).

12 Perioperative and Intensive Care Management

- Physiology: Single ventricle with parallel systemic and pulmonary circulations
- Systemic afterload reduction initiated immediately coming off CPB with milrinone infusion and inotropy with epinephrine infusion
- Chest closure considered if hemodynamically stable and good hemostasis
- Hemodynamic support titrated to reliable systemic oxygen delivery and controlled Qp:Qs:
  - Systemic vascular resistance (SVR) primary target to ensure balanced circulation – lower to promote systemic blood flow and increase to drive pulmonary blood flow
  - Adequate systemic cardiac output: Normal lactate, MVO2 45, ΔAVO2 (arterial-venous oxygen saturation difference) < 30%, cerebral and flank NIRS (near infrared spectroscopy) > 45%.
  - Mean blood pressure > 45 mmHg
  - Systemic oxygen saturation 70–90%
- Delayed chest closure reviewed daily and completed when hemodynamically stable and improvement in myocardial edema
- Hemoglobin target > 140 mg/dL if systemic desaturation

- Modification of PVR is rare and limited to isolated cases in which SVR management is inadequate or clinically significant pulmonary hypertension/high PVR.

13 Outcome

- Operative survival approximately 85–90%
  - Increased risk of postoperative morbidity and mortality if CPR, ECMO, ventricular dysfunction, valvar dysfunction, AKI
- Norwood with RV-PA conduit have increased risk of conduit/PA interventions during the interstage period
- Norwood with BTT shunt have increased risk of shunt obstruction, cardiac arrest and sudden death during the interstage period
- Patients in many institutions (SickKids included) followed closely by dedicated single ventricle team and standardized practice
  - Home oxygen monitoring
  - Home weight measurements
  - Biweekly in person assessments
  - Monthly surveillance echocardiograms
- Aim for completion of bidirectional cavo-pulmonary shunt (BCPS) at 4–6 months in appropriate candidates (evaluated using catheterization and cMRI)
- One-year transplant free survival > 70% with patients and similar longterm outcomes in patients with RV-PA conduit and BTT shunt.

14 Practice Variability

- Preference for primary hybrid procedure as a Norwood alteranative is offered by selective centres
- Primary transplantation for standard risk patients is rare but may be offered at limited number of institutions.

Bibliography

1. Alphonso N, Angelini A, Barron D, et al. Guidelines for the management of neonates and infants with hypoplastic left heart syndrome: The European Association for Cardio-Thoracic Surgery (EACTS) and the Association for European Paediatric and Congenital Cardiology (AEPC) Hypoplastic Left Heart Syndrome Guidelines Task Force. Eur J Cardiothorac Surg. 2020;58(3):416–99.

2. Crucean A, Alqahtani A, Barron D, et al. Re-evaluation of hypoplastic left heart syndrome from developemental and morphological perspective. Orphanet J Rare Dis. 2017;12(1):138.
3. Newburger J, Sleeper L, Frommelt P, et al. Transplantation-free survival and interventions at 3 years in the single ventricle reconstruction trial. Circulation. 2014;129(20):2013–20.
4. Ohye RG, Sleeper LA, Mahony L, et al. Comparison of shunt types in the Norwood procedure for single-ventricle lesions. N Engl J Med. 2010;362(21):1980–92.
5. Tchervenkov CI, Jacobs JP, Weinberg PM, et al. The nomenclature, definition and classification of hypoplastic left heart syndrome. Cardiol Young. 2006;16(4):339–68.

Other Functionally Single Ventricle Lesions

Devin Chetan, Bhavikkumar D. Langanecha, and Rachel D. Vanderlaan

Abstract This chapter outlines a wide morphologic spectrum of single ventricle lesions, a heterogenous group of disorders that exhibit parallel circulations at birth and converge to bidirectional cavopulmonary connection and Fontan palliation. Lesions can be categorized into those with obstruction to pulmonary flow, obstruction to systemic flow, unobstructed bilateral outflows, or balanced circulations. Initial physiology, clinical presentation, initial goals of medical stabilization, and surgical approach are defined by lesion category and the underlying physiology. There is considerable variability in long-term outcomes depending on native anatomy and associated cardiac lesions with estimated 10 to 15 year survival ranging from 50–75% for most patients with a 'typical' risk profile. High risk subgroups include patients with a restrictive atrial septum, associated pulmonary venous anomalies, or those in which the majority of pulmonary blood flow is supplied by aortopulmonary collaterals.

Keywords Single ventricle · Double inlet left ventricle · Tricuspid atresia · Double outlet left ventricle · Congenitally corrected transposition of great arteries · Duct-dependent circulation · Parallel circulation · Obstructed pulmonary blood flow · Obstructed systemic blood flow · Balanced circulation

---

D. Chetan
Division of Cardiology, Labatt Family Heart Centre, The Hospital for Sick Children, Toronto, ON, Canada
e-mail: devin.chetan@sickkids.ca

B. D. Langanecha (✉)
Division of Cardiac Critical Care, Department of Critical Care Medicine, Labatt Family Heart Centre, The Hospital for Sick Children, University of Toronto, Toronto, ON, Canada
e-mail: bhavikkumar.langanecha@sickkids.ca

R. D. Vanderlaan
Division of Cardiovascular Surgery, Department of Surgery, Labatt Family Heart Centre, The Hospital for Sick Children, University of Toronto, Toronto, ON, Canada
e-mail: rachel.vanderlaan@sickkids.ca

© The Author(s), under exclusive license to Springer Nature Switzerland AG 2024

A. I. Dipchand et al. (eds.), *Manual of Cardiac Care in Children*,
https://doi.org/10.1007/978-3-031-70973-9_33

Abbreviations

ASD	Atrial septal defect
AV	Atrioventricular
AVSD	Atrioventricular septal defect
AVVR	Atrioventricular valve regurgitation
BCPS	Bidirectional cavopulmonary shunt
CHF	Congestive heart failure
DILV	Double inlet left ventricle
DKS	Damus-Kaye-Stansel
HLHS	Hypoplastic left heart syndrome
FiO_2	Fraction of inspired oxygen
iNO	Inhaled nitric oxide
LA	Left atrium
LV	Left ventricle
MPA	Main pulmonary artery
PA	Pulmonary artery
PAB	Pulmonary artery band
PA/IVS	Pulmonary atresia / intact ventricular septum
pCO_2	Partial pressure of carbon dioxide
PDA	Patent ductus arteriosus
PFO	Patent foramen ovale
PGE	Prostaglandin
PVR	Pulmonary vascular resistance
Qp	Pulmonary blood flow
Qs	Systemic blood flow
RV	Right ventricle
SV	Single ventricle
T21	Trisomy 21
TAPVC	Total anomalous pulmonary venous connection
TGA	Transposition of the great arteries
TV	Tricuspid valve
VA	Ventriculo-arterial
VSD	Ventricular septal defect

Key Points

- Single ventricle lesions are a heterogenous group of lesions characterized by having a single functional ventricle responsible for systemic and pulmonary blood flow in a parallel configuration and converge to BCPS and Fontan palliation.
- Most common diagnoses include tricuspid atresia, double inlet left ventricle (DILV), PA/IVS, unbalanced AVSD, and DORV. HLHS, Isomerism/Heterotaxy, PA/IVS are discussed separately in Chaps. 32, 35 and 16, respectively.
- At the initial stage, there is complete mixing of systemic and pulmonary venous return
- Underlying physiology is defined by the degree of outflow tract obstruction, systemic and pulmonary venous return, and mixing at atrial or ventricular level.
- Initial priority is to ensure unobstructed systemic blood flow and a source of pulmonary blood flow by establishing ductal patency in patients with duct-dependent circulations
- Subsequent goal of medical management is optimizing the balance of pulmonary and systemic blood flow until palliation

1 Nomenclature and Anatomy

1.1 Types of Single Ventricles

- Most common single ventricle, HLHS, discussed in Chap. 32.

1.1.1 Dominant LV

- Tricuspid atresia (Fig. 1)—situs solitus, absent right AV connection and single left AV connection from LA to LV, rightward and anterior RV connect via VSD, VA connection may be concordant or discordant, variable outflow tract obstruction, ASD or stretched PFO generally unobstructed
- DILV (Fig. 2)—situs solitus, both tricuspid and mitral valves connect predominantly to LV, anterior diminutive RV connected via VSD (may be referred to as bulboventricular foramen) to right or left, VA connection may be concordant or discordant, variable outflow tract obstruction, normal systemic and pulmonary venous return, variable size of ASD
- Unbalanced LV dominant AVSD—situs solitus, AV concordance through a common AV connection, dominant LV, usually concordant VA connection
- PA/IVS (Chap. 16).
- Severe Ebstein anomaly (Chap. 10)—situs solitus, AV and VA concordance, delamination anomaly of the TV with atrialization of RV, functional or structural pulmonary atresia

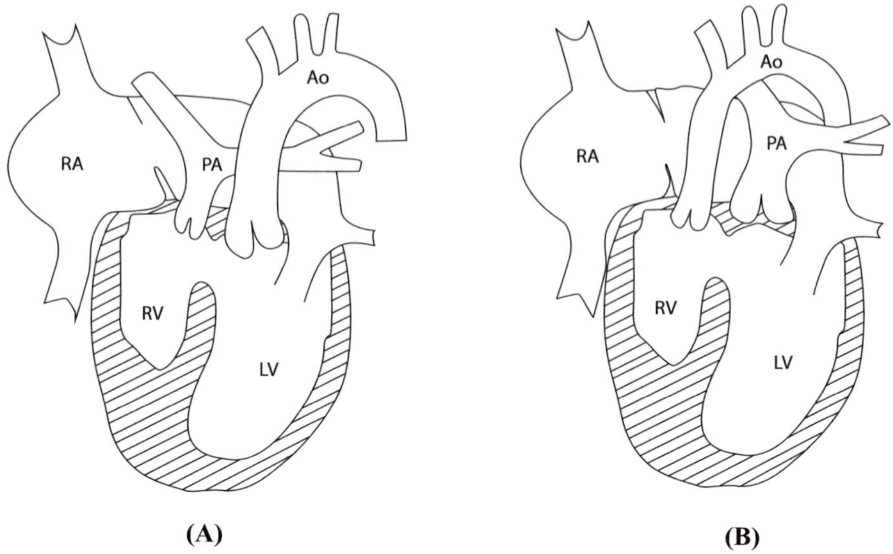

Fig. 1 Spectrum of tricuspid atresia. A) Tricuspid atresia with normally related great vessels. B) Tricuspid atresia with malposed great vessels. Reprinted from Critical Heart Disease in infants and Children, 3rd Edition, Vol 3, Ungerleider RM, McMillian N, Cooper DS, et al., Tricuspid Atresia, portion author Murthy R et al., pages 765–777.e3, 2018, with permission from Elsevier Science and Technology Journals

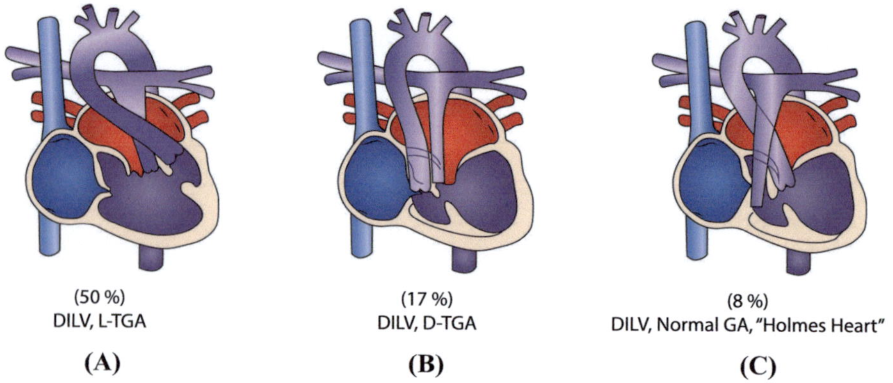

Fig. 2 Spectrum of double inlet-left ventricle (DILV). A) DILV with l-TGA (aorta anterior and leftward of the pulmonary artery). B) DILV with d-TGA (aorta anterior and rightward of the pulmonary artery). C) DILV with normally related great vessels ('Holmes Heart'). Reprinted from Heart, Vol 102, Issue 3, Poterucha JT, Anavekar NS, Egbe AC, et al. Survival and outcomes of patients with unoperated single ventricle, pp 216–222, 2016, with permission from BMJ Publishing Group Ltd

1.1.2 *Dominant RV*

- Unbalanced RV dominant AVSD—situs solitus, AV concordance through a common AV connection, dominant RV, VA connection may be concordant or discordant, variable degree of outflow tract obstruction, possible malalignment of atrial/ventricular septum
- Isomerism/Heterotaxy—Discussed in Chap. 35
- Rarely, may have two well-formed ventricles that cannot be septated and behave as a functional single ventricle—examples include DORV, criss-cross heart (superior-inferior ventricles)
- DORV—rare forms in which one ventricle hypoplastic or VSD remote. Situs solitus, AV concordance, both outflows originate predominantly from RV.

1.1.3 Common to All Single Ventricles

- Wide morphologic spectrum with unifying criteria that the entire AV junction is predominantly connected to a dominant ventricular chamber
- Complete description of the segmental anatomy includes visceral, bronchopulmonary, and atrial situs, cardiac position, atrial morphology, AV connections (including AV valve abnormalities—straddling, overriding), description of ventricular mass, VA connections, ventricular topology
- Dominant ventricular chamber may have right, left, or indeterminant morphology with a diminutive secondary ventricular cavity
- A "true" single ventricle with a single ventricular cavity is very rare
- Description of associated anomalies: systemic or pulmonary venous abnormalities, atrial or ventricular communication, AV valve abnormalities (including straddling, overriding), outflow tract obstruction, relationship of the great vessels, arch sidedness/hypoplasia, ductal anatomy, ventricular function, coronary pattern/arrangement/course

2 Epidemiology

- Most cases are sporadic with polygenic and environmental contributions
- Reported incidence of 54 cases per million live births with more recent estimates being substantially higher
- Tricuspid atresia second most common SV following HLHS (1.5–3% of CHD) followed by DILV (1% of all CHD)
- Possible association with genetic syndromes: Holt-Oram, Noonan, velocardiofacial syndrome, and T21
- Risk to siblings and offspring of affected individuals ranges from 2–5%, with higher concordance rates in some patient groups

3 Clinical Physiology and Presentation

3.1 Physiology

- Wide variety of anatomic lesions that have complete mixing of the systemic and pulmonary venous return
- In most hearts with functionally SV physiology, one outflow is obstructed
- Patients can be classified into four categories:
  - Obstruction to pulmonary blood flow
  - Obstruction to systemic blood flow
  - Unobstructed outflows
  - Balanced circulations (some restriction to pulmonary blood flow)
- Obstruction to outflow may occur at VSD, subvalvar, valvar or supravalvar levels—restrictive VSDs often associated with underdeveloped associated outflow tract
- Main objectives of initial palliation are to ensure unobstructed systemic outflow, controlled source of pulmonary blood flow, unobstructed systemic and pulmonary venous return, unrestrictive communication at the atrial level
- Ventricular output is divided between two parallel circulations
- With complete mixing, saturations in the PA and aorta are the same
- Total ventricular output is the sum of Qp and Qs
- Proportion of ventricular output is determined by relative resistances to flow in the two circuits

3.2 Clinical Presentation

- Majority of patients present in the neonatal period or in early infancy
- Timing and clinical presentation determined by degree of outflow obstruction, associated anomalies, and severity
- May be identified by neonatal screening programs due to systemic desaturation (rarely occurs due to streaming)

3.2.1 Obstruction to Pulmonary Blood Flow

- Severe obstruction to pulmonary blood flow presents in neonatal period with duct-dependent pulmonary circulation
- Cyanosis may be present at or shortly after birth and worsens with ductal closure
- May present as murmur

3.2.2 Obstruction to Systemic Blood Flow

- Weak/absent femoral pulses, mild central cyanosis, and symptoms of high pulmonary blood flow
- If coarctation/arch obstruction is severe, may present with systemic hypoperfusion and shock

3.2.3 Unobstructed Outflows

- Can be asymptomatic at birth
- As the PVR falls, signs of increased pulmonary blood flow become more evident with CHF symptoms: tachypnea, feeding difficulty, hepatomegaly, failure to thrive

3.2.4 Balanced Circulations

- Can appear well with mild central cyanosis
- If the degree of obstruction to pulmonary blood flow increases, cyanosis may become more obvious

4 Natural History

- Have a poor prognosis when left unrepaired
  - ~ 70% of patients with single LV died 16 years after diagnosis (annual attrition rate ~ 4.8%)
  - ~ 50% of patients with single RV died 4 years after diagnosis
  - Highest risk is interval prior to BCPS
- Most common causes of mortality: arrhythmias, CHF, and sudden unexplained death
- Some survivors with lesions that balance their systemic and pulmonary circulations
- Progression in degree of outflow tract stenosis variable

5 Associated Lesions

- Wide spectrum of associated cardiac anomalies

6 Diagnostic Studies

6.1 Echocardiography

- Complete description of the segmental anatomy: atrial situs, cardiac position, atrial morphology, AV connections, description of ventricular mass, VA connections, ventricular topology
- Description of VSD position and size important for diagnosis and treatment
- Description of associated anomalies: systemic or pulmonary venous abnormalities, atrial or ventricular communication, AV valve abnormalities (including straddling, overriding), outflow tract obstruction and how the affected circulation is supplied, relationship of the great vessels, arch sidedness/hypoplasia, ductal anatomy, ventricular function, coronary pattern/arrangement/course

6.2 Fetal Echocardiography

- Over 40–50% of patients are now being diagnosed on fetal echocardiogram
- Important potential benefits: delivery and treatment in specialist centres and potential for improved survival with certain lesions

6.3 CT/MRI

- Is often not needed for complete sequential segmental anatomy for most patients
- Particularly useful in demonstrating distal portions of the PAs, PDA anatomy, ventricular function, delineation of collaterals
- Established a central role in planning for intermediate palliation

6.4 Cardiac Catheterization

- Not usually required for initial diagnosis but may be used for palliation
- Has largely been replaced by non-invasive cross-sectional imaging
- Can be used to assess interventricular communication, ventricular relationship, AVVR, outflow tracts, VA connections, shunt patency, caval venous injections, and aortic arch
- Pulmonary angiography often performed prior to palliation
- Size of the pulmonary arteries, distortion of the PAs, PA stenosis, and/or the pattern of pulmonary venous return

7 Indications for Intervention/Surgery

- Secure unobstructed systemic blood flow, source of pulmonary blood flow, or balance parallel circulations

8 Timing of Intervention and Management Strategy

8.1 Medical and Interventional Management

8.1.1 Obstruction to Pulmonary Blood Flow

- Neonates with cyanosis and duct-dependent pulmonary circulation—rapid improvement with PGE
  - Poor response may indicate obstructed pulmonary venous return (necessitate supportive measures and mechanical ventilation while awaiting urgent repair)
- Catheter-based interventions replacing surgical shunts in many situations
  - Stenting of PDA is preferred over surgical BTT shunt insertion in many institutions
  - Stenting of RV outflow tract is rare in these lesions
  - Pulmonary valve dilation is considered in plate-like atresia or pulmonary valve stenosis with acceptable annulus size (PA/IVS)
  - Hypoxemia secondary to increased pulmonary vascular resistance (PVR) is rare (increase FiO_2, hyperventilation, iNO)

8.1.2 Obstructed Systemic Blood Flow

- May present in critical condition with poor pulses and oliguria—PGE infusion, decreasing SVR and increasing PVR to balance systemic and pulmonary circulations are mainstays of treatment
- Management principles are gentle afterload reduction (once PDA unobstructed), augmenting PVR, and supporting ventricular function
  - PVR can be managed by increasing intrathoracic pressure with mechanical ventilation, permissive hypoventilation/elevated pCO_2, high hematocrit
- Avoid prolonged periods of medical management with unstable physiology; relatively urgent surgical management to a more favorable physiology is indicated
  - With open PDA, urgent MPA or bilateral PA bands may be used as rescue to balance circulations

- Emergent bypass operations possible but generally deferred once PA banded until end-organ injury has resolved

8.1.3 Unobstructed Outflows

- Anti-congestive therapies as PVR drops to improve heart failure symptoms

8.1.4 Balanced Circulations

- If remains well-balanced, no specific medical therapy required

8.1.5 Atrial Septum and Mixing

- Unrestrictive atrial communication that facilitates complete mixing is ideal for most SV lesions
- Right-to-left atrial shunt in setting of right sided SV lesion (tricuspid atresia, PA/IVS) is rarely obstructed but requires ongoing surveillance. Atrial septostomy if presenting with signs of right sided venous congestion and/or associated low cardiac output
- Atrial septostomy indicated to avoid LA hypertension if left atrial egress compromised
- Hypoxemia in setting of restrictive ASD and high LA pressures requires urgent catheter or surgical enlargement of interatrial communication—care taken to avoid or manage rapid increase in pulmonary blood flow following intervention
- Rarely, no atrial mixing tolerated in DILV with good size mitral and tricuspid valves

8.2 Surgical Management

8.2.1 Initial Palliative Surgery

- Initial palliation performed to allow survival and prepare for definitive palliation
- Goals of initial palliation
  - Optimize systemic outflow in those with subaortic or aortic arch obstruction
  - Adequate but not excessive flow through a low-resistance, non-distorted pulmonary vascular bed
  - Ensure systemic and pulmonary vascular returns are unobstructed

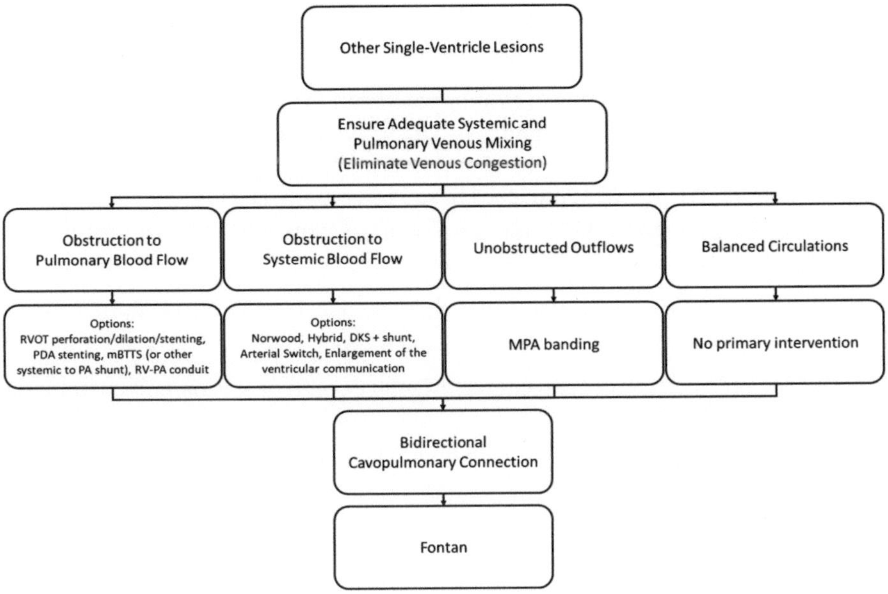

Fig. 3 Management algorithm for patients with other single ventricle lesions

8.2.2 Obstruction to Pulmonary Blood Flow

- Surgical options include modified BTT shunt (or other systemic to PA shunt), RV-PA conduit (Fig. 3)
- Requires CT imaging to confirm PAs (confluent, size) and PDA (tortuosity, insertion site) suitable for intervention.
- Modified BTT shunt (and less commonly, RV-PA conduit) if PDA anatomy not amenable to stenting, proximal PA stenosis or discontinuous PAs, or institutional preference

8.2.3 Obstruction to Systemic Blood Flow

- Arch reconstruction reserved for patients with isolated CoA and hypoplasia of the aortic arch
- Norwood operation required if stenosis at the subvalvar level (including VSD in setting of VA discordance), systemic VA valve, or ascending aorta. Source of pulmonary blood flow (i.e. modified BTT shunt or RV-PA conduit) determined according to ventricular morphology and anatomy of aortic arch branching. Generally, an atrial septectomy is completed to provide unrestrictive mixing.
  - Alternative is hybrid operation with bilateral PA bands to restrict pulmonary blood flow, PDA stent ± atrial septostomy to provide unrestrictive atrial shunting ± reverse modified BTT shunt

- In patients with a dominant LV and VA discordance, development of subaortic obstruction is an indicator of poor prognosis
  - Can manifest at birth or develop in post-natal life following the first stage of palliation i.e., after PA banding in DILV/TGA due to restrictive ventricular septal defect
  - A number of surgical approaches have been employed (Fig. 3):
    1. DKS procedure with modified BTT shunt (our current institutional strategy)

       At initial palliation, isolated interstage operation, or during BCPS operation
    2. Enlargement of the interventricular communication/bulboventricular foramen
    3. Arterial switch operation with arch repair ± modified BTT shunt

8.2.4 Unobstructed Outflows

- Pulmonary arterial banding (PAB) constructed using polytetrafluoroethylene graft trimmed to 2.5 to 3.5 mm width reduces pulmonary blood flow and PA pressure to prevent pulmonary vascular disease (in preparation for BCPS)
- Band size predicted by Trusler's equation (PAB = 20 (biventricular) or 24 (SV) mm + 1 mm for every kg of body weight) depending on patient's anatomy and physiology and partly on surgeon's discretion and individualization based on systemic and pulmonary arterial pressures and systemic arterial oxygen saturations
- Modifications target an echocardiographic peak pressure gradient of at least 25–35 mm Hg or a systolic PA pressure of less than 50% of systemic pressure by direct needle measurement, no increase in AVVR, and preserved ventricular function, and systemic oxygen saturations of approximately 80%
- PAB position is confirmed by echocardiography
- Novel techniques used for percutaneously adjusting PAB in the post-operative period
- Alternative strategy is division of the pulmonary trunk and placement of a systemic-to-PA shunt

8.2.5 Balanced Circulations

- If remains well-balanced, can often have BCPS as first palliation

8.2.6 Anomalies of Pulmonary Venous Return

- Significantly complicate the course of patients at all stages of their care
- Most common in patients with atrial isomerism, TAPVC
- 50% repaired at the time of their initial palliation procedure

8.2.7 Atrial Septostomy or Septectomy

- May be required at the first stage palliation to improve mixing or decrease LA pressure in case of restrictive atrial septum

9 Intensive Care Physiology and Management

9.1 Following Initial Palliation

- Need to account for the effects of the procedure on the myocardium and PVR.
- Following Norwood and DKS procedures, PVR typically transiently elevated and labile
- Cardiac output depressed for 12 to 24 h following surgery because of myocardial ischemia from aortic cross clamping
- Balancing the pulmonary and systemic blood flow (Qp/Qs)
- Routine post-operative management (see Chap. 50, post-operative complications)

10 Outcome

- Wide range of long-term outcomes depending on native anatomy and associated cardiac lesions
  - Estimated 10-to-15-year survival ranges from 50% to 75% for most patients with 'typical' risk profile
- High risk subgroups include patients with restrictive atrial septum, associated pulmonary venous anomalies, majority of pulmonary blood flow being supplied by AP collaterals

Bibliography

1. Fraser CD Jr. Management of systemic outlet obstruction in patients undergoing single ventricle palliation. In: Seminars in thoracic and cardiovascular surgery: pediatric cardiac surgery annual; 2009. p. 70–5.
2. Glatz AC, Petit CJ, Goldstein BH, et al. Comparison between patent ductus arteriosus stent and modified Blalock-Taussig Shunt as palliation for infants with ductal-dependent pulmonary blood flow: Insights from the Congenital Catheterization Research Collaborative. Circulation. 2018;137(6):589–601.

3. Hutter D, Redington AN, et al. The Principles of management, and outcomes for, patients with functionally univentricular hearts. In: Anderson RH, et al., editors. Paediatric cardiology. 3rd ed. Philadelphia: Churchill Livingstone; 2010. p. 687–96.
4. Khairy P, Poirier N, Mercier LA. Univentricular heart. Circulation. 2007;115(6):800–12.
5. Lee JR, Choi JS, Kang CH, et al. Surgical results of patients with a functional single ventricle. Eur J Cardiothorac Surg. 2003;24(5):716–22.
6. Moodie DS, et al. Long-term follow-up in the unoperated univentricular heart. Am J Cardiol. 1984;53(8):1124–8.
7. Nelson DP, Schwartz SM, Chang AC. Neonatal physiology of functionally univentricular heart. Cardiol Young. 2004;14(Suppl 1):52–60.
8. Penny DJ, Anderson RH, et al. Other forms of functionally univentricular hearts. In: Anderson RH, et al., editors. Paediatric Cardiology. 3rd ed. Philadelphia: Churchill Livingstone; 2010. p. 665–86.
9. Petit CJ, et al. Outcomes after decompression of the right ventricle in infants with pulmonary atresia with intact ventricular septum are associated with degree of tricuspid regurgitation: results from the congenital catheterization research collaborative. Circ Cardiovasc Interv. 2017;10(5): e004428.
10. Wernovsky G, Bove EL. Single ventricle lesions. In: Chang AL, Hanley FL, Wernovsky G, et al, editors. Pediatric cardiac intensive care. Lippincott Williams & Wilkins, Baltimore; 1998. p. 271–288.

Borderline Right Ventricles and One and a Half Ventricle Circulation

Bhavikkumar D. Langanecha and Devin Chetan

Abstract One and a half ventricle repair (1.5VR) is a combination of intracardiac repair for hypoplastic subpulmonic ventricle with bidirectional cavopulmonary connection. While this surgery was originally developed to address PA/IVS this procedure is performed when the left ventricle (LV) is functionally normal but the right ventricle (RV) is incapable of handling the entire cardiac output. Common indications include hypoplasia of the RV or tricuspid valve (TV), or well sized RV with acute or chronic dysfunction. 1.5VR decreases the volume load on the suboptimal RV, provides pulsatile pulmonary blood flow, roughly equal systemic and pulmonary flow, and normal systemic oxygen saturations. There has been an improvement in surgical outcome over time with early mortality estimated at 0 to 10% and long-term survival 80.1% and 69.3% at 10 and 20 years, respectively. Patients with 1.5VR have a trend towards higher oxygen consumption (VO_2) when exercising compared to patients with Fontan circulation and there have been no reported complications of high venous pressure like protein-losing enteropathy or chronic liver congestion.

Keywords One and a half ventricle (1.5 ventricle) · Bidirectional cavopulmonary connection · Bidirectional cavopulmonary shunt · Borderline right ventricle (RV) · Fenestrated ASD

Abbreviations

1.5VR One and a half ventricle Repair

B. D. Langanecha (✉) · D. Chetan
Division of Cardiology, Labatt Family Heart Centre, The Hospital for Sick Children, Toronto, ON, Canada
e-mail: Bhavikkumar.langanecha@sickkids.ca

D. Chetan
e-mail: Devin.chetan@sickkids.ca

B. D. Langanecha
Division of Cardiac Critical Care, Department of Critical Care Medicine, Labatt Family Heart Centre, The Hospital for Sick Children, University of Toronto, Toronto, ON, Canada

© The Author(s), under exclusive license to Springer Nature Switzerland AG 2024
A. I. Dipchand et al. (eds.), *Manual of Cardiac Care in Children*,
https://doi.org/10.1007/978-3-031-70973-9_34

ASD	Atrial septal defect
AV	Atrioventricular
BCPS	Bidirectional cavopulmonary shunt
BiV	Biventricular
ccTGA	Congenitally corrected transposition of the great arteries
CHB	Complete heart block
DDD	Dual paced, dual sensed, dual response (pacemaker mode)
DORV	Double outlet right Ventricle
IVC	Inferior vena cava
LSVC	Left SVC
LV	Left ventricle
MV	Mitral valve
OR	Operating room
PA	Pulmonary artery
PAB	Pulmonary artery band
PA/IVS	Pulmonary atresia/intact ventricular septum
PS	Pulmonary stenosis
PVRi	Pulmonary vascular resistance indexed
RA	Right atrium
RV	right ventricle
RVOTO	Right ventricular outflow tract obstruction
SVC	Superior vena cava
TOF	Tetralogy of fallot
TV	Tricuspid valve
VO_2	Oxygen consumption
VSD	Ventricular septal defect

Key Points

- One and a half ventricle repair (1.5VR) is a combination of intracardiac repair and bidirectional cavoplumonary shunt (BCPS) for a subpulmonic ventricle that is unable to exclusively support the pulmonary circulation
- Indications include (i) (most common) hypoplastic subpulmonic ventricle and/or tricuspid valve (TV)—mainly in PA/IVS, (ii) chronic RV dysfunction, (iii) salvage for acute RV failure, and (iv) surgical complexity (e.g. BCPS in complex ccTGA repairs to reduce complication of atrial baffle—LSVC to unroofed coronary sinus)
- While 1.5VR reduces RV volume load and provides pulsatile pulmonary blood flow at roughly equal systemic and pulmonary flow, and normal systemic oxygen saturations, there is competitive flow between the BCPS and subpulmonic forward flow

- A 1.5VR may define the end-state anatomy and physiology or may be included as a palliative procedure to allow for RV growth and rehabilitation for an eventual biventricular repair.
- Complications include chylothorax, pleural effusion, intermittent headache, upper body swelling (SVC syndrome), aneurysmal SVC dilation, and atrial arrhythmias. It is not associated with complications of high venous pressure to lower body, such as protein-losing enteropathy or chronic liver congestion.
- Outcomes have improved over time with early mortality estimates from 0 to 10% and long-term survival of 80% and 69% at 10 and 20 years, respectively

1 Introduction

- One and a half ventricle repair (1.5VR) was introduced by Billingsley et al. in 1989 and initially applied to PA/IVS (Chap. 16) with a well-formed LV and a hypoplastic right ventricle (RV) and/or tricuspid valve (TV) that were not capable of supporting the entire pulmonary circulation.
- Attempting biventricular repair in this group leads to low cardiac output, high systemic venous pressure, and higher mortality. Alternatively, the Fontan circulation is associated with long term attrition risk.
- 1.5VR is defined as a combination of BCPS in association with diverting remaining (inferior) systemic venous return to the pulmonary arterial circulation using the hypoplastic sub-pulmonary ventricle (also referred to as partial biventricular repair) (Fig. 1).
- Hypothetical advantages of 1.5VR are:
  - Complete septation of the pulmonary and systemic circulations—achieving normal systemic oxygen saturations
- Ability to augment cardiac output and better exercise tolerance
- Maintaining pulsatile flow in the pulmonary circulation
- Maintaining low venous pressure in the inferior vena cava (IVC) system
- Ability of the hypoplastic RV to better handle reduced preload

2 Principle

- BCPS reduces the volume load on the RV
- Equal pulmonary (pulmonary flow = combination of antegrade flow from the pulmonary ventricle and BCPS anastomosis) and systemic flow with near normal systemic oxygen saturation.
- In 1.5VR, there is competitive flow between the BCPS and subpulmonic forward flow.
  - Pulmonary blood flow varies during different phases of the cardiac cycle

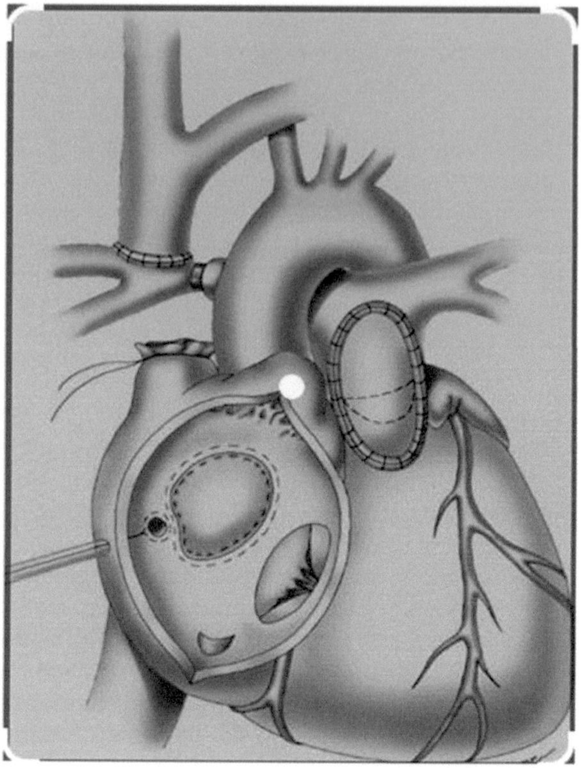

Fig. 1 One and half ventricle repair with right pulmonary artery banding in hypoplastic RVReprinted from The Journal of Thoracic and Cardiovascular Surgery, Vol 117, Issue 4, Kreutzer C, Mayorquin RC, Kreutzer GOA, et al. Experience with one and a half ventricle repair, pp 662–668, 1999, with permission from Elsevier

  - Systole: IVC flow is delivered to pulmonary artery by subpulmonic ventricle contraction
  - Diastole: laminar flow from BCPS anastomosis.
  - Circulation is influenced by TV inflow size, RV compliance, pulmonary vascular resistance, and pulmonary insufficiency
- Decreased volume load on the systemic ventricle due to fully oxygenated blood and absence of major right to left shunt (Table 1).

3 Patients Can Be Stratified According to Their Indications for 1.5VR

- Group A: Small pulmonary ventricle and/or tricuspid valve
  - PA/IVS with hypoplastic RV (Fig. 1)
- Group B: Chronic RV dysfunction
  - Ebstein's Anomaly, Uhl anomaly or PA/IVS with ventricular dysfunction

Table 1 Cardiac Anatomy for 1.5 VR

1.5VR may be Appropriate with:	
• PA/IVS • Ebstein's anomaly • Atypical TOF, hypoplastic TV, RV, ASD • VSD with RVOTO, hypoplastic RV, TV • ccTGA with borderline RV • Inlet VSD with straddling tricuspid valve • Tricuspid stenosis, ASD • D-TGA with VSD and PS	• Complete AVSD with – TOF – DORV – PS – Extreme left ventricular dominance Multiple muscular VSD, hypoplastic RV

Legend ASD—atrial septal defect; AVSD—Atrioventricular septal defect; ccTGA—Congenitally corrected transposition of the great vessels; DORV—Double outlet right ventricle; D-TGA—D looped transposition of great vessels; IVS—Intact ventricular septum; PS—Pulmonary stenosis; RV—Right ventricle; RVOTO—Right ventricular outflow tract obstruction; TOF—Tetralogy of Fallot; TV—tricuspid valve; VSD—Ventricular septal defect

- Group C: Facilitating repair without size or functional problems in the pulmonary ventricle
  - ccTGA with borderline morphological RV (Fig. 2), D-TGA/VSD/PS with smallish RV or straddling TV (Table 2).

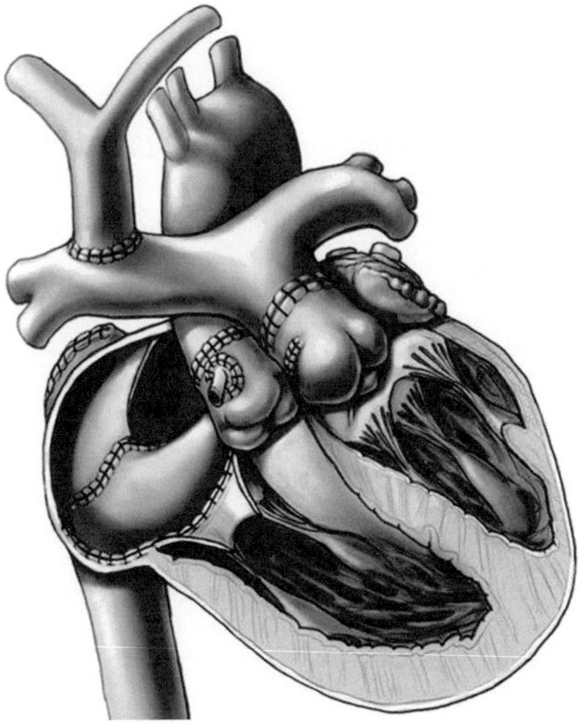

Fig. 2 One and half ventricle repair in congenitally corrected transposition of great arteries (BCPS + Hemi-Senning/Hemi-Mustard + Arterial switch). Reprinted from World Journal for Pediatric and Congenital Heart Surgery 2011 Jan 2(1); pp 64–79; Permission may not be required as per SAGE Journals, email dated July 24th 2023

Table 2 Selection Criteria for 1.5 VR

Anatomical Selection criteria for small pulmonary ventricle and 1.5VR			
Anatomic Criteria	TV Z value	Pulmonary ventricular volume	Surgery recommended
	> − 2	> 80%	Biventricular repair
	< − 2	< 80%	One and a half ventricular repair
	< − 2 and > −5	< 50%	One and a half ventricular repair Consider atrial fenestration
	< − 5	< 30%	Fontan procedure

- Group D: Acute RV dysfunction
  - Acute hemodynamic or functional RV failure after cardiac surgery as a salvage procedure

- Parameters used for decision-making vary across centers—other have also used TV diameter (% of normal), TV:MV ratio and RV morphology in addition to the aforementioned criteria

4 Investigations

4.1 Echocardiogram is Key to the Evaluation for 1.5VR

- Assessment of TV size and function, including TV valve z-score and TV:MV ratio, and TV regurgitation
- RV volume and function
- RV outflow tract and branch PAs
- Atrial communication
- LV ventricular function

4.2 MRI:

- Quantify RV volume and function
- Evaluate RV for endomyocardial fibroelastosis
- Assess systemic ventricular function

4.3 Cardiac Catheterization

- PA pressure (mean PAp less than 15)
- Transpulmonary Gradient
- PVRi (Less than 3WU*m^2)
- Systemic ventricular end diastolic pressure (less than 12 mm Hg)
- RA pressure

5 Surgical Considerations

- Intracardiac repair with SVC anastomosis to PA
- May require RV muscle bundle resection to rehabilitate RV and increase volume
- Performed as staged procedure (BCPS and septation of heart—closure of ASD—achieved with more than one intervention) or primary 1.5VR

6 Special Surgical Concerns Related to 1.5VR

- Pulmonary Insufficiency (PI)
  - Free PI may lead to backflow of blood from the SVC to the RV. It could theoretically further reduce the functional efficiency of an already abnormal RV.

    It may increase volume load on RV and part of the rationale for 1.5VR is lost
  - Free PI may help in increasing RV dimensions and promote RV growth which may help with subsequent biventricular (BiV) repair
- Azygous/Hemiazygos Vein
  - Difference in practices regarding ligation of azygous vein during 1.5VR
  - Advantages of a patent Azygous system include:

    Decompression of SVC or RA in patients with SVC hypertension or severe RV dysfunction without desaturation
    During exercise, it permits blood flow from lower to upper compartment when the RV is incapable of handling the increased systemic venous return
    Only beneficial if TV and RV can accommodate increase in flow
  - Concern for semicircular shunt
- Pulmonary Artery Banding (PAB)
  - Some centers perform an RPA band

  - Rationale is prevention of retrograde SVC flow to RV during diastole and prevention of RV ejection into SVC during systole.
  - Advantages: reducing SVC pulsatility, reducing the amount of regurgitant blood flow from SVC to RV, and decreases the theoretical risk of SVC aneurysmal dilatation.

7 Residual ASD

- Residual atrial communication is considered if flow through TV and RV is limited and unable to tolerate full IVC flow. Would reduce risk of higher RA pressure with low cardiac output; maintains cardiac output at the expense of desaturation and risk of paradoxical embolism. (Sometimes called a 1¼ repair.)
- May create adjustable ASD intraoperatively and determine final physiology at end of OR.
- ASD can later be closed by intervention or spontaneously in most of patients at 10 years follow up.

8 Intensive Care Physiology and Management

- Early extubation if clinical condition permits. Spontaneous ventilation optimizes pulmonary blood flow
- Optimize lung functional residual capacity: Drainage of pleural effusion and opening of collapsed lung
- Maintain AV synchrony. Atrial pacing for junctional rhythm or DDD pacing for complete heart block (CHB)
- Low cardiac output state: Optimization of preload, inotrope/vasopressor support, creating of ASD, mechanical circulatory support

9 Complications

- Chylothorax and pleural effusion
- Intermittent headache and upper body swelling
- Atrial arrhythmia, 8 to 16% (Risk factors are Ebstein's anomaly, systemic ventricular dysfunction, heterotaxy syndrome)
- SVC aneurysmal dilatation
- Reinterventions (takedown of SVC-PA anastomosis, PA plasty, ASD creation/closure)

10 Outcomes

- Very good early outcomes—mortality following 1.5VR ranges from 0 to 10%
- SickKids outcomes: 6.1% operative mortality and 20.2% late mortality. Majority of late mortality is cardiac in nature.
- Good long-term survival with 20-year survival ranging between 69.3% and 91%. Improvement in survival in the recent era
- No reports of protein losing enteropathy.
- Limited exercise tests showed tendency toward the higher maximum oxygen uptake compared to Fontan (similar to biventricular repair)
- Patients with significant PI may have RV dilation with SVC contributing to RV preload (and not PA blood flow) in diastole.

Bibliography

1. Billingsley AM, Laks H, Boyce SW, et al. Definitive repair in patients with pulmonary atresia and intact ventricular septum. J Thorac Cardiovasc Surg. 1989 May;97(5):746–54.
2. Cabrelle G, Castaldi B, et al. Long-term experience with the one-and-a-half ventricle repair for simple and complex congenital heart defects. Euro J Cardiothorac Surg. 2021;59(1):244–52.
3. Chowdhury UK, Airan B, Talwar S, et al. One and one-half ventricle repair: results and concerns. Ann Thorac Surg. 2005;80(6):2293–300.
4. Kim S, Al-Radi O, Friedberg MK, et al. Superior vena cava to pulmonary artery anastomosis as an adjunct to biventricular repair: 38-Year Follow-Up. Ann Thorac Surg. 2009;87(5):1475–83.
5. Talwar S, Siddharth B, Choudhary SK, et al. One and half ventricle repair: rationale, indications and results. Indian J of Thorac Cardiovasc Surg. 2018;34(3):370–80.
6. Van Arsdell GS, Williams WG, Freedom RM. Practical approach to 1 1/2 ventricle repairs. Ann Thorac Surg. 1998;66(2):678–80.

Heterotaxy and Isomerism

Lindsay R. Freud and Shi-Joon Yoo

Abstract Heterotaxy refers to an abnormality of situs or left–right patterning within the body, which is often associated with congenital heart disease and/or arrhythmias. There are two main types: classic right isomerism with asplenia and classic left isomerism with polysplenia. Right isomerism typically involves right ventricular outflow tract obstruction, which is often ductal-dependent, and complete atrioventricular septal defect with ventriculoarterial discordance that is often treated with staged univentricular palliation. The presence of obstructed total anomalous pulmonary venous connection portends a worse outcome. Classic left isomerism with polysplenia, on the other hand, typically manifests with less significant structural congenital heart disease, often amenable to a biventricular repair. However, this form may present with potentially life-threatening bradyarrhythmias, particularly in the fetus. Mixed or disharmonious arrangements may occur in up to 20%. Extracardiac manifestations, such as poor splenic function, intestinal malrotation, and biliary atresia, are common and important to consider for comprehensive management. Outcomes of heterotaxy patients are highly variable; survival is lower compared to non-heterotaxy patients with the same congenital heart defects. Risk factors for mortality from birth include right isomerism/asplenia, obstructed pulmonary venous return, complete atrioventricular septal defect, and common atrioventricular valve regurgitation.

Keywords Heterotaxy · Isomerism · Situs abnormalities · Congenital heart disease · Arrhythmia

L. R. Freud (✉)
Division of Cardiology, Department of Paediatrics, Labatt Family Heart Centre, The Hospital for Sick Children, University of Toronto, Toronto, ON, Canada
e-mail: Lindsay.freud@sickkids.ca

S.-J. Yoo
Department of Diagnostic Imaging, The Hospital for Sick Children, University of Toronto, Toronto, ON, Canada
e-mail: Shi-joon.yoo@sickkids.ca

© The Author(s), under exclusive license to Springer Nature Switzerland AG 2024

A. I. Dipchand et al. (eds.), *Manual of Cardiac Care in Children*,
https://doi.org/10.1007/978-3-031-70973-9_35

Abbreviations

AV	Atrioventricular
AVSD	Atrioventricular septal defect
AVVR	Atrioventricular valve regurgitation
BCPS	Bidirectional cavopulmonary shunt
BiV	Biventricular
CHB	Complete heart block
CHD	Congenital heart disease
DORV	Double outlet right ventricle
IVC	Inferior vena cava
PA	Pulmonary artery
PGE	Prostaglandin
RVOTO	Right ventricular outflow tract obstruction
SA	Sinoatrial
SVC	Superior vena cava
TAPVC	Total anomalous pulmonary venous connection
VA	Ventriculo-arterial

Key Points

- Heterotaxy refers to an abnormality of situs or left–right patterning within the body.
- Two main types: classic right isomerism (asplenia) and classic left isomerism (polysplenia). Mixed or disharmonious arrangements may occur in up to 20%
- Right isomerism typically involves right ventricular outflow tract obstruction (RVOTO) with complete atrioventricular septal defect (AVSD) and ventriculoarterial (VA) discordance and is often treated with univentricular palliation. Obstructed pulmonary venous return portends worse outcome.
- Left isomerism may present with bradyarrhythmia or complete heart block (CHB) in the fetus/neonate, which may be life-threatening. Congenital heart defects (CHD) are typically less severe, and biventricular (BiV) repair is commonly performed.
- Careful evaluation of systemic and pulmonary venous anomalies is critical for surgical planning.
- Comprehensive management also involves attention to extracardiac manifestations, particularly splenic function to determine the need for antibiotic prophylaxis and extended immunizations.
- Outcomes for heterotaxy patients are worse than for non-heterotaxy patients with similar CHD. Right isomerism portends very poor prognosis particularly when early intervention required.

1 Definitions and Nomenclature

- Situs: Arrangement of the internal thoracic and abdominal organs across the left–right axis of the body. Situs is determined at three levels:
  - Abdominal situs (by observing the location of the larger lobe of the liver and stomach, and the presence or absence of the spleen)
  - Bronchopulmonary situs (by observing the relationship between the branch pulmonary arteries and the upper lobar bronchi)
  - Atrial situs (by observing the morphology of the appendages including distribution of the pectinate muscles)
- Types of situs (Fig. 1):
  - Situs solitus (usual arrangement)
  - Situs inversus (mirror-image arrangement)
  - Heterotaxy (neither situs solitus nor situs inversus)

    Classic right isomerism with asplenia
    Classic left isomerism with polysplenia
    Mixed or disharmonious arrangement

1.1 *On-going Debates*

- Van Praagh group: Atrial situs is predominantly determined by the connection of the inferior vena (IVC) to the atrium. Terminology is dictated by splenic appearance (asplenia or polysplenia).
- Anderson group: Atrial situs is determined by the morphology of the atrial appendages and classified into usual arrangement, mirror-image arrangement, right or left isomerism.
- Unresolved problems:
  - Morphological identification of the atrial appendages is often not possible by imaging and, in fact, of little clinical significance.
  - Approximately 20% of cases are not classifiable into right or left isomerism as the organ arrangement shows mixed or disharmonious patterns at three levels.
  - Nevertheless, the concept is helpful to understand the constellation of abnormalities and associated prognosis in most cases.

2 Anatomy

See (Table 1).

Table 1 Key features of right and left isomerism

	Right isomerism	Left isomerism
Structurally normal heart		15%
AV connections	AVSD in 70% Univentricular in 70%	AVSD in > 70% Univentricular in 25%
VA connection	TGA or DORV in > 95%	Concordant in 70%
Pulmonary outflow tract stenosis or atresia	> 90%	30%
Venous connections		
Pulmonary veins	By definition connect anomalously (may be intra/supra/infracardiac)	Normal
SVC	Bilateral SVC in 50%	Bilateral SVC in 50%
IVC	Intact	Interrupted (w/ hemiazygous continuity) in > 80%
Coronary sinus	Absent	Normal
Portal veins	Normal	< 15% Portosystemic shunt
Rhythm issues		
Dual sinus and AV nodes	Common	
Sinus bradycardia		< 40%
Complete heart block		Possible
Hiatal hernia	15%	
Spleen	Absent	Polysplenia
Intestinal malrotation		Common
Biliary atresia		< 10%

- Classic right isomerism (asplenia)
  - Horizontal liver; stomach on either side closer to midline than normal
  - Bilaterally short main bronchi with the descending branches of the pulmonary arteries (PA) located below the upper lobar bronchi (bilateral hypobronchial PAs)
  - Juxtaposition of the IVC and the abdominal aorta on the same side relative to the spine in > 90%
  - Bilateral superior venae cavae (SVC) in 50%
  - Absent coronary sinus in almost all cases
  - Extracardiac total anomalous pulmonary venous connection (TAPVC) in 50%
  - AVSD in 70%; almost always complete
  - Univentricular AV connection in 70%
  - VA connection, not concordant (such as transposition or DORV) in > 95%
  - Pulmonary stenosis or atresia in 90%
  - Paired SA and AV nodes with supraventricular tachycardia in up to 25%

- Classic left isomerism (polsyplenia)
  - Liver, can be symmetric or asymmetric in shape, stomach on either side usually closer to midline than normal
  - Extrahepatic porto-systemic shunt with hypoplasia or agenesis of portal vein, not uncommonly reported
  - IVC on either side or bilateral. Interrupted IVC with azygos or hemiazygos continuation in > 80%
  - Bilateral SVC in 50%
  - Remainder of heart is normal in 15%
  - AVSD in 70%; either partial or complete
  - BiV AV connection in 75%
  - Concordant VA connection in up to 70%
  - Ventricular outflow tract obstruction in two thirds, either pulmonary (one third) or systemic (one third)
  - Bilaterally absent regular SA and AV nodes with discontinuous AV pathway causing sinus bradycardia or CHB in 40%

3 Epidemiology

- ~ 1–2/10,000 births
- 2–4% of CHD seen in infants
- Almost all patients with heterotaxy and classic right isomerism identified; classic left isomerism may not be identified because of lack of functionally significant abnormalities.
- Left isomerism is more frequently seen than right in fetal life because of a high incidence of fetal demise due to congenital CHB and heart failure.

4 Clinical Presentation

- Depends upon individual findings.
- Right isomerism
  - Often presents with cyanosis due to right heart obstruction, (i.e., multi-level pulmonary stenosis or atresia) often ductal-dependent for pulmonary blood flow in the neonatal period.
  - Cyanosis and tachypnea due to TAPVC, particularly with obstruction, may also be the cause for early presentation in up to 25%.
- Left isomerism
  - Commonly presents early in life due to bradyarrhythmia or CHB, which may manifest as hydrops in the fetus and is highly associated with fetal demise.

  - Up to 15% of patients with known left isomerism have structurally normal hearts.

5 Extracardiac Manifestations

- Seen in 15% of cases with a prenatal diagnosis of heterotaxy. More commonly with left than right isomerism.
- Splenic abnormalities, asplenia versus polysplenia
  - Association of right isomerism and asplenia and association of left isomerism and polysplenia in the majority of cases. Note that it is not always the case.
  - When present, a spleen or splenules are always along the greater curvature of the stomach.
  - Splenic function must be confirmed even when splenules are present
- Intestinal malrotation predisposing to volvulus
  - Rule rather than exception.
  - Risk of intestinal obstruction is higher than in non-heterotaxic patients but relatively low.
  - Prophylactic Ladd's procedure is controversial.
- Partial ectopic position of stomach in thorax (also described as hiatal hernia)
  - Reported in up to 15% of heterotaxy with right isomerism.
  - Can be responsible for vomiting and recurrent airway infections.
  - May require fundoplication.
- Biliary atresia
  - In up to 10% of patients with heterotaxy and left isomerism.
  - Heterotaxy patients presenting with jaundice should be investigated.
- Extrahepatic portosystemic shunt
  - Exact incidence, not known
  - 15% of patients with congenital extracardiac portosystemic shunt have polysplenia.
- Primary ciliary dyskinesia in up to 25% of heterotaxy cases and up to 50% of situs inversus cases. The cilia are considered to play a key role in development of right-left asymmetry.

6 Diagnostic Studies

6.1 *Fetal Echocardiogram*

- Accurate diagnosis can be made prenatally and is important for fetal counseling and to prepare for delivery and postnatal management, i.e., need for PGE in right isomerism, pacing in left isomerism.

6.2 *CXR*

- Dextrocardia in 35–40%

6.3 *ECG*

- Right isomerism: Right- and left-sided atrial origins of the P wave may be present at different times, reflecting bilateral SA nodes. Twin AV nodes may also be present, which is a risk factor for re-entrant tachycardia.
- Left isomerism: Sinus rhythm is rare, due to absence of the SA node. Ectopic atrial or junctional rhythm(s) predominate. CHB may occur due to absence of the AV node.

6.4 *Echocardiogram*

- Gold standard to delineate cardiac position, atrial arrangement, and AV and VA relationships and to assess valve regurgitation and ventricular function

6.5 *Cross-Sectional Imaging (CT or MRI)*

- For depiction of complex systemic and pulmonary venous anatomy including pulmonary vein stenosis
- Guide decision-making for BiV and univentricular repair
- Complex VA connection requiring comprehensive 3D modeling and printing

6.6 *Abdominal Ultrasound*

- To establish visceral situs, presence or absence of spleen(s), intestinal malrotation

6.7 Peripheral Blood Smear

- Howell-Jolly bodies or pitted RBC counts to assess splenic function at ≥ 3 months of age

7 Management and Surgical Considerations

7.1 Right Isomerism

- Due to constellation of complex CHD, up to 85% undergo staged univentricular palliation, i.e., intervention to establish pulmonary blood flow, BCPS, and Fontan operations.
- Careful attention needs to be paid to cardiac position, systemic and pulmonary venous return. These anatomical findings may complicate or preclude heart transplantation if univentricular palliation fails.
- Mixed data regarding survival benefit with BiV repair.

7.2 Left Isomerism

- Neonates and children with CHV may require pacemaker placement, particularly in the setting of co-existing CHD.
- Most are amenable to BiV repair.
- When BiV repair is not feasible, Kawashima operation in the presence of an interrupted IVC with azygous continuation and later Fontan completion to mitigate against or manage pulmonary arteriovenous malformation; Kawashima includes BCPS (Chapter 36) when IVC interrupted, and SVC carries all venous return except for hepatic veins and coronary sinus.

7.3 Antibiotic Prophylaxis and Immunizations

- Patients with heterotaxy and asplenia, solitary spleen, and polysplenia are susceptible to bacteremia and septicemia from encapsulated organisms since the solitary spleen or splenules may not function well.
- Antibiotic prophylaxis (amoxicillin 20 mg/kg/day) is recommended for all patients with heterotaxy until 2 years of age, at which time splenic function may be reliably assessed. Prophylaxis should be continued until ≥ 5 years of age if splenic function is impaired.
- In addition to routine pediatric immunizations, patients should receive 23-valent pneumococcal and extended series of meningococcal vaccinations.

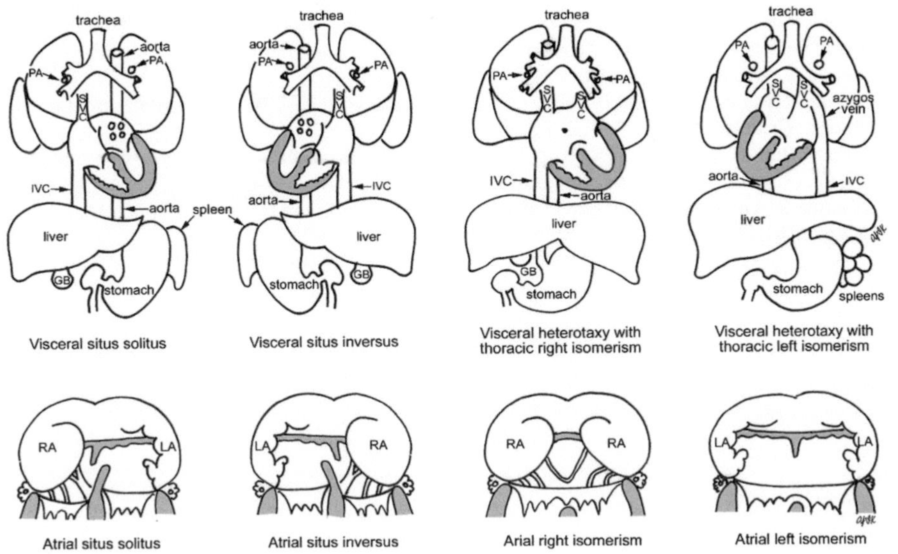

Fig. 1 Types of situs. Heterotaxy is defined as the body organ arrangement other than situs solitus and situs inversus. Although the majority of cases with heterotaxy show either classic right isomerism or classic left isomerism as illustrated, approximately 20% show disharmonious arrangement such as a combination of bronchopulmonary situs solitus, polysplenia and left isomerism

8 Outcomes

- Survival for patients with heterotaxy is worse than for patients with the same congenital heart defects without heterotaxy.
- Overall, 25-year survival from birth is approximately 60%.
  - For right isomerism, 5-year survival from birth is up to 60-and 25-year survival is 50%. Significantly worse outcome if early intervention required.
  - For left isomerism, 5-year survival from birth is 85–95% and 25-year survival is 75%.
- Risk factor for poor prognosis in fetal life is CHB or bradycardia.
- Risk factors for poor prognosis from birth include right isomerism/asplenia, obstructed TAPVC, complete AVSD, and common AVVR.

Bibliography

1. Andrés A, Miño C, Diéguez E, et al. Specific injuries management in the postoperative of congenital heart diseases (II): Univentricular Hearts. Open J Pediatr. 2015;5:67–75.

2. Banka P, Porras D, Mayer JE et al (2014) Single ventricle (Non HLHS) In: Da Cruz EM et al. (eds.) Pediatric and congenital cardiology, cardiac surgery and intensive care, 1st edn. Springer-Verlag, London, p. 1861–1883.
3. George-Hyslop C, Thomas J, Fazari LG. Understanding Stage II Bidirectional Cavopulmonary Shunts. Crit Care Nurse. 2017;37(6):59–71.
4. Luo S, Haranal M, Deng MX, et al. Low preoperative superior vena cava blood flow predicts bidirectional cavopulmonary shunt failure. J Thorac Cardiovasc Surg. 2020;160(6):1529–40.
5. Sharma R. The bidirectional Glenn shunt for univentricular hearts. Indian J Thorac Cardiovasc Surg. 2018;34(4):453–6.

Bidirectional Cavopulmonary Shunt (BCPS)

Constanza Jimenez Navia and Alejandro A. Floh

Abstract The bidirectional cavopulmonary shunt (BCPS) operation connects the upper body venous drainage directly into the right pulmonary artery establishing passive pulmonary blood flow as part of single ventricle palliation. It is generally completed at 4–8 months of age as the second palliative procedure following the Norwood operation, isolated BTT or RV-PA shunt, or main pulmonary artery banding, or first procedure in patients with balanced circulations. The BCPS eliminates the parallel circulations and replaces it with an in-series circulation that offloads volume the heart. Passive pulmonary blood flow is dependent on low pulmonary vascular resistance and transthoracic pressure, and driven by respiratory mechanics of spontaneous breathing. This operation usually serves as a prelude to the total cavopulmonary connection known as the Fontan operation.

Keywords Bidirectional cavopulmonary shunt · Glenn operation · Stage 2 palliation

Abbreviations

AV	Atrioventricular
AVVR	Atrioventricular valve regurgitation
BCPS	Bidirectional cavopulmonary shunt
BTT	Blalock Taussig Thomas
CPB	Cardiopulmonary bypass
DILV	Double inlet left ventricle
DKS	Damus-Kaye-Stansel

C. J. Navia
Cardiac Critical Care Unit, Hospital de Niños Dr. Luis Calvo Mackenna, Santiago, Chile

A. A. Floh (✉)
Division of Cardiac Critical Care Unit, Department of Critical Care Medicine, Labatt Family Heart Centre, The Hospital for Sick Children, University of Toronto, Toronto, ON, Canada
e-mail: alejandro.floh@sickkids.ca

© The Author(s), under exclusive license to Springer Nature Switzerland AG 2024

A. I. Dipchand et al. (eds.), *Manual of Cardiac Care in Children*,
https://doi.org/10.1007/978-3-031-70973-9_36

HLHS	Hypoplastic left heart syndrome
IVC	Inferior vena cava
MPA	Main pulmonary artery
PA	Pulmonary artery
PEEP	Positive end expiratory pressure
PVR	Pulmonary vascular resistance
PVRi	Pulmonary vascular resistance indexed
Qp	Pulmonary blood flow
Qs	Systemic blood flow
RA	Right atrium
RPA	Right pulmonary artery
RV	Right ventricle
SaO_2	Systemic arterial oxygen saturation
SVC	Superior vena cava
SVR	Systemic vascular resistance

Key Points

- Bidirectional cavopulmonary shunt (BCPS), also known as a cavopulmonary shunt, involves the direct connection of SVC flow to pulmonary artery resulting in passive pulmonary blood flow (Fig. 1)
- It serves as the second stage of single ventricle palliation for patients who had undergone a Norwood procedure, isolated BTT or RV-PA shunt insertion, or main pulmonary artery banding. It is the primary stage for single ventricle patients with balanced circulations.
- Unlike alternative operations, BCPS distributes blood flow comparably through both pulmonary arteries
- Reduces the volume load on the single ventricle, resolves the parallel pulmonary and systemic circulations, and may preserve myocardial and AV valve function in setting of a lower and more reliable Qp:Qs.
- Spontaneous breathing and early extubation after surgery reduce the transpulmonary gradient and optimizes hemodynamics
- Postoperative complications include increased pressure—due to anatomic obstruction (intrinsic or extrinsic) or elevated pulomonary vascular resistance (PVR)—in the cavo-pulmonary circuit, hypoxemia and early hypertension.
- Sluggish flow can lead to BCPS thrombosis and/or development of veno-venous decompressing collaterals, pleural effusions, chylothorax

Bidirectional cavopulmonary shunt 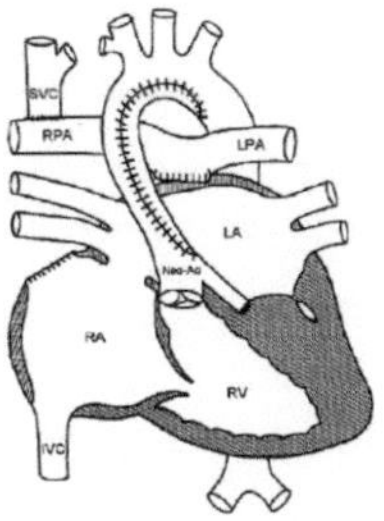 	- End to side anastomosis of the SVC to right PA - SVC is divided at level of branch PA and the cardiac side is oversewn. The cranial side is anastomosed to the superior aspect of the RPA - Provides blood supply to both pulmonary arteries. (thus the term, “bidirectional”)
Hemi Fontan 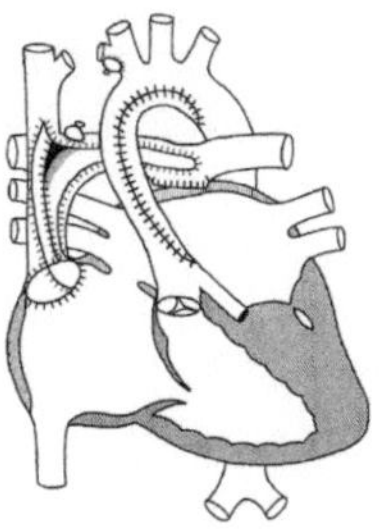	- A confluence of the cardiac end of the SVC, the Right atrium and the RPA is created. – A patch is placed across the superior cavoatrial junction separating SVC blood flow from IVC and coronary sinus blood flow

Fig. 1 Bidirectional cavopulmonary shunt and Hemi-Fontan

1 Timing of Intervention

- Ideal timing of the BCPS is at 4 to 6 months of age, when the pulmonary vascular anatomy and resistance are usually sufficient to allow an appropriate amount of passive pulmonary blood flow at an acceptable pressure.
- Earlier intervention may be required if progressive cyanosis due to shunt (BTT or RV-PA) or pulmonary artery (PA) stenosis in patients with appropriate physiology on preoperative evaluation
- Surgery delayed in patients with bilateral superior vena cava (SVC) and absent connecting vein requiring bilateral BCPS or those undergoing a Kawashima operation
- A Kawashima operation refers to a BCPS in children with an interrupted IVC (usually in setting of heterotaxy) for whom lower limb venous return is diverted into the SVC through the azygous vein—SVC flow carries all but hepatic venous return through pulmonary circulation
- Relevant risk factors include the size of the PAs, the PVR, the SVC size and blood flow, AV valve insufficiency or ventricular dysfunction.

- Hemi-Fontan procedure (Fig. 1) is an alternative approach to achieve a similar physiology—SVC kept intact and flow is baffled from the RA flow directly into RPA

2 Preoperative Evaluation

- Most patients undergo echocardiography, cardiac catheterization, and/or MRI studies
- Increasing use of combined MRI/cath studies to combine flow and pressure data to inform physiologic assessment
- CT is rarely required to delineate anatomy
- Assessment focused on:
  - Pulmonary pressures and PVR—Low PA pressure (< 15 mm Hg) and PVRi < 3 Woods Unit x M^2. Those with high pulmonary blood flow and somewhat elevated pressure may still be acceptable candidates for a BCPS if the PVR is low. Introduction of pulmonary vasodilators considered if PVR elevated.
  - All sources of pulmonary blood flow (antegrade pulmonary blood flow, shunts)
  - Systolic ventricular function—ventricular dysfunction is associated with worse outcome but may improve once volume load reduced following surgery
  - Diastolic ventricular function—Low atrial filling pressures ($\leq$ 10 mm Hg) and end-diastolic ventricular pressure
  - Atrio-ventricular valve regurgitation (AVVR)—May improve with reduction in ventricular volume load but surgical intervention often required if $\geq$ moderate regurgitation. Staging of AV valve surgery prior to BCPS may be required.
  - Unobstructed systemic and pulmonary venous blood return
  - Transplantation at the time of evaluation for BCPS may be considered if any of the above factors preclude moving forward with a BCPS.
  - Assess and quantify aorto-pulmonary collateral flow. Occlude large collaterals.
  - Assess venovenous collaterals and occlude large vessels draining from upper systemic veins
  - Quantify SVC flow. Flow < 1.6 L/min/m2 associated with increased risk of BCPS failure. Overall systemic cardiac output and Qp:Qs must be considered when interpreting value.

3 Surgical Strategy

- The SVC is anastomosed to the superior surface of the right pulmonary artery and the cardiac end of the SVC is oversewn.
- Azygous vein ligated to prevent SVC decompression and systemic desaturation
- Usually performed on cardiopulmonary bypass (CPB) with beating heart—avoiding need for aortic cross-clamp—unless intracardiac interventions required

- The systemic-to-pulmonary artery shunt or PA band(s) previously in place are removed.
- Native flow from the ventricle into the PAs is generally eliminated and the MPA is oversewn. Ventricle-to-PA continuity may be maintained in a limited capacity if increased pulmonary blood flow required
- Preoperative lesions including AVVR or arch narrowing can be addressed if necessary
- May also be combined with DKS in setting of DILV or tricuspid atresia with VA discordance and concern for future restriction of VSD.
- Additional sources of pulmonary blood flow (e.g. controlled forward flow through native/banded PAs) can be used with caution to augment pulmaonry blood flow—results in pulsatile PA flow; varies by institutional and individual anatomy and accepted if PA pressure is not raised.

4 Intensive Care Physiology and Management

- With a BCPS, only cerebral and upper extremity venous blood flow returns to the lungs resulting in a partial in-series circulation with a Qp:Qs < 1.0.
- Physiologic advantage includes a reduction of the volume loading of the single ventricle, reducing the risk of ventricular dysfunction, and providing a predictable Qp:Qs (approximately 0.6 to 0.7). This ratio tends to be higher in young infants due to the relative head size and associated high blood flow that decreases in time; in general, systemic arterial oxygen saturations (SaO_2) are 75% to 85%.
- Early extubation and negative pressure ventilation is beneficial as it increases pulmonary blood flow.
- If postoperative mechanical ventilation necessary, BCPS flow is optimized by ventilating at the lowest mean airway pressure possible while maintaining functional residual capacity
- In the absence of lung disease, PEEP of 3 to 5 cm H_2O maintains functional residual capacity, does not significantly affect PVR or cardiac output, and may improve oxygenation by reducing areas of microatelectasis, and optimizes ventilation/perfusion matching

5 Postoperative Complications

5.1 Elevated BCPS or SVC Pressures

- BPCS pressure is required to drive pulmonary blood flow. Passive pulmonary blood flow is driven by the transpulmonary gradient (PA mean pressure—common atrial mean pressure)

- BCPS pressures may be elevated > 15 mmHg following surgery and slowly decrease to 12–15 in subsequent days
- Malignant or persistently elevated pressure may result from:
  - Anatomical obstruction/thrombus within BCPS circuit (including surgical anastomosis, pulmonary arteries or pulmonary veins)
  - Elevated PVR from pulmonary arterial hypertension or parenchymal lung disease
  - Increased intrathoracic pressure from high airway ventilation pressures, pleural effusion, pneumothorax
  - High distal atrial pressures from AV valve dysfunction (stenosis or insufficiency), elevated ventricular diastolic pressues due to dysfunction (systolic or diastolic) or outflow obstruction, or residual volume load from unaddressed systemic to pulmonary collateral vessels.
- Elevated BCPS pressures manifest as SVC syndrome: Disproportionate swelling of face and upper body, irritability (headache), serous effusions, decompressing subcutaneous collaterals
- Bilateral BCPS are at increased risk for thrombus formation – particulary in PA segment between BCPS. These patients are anticoagulated in the immediate postoperative period with heparin, and then transitioned to chronic anticoagulation therapy (e.g. enoxaparin, oral warfarin, direct oral anticoagulants).

5.2 *Hypertension, Bradycardia and Irritability*

- Common in the immediate postoperative recovery
- Causes:
  - Pain and anxiety
  - Neurohormonal activation and increase in systemic vascular resistance (SVR).
  - Acute decrease in ventricular volume load and subsequent hyperdynamic function response
  - Acute increase in SVC pressure, leading to compensatory increase in systemic blood pressure to mantain cerebral perfusion pressure.
- Management
  - Sedation and analgesia. Dexmedetomidine may be a particularly useful sedative by facilitating extubation, decreasing delirium, and lowering blood pressure.
  - Elevate head of the bed to 30° to 45° and maintain mildline position to aid SVC drainage
  - Systemic vasodilators or beta-blockade as needed. The choice of agent should take the ventricular function into account using caution for beta-blockade in the presence of significant ventricular dysfunction.

5.3 *Marked Hypoxemia and Cyanosis*

- SaO_2 is determined by pulmonary blood flow, lung function, systemic oxygen delivery and consumption.
- Causes of desaturation include:
  - Pulmonary venous desaturation: Atelectasis, parenchymal lung disease/ consolidation, pulmonary edema, pleural effusion, pneumothorax, hemothorax, pulmonary edema
  - Inadequate pulmonary blood flow: Anatomic obstruction (PA stenosis/ distortion) or increased PVR (arterial or venous hypertension, restrictive atrial communication).
  - Veno-venous decompressing collaterals – from SVC system to IVC or pulmonary veins. Often in setting of higher obstruction to pulmonary blood flow (elevation in SVC pressures may be mitigated by large collateral)
  - Hemi-Fontan baffle leak (if applicable)
  - Systemic venous desaturation: Decreased oxygen delivery (anemia, low cardiac output, decreased ventricular function, severe AVVR, pericardial tamponade) or increased oxygen consumption (e.g. sepsis).
  - Intrapulmonary arterio-venous malformations may occur but rare at this stage
- Management:
  - Excessive hypoxemia ($SpO_2 < 70\%$) should be investigated promptly, especially in infants, but borderline saturations may improve with extubation.
  - Increase FiO_2 and lung recruitment to optimize pulmonary vein saturation
  - Evacuate any pleural or pericardial fluid/air
  - Cerebral blood flow is the major determinant of pulmonary blood flow. For cyanotic patients without lung disease, pulmonary blood flow can be augmented in intubated patients by ventilating to respiratory acidosis (pH 7.2–7.25) to increase cerebral blood flow. May be associated with increase in SVC pressure if problems with PVR. Should prompt evalution for reversible causes of cyanosis.
  - Pulmonary vasodilators rarely helpful but should be trialed if concerns of high PVR
  - Transfusion for Hemoglobin target > 140 g/L
- Imaging:
  - Echocardiography: Assess ventricular and AV valve function, BCPS anastomosis and PA anatomy. Upper extremity bubble study may identify decompressing collaterals
  - CT/MRI: cross sectional imaging may be required to ensure BCPS circuit unobstructed
  - Cardiac cath: Diagnostic and interventional. Assess for BCPS pressures/ obstruction, veno-venous collaterals, and ventricular diastolic dysfunction. Device closure of venous collaterals possible.

6 Other Considerations

- Systemic anticoagulation if significant PA plasties or bilateral BCPS, or concern for sluggish BCPS flow

7 Outcome

- BCPS usually associated with short hospitalization
- Surgical mortality is < 5%
- Factors that decrease longer-term survival after a BCPS:
  - High pulmonary artery pressure and PVR
  - Moderate to severe AVVR
  - Poor ventricular function
  - Native cardiac anatomy with RV dominance or HLHS with heterotaxy.

8 Controversies

- Some centres limit pre-operative assessment to MRI in low-risk, uncomplicated pateints and forgo cardiac catheterization
- Maintenance of limited antegrade pulmonary blood flow (through controlled native ventricle-PA connection or conduit) being advocated by centres.

Bibliography

1. Andrés A, Miño C, Diéguez E, et al. Specific injuries management in the postoperative of congenital heart diseases (II): Univentricular Hearts. Open J Pediatr. 2015;5:67–75.
2. Banka P, Porras D, Mayer JE et al (2014) Single Ventricle (Non HLHS) In: Da Cruz EM et al. (eds.) Pediatric and congenital cardiology, cardiac surgery and intensive care, 1st edn. Springer-Verlag, London, p 1861–1883.
3. George-Hyslop C, Thomas J, Fazari LG. Understanding Stage II Bidirectional Cavopulmonary Shunts. Crit Care Nurse. 2017;37(6):59–71.
4. Luo S, Haranal M, Deng MX, et al. Low preoperative superior vena cava blood flow predicts bidirectional cavopulmonary shunt failure. J Thorac Cardiovasc Surg. 2020;160(6):1529–40.
5. Sharma R. The bidirectional Glenn shunt for univentricular hearts. Indian J Thorac Cardiovasc Surg. 2018;34(4):453–6.

Fontan Circulation

Anne I. Dipchand

Abstract Fontan operation (or total cavopulmonary connection, TCPC) is the final palliation for different CHDs with univentricular physiology. It directs the systemic venous return of the lower part of the body to the lung. A number of anatomic and physiologic parameters need to be optimized prior to and/or increase the risk of successful Fontan completion. An extracardiac fenestrated Fontan is most common. Chronically elevated venous pressures and lower cardiac output in a Fontan circulation lead to end-organ consequences and can result in co-morbidities and/or Fontan circulatory failure. Regular surveillance for Fontan-related co-morbidities is recommended. The more common non-cardiac co-morbidities include Fontan-associated liver disease (FALD), educational challenges, learning disabilities, short stature, and thromboembolic events. Cardiac mechanisms of failure include heart failure, cyanosis, atrioventricular valve regurgitation (AVVR), and arrhythmias. Non-cardiac mechanisms are rare and associated with lymphatic abnormalities including protein-losing enteropathy (PLE) and plastic bronchitis. Survival has continued to improve though progressive multisystem changes challenge long term survival.

Keywords Fontan · Extracardiac Fontan · Fenestration · Fontan circulatory failure · PLE

Abbreviations

APCs	Aortopulmonary collaterals
ASA	Aspirin/acetasalicylic acid
AVM	Arteriovenous malformation
AVVR	Atrioventricular valve regurgitation
BCPS	Bidirectional cavopulmonary shunt
BiV	Biventricular

A. I. Dipchand (✉)
Division of Paediatric Cardiology, Department of Paediatrics, Labatt Family Heart Centre, Hospital for Sick Children, University of Toronto, Toronto, ON, Canada
e-mail: anne.dipchand@sickkids.ca

© The Author(s), under exclusive license to Springer Nature Switzerland AG 2024

A. I. Dipchand et al. (eds.), *Manual of Cardiac Care in Children*,
https://doi.org/10.1007/978-3-031-70973-9_37

BTT	Blalock Taussig Thomas
CHD	Congenital heart disease
CPR	Cardiopulmonary resuscitation
CVP	Central venous pressure
DKS	Damus-Kaye-Stansel
DOAC	Direct oral anticoagulant
EP	Electrophysiology
FALD	Fontan associated liver disease
FCF	Fontan circulatory failure
IVC	Inferior vena cava
LV	left Ventricle
PA	Pulmonary artery
PLE	Protein-losing enteropathy
PVR	Pulmonary vascular resistance
RV	right Ventricle
SVC	Superior vena cava
SVT	Supraventricular tachycardia
TCPC	Total cavopulmonary connection
TEE	Transesophageal echocardiogram
VA ECMO	Venous arterial extracorporeal membrane oxygenation

Key Points

- Fontan operation (or total cavopulmonary connection, TCPC) is the final palliation for different CHDs with univentricular physiology. It directs the systemic venous return of the lower part of the body to the lung.
- Operation performed typically around 2.5–4 years of age.
- A number of anatomic and physiologic parameters need to be optimized prior to and/or increase the risk of successful Fontan completion.
- An extracardiac fenestrated Fontan is most common.
- Short- and long-term complications are multifactorial, cardiac and non-cardiac, and require broad diagnostic and therapeutic approaches to manage.
- Fontan circulatory failure results from chronically elevated systemic venous pressures and low cardiac output.

1 Pre-Fontan Completion Considerations

- Final common pathway in appropriate patients with CHD in which biventricular (BiV) repair is not feasible. Can broadly be grouped based on dominant morphologic LV or RV. See individual chapters on univentricular cardiac malformations in this handbook.

- Prior stages include:
  - Possible neonatal surgery to achieve systemic blood flow or supply balanced pulmonary blood flow, and unobstructed venous return/atrial mixing (eg. DKS, BTT shunt; see Chapters 32 and 33). Often referred to as Stage I single ventricle palliation.
  - Bidirectional cavopulmonary shunt (BCPS; Chapter 36). Often referred to as Stage II single ventricle palliation.
- Cumulative survival after aorto-pulmonary shunt or BCPS without completing the Fontan circulation is 89% at 10 and 52% at 20 years.
- Fontan typically completed around age 3 years (2.5–4.0 years).
  - Deferred if suboptimal growth (weight > 12–15 kg preferred), or hemodynamic/anatomic issues that need to be addressed prior to optimize outcomes (see below).
  - No upper age limit for a Fontan—optimizing all pre-Fontan considerations most important
- Low pulmonary vascular resistance (PVR) required to allow passive flow through Fontan circuit and pulmonary vascular bed.
- Determination of extracardiac conduit or lateral tunnel (less frequently used at Sickkids) based on orientation of the heart (mesocardia or dextrocardia) and the relative position of the lower body systemic return (IVC or hepatic veins)
- Acquired lesions that may need to be addressed prior to or at the time of Fontan completion:
  - PA stenosis (related to prior surgeries/patches)
  - Systemic outflow obstruction (in the setting of a DKS or aortic arch reconstruction)
  - BCPS stenosis
  - Venous-venous collaterals
  - Aorto-pulmonary collaterals (APCs)
  - AVVR
  - Semilunar valve regurgitation
  - Ventricular dysfunction
  - Elevated PA pressures/PVR

2 Pre-Fontan Diagnostic Studies

- To assess suitability for the Fontan procedure and resolve acquired lesions that require medical, interventional or surgical management prior to Fontan completion

2.1 *EP Study*

- Considered if pre-existing arrhythmias (postoperative study/ablation challenging through fenestration)

2.2 *Echocardiography*

- Anatomy, function, valvar regurgitation

2.3 *Cardiac Catheterization*

- Hemodynamic assessment: pulmonary pressures, PVR, end diastolic pressure
- Anatomic assessment: PA stenosis: may require interventional procedure (balloon dilatation, stent implantation)
- Assess for APCs and venous-venous collaterals: may require coil occlusion if significant.

2.4 *MRI*

- Assess anatomy, especially if complex CHD (position of IVC, hepatic veins, and pulmonary veins)
- Assess ventricular function, ventricular volumes, valvular function and flow data
- Assess APCs and venous-venous collaterals.

2.5 *CT*

- Rarely indicated (particularly if already have an MRI).

3 Surgical Strategy

- Surgery aims to re-direct all systemic venous return directly into the PAs. Most patients have already undergone BCPS, and so surgery is focused on directing the IVC flow into the PAs.
- Commonest variants are the 'extracardiac TCPC' and the 'lateral tunnel TCPC':

- Extracardiac is the commonest technique worldwide (and is the preferred choice at SickKids, Fig. 1). Performed on bypass but usually on the beating heart. The IVC is disconnected from the atrium and connected to the underside of the PAs using a Gortex conduit of 18–22 mm diameter.
- Lateral tunnel TCPC requires cross clamping to arrest the heart, the atrium is opened and connected to the underside of the PAs, the IVC is then channeled up to the PAs by sewing a baffle within the atrium to create a lateral pathway for the IVC-PA.
- In unusual anatomies (typically isomerism) an intracardiac conduit within the atrial chamber may be required to avoid pulmonary venous obstruction and needs careful pre-op assessment with MRI or CT.
- Both extracardiac and lateral tunnel techniques are widely used and have similar outcomes with in-hospital survival of > 97%. Fenestration is commonly used, creating a 4–6 mm hole in the baffle or in the conduit to communicate with the systemic venous atrium to allow an 'escape' of systemic venous blood that improves pre-load of the systemic ventricle.
- Bilateral chest drains are essential to drain post-operative effusions.
- Off-setting of the SVC and IVC in-flows may reduce power loss in the PAs, Consideration of a Y-graft may improve equal IVC distribution to both lungs but rarely used.
- Additional procedures such as augmentation of localized PA stenosis or AVV repair may be necessary at time of Fontan—performing these as concomitant procedures or prior to Fontan require careful assessment.
- Careful assessment of intraoperative PA pressures and TEE assessment of ventricular function, Fontan flow and unobstructed pulmonary venous return is essential.

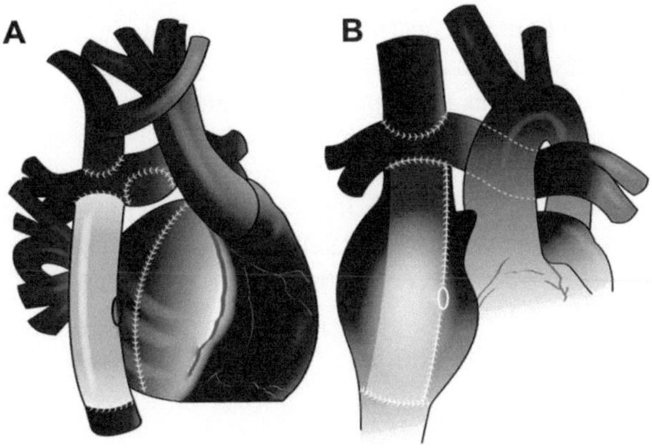

Fig. 1 Type of Fontan operation. A) Extracardiac Conduit with fenestration. B) Lateral Tunnel also called Intracardiac Fontan with fenestration. Reprinted from Circulation, Vol 126, Issue 21, Khairy P, Poirier N. Is the extracardiac conduit the preferred Fontan approach for patients with univentricular hearts? Pp 2516–2525, 2012, with permission from Wolters Kluwer Health, Inc

4 Intensive Care Physiology and Management

- Extubation in the operating room or shortly thereafter is hemodynamically favorable
- If mechanical ventilation is required, ventilate to functional residual capacity and at lowest airway pressure to facilitate venous return through the Fontan circulation
- Avoid fluid collection in potential cavities (pleura, pericardial, peritoneal)—increase can lead to higher intrathoracic pressures, desaturation, and low systemic cardiac output
- SaO_2 often slightly higher than pre-operative (usually > 80%, often > 90%)—residual shunts through fenestration (standard at SickKids) or pulmonary arterio-venous malformations (AVMs)
- Most common cause of hypotension is inadequate filling due to high venous capacitance (even with excellent hemostasis)—volume replacement common
- Target filling pressure usually for CVP pressure between 13–18 mm Hg
- Desaturation due to pulmonary hypertension uncommon in standard risk patient—pulmonary vasodilation therapy not necessary and usually not helpful
- Persistent desaturation should prompt evaluation of for lung disease, Fontan obstruction, PA stenosis, veno-venous collaterals (to pulmonary veins)
- Hemoglobin maintained > 140 g/L (14 g/dL) if desaturated
- Need for inotropic and vasopressor support rare—reassessment of ventricular function, residual lesions, Fontan circuit obstruction
- Anticoagulation with direct oral anticoagulation (DOAC) or coumadin initiated once oral feeds established
- Reduce duration of central venous catheters to avoid venous thrombosis in Fontan circuit
- Persistent and possibly high-volume chest drainage not uncommon, but lower with Fontan fenestration—need for volume replacement rare
- Early mobilization key
- Arrhythmias if not pre-existing are rare
- In case of cardiac arrest, effective CPR is difficult to achieve due to higher intrathoracic pressures limiting passive pulmonary blood flow
- Flows on VA ECMO, if required, can be limited by venous drainage and may need venous cannulation of superior and inferior veins. Central cannulation provides better venous reservoir but dependent on low PVR for adequate pulmonary blood flow.

5 Short-Term Issues

- Prolonged pleural effusions
  - Chylothorax: fluid tested postoperative day 5 if daily volume > 6 mls/Kg/day per tube

- Desaturation (fenestration, collaterals, AVMs, Fontan pathway obstruction, etc.)
- Institutional practice is anticoagulation indefinitely either with a DOAC or if coumadin used initially, then transition to ASA or DOAC at 6 months post-operatively
- Cardiac catheterization between 1–2 years post-operatively to assess for percutaneous closure of the fenestration with device (balloon test occlusion to evaluate).
  - If fenestration closes spontaneously may not be required.
  - If history of tachyarrhythmias that may be amenable to ablation (e.g. SVT), assess need for EP study prior to fenestration closure

6 Long-Term Follow up of a Fontan Circulation

- Chronically elevated venous pressures and lower cardiac output in a Fontan circulation lead to end-organ consequences. Regular surveillance for Fontan-related co-morbidities is recommended (Table 1).
- Cardiac complications
  - Heart failure—2 categories:

    Classic pump/myocardial failure

    Fontan circulatory failure (FCF): symptoms of heart failure may exist despite reasonable ventricular performance of the single ventricle, simply as a consequence of venous hypertension and its end-organ consequences.
  - AVVR due to volume overload, ventricular dilatation, reduced ventricular contractility, and increased postcapillary and CVP.
  - Cyanosis

    Fenestration, collaterals, AVMs, Fontan pathway obstruction

    Saturations typically mid-high 80's, low 90's until fenestration closes or is closed.

    Saturations can drift down over time (months to years) with the development of collaterals or AVMs.
  - Arrhythmias (~40%): most commonly atrial arrhythmias (e.g. atrial flutter/fibrillation)
- Non-cardiac
  - Thromboembolic events (2–25%)
  - Lymphopenia and other immune abnormalities
  - Protein Losing Enteropathy (PLE; 5–12%)

    Abnormal loss of serum proteins into the intestine due to increase in abnormal lymphatic vessels throughout the intestinal tract

Table 1 Fontan Circulation Longterm Surveillance

Timing	Routine
1 year post-Fontan *(if fenestration closes spontaneously may not need)*	Cath + Cardiac MRI *(under GA)* Fenestration closure **Assess need for EP study (if applicable) prior*
Age 10–12 years	**Cardiac & Liver MRI**
Age 16–17 years	**Cardiac & Liver MRI**
Routine f/u Post-Fontan	
Annually	**Cardiology Clinic with Echo and ECG** • Focused History: exercise tolerance, palpitations, syncope, periorbital edema, ankle edema, abdominal distension, stoolingpattern/diarrhea, snoring • weight, height, BMI vs BSA, HR, RR, BP, O2 saturation • Physical exam: edema, venous distension, hepatomegaly, ascites, pitting edema
Q2-3 years **Standard/low risk**: *normal function, mild or less AVVR, normalestimated venous/Fontan pressures, acyanotic, sinus rhythm* **Q1-2 years** **Complex/high risk**: *decreased function, > mild AVVR, elevated Fontan or PA pressures, cyanosis, PLE, plastic bronchitis, arrhythmias,symptoms*	**Routine Blood/Urine Testing** *Bloodwork* Electrolytes,creatinine Calcium, Phosphate ALT, GGT, total and conjugated bilirubin albumin, total protein CBC and differential, INR IgG, IgA, IgE TSH, PTH 25-OH Vit D Iron Studies *(if indicated) Urine* Dip for protein Albumin:CreatinineRatio **Cardiac** 24 hour Holter monitor Bicycle VO_2 Exercise test *(baseline 5 years s/p Fontan; minimum age 8 years)* **Growth assessment** *(obesity, short stature,* etc.*)* **Diet & Exercise Counselling** *(Dietitian/ Physiotherapy)*
Age 10–12 years Age 16–17 years	**Liver ultrasound with Doppler**
q5years	**24 HR ambulatory BP** **Bone Mineral Density**
Age 4–6 years **Age 8–10 years** **Age 12–14 years** ~ 17 years *(if necessary)*	**Neuropsychologyassessments**
Specialized testing/for indication	
Cardiac catheterization	As clinically indicated
EP study ± ablation	As clinically indicated
CT angiogram	As clinically indicated
Event / implantable loop recorder	As clinically indicated

(continued)

Table 1 (continued)

Timing	Routine
Assessment for lymphatic intervention	**Indication: PLE or Plastic bronchitis** Groin ultrasound MRI lymphangiogram
Nuclear medicine GFR	History of AKI ± abnormalities on renal testing screening See Renal Protocol for management of reduced renal function and thresholds for referral to Nephrology
Hepatology Referral	ALT or GGT > 100 INR > 1.5 Splenomegaly by imaging or exam and platelet < 150 Abnormal liver Doppler study (portal vein decreased flow velocity and/or dampened respiratory variation) or other evidence of portal hypertension such as varices Increased liver stiffness by US Liver lesion (e.g. nodules) *Will determine need for and timing of:* Liver elastography with Fibroscan (hepatic stiffness) Upper endoscopy Liver biopsy

AKI Acute kidney injury; *ALT* Alanine aminotransferase; *BMI* Body mass index; *BP* Blood pressure; *BSA* Body surface area; *CBC* Complete blood count; *GGT* Gamma glutamyl transferase; *HR* Heart rate; *INR* International normalized ratio; *PTH* Parathyroid hormone; *RR* Respiratory rate; *TSH* Thyroid stimulating hormone; *US* Ultrasound; VO_2 Oxygen consumption; *25-OH* Twenty-five hydroxy

Results in hypoalbuminemia, failure to thrive, diarrhea
Serum and stool alpha-1-antitrypsin testing confirmatory

- Plastic Bronchitis (<5%)

  Thick, tenacious casts within the airway lumen (spillage of protein-rich lymph through lymphatic-to-bronchial communications)

- Fontan-Associated Liver Disease (FALD)

  Centrilobular hepatic congestion leads to fibrosis and cirrhosis
  Most frequently indolent. Most commonly variable degree of fibrosis and compensated cirrhosis.

- Renal abnormalities: proteinuria (40%), chronic kidney disease
- Osteopenia, low vitamin D, hypoparathyroidism (25–30%)
- Short stature
- Obesity (20–30% in childhood; 40–50% in adulthood)
- Neurodevelopmental challenges

7 Outcomes

- 30 year survival > 80% in the contemporary era
- Institutional outcomes (n = 324, 2000–2013)
  - In hospital mortality: 0.3%
  - Overall mortality: 2.2%
  - Expected survival is 98% and 97.4% at 5 and 10 years respectively.
- 5–10% die or need a heart transplant in childhood

8 Alternative Strategies and Controversies

- In some centres, fenestration is done only in patients at high risk due to increased PVR and reduced ventricular function.
- In some centres, fenestration is not routinely closed.
- The use of mechanical support in the setting of a failing Fontan circulation is challenging but increasing; there is the need for the development of technology meeting the unique needs.

Bibliography

1. d'Udekem Y, Iyengar AJ, Galati JC, et al Redefining expectations of long-term survival after the Fontan procedure. Twenty-five years of follow-up from the entire population of Australia, New Zealand. Circulation. 2014;130(11 Suppl 1):S32–S8
2. Downing TE, Allen KY, Glatz AC, et al. Long-term survival after the Fontan operation: twenty years of experience at a single center. J Thorac Cardiovasc Surg. 2017;154(1):243–53.
3. Gatzoulis MA, Munk MD, Williams WG, Webb GD. Definitive palliation with cavopulmonary or aortopulmonary shunts for adults with single ventricle physiology. Heart. 2000;83(1):51–7.
4. Grosse-Wortmann L, Al-Otay A, Yoo S-J. Aortopulmonary collaterals after bidirectional cavopulmonary connection or Fontan completion: quantification with MRI. Circ Cardiovasc Imaging. 2009;2(3):219–25.
5. Khairy P, Poirier N. Is the extracardiac conduit the preferred fontan approach for patients with univentricular hearts?: The extracardiac conduit is not the preferred fontan approach for patients with univentricular hearts. Circulation. 2012;126(21):2516–25.
6. Pihkala J, Yazaki S, Mehta R, et al. Feasibility and clinical impact of transcatheter closure of interatrial communications after a fenestrated Fontan procedure: medium-term outcomes. Catheter Cardiovasc Interv. 2007;69(7):1007–14.
7. Rychik J, Atz AM, Celermajer DS, et al Evaluation and management of the child and adult with Fontan circulation. A scientific statement from the American Heart Association. Circulation. 2019;140(6):e234–e84.

Infective Endocarditis

Brian McCrindle and Michael Khoury

Abstract Infective endocarditis (IE) is a microbial infection of the endocardial surface of the heart. While rare in the general population, it occurs at a higher frequency in select patient populations at risk, including children with unrepaired, palliated, and repaired congenital heart disease, particularly those with prosthetic valves and residual lesions. About 90% of cases are caused by Gram positive cocci, including alpha-hemolytic Streptococci and Staphylococcus aureus. The clinical presentation can be sub-acute or severe and may include manifestations directly related to the infective illness, the immunologic response to endocarditis, hemodynamic compromise, or manifestations from pulmonary or systemic embolization. The modified Duke criteria are used for diagnosis, and involve pathologic, clinical, laboratory, and imaging elements. Early treatment is crucial, and a low index of suspicion considered for any at-risk patient with an unexplained fever or new illness. Treatment should be targeted to the identified organism, with surgical intervention when indicated. Ultimately, the primary goal is the prevention of IE through good general and oral hygiene and antibiotic prophylaxis when indicated in select circumstances.

Keywords Infective endocarditis · Endocarditis · Streptococci · Staphylococcus aureas · Subacute bacterial endocarditis (SBE) · Duke criteria

Abbreviations

AHA	American heart association
AS	Aortic stenosis
BAV	Bicuspid aortic valve

B. McCrindle (✉)
Division of Cardiology, Department of Paediatrics, Labatt Family Heart Centre, The Hospital of Sick Children, Toronto, ON, Canada
e-mail: Brian.mccrindle@sickkids.ca

M. Khoury
Department of Pediatrics, Stollery Children's Hospital, Edmonton, AB, Canada
e-mail: Khoury1@ualberta.ca

© The Author(s), under exclusive license to Springer Nature Switzerland AG 2024

A. I. Dipchand et al. (eds.), *Manual of Cardiac Care in Children*,
https://doi.org/10.1007/978-3-031-70973-9_38

CHD	Congenital heart disease
IDU	Injection drug user
IE	Infective endocarditis
NBTE	Nonbacterial thrombotic endocarditis
PDA	Persistent ductus arteriosus
S. aureus	Staphylococcal aureas
TEE	Transesophageal echocardiogram
TOF	Tetralogy of fallot
TR	Tricuspid regurgitation
VAD	Ventricular assist device
VSD	Ventricular septal defect

Key Points

- Infective endocarditis should be considered for any patient with underlying heart disease and a febrile or systemic illness.
- The Modified Duke criteria should be used to diagnose infective endocarditis.
- Anti-microbial management ideally should be broad at the outset and then directed at the specific identified pathogen and its sensitivities.
- Surgical intervention may be indicated in addition to medical management.
- Prevention is key. Published guidelines should be used to guide usage of prophylactic antibiotics.

1 Definition

- Microbial infection of the endocardial (endothelial) surface of the heart.
- Heart valves (native or prosthetic) are the most frequently involved sites.
- Can also involve septal defects, mural endocardium, persistent ductus arteriosus (PDA), and intravascular foreign material such as intracardiac patches, surgically constructed shunts, and intravenous catheters.

2 Epidemiology

- Incidence about 0.3:100,000 children per year—mortality 11.6%.
  - In high-risk groups, it is about 300–3,160:100,000 person-years; in moderate risk it is 50–440:100,000 person-years (see below).
- Increasing incidence due to increased survival of patients with cardiovascular disease.

- 30–70% of cases in patients with congenital heart disease (CHD) have had previous cardiac surgery.
  - Bicuspid aortic valve (BAV), aortic stenosis (AS), ventricular septal defect (VSD), and tetralogy of Fallot (TOF) most frequently associated with IE.
- In 8–10% of cases, IE occurs without any structural heart disease or other identifiable risk factors. Usually involves the aortic or mitral valve and is often secondary to Staphylococcus aureus bacteremia.

3 Microorganisms

- Gram positive cocci account for about 90% of infections.
- Most common:
  - Alpha-hemolytic streptococci (viridans group streptococci)—most common overall
  - Staphylococcus aureus (S. aureus)—second most common—may be most common for healthcare associated infections.
  - Coagulase negative staphylococci—less common but increasing especially with prosthetic devices.
  - In prosthetic valve endocarditis, organisms differ depending on timing of IE.

    S. aureus and coagulase negative staphylococcal infections are commonly seeded, regardless of timing.
    Aerobic Gram-negative bacilli and fungal infections may be seeded within the first year of surgery.
    Viridans group streptococci and Enterococcus species may be seeded late (≥ 1) following prosthetic valve replacement.
- Gram negative organisms are rare—increased risk for neonates, immunocompromised patients, and illicit injection drug users (IDUs).
  - Usually demonstrate slow growth. Cultures should be retained for ≥ 2 weeks.
- Fungal endocarditis is rare but can be very severe—seen after cardiac surgery and in immunocompromised individuals and neonates.
  - Incidence is increasing.
  - Survival rates < 20%.
- Approximately 5–10% of patients have negative blood cultures.

4 Pathogenesis

- Propensity for occurrence at sites of pressure gradients and/or turbulent blood flow where there is greater sheer stress, causing trauma to the endothelium.
- Results in formation of platelet rich nonbacterial thrombotic endocarditis (NBTE).
- Transient bacteremia results from trauma of a mucosal surface during various dental, oral, and surgical procedures—however, spontaneous bacteremia may also occur.
- Adherence of bacteria to NBTE → proliferation and formation of a vegetation → adhesion of fibrin and platelets to the vegetation → biofilm formation, encasing the bacteria → rapid proliferation.
- Infection with associated tissue necrosis, particularly with alpha-hemolytic streptococci (less commonly with more virulent bacteria such as S. aureus) leads to destruction of the infected valve, invasion of the myocardium, and/or abscess formation.

5 Clinical Presentation

- General considerations
  - IE should be considered for ***any*** unusual or febrile illness in patients with underlying heart disease.
  - Clinical features depend on the site of infection and may be due to altered hemodynamics or structural changes that are the result of vegetation embolization, immunologic reactions or tissue destruction.
- Emboli
  - Left-sided: systemic embolization leading to ischemia/infarction or mycotic aneurysms.
  - Right-sided: pulmonary embolism.
- Clinical presentation patterns:
  - Fever is the most common finding (except in neonates).
  - Infection with hemolytic streptococci often results in low grade fever, whereas S. aureus infection often results in high, spiking temperature elevations.
  - A subacute clinical picture may include symptoms such as myalgias, arthralgias, headache, loss of appetite and general malaise. May have relapsing or low-grade fever.
  - Acute form: toxic—high fever, hemodynamic compromise, systemic manifestations similar and more pronounced to that seem in the subacute clinical picture.
  - Neonates

Often have relatively few specific symptoms; systemic hypotension, signs compatible with sepsis, focal neurologic findings.
Appear to be particularly prone to septic embolization and the development of satellite infections.

  - New murmurs are often heard, usually related to valvar regurgitation.

- Extracardiac findings:
  - Splenomegaly and/or splenic abscess.
  - Neurologic findings in about 20% (cerebral abscess, infarction, aseptic meningitis).
  - Renal abnormalities: proteinuria, hematuria, leukocyturia—secondary to either emboli or in association with endocarditis-related immune complex deposition.
  - Classically described signs are rare in children.

    Osler nodes—small, tender, raised lesions on pads of fingers and toes.
    Janeway lesions—small, nontender, flat erythematous lesions on palms and soles.
    Roth spots—retinal hemorrhages with white or pale centers.
    Splinter hemorrhages—small, typically linear hemorrhages underneath the nail.

6 Diagnostic Studies

6.1 *Laboratory*

- Positive blood cultures—very common if untreated. Most valuable diagnostic aide.
  - Three separate sets of blood cultures each from separate venipuncture sites over a 24-hour period.
  - When the patient is not acutely ill, if blood cultures remain negative, withholding antibiotics for $\geq$ 48 hours and continuing to obtain cultures may be considered to determine the etiologic microorganism.
- Elevated acute phase reactants—very common.
- Anemia—in most cases.
- Hematuria—in most cases.
- Presence of rheumatoid factor and leukocytosis can be seen but are infrequent.

6.2 Echocardiography

- Transthoracic echocardiography
  - Useful to confirm the diagnosis for those with suspected infective endocarditis, but a negative echocardiogram may not exclude the diagnosis.
  - Detection rate of IE in children > 80%
  - Yield is lower in the absence of positive blood culture(s).
- Transesophageal echocardiography (TEE) often superior to transthoracic; warranted if degree of suspicion for IE is high despite negative transthoracic study.
  - Should be used in presence of prosthetic valves or concern for complicated IE (paravalvular abscess).

7 Other Investigations

- PET/white blood scan: can be useful in identifying distal foci of infection
- MRI/CT—particularly to evaluate for presence and extent of emboli/mycotic aneurysms

8 Diagnostic Criteria

- Modified Duke criteria (Tables 1 and 2)—combination of clinical, microbiologic, pathologic, and echocardiographic findings.
  - Three categories:

    Definite—identified clinically or proven at surgery or autopsy.
    Possible—not meeting the criteria of definite infective endocarditis.
    Not endocarditis.

9 Medical Management

See (Table 3).

- Prolonged antibiotic therapy is required to achieve complete eradication of the infection (4–6 weeks).
- Cessation of bacteremia early following treatment should be documented, with subsequent follow-up cultures to ensure absence of IE relapse.

Table 1 Modified Duke Criteria—Major and Minor Criteria

Major Criteria	1. Blood culture positive for IE: a. Typical microorganisms consistent with IE from 2 separate blood cultures: i. Viridans streptococciStreptococci, Streptococcus bovis, HACEK group, S. aureus; or ii. Community acquired enterocci in absence of primary focus; or b. Persistently positive blood culture: i. Typical organisms: ≥2 positive cultures drawn >12 hours apart; or ii. Organisms that are more commonly skin contaminants: All of 3 or majority of ≥4 cultures positive (first and last sample drawn ≥1 h apart) c. Single positive blood culture for Coxiella burnetii or anti-phase-1 IgG antibody titre >1:800
	2. Evidence of endocardial involvement: a. Echocardiogram positive for IE i. Evidence of vegetation or ii. Abscess; or iii. New partial dehiscence of prosthetic valve b. New valvular regurgitation (increase or change in pre-existing murmur not sufficient)
Minor Criteria	1. Predisposition: predisposing heart condition or IDU 2. Fever, temperature > 38° C 3. Vascular phenomena, major arterial emboli, septic pulmonary infarcts, mycotic aneurysm, intracranial hemorrhage, conjunctivial hemorrhages, and Janeway lesions 4. Immunologic phenomena: glomerulonephritis, Osler nodes, Roth spots, rheumatoid factor 5. Microbiologic evidence: positive blood culture not meeting major criteria or serologic evidence of infection with organism consistent with IE

Reproduced with permission from Li JS, Sexton DJ, Mick N et al. (2000) Proposed modifications to the Duke criteria for the diagnosis of infective endocarditis. Clin Infect Dis 30(4):633–638

Table 2 Modified Duke Criteria—Diagnostic criteria

Definitive IE	1. Pathologic criteria: a. Microorganisms—demonstrated by culture/histology of vegetation or intracardiac abscess or b. Pathologic lesions; vegetation or intracardiac abscess demonstrating active endocarditis by histology
	2. Clinical criteria (see Table 1): a. Two major criteria; or b. One major and three minor criteria; or c. Five minor criteria
Possible IE	1. One major criterion and one minor criterion; or 2. Three minor criteria

Reproduced with permission from Li JS, Sexton DJ, Mick N et al. (2000) Proposed modifications to the Duke criteria for the diagnosis of infective endocarditis. Clin Infect Dis 30(4):633–638

Table 3 Recommended antibiotic therapy for pediatric infective endocarditis

Organism/ Condition	Recommended Antibiotic	Alternative antibiotic	Duration[a]
Empirical therapy/culture negative			
Native valve (community acquired) or prosthetic valve (>1 yr post-surgery)	Ampicillin/sulbactam + gentamicin ± vancomycin For prosthetic valves, add rifampin	Vancomycin + gentamicin	4–6 weeks
Nosocomial associated with vascular cannulae or early prosthetic valve endocarditis (≤1 yr post-surgery)	Vancomycin + gentamicin + cefepime or ceftazidime Add rifampin if prosthetic material present		6 weeks
Streptococci			
Highly susceptible to penicillin G (MBC ≤ 0.1ug/ml)	Penicillin G or ceftriaxone	Vancomycin or first-generation cephalosporin, or ceftriaxone	4 weeks
Relatively resistant to penicillin (MBC ≥ 0.2ug/ml)	Penicillin G (or ampicillin) + gentamicin (for first 2 wk or full course if enterococci)	Vancomycin plus gentamicin for enterococci Ampicillin plus ceftriaxone (for aminoglycoside-resistant enterococci or aminoglycoside-intolerance) Ceftraaxone plus gentamicin (NOT for enterococcal endocarditis)	4 weeks *4–6 weeks for enterococcus (6 weeks if treated with vancomycin)*
Staphylococci			
Susceptible to penicillin G (rare)	Penicillin G	Oxacillin or nafcillin or first-generation cephalosporin or vancomycin	4–6 weeks
Resistant to penicillin G	Oxacillin or nafcillin	Vancomycin or first-generation cephalosporin	4–6 weeks
Resistant to oxacillin	Vancomycin	Daptomycin	6 weeks
Vancomycin resistant or intolerant	Daptomycin		6 weeks

(continued)

Table 3 (continued)

Organism/ Condition	Recommended Antibiotic	Alternative antibiotic	Duration[a]
Prosthetic material present (applies to all staphylococci)	Add rifampin + gentamicin (for first 2 weeks)		At least 6-weeks
Gram-negative bacilli	Ceftazidime, cefepime, cefotaxime, or ceftriaxone Plus gentamicin (or tobramycin or amikacin, based on susceptibility)	Broad-spectrum penicillin plus gentamicin (or tobramycin or amikacin)	At least 6 weeks
HACEK group	Ceftriaxone or cefotaxime OR ampicillin-sulbactam	Ampicillin (if susceptible) + aminoglycoside	4 weeks, including if prosthetic material
Fungi (Candida, Aspergillus)	Surgical resection plus amphotericin B ± flucytosine	Amphotericin B followed by imidazole for suppression if surgery cannot be performed	In consultation with infectious disease

[a] If prosthetic material present, treat for at least 6 weeks, except for hacek group

Information adapted from content in Baltimore RS, Gewitz M, Baddour LM et al. (2015) Infective Endocarditis in Childhood: 2015 Update: A Scientific Statement from the American Heart Association. Circulation 132(15):1487–515.

Reproduced with Permission from Circulation. 2015;132:1487–1515; (©2015 American Heart Association, Inc

- Initial empiric antibiotic therapy should subsequently be tailored to the sensitivities of the identified organism.

10 Complications

- Embolic events and the formation of mycotic aneurysms.
- Numerous clinical situations can place the patient at high risk for complications including:
  - Prosthetic cardiac valves
  - Left-sided IE
  - Staphylococcus aureus IE
  - Fungal IE
  - Previous IE
  - Prolonged clinical symptoms (>3 months)
  - Cyanotic CHD
  - Patients with systemic-to-pulmonary shunts
  - Poor clinical response to antimicrobial therapy

11 Indications for Surgical Intervention

- Features that may suggest the need for surgical intervention may be stratified by right-sided versus left-sided IE:

11.1 Left-Sided IE

- Fungal IE or highly resistant organisms (vancomycin-resistant *enterococcus,* multi-drug resistant bacteria)
- Uncontrolled infection: persistent fever/bacteremia ≥ 5–7 days following initiation of antimicrobial therapy. An increasing vegetation size after 4-weeks of antimicrobial therapy may also indicate an uncontrolled infection.
- Heart failure secondary to valvular dysfunction
- High-grade (grade II or III) conduction disease.
- Annular or aortic abscess.
- Destructive penetrating lesions.
- High embolic risk, including recurrent emboli, persistent or enlarging vegetations despite antimicrobial therapy, severe valvar regurgitation, mobile vegetation ≥ 10 mm or a mobile vegetation > 10 mm with anterior mitral valve leaflet involvement or in the setting of other relative indications for surgery. IE of the mitral valve secondary to S. aureus may indicate a higher embolic risk.
- In the setting of prosthetic valve endocarditis, the same indications apply. Early surgical intervention should also be considered in those patients with relapsing prosthetic valve endocarditis.

11.2 Right-Sided IE

- Uncontrolled infection: persistent fever/bacteremia ≥ 5–7 days following initiation of antimicrobial therapy.
- Right-heart failure secondary to severe TR that is refractory to medical therapy.
- Drug-resistant organisms, including fungal infections and multidrug resistant bacteria
- High embolic risk: vegetations ≥ 20 mm or recurrent pulmonary embolisms despite antimicrobial therapy.

11.3 Timing for Surgical Intervention

- Timing for surgical intervention must consider the risk of imminent embolization and the presence or absence of neurologic complications. In the presence of such neurologic complications, neurosurgical and/or neurologic consultation is required to facilitate a balanced decision-making approach regarding timing of surgical intervention.

  - In the setting of left-sided IE warranting surgical intervention, screening for neurologic complications (including cerebral emboli, mycotic aneurysms, intracranial hemorrhage) should be routinely performed prior to surgical intervention.
  - Untreated mycotic aneurysms pose the risk of rupture during routine heparinization during cardiac surgery.

- In those without neurologic complications, prompt intervention during the initial hospitalization and prior to completion of the full therapeutic antibiotic course is warranted.
- In those with ischemic strokes without major neurologic deficits, imminent surgical intervention may be considered; however, a delay of 1–2 weeks may also be warranted.
- In those with major neurologic deficits or intracranial hemorrhage, surgical delay of ≥ 4 weeks is typically required.
- Typically, surgical intervention involves removal of the vegetation along with replacement of the infected and diseased valve or conduit. In more rare circumstances, valve repair rather than replacement may be suitable.

12 Prevention

- Repairing underlying cardiac defect without residual lesions reduces the likelihood of IE developing.
- Preventative measures to reduce the likelihood of bacteremia (e.g., good general and oral hygiene); more important than prophylactic antibiotics for a dental procedure.
  - Note: poor dental hygiene and periodontal or periapical dental infections may produce bacteremia in the absence of dental/oral procedures. Therefore, it is important to maintain good oral health as an important factor in preventing endocarditis.
- Recommendations from the AHA, similar to guidelines internationally, have restricted which patients are eligible for IE prophylaxis:
  - Prophylaxis for patients with cardiac conditions associated with the highest risk of adverse outcomes from IE (Table 4).
  - Prophylaxis limited to dental procedures that involve manipulation of gingival tissue or the periapical region of teeth or perforation of the oral mucosa.
  - No prophylaxis recommended for most procedures involving the respiratory, gastrointestinal, and genitourinary tract.

Table 4 Cardiac conditions where antibiotic prophylaxis is suggested

Prosthetic cardiac valve or material Including: Transcatheter implantation of prosthetic valves Cardiac valve repair using devices VAD therapy
CHD • Unrepaired cyanotic CHD, including shunts and conduits • Repaired CHD with prosthetic material or device within the first 6mo of procedure • Repaired CHD with residual defects at the site or adjacent to prosthetic patch/device • Surgical/transcatheter pulmonary artery valve or conduit, including Melody valve and Contegra conduit
Cardiac transplant recipients who develop cardiac valvulopathy

Adapted from: Wilson WR, Gewitz M, Lockhart PB et al. (2021) Prevention of Viridans Group Streptococcal Infective Endocarditis: A Scientific Statement From the American Heart Association. Circulation 143(20):e963–e978. Reproduced with permission from Circulation 2021; 143:e963–e978. ©2021 American Heart Association, Inc

If there is an established respiratory infection and they are undergoing a respiratory tract procedure, then the antibiotic given should cover organisms that could potentially cause IE.

If the patient is undergoing a gastrointestinal/genitourinary procedure where there is an established infection, or for those who are getting antimicrobial therapies to prevent wound infection or sepsis associated with the procedure, then the patient should get a regimen that is effective against enterococci.

  – No prophylaxis recommended for tattoos.

- Antibiotic prophylaxis should be administered as a single dose 30–60 minutes before the procedure.
- Amoxicillin is the drug of choice, with alternatives available when necessary.
- If patient already on an antibiotic and requires prophylaxis, then the patient should receive one from a different class.

Bibliography

1. Baddour LM, Wilson WR, Bayer AS, et al. Infective endocarditis in adults: diagnosis, antimicrobial therapy, and management of complications: a scientific statement for healthcare professionals from the american heart association. Circulation. 2015;132(15):1435–86.
2. Baltimore RS, Gewitz M, Baddour LM, et al. Infective endocarditis in childhood: 2015 update: a scientific statement from the American heart association. Circulation. 2015;132(15):1487–515.
3. Day MD, Gauvreau K, Shulman S, Newburger JW. Characteristics of children hospitalized with infective endocarditis. Circulation. 2009;119(6):865–70.

4. Gewitz M, Taubert K. Chapter 63. Infective endocarditis and prevention. moss and adams' heart disease. In: Infants, children, and adolescents. including the fetus and young adult. 9th ed. Lippincott Williams & Wilkens; 2016.
5. Li JS, Sexton DJ, Mick N, et al. Proposed modifications to the Duke criteria for the diagnosis of infective endocarditis. Clin Infect Dis. 2000;30(4):633–8.
6. Martin JM, Neches WH, Wald ER. Infective endocarditis: 35 years of experience at a children's hospital. Clin Infect Dis. 1997;24(4):669–75.
7. Pasquali SK, He X, Mohamad Z, et al. Trends in endocarditis hospitalizations at US children's hospitals: impact of the 2007 American Heart Association Antibiotic Prophylaxis Guidelines. Am Heart J. 2012;163(5):894–9.
8. Saiman L, Prince A, Gersony WM. Pediatric infective endocarditis in the modern era. J Pediatr. 1993;122(6):847–53.
9. Wilson WR, Gewitz M, Lockhart PB, et al. Prevention of viridans group streptococcal infective endocarditis: a scientific statement from the american heart association. Circulation. 2021;143(20):e963–78.

Myocarditis

Alyssa Power and Emilie Jean-St-Michel

Abstract Myocarditis is an inflammatory disease of the myocardium that is often a consequence of infection, toxin exposure, or autoimmune disorder. The presentation varies from mild self-limited disease to sudden cardiac death. The diagnosis of myocarditis cannot be confirmed with one specific test and requires a detailed history, physical examination and targeted cardiac testing such as electrocardiogram and echocardiogram. The role of cardiac magnetic resonance as a diagnostic aid is becoming clearer in pediatrics. Immunosuppression is recommended only in suspected giant cell myocarditis with presence of frequent ectopy or varying degree of heart block, or with proven autoimmune myocarditis. In most cases there is complete functional recovery, but about 30% of patients will progress to chronic, dilated cardiomyopathy. Guideline-directed heart failure therapy with reverse remodeling agents should be initiated if ventricular dysfunction persists.

Keywords Inflammation · Viral infection · Cardiac magnetic resonance · Biopsy

Abbreviations

ALCAPA	Anomalous left coronary artery from the pulmonary artery
CMRI	Cardiac magnetic resonance imaging
ECMO	Extracorporeal membrane oxygenation
LA	Left atrium
LGE	Late gadolinium enhancement
LV	Left ventricle
NT-proBNP	N-terminal prohormone of brain natriuretic peptide

A. Power (✉)
Division of Cardiology, Labatt Family Heart Centre, Hospital for Sick Children, Toronto, ON, Canada
e-mail: Alyssa.power@sickkids.ca

E. Jean-St-Michel
University Hospital for Northern British Columbia, Prince George, BC, Canada
e-mail: Emilie.JeanStMichel@northernhealth.ca

© The Author(s), under exclusive license to Springer Nature Switzerland AG 2024

A. I. Dipchand et al. (eds.), *Manual of Cardiac Care in Children*,
https://doi.org/10.1007/978-3-031-70973-9_39

PCR	Polymerase chain reaction
VAD	Ventricular assist device

Key Points

- Myocarditis is a condition that results from inflammation of the heart muscle.
- Most cases in children are a consequence of viral or bacterial infection, toxin exposure, and rarely autoimmune disease.
- Symptoms vary broadly and diagnosis may be challenging - all patients should undergo a detailed history, physical examination, electrocardiogram, and echocardiogram on presentation
- Cardiac magnetic resonance imaging (CMRI) should be considered in all patients who do not need general anaesthesia. It should not be considered in life-threatening situations.
- Immunosuppression is recommended only in suspected giant cell myocarditis with presence of frequent ectopy or varying degree of heart block, or with proven autoimmune myocarditis.
- Most patients will have complete functional recovery. Guideline-directed heart failure therapy with reverse remodeling agents should be initiated if ventricular dysfunction persists.

1 Definition

- Inflammatory disease of the myocardium with a heterogeneous presentation.
- 4 diagnostic strata: biopsy-proven myocarditis, CMRI-confirmed myocarditis, clinically suspected myocarditis, and possible myocarditis.
- Can also be defined by clinical features: fulminant, acute, subacute (including chronic active with persistent inflammation) or chronic persistent without persisting inflammation.
- Fulminant myocarditis is characterized by a rapid progressive decline in cardiac function or emergence of malignant arrhythmias with severe hemodynamic compromise and a high acute mortality rate.

2 Epidemiology

- The incidence of myocarditis is difficult to establish because of the lack of a gold standard for diagnosis and the diverse possible presentations.

3 Etiology

- The most common etiology in children is viral infection. Immune response to virus results in direct myocardial inflammation and injury.
- Table 1 presents a non-comprehensive overview of the etiologies of myocarditis.
- Emerging understanding of oncological-drug induced myocarditis.
- Giant cell myocarditis is very rare in children. It is characterized by widespread inflammation and myocyte necrosis and has multiple etiologies (viral, autoimmune, etc.). It is commonly associated with ventricular ectopy and heart block. It is frequently fatal.

4 Pathogenesis

- Myocyte damage is the first step leading to cytokine release and immune system activation including macrophage activation followed by lymphocyte infiltration.
- Inflammation is often patchy and may be missed on myocardial biopsy.
- This process can eventually result in myocardial healing with resolution of the process, but it can also lead to ongoing inflammation.

5 Clinical Presentation

- The clinical presentation varies greatly. It will range from:
  - Non-specific symptoms such as myalgia, fever, chest pain
  - Abdominal symptoms—pain, nausea, vomiting—are common in children
  - Rhythm disturbance (ectopy and varying degree of heart block)
  - Congestive heart failure (See Chapter 41)
  - Sudden death
- The presentation varies between a stable acute child (similar to presentation of pericarditis) to acute decompensated heart failure in a previously well child requiring advanced cardiac therapies including inotropic support, anti-arrhythmic therapy, ventricular pacing, and/or mechanical circulatory support.
- Autopsy studies in the UK and Australia suggest that between 8–12% of sudden deaths could be linked to myocarditis.
- History of recent viral prodrome is present in about 2/3 of patients.

Table 1 Major Etiologies of Myocarditis

INFECTIOUS ETIOLOGIES	INFECTIOUS ETIOLOGIES CONT'D
Viral	*Protozoal*
- Enterovirus (Coxsackie A and B)	- Chagas disease
- Adenovirus	- Toxoplasmosis
- Herpes simplex virus (HSV)	- Malaria
- Influenza A and B	*Helminthic*
- Coronavirus (including COVID-19)	- Echinococcosis
- Parvovirus B19	- Trichinosis
- Cytomegalovirus (CMV)	- Schistosomiasis
- Epstein-Barr virus (EBV)	- Strongyloidiasis
- Respiratory syncytial virus (RSV)	
- Human immunodeficiency virus (HIV)	*NON-INFECTIOUS ETIOLOGIES*
- Rubella	*Drugs/Cardiotoxins*
- Rubeola	- Anthracyclines
Bacterial	- Cyclophosphamide
- Diphtheria	- Heavy metals (copper, lead, iron)
- Meningococcus	- Alcohol
- Tuberculosis	- Cocaine
- Staphylococcus	- Vaccines (including COVID-19)
- Streptococcus	*Immunologic*
- Meningococcus	- Systemic lupus erythematosus
- Pneumococcus	- Kawasaki disease
- Mycoplasma	- Multisystem inflammatory syndrome
Spirochetal	- Inflammatory bowel disease
- Lyme disease	- Celiac disease
Mycotic	- Thyrotoxicosis
- Candidiasis	- Giant cell myocarditis
- Aspergillosis	*Hypersensitivity*
- Histoplasmosis	- Hypereosinophilia
Rickettsial	- Antibiotics
- Typhus	- Diuretics
- Rocky Mountain Spotted Fever	- Anticonvulsants
	Radiation

6 Diagnosis

- The diagnosis of myocarditis cannot be confirmed with one specific test. A combination of history, physical exam, and imaging is required. Histopathological information via endomyocardial biopsy can be helpful in some cases.

6.1 Detailed History and Physical Exam

- Even though it has limited specificity, a good history and physical examination remains crucial.
- The clinical presentation can be helpful: fever, new onset chest pain, right/left heart failure symptoms, unexplained arrhythmia, syncope, aborted sudden cardiac death.
- To recognize chronic heart condition (ex: stunted growth/chest bulge).
- To identify associated abnormality to point toward other diagnoses (ex: developmental delay/family history).
- To help identify a particular etiology of myocarditis (ex: symptomatology consistent with a particular viral illness).

6.2 Laboratory Testing

- No laboratory testing or biomarker can differentiate myocarditis from other etiologies of ventricular dysfunction.
- Serum cardiac troponin, creatinine kinase and N-terminal prohormone of brain natriuretic peptide (NT-proBNP) are usually elevated.
- Fulminant myocarditis may see elevation of troponin several hundred-fold higher than other etiologies.
- An evaluation of end organ function (renal and hepatic) is important.
- A screen for inborn errors of metabolism should be considered in neonates, infants and younger children or if the history/physical exam are suggestive of a specific disorder in an older child.
- Should perform testing to rule out reversible causes of ventricular dysfunction such as vitamin D deficiency, carnitine deficiency, and hypo/hyperthyroidism.
- Nasopharyngeal, gastrointestinal, and serum viral PCR or serology are nonspecific tests and it is unclear if a positive PCR increases the likelihood of myocarditis. Routine viral serology is not recommended in adult guidelines due to poor correlation with biopsy results (contrary to viral PCR done on endomyocardial biopsy).

6.3 Electrocardiogram

- Common findings are sinus tachycardia, PR depression, ST/T wave changes, and low QRS voltages.
- Required to assess for atrioventricular block, atrial or ventricular ectopy/arrhythmia (commonly seen with fulminant myocarditis or giant cell myocarditis).

6.4 Chest X-ray

- Usually completely normal with narrow cardiothoracic ratio
- Possibly plethoric lung fields secondary to interstitial edema

6.5 Echocardiogram

- There is no classic appearance of myocarditis by echocardiogram.
- It is used to assess ventricular size, wall thickness, ventricular function, regional wall motion abnormalities, pericardial effusion, atrial or ventricular thrombus.
- As a general rule, children with myocarditis are more likely to have a normal ventricular size, in contrast to children with dilated cardiomyopathy who are more likely to have a dilated ventricle. However, a variable degree of ventricular dilation can be seen in myocarditis.
- Important to rule out other treatable causes of ventricular dysfunction such as ALCAPA, coarctation or severe aortic stenosis.
- Increased wall thickness can be seen with presence of wall edema.

6.6 Cardiac Magnetic Resonance Imaging

- Growing evidence but still lacking large scale multi-center trials and pediatric studies.
- Gold standard for functional measurements such as ventricular dimension, wall thickness, and ventricular function.
- Used for tissue characterisation:
  - Myocardial edema is measured using high signal intensity on T2-weighted imaging and elevated T1 times denoting increased extracellular volume fraction (Fig. 1).
  - Capillary leak (regional myocardial vasodilatation) is detected by an increase volume of gadolinium distribution in the early washout period.
  - Fibrosis is detected by the finding of myocardial late gadolinium enhancement (LGE).

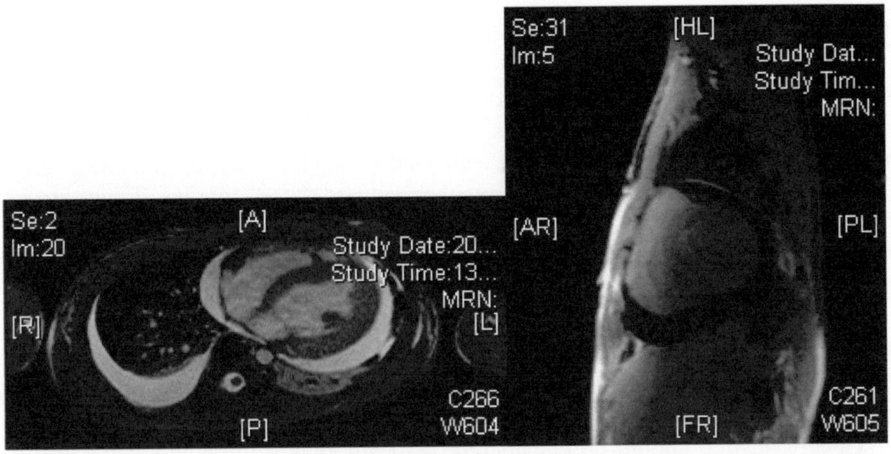

Fig. 1 Cardiac magnetic resonance imaging for 15-year-old patient with clinically suspected myocarditis. Severe myocardial edema causing increased wall thickness with pericardial effusion. T1 mapping (short axis of LV) at septum was 1303 ms with extracellular volume fraction of 46% at the base and 1290 ms with extracellular volume fraction of 47% at the mid septum

- Lake Louise Criteria: at least 2 of the following must be present:
  - Evidence of edema on T2-weighted imaging.
  - Evidence of hyperemia with gadolinium-enhanced T1-weighted imaging.
  - Evidence of late gadolinium enhancement (LGE).
- Ventricular dysfunction or pericardial effusion provide only supportive evidence to the Lake Louise criteria.

6.7 Endomyocardial Biopsy

- The usefulness of a biopsy for diagnostic purposes remains questionable because of variability in sampling and in the interpretation of the biopsy samples.
- The Dallas criteria was first described in 1987 and provided a histopathological categorization of myocarditis. It requires:
  - An inflammatory infiltrate.
  - Myocyte damage or necrosis that cannot be explained by another diagnosis.
- In our center, biopsy is not frequently performed and is reserved for unique cases. Certain forms of acute myocarditis, including giant cell myocarditis and eosinophilic myocarditis, are diagnosed by biopsy.

7 Prognosis

- The prognosis associated with myocarditis varies depending on the etiology. Most patients will recover within weeks.
- Fulminant myocarditis associated with > 90% long term survival and heart function recovery, even after requiring mechanical circulatory support, if they survive the acute event.
- Up to 30% of patients with biopsy-proven myocarditis will progress to dilated cardiomyopathy. In addition, for children with biopsy-proven myocarditis, the transplant-free survival at 2 years is about 80%.
- A lifetime recurrence rate of 10% has been described. Recurrence is more likely in patients with prolonged (> 7 days) initial admission, with ventricular arrhythmia on initial presentation, and with inflammatory bowel disease.
- Genetic testing should be considered, as desmoplakin mutations can cause an inflammatory cardiomyopathy described by recurrent episodes of myocardial injury.

8 Treatment

- Initial monitoring in an intensive care setting should be strongly considered. Acute myocarditis can rapidly progress to cardiovascular shock and cardiac arrest.
- Acute myocarditis management largely supportive—including invasive ventilation, inotropic/vasoactive therapy, and mechanical circulatory support.
- Mechanical support should be considered as a bridge to recovery or transplant in severe cases. Patients who present in extremis may need urgent ECMO cannulation (Chapter 57). Standard cannulation (neck or femoral according to age) may be sufficient but it is important to ensure adequate LV decompression in cases with very poor function, which may require LA venting or creation of an atrial communication in the cath lab. Mechanical support is usually only temporary and so ECMO or Impella systems are those most commonly used. Patients who fail to recover function may have to be considered for conversion to durable VAD (Chapter 42).
- Intense or competitive exercise may be restricted during the first few months after myocarditis presentation depending on the clinical severity and trajectory of heart function recovery. A slow and cautious return to exercise may be advised. This does not apply to return to routine activities.
- Cardiac reverse remodeling therapies should be implemented according to the current guidelines for patients with persistent ventricular dysfunction (Chapter 41). Timing is a clinical decision that factors in the acuity of the illness, remodeling of the cardiac chamber sizes, and ongoing ventricular and valve function. Can be considered as early as 2 weeks after diagnosis but more often initiated around 4 to 6 weeks if there is the clinical impression of a conversion to a more chronic disease.

- Heart transplant should be delayed in the acute phase if possible, since recovery may occur (Chapter 43), in addition to suboptimal outcomes post-heart transplant in the setting of acute myocarditis.
- Immunosuppression is not a routine treatment in myocarditis. It is usually recommended only in suspected giant cell myocarditis with presence of frequent ectopy or varying degree of heart block or with proven autoimmune myocarditis. However, due to the equipoise in the literature, treatment of all patients with suspected myocarditis with steroids *could* be considered.
- Intravenous immunoglobulin: There is no data supporting the use of this therapy in this population.
- Long-term follow-up is recommended in all patients with myocarditis, even after complete recovery.

Bibliography

1. Caforio ALP, Calabrese F, Angelini A, et al. A prospective study of biopsy-proven myocarditis: prognostic relevance of clinical and aetiopathogenetic features at diagnosis. Eur Heart J. 2007;28(11):1326–33.
2. Caforio ALP, Pankuweit S, Arbustini E, et al. Current state of knowledge on aetiology, diagnosis, management, and therapy of myocarditis: a position statement of the European Society of Cardiology Working Group on Myocardial and Pericardial Diseases. Eur Heart J. 2013;34(33):2636–48.
3. Cooper LT, Berry GJ, Shabetai R Idiopathic giant-cell myocarditis - natural history and treatment. For the multicenter giant cell myocarditis study group investigators. N Engl J Med 1997;336(26): 1860–6.
4. Foerster SR, Canter CE, Cinar A, et al. Ventricular remodeling and survival are more favorable for myocarditis than for idiopathic dilated cardiomyopathy in childhood: an outcomes study from the Pediatric Cardiomyopathy Registry. Circ Heart Fail. 2010;3(6):689–97.
5. Friedrich MG, Sechtem U, Schulz-Menger J, et al. Cardiovascular magnetic resonance in myocarditis: A JACC White Paper. J Am Coll Cardiol. 2009;53(17):1475–87.
6. Kytö V, Sipilä J, Rautava P. Rate and patient features associated with recurrence of acute myocarditis. Eur J Intern Med. 2014;25(10):946–50.
7. Law Yuk M, Lal Ashwin K, Sharon C, et al. Diagnosis and management of myocarditis in children: a scientific statement from the American Heart Association. Circulation. 2021;144(6):e123–35.
8. Parrillo A, Cunnion RE, Epstein SE, et al. Prospective, randomized, controlled trial of prednisone for dilated cardiomyopathy. N Engl J Med. 1989;321(16):1061–8.
9. Pollack A, Kontorovich AR, Fuster V, Dec GW. Viral myocarditis- diagnosis, treatment options, and current controversies. Nat Rev Cardiol. 2015;12(11):670–80.

Hypertrophic Cardiomyopathy

Áine Lynch and Aamir Jeewa

Abstract Hypertrophic cardiomyopathy (HCM) is the second most common cardiomyopathy in children. It is characterized by myocyte hypertrophy and disarray resulting in left ventricular hypertrophy most often affecting the basal interventricular septum. HCM is often asymptomatic until adulthood but may manifest with symptoms of left ventricular outflow tract obstruction (LVOTO), heart failure, or ventricular arrhythmias. Diagnosis is based on maximal left ventricular wall thickness z score ≥ 2.5 on echocardiogram or magnetic resonance imaging (MRI). Serial echocardiogram is the mainstay of clinical follow up assessment with special attention to wall thickness, outflow tract obstruction, mitral valve abnormalities, systolic and diastolic function. Regular ECG and Holter testing are also recommended for arrhythmia surveillance. Existing management is focused on alleviating symptoms and preventing disease complications such as arrhythmias and sudden cardiac death. For those with symptoms of LVOTO, medical management is recommended, with myectomy reserved for those with symptoms refractory to medications. For those with risk factors for sudden cardiac death (SCD), shared decision making with patients and families should guide Implantable cardioverter defibrillator (ICD) insertion. Given the inheritance risk in families, clinical screening is recommended for all first-degree relatives with consideration for genetic testing in those families in whom the index case is known to harbor a pathogenic variant.

Keywords Hypertrophic cardiomyopathy · Left ventricular outflow tract obstruction · Diastolic dysfunction · Heart failure · Sudden cardiac death · Myectomy · Implantable Cardioverter defibrillator

---

Á. Lynch
Columbia University Vagelos College of Physicians and Surgeons, Morgan Stanley Children's Hospital of New York Presbyterian, New York, NY, USA
e-mail: al4599@cumc.columbia.edu

A. Jeewa (✉)
Division of Cardiology, Department of Paediatrics, The Hospital for Sick Children, Labatt Family Heart Centre, University of Toronto, Toronto, ON, Canada
e-mail: aamir.jeewa@sickkids.ca

© The Author(s), under exclusive license to Springer Nature Switzerland AG 2024

A. I. Dipchand et al. (eds.), *Manual of Cardiac Care in Children*,
https://doi.org/10.1007/978-3-031-70973-9_40

Abbreviations

ACE	Angiotensin converting enzyme
AHA	American heart association
ARB	Angiotensin receptor blocker
CCB	Calcium channel blocker
ECG	Electrocardiogram
HCM	Hypertrophic cardiomyopathy
HF	Heart failure
HR	Heart rate
ICD	Implantable cardioverter defibrillator
LVOT	Left ventricular outflow tract
LVOTO	Left ventricular outflow tract obstruction
LV	Left ventricle
LVH	Left ventricular hypertrophy
MR	Mitral regurgitation
MRI	Magnetic resonance imaging
MV	Mitral valve
NSVT	Non-sustained ventricular tachycardia
RV	Right ventricle
RVSP	Right ventricular systolic pressure
SAM	Systolic anterior motion
SCD	Sudden cardiac death

Key Points

- Hypertrophic cardiomyopathy (HCM) is characterized by myocyte hypertrophy and disarray.
- HCM is associated with left ventricular hypertrophy, outflow tract obstruction, diastolic dysfunction, arrhythmia and risk of sudden cardiac death (SCD). Systolic heart failure occurs less frequently.
- Most cases relate to inherited defects in genes coding for sarcomeric proteins, but infantile cases may result from RASopathy, neuromuscular disease or inborn errors of metabolism.
- Most cases are asymptomatic, but patients may experience chest pain and syncope.
- First-line therapies for children and adolescents with symptomatic left ventricular outflow tract obstruction (LVOTO) are beta blockers, calcium channel blockers and disopyramide. Myectomy should be considered for those with symptoms refractory to medical management.
- Risk factors for SCD have been identified; non-sustained ventricular tachycardia, syncope, family history SCD, massive left ventricular hypertrophy (LVH), systolic

Table 1 Sarcomeric genes associated with HCM

Gene	Protein	% HCM caused
MYBPC3	Myosin binding protein C	50%
MYH7	β myosin heavy chain	30%
TNNI3	Cardiac troponin T	5%
TNNT2	Cardiac troponin I	4%
TPM1	α tropomyosin	< 3%
ACTC1	Cardiac actin	< 3%
MYL2	Myosin light chain 2	< 3%
MYL3	Myosin light chain 3	< 3%
PLN	Phospholamban	< 3%

dysfunction and late gadolinium enhancement on MRI. Recent data also suggests ischemic changes on exercise testing have also been associated with SCD. ICD insertion should be guided by a shared decision-making process with patients and families, taking into account the risk–benefit of both SCD prevention and device related complications.

1 Epidemiology

- Second most common cardiomyopathy in childhood
- Annual incidence of 0.51–3.2 per 10,000 live births in children.
- Primary HCM is a single gene disorder with autosomal dominant inheritance and variable penetrance, attributed to defects in genes encoding sarcomere proteins (Table 1). At least 11 genes have been implicated, most commonly *MYBPC3* and *MYH7*, accounting for 30–60% of familial or sporadic HCM. To date, there is no convincing evidence of genotype-phenotype correlation in this cohort.
- Secondary HCM related to underlying defects in the RAS-MAPK pathway, neuromuscular disease or inborn errors of metabolism accounts for a majority of infantile onset HCM. RASopathy associated HCM results from genetic defects in intracellular proteins that regulate cell cycle progression and cellular growth. Patients with secondary HCM are more likely to present in infancy with heart failure and are at increased risk of early mortality.

2 Anatomy

See (Fig. 1).

- Characterized by LVH with a non-dilated left ventricle (LV), not explained by loading conditions

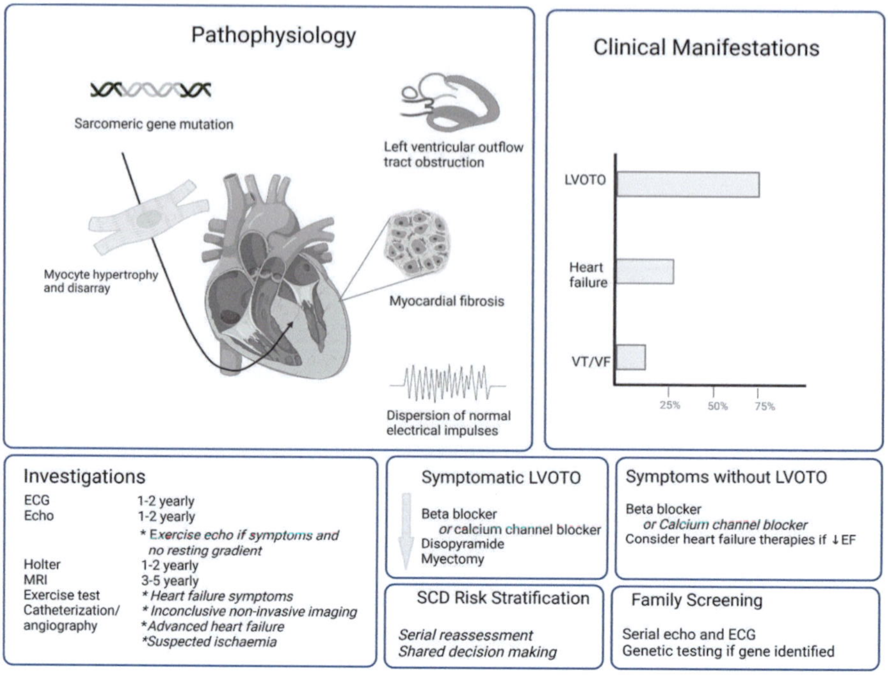

Fig. 1 Overview of Hypertrophic cardiomyopathy

- LVH is typically asymmetric and usually involves, but not limited to, the basal interventricular septum. A subgroup of patients have apical HCM with 'spade-like' configuration of the LV cavity (often missed on echocardiogram and may require MRI).
- Often associated with structural abnormalities of the mitral valve (MV).
- Thickening of the anterior leaflet may occur due to repeated contact with the hypertrophied interventricular septum.

3 Pathophysiology

See (Fig. 1).

- Myocyte hypertrophy and disarray is the histologic hallmark; this disorganized muscle architecture causes dispersion of electrical impulses and may contribute to dysfunction and arrhythmia risk.
- Septal hypertrophy results in LVOTO at rest in approximately one-third of patients, an additional one-third have provokable LVOTO. Hypertrophied LV is often hyperdynamic, which may result in systolic anterior motion (SAM) of the MV during ejection, further contributing to outflow tract obstruction.

- Intramural coronary arteries are also involved with intimal and medial thickening resulting in luminal narrowing predisposing to subclinical ischemia and replacement fibrosis in adjacent myocardium. A myocardial bridge is a segment of myocardium that overlays an epicardial coronary artery and can cause systolic compression of the vessel that can persists into diastole with the potential to disrupt coronary blood flow. The clinical impact of myocardial bridges are still unclear.
- Diastolic dysfunction is common independent of degree of hypertrophy. Active relaxation is impaired by abnormal sarcomere function and calcium homeostasis at a cellular level. Passive stiffness is also increased related to increased LV mass, subendocardial ischemia and replacement fibrosis.

4 Clinical Physiology and Presentation

See (Fig. 1).

- Influenced by underlying etiology.
- Infantile presentation is associated with increased risk of mortality within the first year of life (up to 14% at 1-year), with most deaths related to heart failure; most often associated with secondary causes of HCM.
- Presentation outside of infancy is variable
  - Most paediatric HCM patients remain asymptomatic into adulthood.
  - Exercise intolerance with or without chest pain or syncope is the most common complaint and may relate to LVOTO or microvascular ischemia.
  - SCD occurs at a rate of 1–2% per year.

4.1 Symptomatology

4.1.1 LVOTO

- Dynamic obstruction of the LVOT is the most common clinical manifestation, occurring in up to 75% of patients.
- Peak LVOT gradient > 30 mmHg is consistent with obstruction with pharmacologic or surgical intervention threshold of > 50 mmHg at rest or provoked.

4.1.2 Heart Failure

- Clinical heart failure may occur as a consequence of diastolic or systolic dysfunction and is further contributed to by LVOTO with resultant increased ventricular end-diastolic pressure and mitral regurgitation (MR); this leads to progressive left atrial dilation and pulmonary oedema.

- In a small subgroup of HCM patients (~5% in adult cohorts), myocardium becomes fibrosed resulting in myocardial thinning and systolic dysfunction ('burnt out' myocardium).

4.1.3 Arrhythmia and SCD

- The combination of myocardial fibrosis and ischemia interferes with usual conduction and predisposes to ventricular arrhythmias and SCD.
- Although degree of LVH has been associated with arrhythmia risk; recent data has shown this is likely due to overlap with other risk factors.
- Up to 10% of pediatric patients experience ventricular arrhythmias.
- Atrial arrhythmias (most commonly atrial fibrillation) are more commonly seen in adults with up to 20% by age 40 years.
- ECG findings of pre-excitation are seen in up to 5%, however pre-excitation pattern on ECG does not always infer accessory pathway in HCM patients, and 'pseudo pre-excitation' has been demonstrated related to abnormalities in atrioventricular nodal and His Purkinje conduction.

4.2 Physical Findings

- Systolic ejection crescendo-decrescendo murmur which decreases with increases in preload (squatting), or afterload (handgrip) and increases with decrease in preload (Valsalva).
- Less common findings include pulsus bisferiens (double carotid pulse), laterally displaced apical impulse, S4 and holostolic murmur (MR).
- Dysmorphic features associated with secondary HCM syndromes

5 Diagnostic Studies

See (Table 2 and Fig. 2).

6 Management

- While disease modifying agents are currently under investigation, existing management priorities involve symptom management and prevention of complications.

Table 2 Diagnostic tests and investigations in paediatric HCM

Investigation	Indication	Findings
Chest Xray		– Cardiomegaly – Left atrial enlargement – Pulmonary edema
ECG	– Diagnosis – 1–2 yearly – Clinical concern **Abnormal in up to 90%*	– Voltage criteria for LVH – T-wave inversion (LV strain) – ST-T wave changes – LA enlargement – Pre-excitation or pseudo pre-excitation
Echo	– Diagnosis **LV wall z score ≥ 2.5 in those without family history or ≥ 2 in those with family history* – 1–2 yearly – Clinical Concern	– Full anatomic assessment – Ventricular wall thickness (2D) – LVOT assessment in 2D, Doppler, and colour *Aim to identify etiology and extent and level of obstruction* – LV systolic and diastolic function *M-mode, Simpsons biplane, strain, LA diameter and volume, pulse Doppler of mitral inflow and pulmonary vein, tissue Doppler* – RV size, function and RVSp
MRI	– Diagnosis *Exclude secondary cause* – 3–5 yearly – Challenging echo windows – Clinical Concern	– Wall thickness – Ventricular function – Increased T1 signaling **Myocardial fibrosis is independently associated with increased SCD risk* – Late gadolinium enhancement
Holter	– Diagnosis – 1–2 yearly – Clinical Concern	– Atrial and ventricular arrhythmias
Cardiopulmonary Exercise Test	– Advanced HF despite max medications *Quantify functional limitations*	– Ischemia – Exercise induced arrhythmias
Exercise echocardiography	– Symptoms without LVOTO > 30 mmHg ar rest	
Cardiac Catheterization	– Inconclusive non-invasive imaging in symptomatic patient – Advanced HF – Suspected ischemia	– Hemodynamic assessment – Coronary origins and course including myocardial bridging

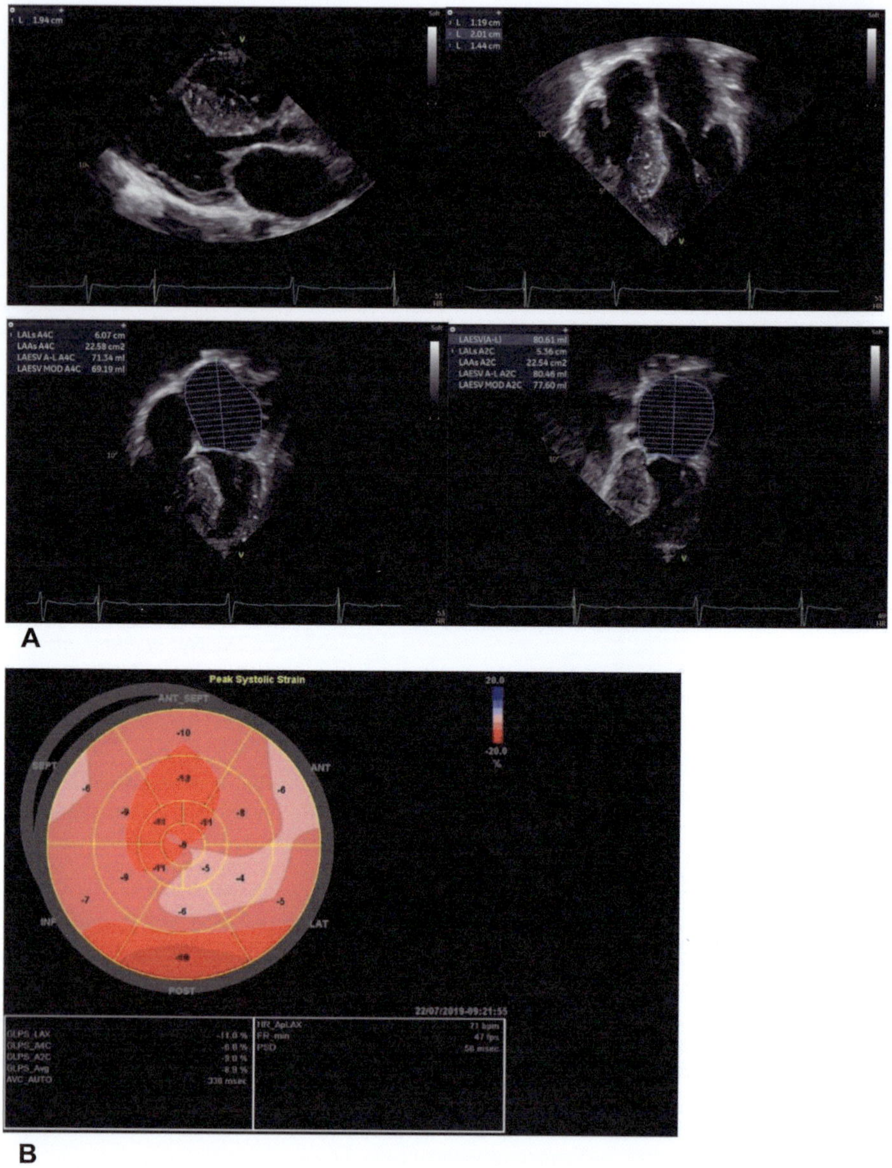

Fig. 2 (A) Severe asymmetric LVH with dilated left atrium in child with gene elusive familial HCM. (B) Reduced longitudinal strain and end-diastolic volume in teenager with HCM; (C) ECG of teenager with HCM showing left ventricular hypertrophy with strain (inferolateral T wave inversion and ST depression)

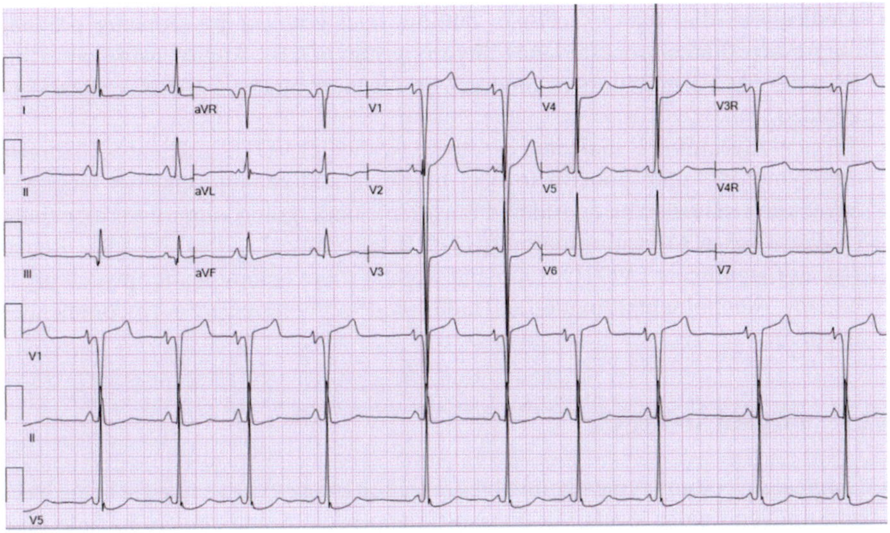

C

Fig. 2 (continued)

6.1 Acute Hypotension

- Goals are to reduce outflow tract gradient by optimizing preload and afterload, while avoiding increasing HR and contractility.
- Interventions include fluid resuscitation, and intravenous vasoconstrictors including phenylephrine. Beta blocker use may be used with caution once stabilized.

6.2 Symptomatic LVOTO

- Currently no licensed disease modifying medications in paediatrics.
- Pharmacotherapy is indicated only for symptom relief (exertional chest pain, dyspnea, syncope or pre-syncope).
- Echocardiographic measures of LVOTO severity have not been shown to correlate with symptoms.
- First line therapy includes non-vasodilating beta-blockers titrated to symptom improvement.
- Non-dihydropyridine calcium channel blockers (CCB) may be used as an alternative if intolerant of beta-blockers.
- Disopyramide, an antiarrhythmic, can be used instead of CCB for the amelioration of the LVOTO.

- Medications that may exacerbate outflow tract gradient by reducing pre-load (aggressive diuresis) or afterload (dihydropyridine CCBs, Angiotensin Converting Enzyme (ACE) inhibitors or angiotensin receptor blockers (ARB)s) should be avoided.
- Surgical myectomy is indicated in select cases with LVOTO gradient > 50 mmHg and symptoms unresponsive to beta blockade and calcium channel blockade. Myectomy may also be considered in patients undergoing surgery for associated cardiac disease. Operative mortality is < 1% and clinical success 90–95%. Recurrence of significant LVOTO is rare but slightly more common after myectomy in infancy. Alcohol septal ablation and radiofrequency ablation are not recommended in children.

6.2.1 Surgical Strategy

- Surgical myectomy typically involves resection of obstructive muscle at the basal and midventricular levels via transaortic approach. Some centers include revision of the anterior leaflet of the mitral valve to further reduce risk of mitral regurgitation due to systolic anterior motion of the valve.
- Surgical complications include iatrogenic ventricular septal defect (0.1%), damage to conduction system including bundle branch block with risk of future arrhythmias, heart block (2), and injury to mitral (2%) or aortic valves (5%).
- The transaortic approach is particularly challenging in small children due to aortic valve size, and apical ventriculotomy may be required to relieve midventricular or apical obstruction.

6.3 Symptomatic Non-obstructive HCM

- May present with similar symptoms of chest pain and dyspnea due to diastolic dysfunction, increased oxygen requirements of hypertrophied myocardium, or microvascular disease.
- Similar to obstructive HCM, beta blockers or non-dihydropyridine calcium channel blockers may alleviate symptoms by reducing HR, LV filling pressures and myocardial oxygen demand.
- Significant diastolic heart failure may benefit from cautious use of diuretics.

6.4 Heart Failure

- Symptoms of heart failure should be managed with conventional heart failure therapy; diuretic use should be guided by volume status and symptomatology.
- Those who develop systolic dysfunction should be initiated on guideline directed medical therapy for heart failure.

6.5 Ventricular Arrhythmias

- Documented sustained ventricular arrhythmias should be referred for ICD consideration (see SCD risk management).
- Ventricular arrhythmias or recurrent ICD shocks on optimal beta-blocker dosing: antiarrhythmic therapy should be initiated.
- MRI imaging prior to ICD placement should also be considered; however, MRI compatible ICDs may allow for ongoing imaging with modality in the future.

6.6 SCD Risk Management

- Risk stratification and consideration for ICD insertion in HCM patients remains a challenge.
- Contributing risk factors include syncope, family history SCD, massive LVH, systolic dysfunction, diffuse LGE in MRI and documented non-sustained ventricular tachycardia (NSVT).
- A shared decision process making for ICD insertion should be offered to patients and parents regarding risks of SCD versus ICD insertion and associated complications.
- Risk prediction models have been developed and are linked below.
  https://primacycalculator.com/
  https://hcmriskkids.org/
- Additional adult risk calculators are validated in patients > 16 years of age
  https://qxmd.com/calculate/calculator_303/hcm-risk-scd

6.7 Atrial Fibrillation

- Anticoagulation with direct anti-thrombin agents or warfarin should be initiated in patients with atrial fibrillation to reduce the risk of thromboembolism.

6.8 Lifestyle Considerations

- A heart healthy lifestyle including mild-moderate physical activity is encouraged. Higher activity levels than this are not absolutely contraindicated, but should rather be approached on a case-by-case basis and with a shared-decision making model after risk stratification is completed.

7 Family Screening and Genetic Testing

- Clinical screening with echocardiogram and ECG is recommended for all first-degree relatives of phenotype-positive HCM patients and should be repeated every 1–2 years during childhood and adolescence.
- Sarcomere gene mutations are inherited in an autosomal dominant fashion, and cascade screening should be performed in families in whom a pathogenic variant is identified.
- Genetic counselling is of benefit for families with HCM.
- Follow-up clinical screening is not indicated in first degree relatives who do not harbor the familial pathogenic variant. However, it is important that genetic testing results are reviewed regularly for reclassification.

8 Natural History and Outcomes

- Often compatible with normal lifespan however patients presenting at young age may be at increased risk.
- Existing data suggesting mortality rates of 5% at 10 years after diagnosis.
- 30–40% will experience major cardiac events during their lifetime including SCD, symptomatic LVOTO, and systolic or diastolic heart failure.
- SCD is the most prominent cause of death later in childhood and adolescence.

9 Controversies

- The complex interplay of lifestyle mediated risk factors and disease related risk factors for cardiac events in HCM patients presents challenges to the establishment of definitive criteria for exercise restriction and ICD insertion. This is further added to by lack of data on effects of high-intensity exercise in HCM.
- Despite recently developed risk prediction models, positive predictive value for SCD events remains low. The most recent AHA guidelines advocate for a shared decision-making model with patients and families regarding ICD insertion and exercise restriction, facilitating patient autonomy.

10 Alternative Strategies

- Recent adult trials have demonstrated encouraging results with use of the novel cardiac myosin inhibitor, Mavacamten, in relieving symptomatic LVOTO in HCM. Additionally, it has been shown to result in a dose dependent reduction in NT proBNP and Troponin, and favorable effects on indexed LV wall thickness and wall stress. Paediatric data is pending.

Bibliography

1. Alexander PMA, Nugent AW, Daubeney PEF, et al. Long-term outcomes of hypertrophic cardiomyopathy diagnosed during childhood: results from a national population-based study. Circulation. 2018;138(1):29–36.
2. Altarabsheh SE, Dearani JA, Burkhart HM, et al. Outcome of septal myectomy for obstructive hypertrophic cardiomyopathy in children and young adults. Ann Thorac Surg. 2013;95(2):663–9.
3. Bilen O, Saberi S, Jacoby D, Masri A Mavacamten-induced cardiac remodeling in HCM. Am College Cardiol. 2021 Epub
4. Colan SD, Lipshultz SE, Lowe AM, et al. Epidemiology and cause-specific outcome of hypertrophic cardiomyopathy in children: Findings from the Pediatric Cardiomyopathy Registry. Circulation. 2007;115(6):773–81.
5. Fogel MA, Anwar S, Broberg C, et al. Society for cardiovascular magnetic resonance/European society of cardiovascular imaging/American society of echocardiography/society for pediatric radiology/north American society for cardiovascular imaging guidelines for the use of cardiac magnetic resonance in pediatric congenital and acquired heart disease: endorsed by the American heart association. Circ Cardiovasc Imaging. 2022;15(6): e014415.
6. Miron A, Lafreniere-Roula M, Steve Fan CP, et al. A validated model for sudden cardiac death risk prediction in pediatric hypertrophic cardiomyopathy. Circulation. 2020;142(3):217–29.
7. Norrish G, Ding T, Field E, et al. Development of a novel risk prediction model for sudden cardiac death in childhood hypertrophic cardiomyopathy (HCM Risk-Kids). JAMA Cardiol. 2019;4(9):918–27.
8. Norrish G, Kolt G, Cervi E, et al. Clinical presentation and long-term outcomes of infantile hypertrophic cardiomyopathy: a European multicentre study. ESC Hear Fail. 2021;8(6):5057–67.
9. Norrish G, Ding T, Field E, et al. Relationship between maximal left ventricular wall thickness and sudden cardiac death in childhood onset hypertrophic cardiomyopathy. Circ Arrhythm Electrophysiol. 2022;15(5): e010075.
10. Ommen SR, Mital S, Burke MA, et al. AHA/ACC Guideline for the diagnosis and treatment of patients with hypertrophic cardiomyopathy: a report of the American college of cardiology/American heart association joint committee on clinical practice guidelines. Circulation. 2020;142(25):e558–631. Erratum in: Circulation. 2020 142(25):e633.

Heart Function

Kathryn R. Armstrong and Aamir Jeewa

Abstract Heart failure is a clinical syndrome that manifests from the failure of the heart to supply blood to the systemic circulation with or without elevated central venous filling pressures and resulting in classical signs and symptoms. Echocardiography is the key initial diagnostic modality. Further investigations are guided by the suspected underlying etiology. Etiologies can be congenital or acquired but are multiple and diverse. The approach to the child with heart failure should be considered in a stepwise fashion in terms of both investigation and treatment. The common underlying pathophysiology of activation of the renin–angiotensin–aldosterone system (RAAS) leading to a combination of myocardial injury and maladaptive process in response to neurohormonal activation also leads to the common treatment strategies. Medical heart failure therapy includes establishment of guideline directed medical therapy (GDMT) to promote reverse remodeling with a goal to improve quality of life and survival. Acute decompensated heart failure (ADHF) may require short-term intravenous inotropic support, non-invasive or invasive ventilation and/or mechanical support as a bridge to recovery or decision-making.

Keywords Heart failure · Pediatric · Cardiomyopathy · Guideline directed medical therapy

Abbreviations

ADHF	Acute decompensated heart failure
ARNI	Angiotensin receptor-neprilysin inhibitor

K. R. Armstrong
Division of Cardiology, Department of Pediatrics, University of British Columbia, British Columbia Children's Hospital, Vancouver, BC, Canada
e-mail: kathryn.armstrong@cw.bc.ca

A. Jeewa (✉)
Department of Paediatrics, Division of Cardiology, Labatt Family Heart Centre, The Hospital for Sick Children, University of Toronto, Toronto, ON, Canada
e-mail: aamir.jeewa@sickkids.ca

© The Author(s), under exclusive license to Springer Nature Switzerland AG 2024
A. I. Dipchand et al. (eds.), *Manual of Cardiac Care in Children*,
https://doi.org/10.1007/978-3-031-70973-9_41

AV	Atrioventricular
AVC	Arrhythmogenic cardiomyopathy
BIPAP	Bilevel positive airway pressure
BNP	B-type natriuretic peptide
CHD	Congenital heart disease
CPAP	Continuous positive airway pressure
CPET	Cardiopulmonary exercise test
CRP	C reactive protein
CRT	Cardiac resynchronization therapy
DCM	Dilated cardiomyopathy
DOAC	Direct oral anticoagulant
ECMO	Extracorporeal membrane oxygenation
EF	Ejection fraction
GDMT	Guideline directed medical therapy
HCM	Hypertrophic cardiomyopathy
HF	Heart failure
HFpEF	Heart failure with preserved ejection fraction
HFrEF	Heart hailure with reduced ejection fraction
LCOS	Low cardiac output syndrome
LMWH	Low molecular weight heparin
LV	Left ventricle
LVEDP	Left ventricular end-diastolic pressure
NPPV	Non-invasive positive pressure ventilation
NT-proBNP	N-terminal prohormone of brain natriuretic peptide
Qp	Pulmonary blood flow
Qs	Systemic blood flow
RAAS	Renin-angiotensin-aldosterone system
RCM	Restrictive cardiomyopathy
RV	Right ventricle
SCD	Sudden cardiac death
SGLT2i	Sodium glucose cotransporter-2 inhibitor
VO2	Oxygen consumption
VAD	Ventricular assist device

Key Points

- Etiologies of pediatric heart failure (HF) include acquired (ie. myocarditis) and congenital causes (ie cardiomyopathies or congenital heart disease).
- Pediatric HF carries a high morbidity and mortality and is a growing issue.
- Early recognition is key to initiating appropriate treatment and may optimize outcome.

- Electrocardiogram, chest radiography, and echocardiography should be considered as the first line investigations.
- Afterload reducing agents and other medications that modify the neurohormonal activation of HF are often used as first line agents in stable pediatric HF and form the basis for "guideline directed medical therapy" (GDMT).
- Diuretics should be reserved for patients presenting with fluid overload or congestion.
- Approach to the child with HF should be considered in a stepwise fashion in terms of both investigation and treatment.

1 Definition

- HF in children is defined as the clinical syndrome that manifests from the failure of the heart to supply blood (ie low output) to the systemic circulation with or without elevated central venous filling pressures. This results in the classical signs and symptoms of HF secondary to the adverse effects on the heart, the circulation and the patient.
- HF can be further differentiated by descriptors based on ventricular function such as Heart Failure with reduced Ejection Fraction (HFrEF) and Heart Failure with preserved Ejection Fraction (HFpEF).

2 Terminology

- Acute decompensated heart failure (ADHF) is characterized by an abrupt presentation, such as cardiogenic shock, either at initial presentation or as a deterioration of pre-existing symptoms, commonly with no identifiable precipitating event or illness.
- Chronic HF implies the presence of structural remodeling of heart and may be present irrespective of current symptoms.

3 Epidemiology

- The incidence of pediatric HF is unknown due to diverse etiologies. Primary cardiomyopathies and congenital heart disease (CHD) are the principal causes.
- The incidence of dilated cardiomyopathy (DCM), one of the more common causes of pediatric HF, is estimated to be around 0.57 per 100,000.
- CHD contributes to 60–70% of HF admissions in children.

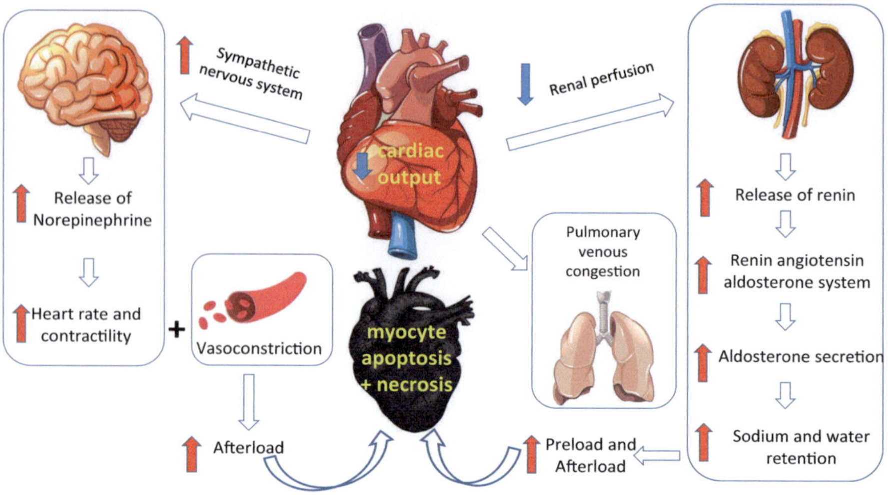

Fig. 1 Overview of the pathophysiology of heart failure in children

4 Pathophysiology of Heart Failure

- A combination of myocardial injury and maladaptive processes, that are in response to the neurohormonal activation of the renin-angiotensin aldosterone system (RAAS) and increase in sympathetic and adrenergic activity, leading to systemic vasoconstriction, myocyte apoptosis and necrosis.
- The cause of myocardial injury can be due to intrinsic abnormalities of the myocardium (cardiomyopathies or congenital), exposure to cardiotoxic agents or other acquired causes.
- See Fig. 1.

5 Etiology

- Intrinsic cardiomyopathies
  - Dilated cardiomyopathy (DCM): dilated LV with systolic dysfunction in the absence of an identifiable hemodynamic cause (e.g., sepsis, aortic stenosis, ischemia) (Table 1).
  - Hypertrophic cardiomyopathy (HCM; see Chap. 40).
  - Restrictive cardiomyopathy (RCM): primary diagnosis is abnormal myocardial compliance without a DCM or HCM phenotype (Table 2).

– Non-compaction cardiomyopathy: based on the appearance of prominent LV trabeculations and deep intratrabecular recesses detected on imaging or pathology. Most commonly due to sarcomeric or other genetic mutations (e.g., ZASP, HCN4), or metabolic causes (e.g., Barth Syndrome).

Sarcomeric
Metabolic disorder
Barth syndrome
Other genetic
ZASP
HCN4
α-Actinin-2

– Arrhythmogenic cardiomyopathy (AVC): autosomal-dominantly inherited heart disease with fibrofatty replacement of the myocardium and ventricular arrhythmias as well as by impaired ventricular systolic function.

- Congenital cardiac malformations: leading to volume/pressure overload, atrioventricular/semilunar valve insufficiency, single ventricle physiology.
- Coronary artery abnormalities leading to myocardial ischemia and dysfunction.
- Arrhythmias/dyssynchrony-induced: tachycardia (acute or incessant), bradycardia, preexcitation, pacing-induced.
- Acquired conditions: myocarditis, toxin/drug related, anemia, thyrotoxicosis (Table 3).

6 Clinical History (Table 4)

- Timing of onset of symptoms and if they are progressive or worsening.
- Detailed family history that includes questions about consanguinity, prior childhood cardiac disease (especially in first degree relatives), sudden cardiac death (SCD) or aborted SCD, other congenital malformations.
- Other relevant points: Sudden infant death/miscarriages, developmental and growth history, infectious or toxic exposures, previous surgeries or interventions, travel

7 Physical Examination

- Four classic patterns of presentation based on presence of low perfusion and/or congestion (Fig. 2).

Table 1 Causes of DCM

Primary DCM
Familial/genetic
Sarcomeric
Mitochondrial diseases
Neuromuscular disorders
Laminopathies
Secondary DCM
Inflammatory
Toxins
Iron
Lead
Cobalt
Arsenic
Anthracycline
Radiation
Metabolic disorders
Endocrinopathies
Thyroid disorders
Catecholamine-secreting tumor
Parathyroid disease
Diabetes mellitus
Fatty acid oxidation disorders
Carnitine deficiency
Malonyl coenzyme decarboxylase deficiency
Glycogen Storage Diseases (GSDs)
GSD type II (Pompe disease)
GSD type IV (Andersen disease)
Lysosomal storage disorders
Gaucher disease
Mucopolysaccharidoses
Sphingolipidoses
Nutritional disorders
Thiamine deficiency
Selenium deficiency
Protein energy malnutrition
Structural heart diseases
Valvular heart disease
Ischemia: coronary artery anomalies, coronary artery injury

(continued)

Table 1 (continued)

Primary DCM
Single ventricle
Pulmonary diseases

Reprinted from Circulation, Vol 140, Lipschultz SE, Law YM, Asante-Korang A, et al., AHA Scientific Statement: Cardiomyopathy in Children: Classification and Diagnosis, Page e17, Table 2—Causes of DCM, e9-e68, 2019, with permission from © American Heart Association, Inc.

Table 2 Causes of RCM

Primary RCM
Genetic
Sarcomeric
Desmin
Filamin-C
Secondary RCM
Infiltrative
Amyloidosis
Lysosomal storage disorder
Anderson-Fabry disease
Iron overload
Endomyocardial fibrosis
Parasitic infection
Autoimmune disorders
Malignancy with hypereosinophilia
Possible dietary deficiencies or ingested toxins in certain areas of endemic disease

Reprinted from Circulation, Vol 140, Lipschultz SE, Law YM, Asante-Korang A, et al., AHA Scientific Statement: Cardiomyopathy in Children: Classification and Diagnosis, Page e43, Table 11—Causes of RCM, e9-e68, 2019, with permission from © American Heart Association, Inc.

- Tachycardia.
- Signs of poor perfusion
  - Cool/mottled peripheries,
  - Prolonged capillary refill time,
  - Decreased peripheral pulses,
  - Decreased urine output,
  - Low systemic blood pressure,
  - Narrow pulse pressure,
  - Decreased level of consciousness, obtunded.
- Pulmonary Congestion

Table 3 Causes of inflammatory cardiomyopathy

	Causal agent or exposure
Commonly reported	
Infectious causes	
Bacterial	
Fungal	
Viral	Adenoviruses, enteroviruses, herpes simplex virus, varicella-zoster virus, human cytomegalovirus, Epstein-Barr virus, human herpesvirus 6, influenza A and B viruses, HIV, parvovirus B19
Rickettsial	
Spirochete	*Borrelia burgdorferi*
Noninfectious causes	
Autoimmune diseases	
Hypersensitive reactions	Dermatomyositis, hypereosinophilic syndrome, Kawasaki disease, lupus erythematodes, rheumatoid arthritis
Drug reactions	
Toxic reactions to drugs	Penicillin, ampicillin, cephalosporins, tetracyclines, sulfonamides, anthracyclines
Other exposures	
Rarely reported	
Infectious causes	
Bacterial	Chlamydia, Corynebacterium diphtheria, legionella, Mycobacterium tuberculosis, mycoplasma, staphylococcus, Streptococcus A, Streptococcus pneumonia
Fungal	Actinomyces, aspergillus, candida, Cryptococcus helminthic: Echinococcus granulosus,
Viral	Variola virus, vaccinia virus, mumps virus, measles virus, rubella virus, hepatitis C virus,
Rickettsial	Coxiella brunetti, Rickettsia typhi
Spirochete	Leptospira, Treponema pallidum
Noninfectious causes	
Autoimmune diseases	Celiac disease, Churg-Strauss syndrome, Crohn disease, giant-cell
Hypersensitive reactions	Antiphlogistics, benzodiazepines, clozapine, loop and thiazide diuretics
Drug reactions	
Toxic reactions to drugs	Amphetamines, catecholamines, cocaine, cyclophosphamide, 5-fluorouracil, phenytoin, trastuzumab, ethanol
Other exposures	Arsenic, copper, iron, radiotherapy, thyrotoxicosis

Reprinted from Heart Failure Clinics, Vol 6, Issue 4, Kuhl W, Schultheiss HP, Myocarditis in children, pp 483–496 viii–ix, 2010, with permission from Elsevier Science & Technology Journals

Table 4 Approach to Child with Heart Failure presentation

	Common Symptoms	Uncommon symptoms
Infants	Failure to thrive/feeding difficulties (vomiting, refusal, gastroesophageal reflux, tachypnea, tachycardia, diaphoresis pallor)	Cyanosis, palpitations, syncope, facial/ dependent edema, ascites
Children/ Adolescents	Fatigue, exercise intolerance, tachycardia dyspnea/orthopnea, abdominal pain/nausea pipinppain/Nausea/Vomiting	Palpitations, chest pain, dependent edema, ascites

  - Tachypnea,
  - Use of accessory respiratory muscles, grunting, nasal flaring, wheeze.
- Systemic Congestion
  - Hepatomegaly,
  - Jugular venous distention.
- On auscultation—S3, S4 (gallop rhythm), diastolic rumble

8 Investigations and Common Findings

8.1 First Line

- CXR
  - Cardiomegaly, signs of pulmonary congestion
- ECG
  - Sinus tachycardia, LV hypertrophy, low QRS voltages (myocarditis), ST-T wave changes, ischemic changes such as presence of Q waves, 1st/2nd/3rd degree AV Block or be non-specific.
- Laboratory Investigations
  - Renal/liver function, complete blood count, inflammatory markers (CRP, ESR), venous gas and lactate, blood cultures or studies for viral infections (i.e., polymerase chain reaction and serology) if suspected myocarditis.
- Cardiac Biomarkers
  - BNP (B-type natriuretic peptide) or N terminal pro-B natriuretic peptide (NT-proBNP)

    If elevated supports systolic dysfunction.

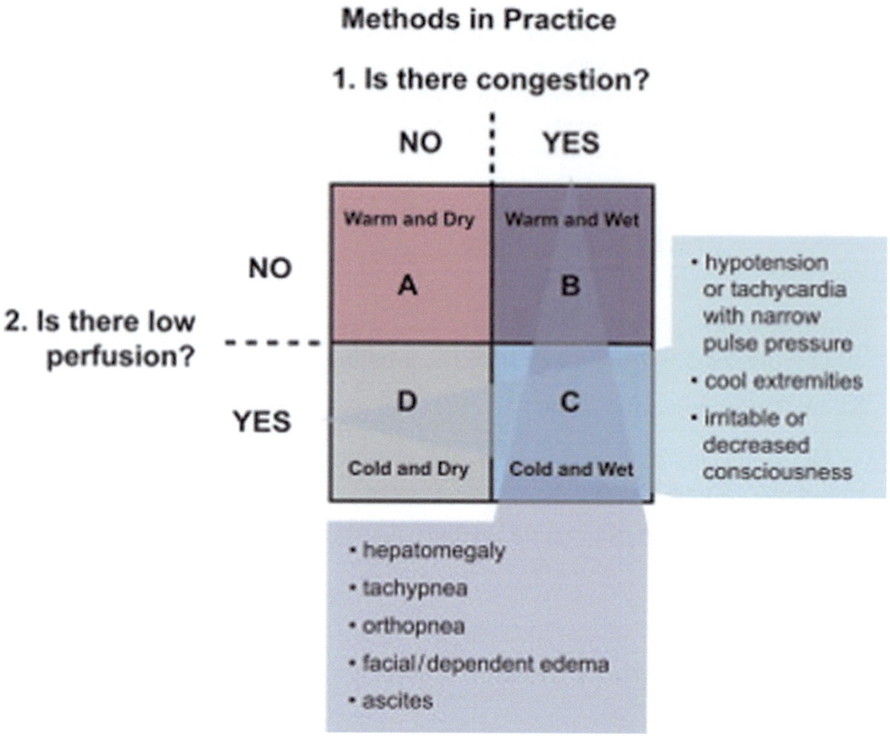

Fig. 2 Patterns of presentation recognized in acute decompensated heart failure. Reprinted from Canadian Journal of Cardiology, Vol 29, Issue 12, Kantor PF, Lougheed J, Dancea A, et al., Presentation, diagnosis and medical management of heart failure in children: Canadian Cardiovascular Society Guidelines, pp 1535–1552, 2013, with permission from Elsevier

Can be useful to follow serially to determine response to treatment and fluid status.

- Troponin is a sign of myocardial injury and may be elevated in both acute and chronic HF.

- Echocardiography
    - First line investigation in the assessment of HF.
    - Confirms cardiac anatomy to rule out structural causes contributing to dysfunction—coronaries, LV outflow, arch.
    - Assessment of intracardiac thrombus and pericardial effusion.
    - Complete evaluation of LV dimensions, wall thickness, fractional shortening and ejection fraction by M Mode, compaction.
    - 2-dimensional measurements of ejection fraction (EF) by modified Simpson's method; 3-dimensional measurements of function (if available).

- Tissue Doppler measurements of longitudinal function, detection of dyssynchrony.
- Strain imaging for the evaluation of dyssynchrony.

8.2 Second Line

- 24 /48 Hour Holter monitor
  - Arrhythmias/tachycardia; Ventricular ectopy.
- Metabolic Screening.
- Nutrient/Vitamin Deficiency
  - Evaluate for reversible causes (carnitine, vitamin D, selenium deficiency).
- Genetic Screening
  - See Chap. 46.
  - Recommended for patients with all forms of cardiomyopathy
  - Consider DNA banking on initial evaluation and ideally prior to blood transfusion.

8.3 Additional Testing

- Cardiopulmonary Exercise testing
  - A cardiopulmonary exercise test (CPET) with measurement of peak oxygen consumption (VO2) in ambulatory children
  - Peak V02 < 50% predicted indicative of severe HF. In children unable to perform a CPET, a 6-min walk test may provide adequate information with regards to functional capacity.
- Cardiac CT
  - May be used to delineate cardiac, vascular, and/or coronary artery anatomy.
  - Has higher spatial resolution than MRI, however exposure to radiation and lack of functional information limit its use.
  - May be required in the setting of operative planning for mechanical support (Chaps. 42 and 57).
- Cardiac MRI
  - The reference standard for measuring ventricular volumes and non-invasive assessment of cardiac output.
  - Late gadolinium enhancement for presence of fibrotic scar or interstitial fibrosis or edema.

  - Patient age limits use as younger children or children with developmental delays may require general anesthesia.
- Cardiac catheterization
  - Assessment of coronary artery anatomy, direct measurement of intracardiac filling pressures (such as the left ventricular end-diastolic pressure or LVEDP), and calculation of systemic and pulmonary vascular resistance.
  - In children with CHD and HF, catheterization will aid in the quantification of shunt lesions (Qp:Qs ratio), burden of collateral vessels, and other relevant hemodynamic data secondary to the structural heart disease.
- Endomyocardial Biospy
  - Not commonly performed; reserved for unique cases with specific indications (see Chap. 39 on myocarditis).

9 Medical Treatment

- Introduction of medications that alter the neurohormonal and renin-angiotensin aldosterone systems (RAAS) that are activated in HF and decongestive therapies (diuretics) if indicated.
- This can be done concurrently or in a step-wise fashion. The goal of therapy should be to relieve symptoms, reverse remodel ventricular function from the maladaptive changes, and ultimately to reduce morbidity and improve quality of life and survival
- Limited evidence exists for almost all medical therapies used in management of HF in children
- The vast majority of therapies are geared towards the improvement of HF secondary to systolic dysfunction. Diastolic HF, such as that seen in HFpEF states, have limited evidence based medical therapies in children and are largely based around management of symptoms with diuretics.

10 Heart Failure Therapies

- See Fig. 3
  - The goal is to establish combination therapy with longer acting oral agents referred to as GDMT and based on the adult HF experience.
  - GDMT forms the basis for management of chronic HF.
- Diuretics:
  - First line therapy in patients with symptomatic congestive HF.

  - Reduce extracellular fluid with an associated decrease in hydrostatic pressure in the peripheral, hepatic and pulmonary vascular bed.
  - In adults, have been shown to improve cardiac functional class, symptoms and exercise tolerance.
  - Should be initiated as early as possible, even in the emergency room, in symptomatic patients.
  - For first line therapy consider loop diuretics, i.e., furosemide (PO or IV).
  - Caution is required in patients with hypertrophic cardiomyopathy (HCM) or a restrictive physiology (preload dependent).
  - Augmentation may be required with thiazide type diuretics, i.e. metolazone or hydrochlorothiazide.
  - Use of diuretics requires monitoring of electrolyte levels, i.e. hyponatremia, hypo/hyperkalemia, hypomagnesemia and hypocalcemia.

- Angiotensin Converting Enzyme Inhibitors (ACEi):

  - Afterload reduction, reduce systolic wall stress of the failing ventricle, limit the negative effects of the RAAS up-regulation.
  - Captopril, Enalapril, Ramipril, Perindopril
  - Test dose required and then uptitrated

- Monitor for hypotension, renal dysfunction (especially in neonates and ACEi therapy generally avoided in this age group), and angioedema
- Angiotensin Receptor Blocker Antagonists (ARBs):

  - Similar effects on the RAAS up-regulation as ACE inhibitors.
  - Losartan, irbesartan.
  - Currently available in a combination drug that includes a neprilysin inhibitor, which promoted further natriuresis.
  - Sacubitril-Valsartan is the first in this class of Angiotensin receptor-neprilysin inhibitor (ARNI) and is available for use in children.

- Beta-Blockers:

  - Neurohormonal inhibition. The class of medication shown to have the highest mortality benefit over other medications in adults with HF.
  - Carvedilol, Metoprolol, Propranolol, etc.
  - Monitor for hypotension, bradycardia, and hypoglycemia especially in infants.

- Aldosterone Antagonist:

  - Exhibit antifibrotic effects and promote reverse remodeling of the myocardium.
  - Spironolactone, Eplerenone.

- Potential Adjuvant Heart Failure Medications

  - Digoxin**:** A cardiac glycoside that is less commonly used in pediatric HF. Conflicting evidence for its use in HF but may have some adjuvant role in those with symptomatic heart failure.

  - SGLT2 inhibitor: a new class of medications that target the sodium glucose cotransporter-2 inhibition with very limited experience in children to date. Examples are Dapagliflozin and Empagliflozin.
  - Ivabradine**:** An inhibitor of the I_f, or funny current, and is used to slow the heart rate. Can be used in patients unable to tolerate beta blockers due to hypotension. Limited experience in pediatric HF.
  - Vericiguat: Novel soluble guanylate cyclase (sGC) inhibitor which promotes the release of endogenous nitric oxide and resulting vascular smooth muscle relaxation.

- Inotropic Agents:

  - Improve end organ perfusion in patients with low cardiac output. Should only be initiated in the setting of ADHF requiring symptomatic HR unresponsive or intolerant to the initiation of oral HF therapies or as acute treatment in the setting of ADHF.
  - Acute treatment only as rescue in ADHF—long term treatment associated with increased mortality.
  - Epinephrine/Norepinephrine: alpha- and beta-adrenergic receptor agonists that have dose responsive effects to systemic circulation and can increase heart rate, stroke volume and cardiac contractility. Often used in ADHF states to rescue from cardiogenic shock.
  - Milrinone: Phosphodiesterase 3 inhibitor improves myocardial contractility and causes both systemic and pulmonary vasodilatory effects. Shown to improve low cardiac output syndrome (LCOS) in children after cardiopulmonary bypass.

    Given to improve low cardiac output and/or help with diuresis and symptoms in severe refractory HF patients.
    May be considered for home IV inotropic support if unable to transition to oral HF medications.

  - Levosimendan: Increases cardiac contractility by calcium sensitization of troponin C, reduces cardiac afterload (not currently licensed in Canada or North America).
  - Dobutamine (a beta-1 adrenergic agonist) and Dopamine (a dopaminergic agonist) are rarely used in the contemporary management of pediatric HF.

11 Anticoagulation

- Children with reduced systolic function are at increased risk of thromboembolism and intracardiac thrombus formation.
- Aspirin: First line choice in infants and children with severely reduced LV function (i.e. EF less than 20%).

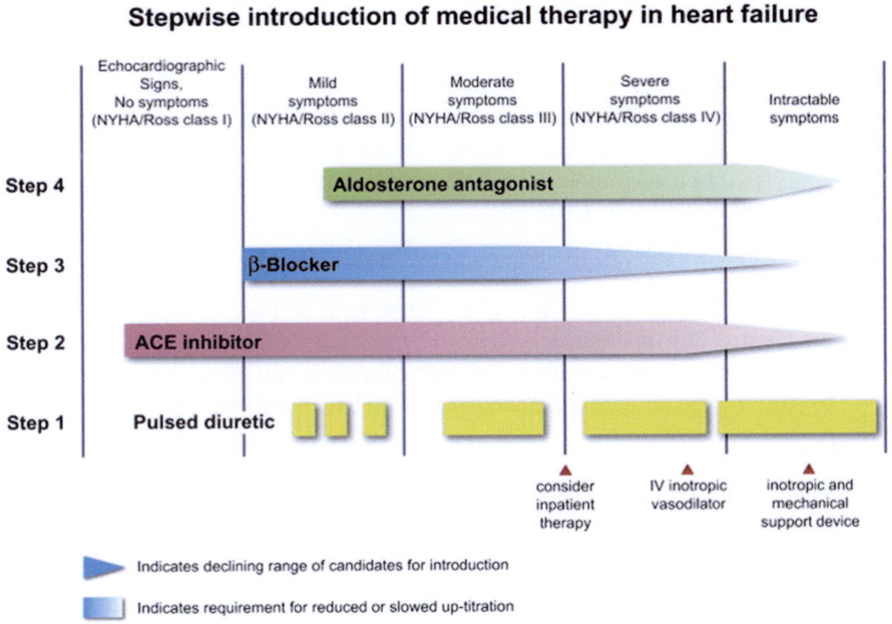

Fig. 3 A symptom-based guide to the introduction of oral maintenance therapy for children with chronic heart failure (HF). Lighter shading for each drug indicates when the possibility of a lower target dose, or slower increment than usual is needed, because of advanced HF with severely compromised systolic function. Narrowing of the bars indicates the possibility that fewer patients will tolerate the introduction of that agent at that given symptomatic stage. Note the preferred use of pulsed diuretic therapy, which becomes more frequent as symptoms advance. Red arrows indicate the point at which admission to hospital and additional support therapies might be required. ACE, angiotensin-converting enzyme; IV, intravenous; NHYA, New York Heart Association. Reprinted from Canadian Journal of Cardiology, Vol 29, Issue 12, Kantor PF, Lougheed J, Dancea A, et al., Presentation, diagnosis and medical management of heart failure in children: Canadian Cardiovascular Society Guidelines, pp 1535–1552, 2013, with permission from Elsevier

- Low molecular weight heparin (LMWH)/Warfarin: In patients with a prior history of an intracardiac thrombus, central venous catheter, or an inability to tolerate Aspirin—consideration should be given for LMWH or warfarin use.
- Direct oral anticoagulants (DOAC) have not been studied extensively in this group of patients.

12 Supportive Therapies

- Growth/Nutrition/Weight

  - Adequate growth and nutrition is necessary for management of HF but tolerance of enteral nutrition is also a prognostic feature used in response to therapy and transplant listing decision.
  - Caloric supplementation/enteral feeds (nasogastric tube, gastrostomy tube, nasojejunal tube, gastrojejunostomy feeding tube).
  - Daily weight measurement can help guide diuretic therapy and fluid management especially in the early phase of care.

- Anemia—commonly observed in pediatric HF.
  - Iron studies confirm iron deficiency. Treatment with iron supplementation in the context of iron deficiency.
  - Blood transfusion is considered if Hemoglobin < 100 g/L.
  - Erythropoietin stimulating agents may also be considered.

- Rehabilitation
  - Plays a role in the management of HF utilizing the expertise of physiotherapists, occupational therapists, and other multi-disciplinary staff.
  - Also has a prognostic role as the inability to perform activities of daily living or have an adequate exertional tolerance will reflect a need to escalate HF therapies.

13 Additional Therapy

- Cardiac Resynchronization therapy (CRT)—consider in symptomatic children who are optimized on medical HF management but with ongoing systemic LV/RV dysfunction and an EF < 35%, complete right/left bundle branch block pattern, QRS (native/paced) > upper limit of normal for age. Echocardiography may be used for the assessment of dyssynchrony and aide decision-making. (see Chap. 56).
- Implantable Cardioverter Defibrillator– Can be implanted in patients who are at risk for sudden cardiac death or life-threatening arrhythmias. No absolute EF number cut off for implantation in children. (In adults implanted for LVEF $\leq$ 35%). Can also be combine with a CRT device. (See Chap. 56).
- Ablation Therapy—Patients with tachycardia induced cardiomyopathy when medical therapy has failed.

14 Mechanical Ventilation

- Non-invasive positive pressure ventilation (NPPV) such as CPAP or BiPAP may be considered to potentially reduce afterload on the LV.

   - May help with symptom relief of pulmonary edema/increased work of breathing and from apneic episodes. Need to be cautious in the use of those with significant RV dysfunction. Should be instituted initially in the Cardiac Critical Care Unit.
- Invasive ventilation should be considered in patients with ADHF and respiratory compromise
   - Should be performed in a controlled setting by experienced ICU or Anesthesia staff due to the high risk of cardiac arrest at the time of intubation and sedation

15 Advanced Heart Failure Therapies: Mechanical Circulatory Support (MCS)

- Extracorporeal membrane oxygenation (ECMO, Chap. 57): In ADHF allows for short term cardiopulmonary circulatory support that can be rapidly instituted ideally for reversible causes of HF such as post cardiopulmonary bypass or myocarditis.
- Ventricular Assist Device (Chap. 42): Increasing over time as a bridge to transplant, recovery, or possibly as long-term decision making and destination therapy. Can be further divided into temporary or durable.
- Heart Transplant (Chap. 43).

Bibliography

1. Heidenreich PA, Bozkurt B, Aguilar D, et al. AHA/ACC/HFSA guideline for the management of heart failure: a report of the American college of cardiology/American heart association joint committee on clinical practice guidelines. Circulation. 2022;145(18):e895–1032.
2. Kantor PF, Lougheed J, Dancea A, et al. Presentation, diagnosis, and medical management of heart failure in children: canadian cardiovascular society guidelines. Can J Cardiol. 2013;29(12):1535–52.
3. Lasa JJ, Gaies M, Rossano J, et al. Acute decompensated heart failure in the pediatric population: a report from the pediatric cardiac critical care consortium (PC^4). J Heart Lung Transplant. 2018;37(4):S157–8.
4. Lipshultz SE, Sleeper LA, Towbin JA, et al. The incidence of pediatric cardiomyopathy in two regions of the United States. N Engl J Med. 2003;348(17):1647–55.
5. Loss K, Shaddy RE, Kantor PF. Recent and upcoming drug therapies for pediatric heart failure. Front Pediatr. 2021;9:681224.
6. Lytrivi ID, Blume ED, Rhodes J, et al. Prognostic value of exercise testing during heart transplant evaluation in children. Circ Heart Fail. 2013;6(4):792–9.
7. Shaddy R, Canter C, Halnon N, et al. Design for the sacubitril/valsartan (LCZ696) compared with enalapril study of pediatric patients with heart failure due to systemic left ventricle systolic dysfunction (PANORAMA-HF study). Am Heart J. 2017;193:23–34.

Ventricular Assist Devices

Andrea Maurich and Aamir Jeewa

Abstract Ventricular assist devices (VADs) have become a mainstay therapy for children with end-stage heart failure, most often as a bridge to heart transplantation. Over the past decade, a number of devices have entered the market with the ability to support small infants to adult-sized adolescents. Despite excellent outcomes, providers need to be aware of the indications for VAD support, timing of implantation, intra and post-operative management, and known complications such as neurologic injury, bleeding, and infection. Though the development of these adverse events have improved over time, they still represent the major cause for significant mortality and morbidity in children supported with a VAD. In addition, emerging concepts are the evolution from sole use as a bridge to transplant towards bridge to recovery and possibly destination therapy. The focus of this chapter will be on long-term or durable support VADs.

Keywords Ventricular assist devices · Pediatric mechanical circulatory support · Heart failure

Abbreviations

ACE	Angiotensin converting enzyme
ADL	Activity of daily living
ASA	Aspirin/acetasalicylic acid
ARNI	Angiotensin receptor-neprilysin inhibitor
ASD	Atrial septal defect

https://www.actionlearningnetwork.org/

A. Maurich · A. Jeewa (✉)
Division of Paediatric Cardiology, Department of Paediatrics, Labatt Family Heart Centre, Hospital for Sick Children, Toronto, ON, Canada
e-mail: aamir.jeewa@sickkids.ca

A. Maurich
e-mail: andrea.maurich@sickkids.ca

© The Author(s), under exclusive license to Springer Nature Switzerland AG 2024

A. I. Dipchand et al. (eds.), *Manual of Cardiac Care in Children*,
https://doi.org/10.1007/978-3-031-70973-9_42

AVV	Atrioventricular valve
BIVAD	Biventricular assist device
BSA	Body surface area
CHD	Congenital heart disease
CNS	Central nervous system
CPB	Cardiopulmonary bypass
CVP	Central venous pressure
DTI	Direct thrombin inhibitor
ECMO	Extracorporeal membrane oxygenation
EFE	Endocardial fibroelastosis
HF	Heart failure
INR	International normalized ratio
LVAD	Left ventricular assist device
MCS	Mechanical support
NT-proBNP	N-terminal prohormone of brain natriuretic peptide
NYHA	New york heart association
PI	Pulsatility index
POD	Post-operative day
PTT	Prothrombin time
QOL	Quality of life
RV	Right ventricle
RVAD	Right ventricular assist device
RVSP	Right ventricular systolic pressure
SVAD	Systemic ventricular assist device
TAH	Total artificial heart
VAD	Ventricular assist device
VSD	Ventricular septal defect

Key Points

- Ventricular Assist Devices (VADs) have evolved as an important therapeutic option in supporting cardiac function as a bridge to transplant, recovery/remission, decision and destination.
- Durable VADs are largely in the form of extracorporeal pulsatile devices (e.g., the Berlin Heart EXCOR®) wherein the pump resides outside of the body, and intracorporeal continuous flow devices (e.g., the HeartMate 3™) in which the pump is implanted within the chest. Other centres may use an extracorporeal continuous flow pump (e.g., CentriMag™) for long-term support with Berlin Heart cannulae.
- VADs can also be configured in left sided support only (LVAD) and biventricular support (BIVAD). As well, in single ventricle physiologies, VAD implant is

often referred to as systemic VAD (SVAD). The incidence of BIVAD support has dramatically decreased over the years with increased centre volume experience.
- Over the last decade there has been a reduction in the known major associated complications. Almost 60% of implants are for children with cardiomyopathy. A positive outcome (transplant, recovery, or still on device) is seen in 84% of children at 6 months post implant.
- VAD support has the ability to improve quality of life (QOL) through assisting in restoring end-organ function, allowing patients to meet nutritional and physical rehabilitation goals, maximize growth and development, and in the setting of intracorporeal VADs allow for eventual discharge from hospital.
- Demonstration of improved waitlist/post-transplant survival and rehabilitation are significant outcomes for children supported with VADs.

1 Indications for VAD Candidacy

- End-stage heart failure (HF) refractory to medical management
  - Only long-term durable option for managing a failing circulation.
  - Timely implantation of a VAD can lead to better outcomes through reversal of end-organ dysfunction which is known to be associated with poor outcomes following transplantation.
  - Intermacs profiles (see Table 1) were generated to further discern the level of illness.
  - Implantation with a Intermacs Level 1 is associated with lower overall survival than at a Level 2 or Level 3.
- Inadequate cardiac output and/or congestion
  - Consider VAD implant when there is a dependency on inotropes with the inability to wean successfully or clinical concern of further deterioration.
  - Appropriate timing of implant can lead to reversal of end-organ dysfunction and more favourable outcomes.
  - End-organ dysfunction that typically prompts VAD consideration may include but are not limited to:

    Respiratory failure/decompensation
    Liver dysfunction
    Kidney injury
    Feeding intolerance leading to poor weight gain or weight loss
    Increasing central nervous system (CNS) symptoms (somnolence or irritability)
- Inability to separate from other temporary mechanical circulatory support (MCS)/ECMO or cardiopulmonary bypass (CPB)

Table 1 Intermacs profiles

Profile	Title	Description
1	Critical cardiogenic shock	Life-threatening hypotension refractory to IV inotropes "Crash and burn"
2	Progressive decline	IV inotropes required with worsening end-organ function "Sliding on inotropes"
3	Inotrope dependent	Stable blood pressure and end-organ function but failure to wean from IV inotropes "Dependent stability"
4	Resting symptoms	Daily symptoms of congestion at rest or with ADLs. High doses of diuretics
5	Exertion intolerant	Unable to engage in any activity above ADLs
6	Exertion limited	Can participate in minor activities but quickly fatigues "Walking wounded"
7	Advanced NYHA III	Comfortable with meaningful activity, limited to mild exertion

Three modifiers: TCS temporary circulatory support, A arrhythmia, FF frequent flyer
Adapted from Stevenson et al. (2009)

2 Contraindications to VAD Insertion

- Mismatch in size and device availability may be limiting for some patients
- Irreversible end-organ dysfunction
- Extreme prematurity/weight < 3 kg
- Severe neurologic injury
- Active malignancy
- Congenital anomalies with poor prognosis
- Severe genetic/chromosomal abnormalities
- Anatomical/circulatory condition incompatible with mechanical assistance
- Multisystem organ failure
- Inability to be anticoagulated
- Active systemic infection (especially fungal infection)

3 Left Ventricular Assist Device versus Biventricular Ventricular Assist Device

- The majority of VAD implants can be managed with an LVAD alone.
- The need for an RVAD should be based on the inability to separate from CPB following LVAD implantation, despite strategies for right heart optimization such as inotropes, pacing, and inhaled nitric oxide.

- In the post-operative VAD patient, the right ventricular function is often not normal by echocardiogram but has the sole role of providing enough preload to the LVAD to adequately fill the pump and support cardiac output, all at a reasonable central venous pressure (CVP). The appropriate CVP may vary between patients but should ideally be less than the pre-implant state.
- Right heart failure that develops post-operatively as evidenced by renal or hepatic failure may also warrant RVAD implant.
  - Consideration should be given to those with an underlying myopathy of the right ventricle (RV), such as arrhythmogenic cardiomyopathy or in children with congenital heart disease (CHD).
  - Other indications may include those with restrictive physiology such as restrictive cardiomyopathy that may have elevation in their pulmonary vascular resistance.
- In some instances, there may be need for a Total Artificial Heart (TAH).
  - Failing post heart transplant graft, often due to cardiac allograft vasculopathy, where ongoing immunosuppression can be stopped.
  - Failing Fontan circulation to substantially decrease CVP, and improve Fontan complications, such as protein losing enteropathy, but also allow for a potential discharge from hospital.
  - A major limitation of this support is size as the smallest size of pumps are most suitable for a small adult (~BSA > 1.2 m^2).
- Single ventricle physiology and end-stage HF secondary to ventricular dysfunction may require SVAD support as a bridge to transplantation.
  - Approximately 15% of VAD implants are SVADs with a positive outcome in 67% at 6 months.

4 Therapeutic Goals for VAD Implantation

- Bridge to Transplant
  - Most common indication for long-term VAD support.
  - Lowers risk of death on waitlist.
- Bridge to Eligibility/Decision
  - Unsure of long-term goals.
  - More common in children with malignancies.
- Bridge to Recovery/Remission
  - Temporary support while the heart regains function.
  - Ability to explant device.

Table 2 Ventricular Assist Devices currently used at SickKids

Device	Manufacturer	Type of support
Durable long-term support devices		
Berlin Heart EXCOR® Pediatric	Berlin Heart GmbH	Pulsatile
HeartMate 3™ Left Ventricular Assist System	Abbott	Centrifugal
Total Artificial Heart (TAH-t)	SynCardia	Pulsatile
Temporary support devices		
CentriMag™ and PediMag™	Abbott	Centrifugal
Rotaflow	Getinge	Centrifugal
Impella®	Abiomed	Axial Flow

Note: Centrifugal and axial flow VADs both represent types of continuous flow pumps but with different hydrodynamic properties

- Destination
  - VAD implanted indefinitely to support quantity and QOL. This mode of support is only appropriate for intracorporeal VADs that allow for discharge from hospital.
  - Uncommon in children but possible.

  Table 2 outlines the types of VADs currently used at SickKids.

5 Pre-implantation Assessment

- Clinical history and physical examination:
  - Assessment for severity of HF and end-organ function
  - Baseline neurologic evaluation
  - Assessment for active systemic infection
- Pre-implantation bloodwork:
  - Chemistry and Microbiology

    Comprehensive metabolic panel
    C-reactive protein
    NT pro-BNP
    Infectious screening if clinically indicated
    Additional testing required for specific patient concerns

  - Hematology

    Type and screen
    CBC and differential

PTT/INR
LDH
Fibrinogen
Anti-Xa (if on Heparin/LMWH)
Plasma-free hemoglobin
D-dimer

- Ancillary studies:
  - ECG and echocardiogram
  - Consider head CT if concerns with or unable to obtain reliable neurological exam
- Consultation of additional services:
  - Palliative care service
  - Pre-implant Neurology, Hematology and Thrombosis team consults
  - Services based upon clinical indication (e.g., Infectious Diseases)
  - Cardiac Radiology (in regard to virtual fit testing and cross-sectional imaging)

6 Intra and Peri-Operative Considerations

- Transesophageal echocardiogram and/or epicardial echocardiogram to assess the site of the apical (or less commonly atrial) cannula position prior to implantation. Epicardial studies are done especially in the setting of complex CHD. Imaging will also delineate the atrioventricular valve (AVV) function and mechanism of valve regurgitation.
- It is important to identify and close sources of shunt at the atrial and ventricular level (e.g., ASDs and VSDs). Residual shunts can potentially lead to sources of right to left shunt once on VAD support.
- Intra-operative repair or annuloplasty of AVV may need needed especially if there is significant regurgitation once off CPB.
- Right heart failure in the intra-operative setting is most often defined by the inability to wean from CPB and manifest with poor or suboptimal LVAD filling/performance. Strategies to optimize RV function include:
  - Inotropes such as moderate to high dose epinephrine
  - Pacing the RV with temporary pacing wires
  - Volume replacement
  - Inhaled nitric oxide
  - Early extubation (if reasonable hemodynamics)
- However, with poor hemodynamics and despite the above maneuvers, consideration for RVAD placement (BIVAD) may be necessitated. This can be in the form of temporary MCS or with durable VAD support. Prior to placing an RVAD, further

imaging of the LVAD cannula is warranted to ensure there are no mechanical sources for obstruction.

7 Berlin Heart EXCOR® (Fig. 1)

- The Berlin Heart EXCOR® is a pneumatically driven pulsatile paracorporeal pump that can be used to support the RV or LV for univentricular support or both ventricles for BIVAD support.
- LVAD configuration: inflow cannula from the LV apex to the pump and outflow cannula from the pump to the aorta.
- BIVAD configuration: addition of right atrium to pulmonary artery cannulae set up.
- Although not commonly done, it is possible to create a left atrium to aorta configuration.
- There are a number of pump sizes available for the Berlin Heart EXCOR® (10–60 cc).
- Alternating positive and negative driving pressures provided by the driving unit called the IKUS or Active moves the membrane within the blood pump(s) to fill and empty the pump(s).
- Used to support patients 3.5-20 kg (BSA > $0.6m^2$).
- Table 3 summarizes the Berlin Heart EXCOR® unique clinical events.

7.1 Parameters

- Systole
  - Positive pressure set to eject blood from the pump (pump emptying)
  - Pump ejection should always be 100%

    Incomplete pump emptying increases risk of thrombus formation
    Incomplete pump emptying may be caused by increased systemic vascular resistance, outflow cannula obstruction or tamponade
- Diastole
  - Negative pressure set to fill the blood pump
  - Complete pump filling defined as 75–100%

    Incomplete pump filling may be caused by issues affecting preload, cannula obstruction, tamponade, or effusion

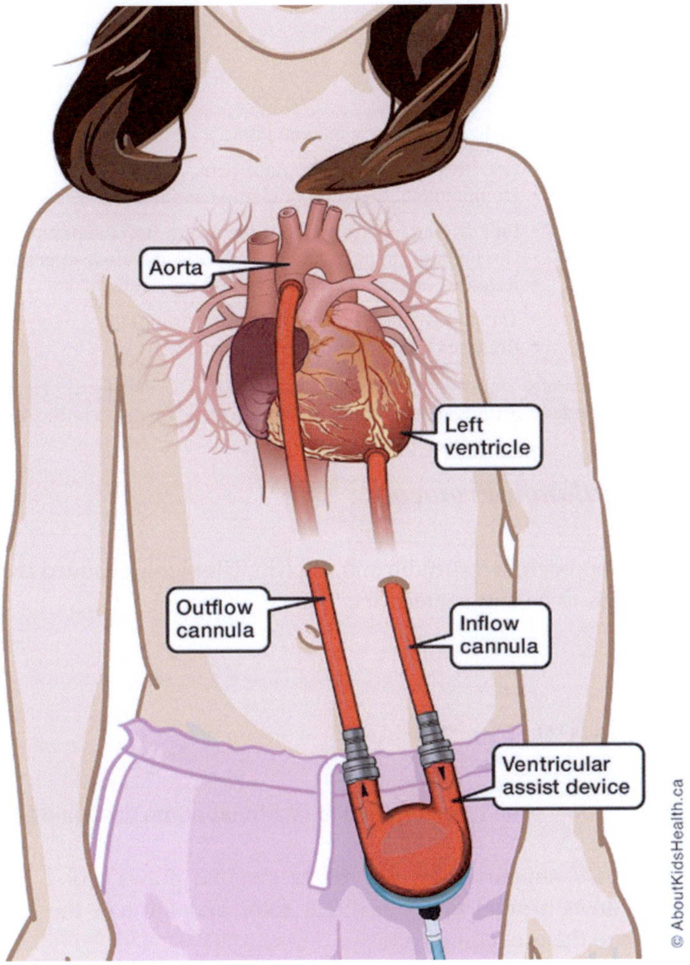

Fig. 1 Berlin heart EXCOR®

- Rate (beats per minute)
  - Blood pump(s) deliver a fixed stroke volume
  - Adjustment of rate contributes to achieving sufficient blood flow and cardiac index
- % Systole
  - Relative systolic duration
  - Amount of time the blood pump(s) spend in systole

    May be increased to improve systole
    May be decreased to improve diastole

Table 3 Unique clinical events

Berlin heart EXCOR®: unique clinical events	
Problem	Actions to take
IKUS/Active failure	• Utilize emergency manual pump
Membrane defect	• Requires urgent pump replacement • Do not manually pump or clamp cannulae
Cannula disruption	• Pull driving tube from IKUS/Active to stop the pump • Clamp both cannula above disruption and close to patient • Requires emergent cannulae/pump replacement
Cracked driving tube	• Temporarily cover crack with waterproof tape • Requires urgent driving tube exchange

Advanced Cardiac Therapies Improving Outcomes Network (ACTION) Berlin Heart emergency algorithms and care guide https://myactioneducation.org/emergencycare-berlinheart/

7.2 Anticoagulation Protocol

- Institutional approach: Bivalirudin and Aspirin; Clopidogrel added if antiplatelet inhibition needs to be augmented. See Table 4.

8 HeartMate 3™ (Fig. 2)

- The HeartMate 3™ is an intracorporeal centrifugal pump designed to offload the LV.
- Designed for LV support only, the inflow cannula draws blood from the LV apex which flows around the centrifugal rotor and through the outflow graft anastomosed to the ascending aorta.
- The pump contains a magnetically levitated rotor that is not dependant on hydrodynamic or mechanical bearings.
- A pump cable is tunnelled through the abdomen and connects to a system controller which monitors pump performance and supplies power to the pump.
- Used in patients > 20 kg (BSA > 1.0m^2).

8.1 Parameters

- Flow (litres per minute, lpm)
  - Estimated based on power
  - Directly related to pressure across the pump
  - Difference between aortic and LV pressures

Table 4 Anticoagulation dosing guidelines

BIVALIRUDIN	
• Bivalirudin is a direct thrombin inhibitor (DTI) with a half-life of approx. 25 min in patients with normal renal function • It has an on-set of 2 min and does not require antithrombin III (ATIII) for activity • There is no reversal agent for Bivalirudin	
Timing • POD 1 – 12–24 h post implant – Chest tube output < 2 ml/kg/h for 4 h – No other sources of active bleeding	
Initial Dosing	
Goal: aPTT *Standard risk (of bleeding)*: aPTT 60–90 (~2–3 × baseline), INR < 1.3, Fibrinogen > 10, Platelet count > 100 *High risk (of bleeding):* aPTT 50–60 (~1.5–2 × baseline)	
Renal function	**Initial dosing**
Normal (>60 ml/min/1.73 m2)	0.3 mg/kg/hr IV infusion
Mild-moderate (30–60 ml/min/1.73 m2)	0.2 mg/kg/hr IV infusion
Severe (<30 ml/min/1.73 m2)	0.1 mg/kg/hr IV infusion
Maintenance Bivalirudin Titration *Initial aPTT target 60–80 unless determined otherwise by VAD Team	
Goal: aPTT *Standard risk (of bleeding):* aPTT 60–90 (~2–3 × baseline) *High risk (of bleeding):* aPTT 50–60 (~1.5–2 × baseline)	
If aPTT 5–15 s out of range: • Increase or decrease by 10% (round up to closest 2nd decimal) • Recheck 4 h after dose change	
If aPTT in target range, no change: • Recheck in 4 h, then can decrease frequency when stable	
If aPTT ≥ 15–30 s out of range: • Increase or decrease by 25% (round up to closest 2nd decimal) • Recheck 4 h after dose change	
If aPTT > 3 × baseline or ~ 120 s: • With normal renal function: hold 15 min and reduce by 30% • With mild to moderate renal dysfunction: hold for 45 min and reduce by 40% • With severe renal dysfunction: hold 2 h and recheck PTT before restarting	
ASPIRIN or ASA (Acetylsalicylic Acid)	
• ASA induces platelet inhibitory effect via COX-1 inhibition • The effect of ASA is irreversible for life of platelets exposed (7–10 days) and even shorter with inflammation or exposure to extracorporeal circuits	
Timing • POD 3–4 – Chest tubes and pacing wires out preferably – May need GI prophylaxis	

(continued)

Table 4 (continued)

Dosing • Initial starting dose: 4–5 mg/kg/day • Consider BID dosing if: – Significant thrombocytosis – Significant fibrin burden
CLOPIDOGREL (Plavix)
• Clopidogrel prevents platelet activation and aggregation • Half-life of the parent drug 6 h and half-life of active metabolite 30 min
Timing • Consideration in children if: – High risk for thromboembolic event (<5 kg patient, CHD, atrial cannulation, significant fibrin burden) – To be determined by the VAD team
Dosing • Initial starting dose: 0.1 mg/kg/day
WARFARIN (Coumadin)
• Warfarin is a vitamin K antagonist which acts to inhibit the production of vitamin K • The active half-life of warfarin is 20–60 h
Timing • POD 3–5 – Chest tubes and pacing wires must be out
Dosing • Initial starting dose: As per institutional formulary recommendations for Warfarin initiation
Target • INR 2–3

Adapted from the Advanced Cardiac Therapies Improving Outcomes Network (ACTION) direct thrombin inhibitor (DTI) harmonization protocol for VADs (2020). https://myactioneducation.org/wp-content/uploads/2023/12/ACTION-DTI-Harmonization-Protocol-12_19_23.docx

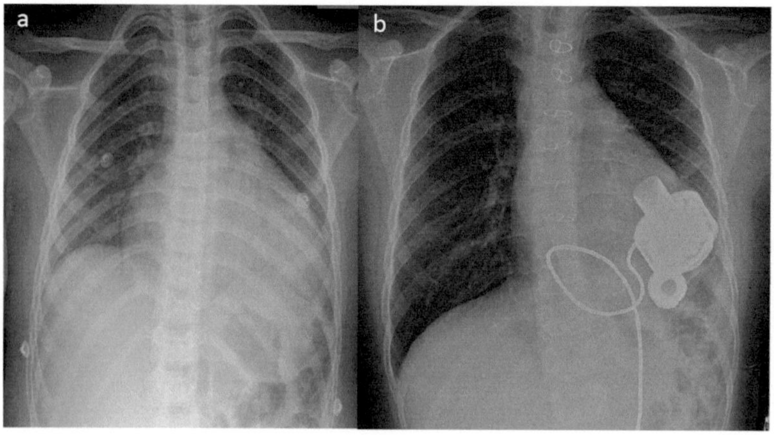

Fig. 2 HeartMate 3™: A) Chest x-ray pre HeartMate 3™ implant, B) Chest x-ray 3 months post HeartMate 3™ implant

Outflow aortic pressure minus inflow LV pressure
Fluctuates throughout the cardiac cycle

- Inversely related to resistance

  ↑Pressure gradient → ↓Flow
  ↓Pressure gradient → ↑Flow

- Power (watts, w)
  - Direct measurement of pump motor voltage required to rotate the rotor and generate blood flow, with an ideal target between 3–6 w
  - Pump power affected by

    Speed
    Flow
    Physiological demand

    ↑Speed → ↑Power
    ↑Flow → ↑Power

  - Notable increase in power

    Aortic insufficiency
    Pump thrombus

  - Notable reduction in power

    Obstruction of flow

- Speed (revolutions per minute, rpm)
  - Only parameter that can be adjusted
  - Clinical speed range: 4800–6200 rpm (changes made in 100 rpm increments)
- Pulsatility Index (PI)
  - Calculation based on power

    PI = Power Max.—Power Min./Power Avg.
    Measured over 15 second intervals
    Values range from 1 to > 10 with an ideal target between 2 and 6

  - Magnitude of PI is related to the amount of contractility provided by the native heart as well as the preload entering the LVAD

    Higher values indicate more ventricular filling and higher pulsatility (less support provided by the pump)
    Lower values indicate less ventricular filling and lower pulsatility (more support provided by pump for ventricular unloading)

- PI Event

    Triggered when power consumption differs by > 45% over 15 seconds
    Pump speed decreases to set low speed limit, then gradually increases to the set fixed speed
    No audible alarm
    May be caused by acute changes in preload or afterload

        Suction event, arrhythmias, coughing, sneezing, and blood pressure

8.2 Anticoagulation Protocol (Table 4)

- Recommendations based on industry guidelines and instructions for use (IFU); historically Heparin as a bridge to Warfarin and ASA.
- ACTION DTI Protocol has become favourable with increasing experience and comfort with Bivalirudin as a bridge. Close monitoring of PTT and INR needed during transition from Bivalirudin to Warfarin.

9 Assessment for Recovery

- Recovery or remission from HF has been seen in children on VAD support.
- Factors that influence the potential for recovery include severity and etiology of HF (CHD or biventricular HF), presence of a pathogenic mutation, EFE seen on pathology, evidence or presentation consistent with myocarditis, and age at presentation.
- The recovery pathway for pediatric patients on VAD support includes:
  - Optimization of guideline directed medical therapy (ACEi/ARNI, beta blocker, and Spironolactone).
  - Improvement in rehabilitation state, chest radiograph, end-organ function, nutrition, and NTpro-BNP or BNP.
  - Significant improvement of ventricular function on echocardiogram at baseline (e.g., EF > 45%).
  - Completion of a wean echocardiogram: reduction of either RPM (HeartMate 3) or rate (Berlin Heart) during echocardiogram with detailed assessment of ventricular function, AVV regurgitation, RVSP, and semi-lunar valve function.
  - If the above is reassuring at reduced support, then proceed with elective cardiac catheterization for hemodynamic assessment, mixed venous, ABG, and lactate at baseline and at reduced support.

- Once available data is obtained and hemodynamics are consistent with myocardial recovery, consideration for VAD explantation can be made. This is a shared decision as the risk is unclear as to the potential relapse of HF after device removal.

10 Adverse Events

- Neurologic injury in the form of ischemic and hemorrhagic stroke:
  - Original incidence of stroke was almost 30% and a significant contributor to the mortality. Majority of these were thromboembolic in nature.
  - Switch to Bivalirudin has led to a decrease in the stroke rate to 12%.
- Bleeding complications (post surgical):
  - Most common in the first 2 weeks after implant.
  - Most common type is epistaxis.
- Infection of the driveline and cannulae sites.
- Gastrointestinal bleeding:
  - Reported more in the adult experience.
  - Thought to be secondary to hemolysis and an acquired von Willebrand deficiency.
  - Rare occurrence in children.
- Less common: arrhythmias, late right heart failure, and device malfunction.

Bibliography

1. Adachi I, Peng DM, Hollander SA, et al. Sixth annual pediatric interagency registry for mechanical circulatory support (pedimacs) report: the society of thoracic surgeons pedimacs annual report. Ann Thorac Surg. 2022;115(5):1098–108.
2. Advanced Cardiac Therapies Improving Outcomes Network (ACTION). Direct thrombin inhibitor (DTI) harmonization protocol for VADs; 2020. https://myactioneducation.org/wp-content/uploads/2023/12/ACTION-DTI-Harmonization-Protocol-12_19_23.docx. Accessed 08 Jul 2024.
3. Advanced Cardiac Therapies Improving Outcomes Network (ACTION) Berlin Heart Emergency Algorithms & Care Guide. https://myactioneducation.org/emergencycare-berlinheart/. Accessed 08 Jul 2024
4. Berlin Heart GmbH. EXCOR® VAD ventricular assist device: Ikus stationary driving unit instructions for use. Berlin, Germany: Berlin Heart;. 2018. https://www.fda.gov/media/102611/download. Accessed 28 Jun 2023
5. Dipchand AI, Kirk R, Naftel DC, et al. Ventricular assist device support as a bridge to transplantation in pediatric patients. J Am Coll Cardiol. 2018;72(4):402–15.

6. Jeewa A, Price JF, Adachi I. Mechanical circulatory support in children. In: Shaddy RE, editor. Moss & Adams' heart disease in infants, children and adolescents including the fetus and young adult. Lippincott Williams & Wilkins; 2021. p. 678–88.
7. Joong A, Gossett JG, Blume ED, et al. Variability in clinical decision-making for ventricular assist device implantation in pediatrics. Pediatr Transplant. 2020;24(8):e13840.
8. Lorts A, Conway J, Schweiger M, et al. ISHLT consensus statement for the selection and management of pediatric and congenital heart disease patients on ventricular assist devices endorsed by the American Heart Association. J Heart Lung Transplant. 2021;40(8):709–32.
9. Rossano JW, VanderPluym CJ, Peng DM, et al. Fifth annual pediatric interagency registry for mechanical circulatory support (Pedimacs) report. Ann Thorac Surg. 2021;112(6):1763–74.
10. Thoratec Corporation. HeartMate 3 left ventricular assist system: instructions for use. Thoratec Corporation. Available via DIALOG. 2017. https://www.accessdata.fda.gov/cdrh_docs/pdf16/P160054C.pdf. Accessed 28 Jun 2023.

Heart Transplantation

Kathryn R. Armstrong and Anne I. Dipchand

Abstract Pediatric heart transplantation is the treatment of choice for children with end-stage heart disease. For patients who are carefully selected through the transplant evaluation process, transplantation offers an improved survival and quality of life. This chapter reviews the indications for transplantation, transplant candidacy and the pre transplant evaluation process including the investigations and evaluations involved. The unique concept of ABO incompatible transplant in the pediatric population is introduced. The process for transplant listing, waitlist mortality along with strategies to optimize medical and psychosocial needs as patients wait are discussed. As part of the surgical strategy, donor considerations are reviewed along with induction immunosuppression alongside intensive care support. Finally post-transplant surveillance and monitoring for rejection and cardiac allograft vasculopathy along with screening for common co morbidities such as renal insufficiency, infection and post-transplant lymphoproliferative disease are reviewed. Long term outcomes for transplant are put forward.

Keywords Heart transplantation · Waiting list · Immunosuppression · Survival · Children · Pediatric

Abbreviations

ABO-i	ABO-incompatible
ACEi	Angiotensin converting enzyme inhibitor
ACR	Acute cellular rejection
AMR	Antibody-mediated rejection

K. R. Armstrong
British Columbia Children's Hospital, Vancouver, BC, Canada
e-mail: kathryn.armstrong@cw.bc.ca

A. I. Dipchand (✉)
Division of Paediatric Cardiology, Department of Paediatrics, Labatt Family Heart Centre, Hospital for Sick Children, Toronto, ON, Canada
e-mail: anne.dipchand@sickkids.ca

© The Author(s), under exclusive license to Springer Nature Switzerland AG 2024

A. I. Dipchand et al. (eds.), *Manual of Cardiac Care in Children*,
https://doi.org/10.1007/978-3-031-70973-9_43

CAV	Cardiac allograft vasculopathy
CHD	Congenital heart disease
CKD	Chronic kidney disease
CM	Cardiomyopathy
CMV	Cytomegalovirus
CNI	Calcineurin inhibitor
CPR	Cardiopulmonary resuscitation
CVP	Central venous pressure
DCD	Donation after cardiac death
DSA	Donor specific antibody
EBV	Ebstein Barr virus
ECMO	Extracorporeal membrane oxygenation
HLA	Human leukocyte antigen
HTx	Heart transplant
ISHLT	International society of heart and lung transplantation
IS	Immunosuppression
IVC	Inferior vena cava
MCS	Mechanical support
MMF	Mycophenolate mofetil
MPA	Mycophenolic acid
mTORi	Mammalian target of rapamycin inhibitors
NSAIDs	Non-steroidal anti-inflammatory drugs
PCR	Polymerase chain reaction
PTLD	Post-transplant lymphoproliferative disorder
PVR	Pulmonary vascular resistance
RV	Right ventricle
TDM	Therapeutic drug monitoring
VAD	Ventricular assist device
VO2	Oxygen consumption

Key Points

- Heart transplantation (HTx) is the standard of care for children with end-stage heart disease refractory to medical and surgical interventions; though not a cure, it is expected to provide children with an improved quality of life and survival.
- Patient selection for listing is one of the most important factors influencing post-transplant outcomes; the decision is made following a comprehensive evaluation and multidisciplinary committee review.
- Significant complications include rejection, infection, malignancy, renal dysfunction and cardiac allograft vasculopathy.
- Survival post pediatric HTx continues to improve.

1 Epidemiology

- Numbers of HTx procedures are limited by donor organ availability and need continues to exceed supply.
- Waitlist mortality ranges from 5–25% and is highest in the infant age range.
- Waiting time varies predominantly by age and size and is impacted by recipient medical acuity (ability to wait).
- In infants, congenital heart disease (CHD) followed by cardiomyopathy (CM) are the commonest reasons for transplant; in adolescents CM remains the leading cause.
- Transplant assessment should be considered when life expectancy of the patient with HTx is greater compared to their current situation.
- ABO incompatible (ABO-i) HTx has led to a significant decrease in waiting time in eligible patients.

2 Transplant Candidacy

2.1 Indications

- Endstage myocardial failure despite maximal medical therapy.
- Complex CHD with no options for surgical palliation at an acceptable risk.
- Malignant arrhythmias refractory to medical or device management.
- Unresectable cardiac tumours causing obstruction or ventricular dysfunction (systolic or diastolic) or refractory arrhythmias.
- Progressive cyanosis in the presence of complex CHD that is not amenable to surgical repair or palliation or for which surgery is associated with unacceptable mortality.
- Excessive disability, unacceptably poor quality of life, or long-term morbidity in the setting of failing myocardial function, complex CHD, or after failed surgical palliation.
- Advanced functional class and/or heart failure stage (Class III, IV or Stage D).
- Low or deteriorating peak VO2 predicted for diagnosis, age, sex, and body size.
- Progressive pulmonary hypertension that could preclude HTx at a later date.

2.2 Contraindications

- Institutional practice: MCS with ECMO or temporary VAD and identified risk factors that preclude reasonable survival to hospital discharge including but not exclusive to: (1) complex CHD at any stage of palliation, (2) moderate to severe renal insufficiency, (3) age < 1 year, (4) instability on mechanical support, (5) fungal infection, (6) ventilator dependency for oxygenation and/or requiring high pressures. (Some centers continue to offer HTx in these high risk settings.)

- Anatomic: pulmonary vein atresia or progressive stenosis, severe hypoplasia of the branch pulmonary arteries, severe hypoplasia of the thoracic aorta. (consideration may be given to heart–lung transplantation).
- High HLA sensitization in the setting of other cumulative risk factors.
- Pulmonary hypertension: relative contraindication based on patient age, underlying disease/heart defect and response to aggressive testing in cardiac catheterization laboratory for evidence of reactivity if warranted.
- Progressive or refractory multisystem organ failure.
- Progressive systemic disease with early mortality (e.g., genetic/metabolic, idiopathic, mitochondrial, syndromic).
- Inability to undergo post-transplant rehabilitation in severely debilitated patients.
- Morbid obesity.
- Diabetes mellitus with evidence of end-organ damage.
- Severe chromosomal, neurologic, neuromuscular or syndromic abnormalities.
- Active infection: patients should be assessed on an individual basis, especially if it is being appropriately treated with good clinical response.
- Malignancy: Patients in remission should be assessed on an individual basis based on the prognosis of individual malignancy.
- Psychosocial and/or social circumstances that jeopardize post-HTx care and survival in the opinion of the interdisciplinary team following appropriate assessment and intervention.

3 Transplant Assessment (Table 1)

- Allows the multidisciplinary team and family to gain the knowledge needed to make an informed decision about moving forward with HTx listing.
- Consideration should be given to potential medical, interventional and/or surgical procedures that may mitigate the need for HTx and/or optimize a patient to wait for HTx.
- At the end of the assessment, listing and transplant considerations should be reviewed and summarized by the multidisciplinary team including recipient considerations, donor considerations, estimated outcomes, and resuscitation status. (Box 1)

Box 1: Transplant Assessment Summary and Considerations

Patient Considerations

Anticoagulation reversal: ***

Bleeding Risk: ***

Table 1 Heart Transplant Assessment Investigations

Category of assessment	Specific testing or consult
Cardiac investigations	CXR/echocardiogram/ECG/holter/exercise test or 6 min walk
	Cardiac catheterization (PVR, collaterals, residual lesions, etc.)
	Cardiac CT/MRI
Laboratory	Renal/Liver function/Lipid profile/CBC/Coagulation/Blood group/ Immunoglobulins
	Immunology Human leukocyte antigen (HLA) to determine recipient/donor compatibility Isohemagglutinins (to determine eligibility for ABO-I HTx)
	Virology/serology EBV/CMV/Hepatitis ABC/Varicella, Toxoplasma
Abdominal ultrasound (renal/liver)	
Pulmonary function tests	
Vascular ultrasound (upper and lower vascular patency)	
Glomerular filtration rate (GFR)	
Bone mineral density (BMD)	
CT brain/cranial USS (if mechanical circulatory support being considered)	
Consulting services	**Mandatory** Cardiac anesthesia Cardiothoracic surgery Palliative care Social work Physiotherapy Occupational therapy Dietician Transplant nursing **As needed** Electrophysiology Nephrology Hepatology Child life specialist Adolescent medicine Speech and language pathology Neuropsychology Pharmacy/clinical pharmacology Other (as necessary)

ABO-incompatible candidate: ***
HLA sensitization: ***
Anatomic considerations: ***
PVRi: ***
Sternal re-entry risk: ***

Vascular access: ***
Concurrent Surgery: ***
Pacemaker/ICD/VAD removal: ***
Samples/specimens at the time of transplant: ***
Renal considerations: ***
Liver considerations: ***
Pharmacogenetic considerations: ***
Nutritional issues: ***
Psychosocial issues: ***
Immunizations: ***
Other: ***

Donor Considerations
Distance: ***
Specific Harvest Needs: ***
Donor Weight Range: ***—***
Upper Age Limit: ***

Estimated Outcomes
Waitlist mortality: ***%
Surgical Mortality: ***%
Perioperative Transplant Mortality: ***%
1 year post-transplant survival: ***%
10 years post-transplant survival: ***%

Code Status
Cpr: ***
Vad: ***
Ecmo: ***

Listing Information
Status: ***
ABO-incompatible: Y/N
Tx across a positive crossmatch: Y/N

4 Listing for Transplantation

- Patient can be listed for HTx only if it has been deemed to be in the patient's best interest, and both the physicians and parents/patient agree to proceed
- HTx listing systems vary by country; patients are listed by criteria based on disease severity (Status 1–4) with those listed as Status 4 in Canada being the sickest.

5 Waitlist Mortality

- Waitlist mortality remains higher than for any other solid organ transplant.
- Extracorporeal membrane oxygenation (ECMO) support, ventilator support, CHD, dialysis support, non-white race and higher medical acuity status are associated with increased wait list mortality.

6 Pre-transplant Management Principles

- Optimize medical, surgical, nutritional and psychosocial needs
- Ventricular assist devices (VAD) have improved survival to HTx although options for those < 10 kg remain limited (see Chap. 42).
- Optimize immunizations on an accelerated schedule (consult local public health guidelines for the most up-to-date immunization schedule)
- Monitor anti-A and or anti-B isohemagglutinin titres monthly for those who are listed for ABO-i HTx (Table 2)
- Monitor Anti HLA antibodies every 3 months or following a sensitizing event
- Desensitization (interventions for any pre-formed antibodies) is not routine institutional practice (remains controversial, treatment modalities have been used to reduce the amounts of circulating anti-HLA antibodies with varying degrees of success).

7 The Heart Transplant Operation

7.1 Donor Considerations

- Characteristics of both donor and recipient are important when accepting a donor heart.
- Acceptable donor size, distance, blood type, and thresholds for donor-specific antibodies are determined at time of listing (see Box 1)
- Donor risk factors may include age, mechanism of death, heart function, vasoactive medications, infectious concerns, amongst others.
- Ischemic time (travel time, complexity of surgery) and older age of donor may have an impact on outcome in older heart recipients.
- Paediatric experience is increasing with donor organs retrieved using ex vivo perfusion or in the setting of donation after cardiac death (DCD).

Table 2 Blood product guidelines for ABO-incompatible heart transplantation

Patient's group	Donor's group	SAGM red cells	FP/FFP	Cryo	Platelets
O	A	O	A	A AB B O	A or AB B or O concentrated
O	B	O	B	B AB A O	B or AB A or O concentrated
O	AB	O	AB	AB A B O	AB A or B concentrated O concentrated
A	B	A	AB	AB B A O	AB B concentrated A or O concentrated
A	AB	A	AB	AB A B O	AB A or B concentrated O concentrated
B	A	B	AB	AB A B O	AB B or O concentrated
B	AB	B	AB	AB A B O	AB A or B or O concentrated

Note Group AB cryoprecipitate is very rarely available. Cryoprecipitate is a small volume product and group O is acceptable

8 Surgical Strategy

- Reviewed and planned for prior to HTx at the time of assessment including re-entry risk, cannulation strategy, need for additional reconstruction, and/or VAD/pacemaker explant.
- Minimize the total ischemic time (starts at the time of crossclamp in the donor), but more specifically the warm ischemic time (starts when the donor organ is removed from ice).
- May need to harvest pulmonary arteries, aorta, IVC at time of donor heart retrieval, particularly for recipients with CHD with complex surgical considerations.
- Two surgical approaches: bicaval (preferred) and, less commonly, biatrial anastomosis

- Bicaval anastomosis has been reported to be associated with better hemodynamics, less TR and less arrhythmias than the biatrial approach

9 Induction Immunosuppression

- Immunosuppression (IS) administered in the peri-operative period.
- Peri-operative steroids (10–15 mg/kg) administered in the OR on induction of anaesthesia and just prior to cross clamp removal.
- Institutional practice is anti-thymocyte globulin for 2–5 days (1.5 mg/kg/dose); duration based on immunologic risk and clinical status post-operatively.
- Consider antibody removal strategies (e.g. plasma exchange on pump) if (1) ABO-i HTx, or (2) highly sensitized with positive virtual crossmatch or until crossmatch results available.

10 Intensive Care Management

- First 72 h: IS is initiated, the ischemic heart has been reperfused, the new heart is exposed to varying levels of pulmonary vascular resistance
- Post operative management strategies include:
  - Isoproterenol and/or pacing may be required to optimize heart rate due to denervation of the transplanted heart and reduce risk of sudden bradycardic events
  - Optimizing preload to the ischemic and dilated RV by limiting the circulating volume and CVP – may require aggressive diuresis or early renal replacement therapy if transient acute kidney injury
  - Early extubation (ideally in OR) if hemodynamically stable and good hemostasis to reduce RV afterload and need for sedation
  - Reducing RV afterload and pulmonary vascular resistance
  - Providing early mechanical assistance to facilitate recovery of transplanted heart
  - Systemic vasopressors may be required for poorly controlled heart failure or for those with CHD, particularly for those with failing Fontan.

11 Post-transplant Care and Surveillance

- Care is marked by routine surveillance testing with meticulous attention to detail for the development of morbidities and aggressive prophylactic, pre-emptive, or treatment strategies.
- Centre approach summarized in Table 3.

12 Immunosuppression (IS)

- Individualized maintenance IS to prevent rejection but to minimize morbidities (balance remains challenging)
- Mainstay of IS consists of a calcineurin inhibitor (CNI) (tacrolimus) and an adjunctive anti-metabolite agent (mycophenolate mofetil, MMF) though CNI monotherapy is achieved in 30–40% institutionally
- Antiproliferative mTor inhibitors such as sirolimus are used for secondary considerations including chronic kidney disease and cardiac allograft vasculopathy (CAV).
- Maintenance steroids are not institutional practice.

13 Post-transplant Complications

13.1 Rejection

- Incidence is low and most common within the first year post-HTx
- Clinical signs and symptoms are rare and echocardiogram is generally unremarkable
- Diagnosed on endomyocardial biopsy and may be acute cellular (ACR) or antibody medicated rejection (AMR); ISHLT standardized grading system used.
- ACR treatment depends on grade of rejection and presence of symptoms or functional changes by echocardiogram; in general, only moderate or greater rejection requires treatment; usually an oral steroid pulse and modification of maintenance IS.
- AMR treatment may include steroids, optimizing maintenance IS, immunoglobulin, plasmapheresis and anti B cell therapies; focuses on suppressing/eliminating DSA responsible for damage to the allograft

13.2 Cardiac Allograft Vasculopathy (CAV)

- Leading cause of morbidity and mortality with increasing time post-transplant.
- Low to moderate risk: screening with coronary angiography at 5 and 10 years post-transplant; frequency may be increased with risk factors and/or clinical concerns.
- Higher risk: reassessment every 2 years (e.g. AMR or abnormal cardiac testing).

Table 3 SickKids post-heart transplant ambulatory surveillance schedule

Schedule at a glance	Post-transplant ambulatory surveillance protocol
Clinic visits	May be modified depending on clinical status but in general: Twice a week for up to 3 weeks Weekly for 4 weeks Biweekly for 4 weeks Monthly for 3 months Q3-4 months up to 2 years post-transplant > 2 yrs post-transplant: q6-12 months
ECG	Pre-discharge 6–12 months post-HTx (with Holter) Annually thereafter
Holter monitor	6–12 months post-Tx (with ECG) Biennially unless otherwise clinically indicated
Echocardiogram (Echo)	Intra-op TEE Day 1 and/or Day 2 post-HTx Weekly to 2 months post-HTx Q2 weeks to 3 months post-HTx Q4 weeks to 6 months post-HTx Q8 weeks to 1 year post-HTx Q3-4 months to 2 years post-HTx Longterm: 2–3 per year May be modified based on clinical status
Endomyocardial biopsy (EMBx) with right heart hemodynamics	7–21 days post-HTx for first biopsy Infants in general are not biopsied until > 10 kg *Frequency based on time post-HTx and risk factors for rejection* 1–6 months: 8 weeks then 5–6 months post-HTx 6–12 months: 1 year post-HTx 1 y-3y: qannually > 3 y: q12 months or consider no further biopsies
Glomerular filtration rate (GFR)	6–12 months post-HTx Annual if abnormal Biennial if normal or mildly reduced
Bone mineral density (BMD)	Age > 5 years; Initial study 1 year post-HTx Q1-2 years if abnormal Every 5 years if normal

(continued)

Table 3 (continued)

Schedule at a glance	Post-transplant ambulatory surveillance protocol
24 h ambulatory blood pressure monitoring (ABPM)	Weight > 15 kg; able to cooperate At 6 months post-HTx if hypertensive or on antihypertensive medications, otherwise at 1 year post-HTx Biennially thereafter if normal renal function Annually if decreased renal function, on maintenance steroid, sirolimus, and/or antihypertensives
Graded exercise test (GXT) with VO2 With MIBI	One year post-transplant then biennially *(age/size appropriate [Ht 117 cm] and physically capable)* Supplementary test—if clinically indicated
Exercise echocardiography	Supplementary test—if clinically indicated *(age/size appropriate [Ht 140 cm] and physically capable)*
Dobutamine stress echo (DSE)	Patients incapable of exercise testing or if clinically indicated
Coronary angiography Intravascular ultrasound (IVUS)	Low—moderate risk: q5years High risk: q2-3y post-HTx Supplementary test—if clinically indicated
Neurodevelopmental assessment	For children < 3 years at the time of HTx: 6 months post-HTx 12 months post-HTx Pre-school assessment at 3.5–5 years of age *(if age < 2 y at HTx)* Includes: Ages and Stages Questionnaire (ASQ) Gross and Fine Motor Evaluation (AIMS and/or PDMS II) Clinical assessment of sensorineural and neuromuscular systems Beery-Buktenica Developmental test of Visual Motor Intergration
Neuropsychology assessment	If clinically indicated
Speech and language pathology	If clinically indicated
Adolescent medicine	If clinically indicated *(e.g. non-adherence, susbtance abuse, eating disorder, mood disorders,* etc.*)*
Psychiatry	If clinically indicated

(continued)

Table 3 (continued)

Schedule at a glance	Post-transplant ambulatory surveillance protocol
Quality of life	Recipient Age 5–17 years: Annually post-HTx Parent/guardians of recipients 2–17 years of age: Annually post-HTx
BLOODWORK	
First month post-Tx	TCO_2, electrolytes, creatinine weekly CBC and diff, magnesium: q2weeks TDM (Tacrolimus/Sirolimus/MPA) individualized EBV PCR and CMV PCR weekly
ABO-incompatible patients	Isohemagglutinins: Daily × 3–4 days Weekly × 3 weeks *(to 4 weeks post-HTx)*
Q monthly up to 6 months post-Tx then q3 months to 1 year post-Tx	CBC and diff TCO_2, electrolytes, creatinine TDM (determined by individual response and target levels) Magnesium to 3 months post-HTx EBV PCR AND CMV PCR: Q2wks until 3 months post-HTx Qmonthly to 6 months post-HTx Q3monthly until 1 year post-HTx
ABO-incompatible patients	Isohemagglutinins *(beyond the 1st month):* Q2weekly to 3 months post-HTx Monthly to 6 months post-HTx
Q3months up to 1 year post-Tx	ALT, alkaline phosphatase, bilirubin(s), Ca, phos, albumin
> 1 years post-Tx: Q3-6 months *(frequency equivalent to routine clinic visits)*	CBC and diff TCO_2, electrolytes, creatinine, ALT Ca, phos, albumin, alkaline phosphatase, 25(OH) Vit D, PTH q6months *if on Ca or Vit D suppls or decreased BMD* Urine dip for protein q12 months if normal otherwise q6 months Spot urine for albumin/creatinine ratio q12 months if normal (no proteinuria) otherwise q6 months TDM *(frequency may change depending on result)* EBV PCR AND CMV PCR
ABO-incompatible patients Diabetic patients	Isohemagglutinins (q6-12 months) HbA1c *(as needed)*
Patients on statin therapy	CK, ALT: Baseline at start of therapy 3–4 weeks after start/change of therapy Annually

(continued)

Table 3 (continued)

Schedule at a glance	Post-transplant ambulatory surveillance protocol
At 1 year post-Tx then annually	nt-proBNP EBV and CMV serology *(seronegative)* Toxoplasma serology *(seronegative)* Varicella serology *(seronegative)* Non-fasting blood glucose Non-fasting lipid level: HDL, total cholesterol (TC) and calculated non-HDL Calcium, phosphorus, albumin, alkaline phosphatase, 25(OH) Vit D, PTH *(fall months preferred)* Albumin, total protein, bilirubin(s) IgG/A/M Lymphocyte immune-phenotyping CD45 Ra/Ro Spot urine for calcium to creatinine ratio (age 12 to 18 years)
ABO-incompatible patients	Isohemagglutinins
6–12 months after immunization	Hepatitis B Titres
Anti-HLA antibody testing	*Not sensitized* q3months then annually *Sensitized with negative donor-specific crossmatch* Q biopsy for the 1st year post-HTx then annually if no development of donor-specific antibody (DSA) *Sensitized with positive donor-specific crossmatch* Q biopsy unless no further biopsies then annually With first biopsy following completion of chemotherapy
nt-proBNP	6 months post-Tx (baseline) then Annually Q Biopsy (beyond 6 months post-Tx) Any clinical suspicion for rejection

13.3 Infection

- 12% of deaths during the first year post-HTx.
- Common bacterial infections: staphylococcus, pseudomonas, and enterobacter cloacae.
- CMV is the most common viral infection with a peak incidence at 6–8 weeks post-HTx
  - Prophylactic and pre-emptive strategies exist using valganciclovir for the first 3 months in high risk patients.
- Fungal infections while rare have a high mortality rate in the first six months post-HTx

13.4 Post Transplant Lymphoproliferative Disorder (PTLD)

- Incidence at 5 and 10 years post-HTx is about 5% and 10% respectively.
- Ranges from benign lymphoid hyperplasia to aggressive B or T cell lymphoma.
- Typically an abnormal proliferation of B cells; most often linked to EBV.
- Donor to recipient EBV mismatch and EBV viral load are risk factors for the development.
- Treatment involves reduction in IS and may warrant chemotherapy

13.5 Chronic Kidney Disease (CKD)

- Multifactorial (pre-HTx chronic heart failure, nephrotoxicity secondary to CNIs)
- Multiple possible manifestations including decreased creatinine clearance, hyperkalemia, hypomagnesemia, renal tubular acidosis, proteinuria, etc.
- Renal function and renal protective measures (e.g., minimum fluid intake; avoid NSAIDS, modify IS to renal-sparing strategy, etc.)

13.6 Neurodevelopmental Outcomes

- In the low-normal range with an increased incidence of language, fine motor and cognitive/intellectual delay in children transplanted as infants, particularly those with CHD; also have an increased incidence of abnormal neurologic exam including hypo- or hypertonia.
- Provision of neurodevelopmental assessment and multidisciplinary functional interventions (e.g., occupational/physiotherapy, speech language pathology, educational assistant, etc.) maintain and/or improve developmental milestones.

13.7 Hypertension

- An adverse effect of CNIs.
- Angiotensin converting enzyme inhibitors (ACEi) are first line treatment.

13.8 Nutrition

- Goal is to normalize feeding and growth according to developmental and functional level.
- Impacts multiple post-HTx co-morbidities including hypertension, bone health, infectious risk, bone health, neurodevelopmental outcomes, amongst others.

13.9 Bone Health

- Decreased bone density can be associated with fractures and avascular necrosis.
- Weight bearing exercises, calcium and Vitamin D supplementation are first line treatment.

13.10 Hyperlipidemia

- Higher lipid levels than aged matched controls, thought to be related to direct effects of immunosuppressant therapy
- Early treatment with statin therapy is felt to be protective against the development of CAV.

13.11 Adherence

- Medication non adherence may result in life threatening events and decreased long-term survival.
- Teenagers remain at highest risk of non-adherence.
- Identifying patients at risk for non-adherence early on may help with strategies to mitigate.

14 Outcomes

- Current graft survival rates are based on multiple factors and age at time of HTx.
- The most recent analysis from ISHLT registry shows a median survival of
  - 24.5 years for those < 1 year at time of HTx
  - 20.2 years for those 1–5 years at time of HTx
  - 15.0 for those 6–10 years at time of HTx
  - 14.3 years for those > 11 at time of HTx.

Bibliography

1. Almond CS, Thiagarajan RR, Piercey GE, et al. Waiting list mortality among children listed for heart transplantation in the United States. Circulation. 2009;119(5):717–27.
2. Canadian Cardiac Transplant Network. Paediatric heart transplant listing criteria in Canada; 2021. https://ccs.ca/app/uploads/2022/01/PEDS-Cardiac-Transplant-Eligibility-and-Listing-Criteria-Aug-9-2021-APPROVED.pdf. Accessed 08 Sep 2023.

3. Chinnock RE, Catherin Freier M, Ashwal S, et al. Developmental outcomes after pediatric heart transplantation. J Heart Lung Transplant. 2008;27(10):1079–84.
4. Conway J, Chin C, Kemna M, et al. Donors' characteristics and impact on outcomes in pediatric heart transplant recipients. Pediatr Transplant. 2013;17(8):774–81.
5. Dipchand A. Current state of pediatric cardiac transplantation. Ann Cardiothorac Surg. 2018;7(1):31–55.
6. Dipchand AI, Kirk R, Edwards LB, et al. The registry of the international society for heart and lung transplantation: sixteenth official pediatric heart transplantation report–2013; focus theme: age. J Heart Lung Transplant. 2013;32(10):979–88.
7. Rossano JW, Singh TP, Cherikj WS, et al. The international thoracic organ transplant registry of the international society for heart and lung transplantation: twenty-second pediatric heart transplantation report—2019; Focus theme: donor and recipient size match. J Heart Lung Transplant. 2019;38(10):1028–41.

Cardiac Tumors

Alejandro A. Floh and Robert Hamilton

Abstract Cardiac tumors are rare in children and represent only 0.03–0.2% of all cardiac consultations. Rhabdomyomas are the most common tumor in children with a peak incidence in the first year of life. Diagnosis is often made during routine prenatal screening and most regress postnatally without need for interventions. Fibromas are isolated growths and the second most common pediatric tumor. Other tumors include atrial myxomas, hemangiomas, and malignant rhabdomyosarcomas. Echocardiography and cross-sectional imaging are useful to delineate tumor size, location, and associated findings; MRI is the best modality for tissue characterization. The management of a tumor depends on whether it is causing obstruction or arrhythmia, and whether it has malignant potential. Medical treatments, including tumor suppression therapy (sirolimus), are directed to address symptoms or arrhythmias. Interventions are limited to tumors causing hemodynamic compromise, intractable arrhythmias, or at risk for complications.

Keywords Cardiac tumor · Rhabdomyoma · Fibroma · Myxoma

Abbreviations

ASD	Atrial septal defect
AV	Atrioventricular
CNS	Central nervous system
LV	Left ventricle
RV	Right ventricle

A. A. Floh
Department of Critical Care Medicine, Division of Cardiac Critical Care Unit, Labatt Family Heart Centre, The Hospital for Sick Children, University of Toronto, Toronto, ON, Canada
e-mail: alejandro.floh@sickkids.ca

R. Hamilton (✉)
Division of Cardiology, Department of Paediatrics, Labatt Family Heart Centre, Hospital for Sick Children, University of Toronto, Toronto, ON, Canada
e-mail: robert.hamilton@sickkids.ca

© The Author(s), under exclusive license to Springer Nature Switzerland AG 2024

A. I. Dipchand et al. (eds.), *Manual of Cardiac Care in Children*,
https://doi.org/10.1007/978-3-031-70973-9_44

Key Points

- Cardiac tumors are rare with the most common being rhabdomyomas and fibromas
- Clinical presentation dependent on size, location and resultant impact on hemodynamics
- Arrhythmias are frequent manifestations and may be difficult to control.

1 Overview

- Cardiac tumors are being increasingly recognized, although this is likely related to the improvement of imaging modalities rather than a true change in the prevalence of disease.
- The most common cardiac tumor in childhood is rhabdomyoma, followed by fibroma and other rarer conditions.

2 Presentation

- Up to 40% of tumors are diagnosed during fetal exam
- Mode of presentation otherwise dependent on tumor type, size, number, position within the heart (particularly in relation to valve structures), and degree of extension.
  - May present as incidental finding if benign (~25%), clinical symptoms due to obstructive symptoms or valve dysfunction (~50% of cases), arrhythmia, or sudden death

3 Clinical Presentations

3.1 Low Cardiac Output Syndrome

- Low preload to right or left ventricle—size of mass can impede inflow into either ventricle or reduce the ventricular cavity size and/or ventricular compliance. Inadequate ventricular filling results in low stroke volume.
- Obstruction to outflow—mass may obstruct pulmonary or systemic outflow leading to low stroke volume. Increased afterload can result in ventricular dysfunction and failure.
- Pericardial effusion and tamponade.
- Leads to poor exercise tolerance, syncope, sudden death.

3.2 *Cyanosis*

- Right ventricular outflow obstruction resulting in ASD level (right to left) shunt or postnatal duct dependent pulmonary circulation.

3.3 *Venous Congestion*

- Pulmonary congestion if left sided mass obstructing pulmonary venous return: tachypnea, hyperpnea, orthopnea, pulmonary edema.
- Systemic congestion if obstructing systemic venous return: edema, hepatomegaly, ascites.

3.4 *Arrhythmia*

- Arrhythmias are a frequent manifestation of cardiac tumors and may be difficult to control
- Associated supraventricular tachycardias are thought to be due to rhabdomyoma invasion of the atrioventricular (AV) ring functioning as accessory pathways, producing manifestations of either pre-excitation, AV reentrant tachycardia, or both.
- Atrial rhabdomyomas may be associated with atrial ectopic tachycardia, and ventricular rhabdomyomas may be associated with potentially lethal ventricular tachycardias.
- Complete heart block is a rare manifestation.

3.5 *Systemic Manifestations*

- Constitutional: fevers, anorexia, malaise, myalgia and arthralgia
- Embolism
  - Systemic embolization of particles or related thrombi reported with left atrial myxomas.
  - Pulmonary embolization from right sided masses.

4 Diagnostic Investigations

4.1 ECG

- Nonspecific ST-T wave changes
- Pre-excitation can be seen
- Mostly useful to diagnose associated arrhythmia.

4.2 Echocardiogram

- Transthoracic echocardiograms are the primary diagnostic modality
  - Can detect all important diagnostic characteristics of tumor, including number, location, size, shape, capsule, consistency (solid, cystic, combination), and base.
  - Detect presence of pericardial effusion
  - Performs best for endocardial growths and less effective for pericardial growths and mediastinal extension.
  - Allows for surveillance without sedation or radiation risk.
- Trans-esophageal echocardiography
  - Intraoperative use to direct resection or visualization of left atrial appendage.
- Fetal echocardiography
  - Prenatal detection as part of usual screening
  - May guide postnatal management.

4.3 Catheterization

- Rarely required to assess hemodynamic consequences of cardiac tumors, coronary angiography to ensure patency, or for endomyocardial biopsy.

4.4 Computed Tomography and MRI

- Assess effect of growth on mediastinum, vascular and/or airway tissues.
- CT best suited to detect calcification.
- MRI for tissue differentiation (vascular tumors from rhabdomyomas), detection of coexisting thrombi, assess pericardial involvement.
- Particularly helpful for apical tumors.

5 Overall Incidence

- Varies across studies and age groups
- Nearly half are single growths
- Majority benign growths within ventricular mass (90%)—RV, LV, intraventricular septum.

6 Tumors

6.1 Rhabdomyomas

- Type of hamartoma—growths caused by abnormal formation of normally occurring cells.
- Most common pediatric tumor with incidence highest in first year of life. (Fig. 1)
- 90% of cases have multiple cardiac tumors, particularly if related to tuberous sclerosis complex
- Well circumscribed but not encapsulated usually isolated to ventricular wall or cavity

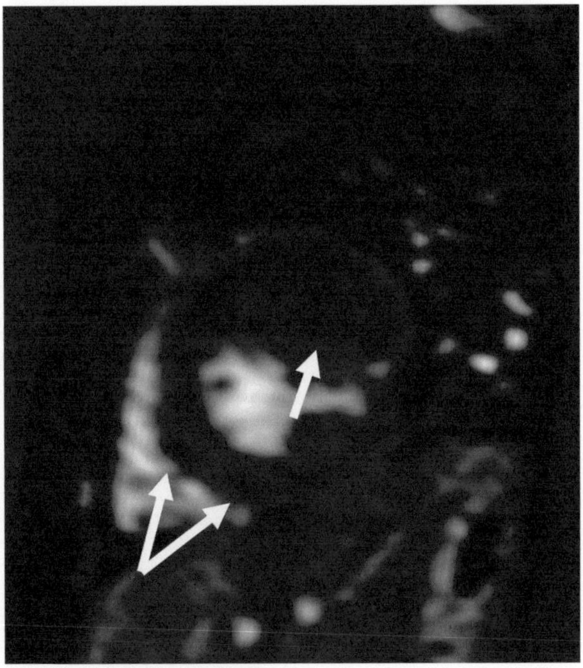

Fig. 1 MRI demonstrating multiple (arrows: one large, two small) rhabdomyomas without significant early enhancement. Reproduced with permission from Dr. Christopher Lam

- Appear as echogenic, homogenous masses—not usually associated with pericardial effusions.
- Resolve spontaneously following birth—surgical intervention required only if hemodynamic compromise
- Occasionally, myocardium may become infiltrated with cells like those of classical congenital rhabdomyoma: a condition called rhabdomyomatosis
- Everolimus may have a role in promoting tumor regression or control of tumor-mediated arrhythmias.
- Tuberous sclerosis complex
  - 60–90% have Tuberous sclerosis—associated with other hamartomas of skin, CNS, kidney, retina
  - Caused by mutations of either the TSC1 (Hamartin, 33%) or TSC2 (Tuberin, 67%) gene.
  - This molecular understanding provides for novel therapies in tuberous sclerosis (such as sirolimus and everolimus).

6.2 *Fibromas*

- Tumor from abnormal fibrotic tissue: collagen, fibroblast, elastic tissue.
- Second most common tumor in pediatric age group; mostly seen in younger children.
- Single, firm, non-encapsulated mass but may have satellite growths. (Fig. 2)

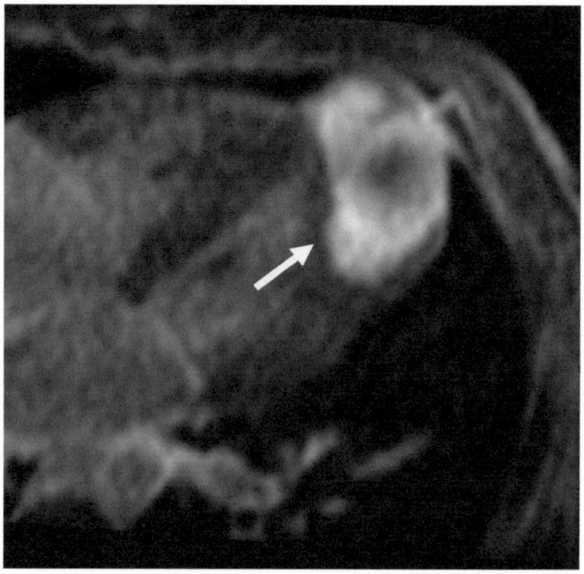

Fig. 2 MRI of single fibroma (arrow) at the left ventricular apex showing pathognomonic features of avid delayed peripheral enhancement with central dark core. Reproduced with permission from Dr. Christopher Lam

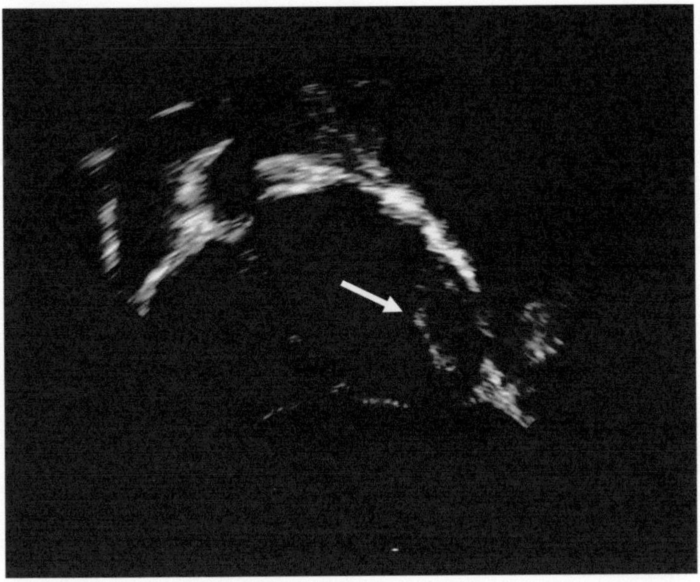

Fig. 3 Echocardiogram of single fibroma (arrow) in at the apex of the left ventricle. Reproduced with permission from Dr. Christopher Lam

- Slow growing but have potential of invasive spread.
- Bright on echocardiography; can have calcification and cystic degeneration. (Fig. 3)
- Difficult to differentiate from rhabdomyomas, workup for TS if uncertain.
- Resection rare, transplantation reported.
- Do not change in size over time.
  - In rare instances they may be part of the nevoid-basal cell carcinoma (Gorlin) syndrome, an autosomal dominant condition due to mutations of the PTCH gene strongly characterized by a predisposition to non-*melanoma skin cancers; ca*rdiac fibromas occur in 10% of cases.

6.3 Myxomas

- Benign tumor of mesenchymal cells in myxoid background.
- Half of all cardiac tumors but rare in children (not seen in infancy).
- High familial recurrence
- Arise from atrial septum: single left atrium mass (75%), remainder single right atrial masses
- Pedunculated, gelatinous masses

- Symptoms usually result from inflow obstruction of atrioventricular valves, systemic/pulmonic emboli (tissue or thrombi), or rarely constitutional systemic symptoms (immunologic response—IL6 implicated.)
- Rarely locally invasive.
- May be associated with endocrinopathies.
- Require surgical excision.
- Recurrence can be seen after 3 years.
- Approximately 7% of cardiac myxomas are associated with Carney complex.
  - *Autosomal dominant* condition caused by mutations in the PRKAR1A gene which lead to *myxomas* of heart and skin, hyperpigmentation of the skin (*lentiginosis*), and *endocrine* overactivity.

6.4 Pericardial Teratomas

- Rare, benign tumor usually found at base of the heart during fetal development and infancy.
- Tissue arises from all germ layers.
- Single, encapsulated masses. (Fig. 4)
- Pericardial effusions common, may precipitate decompensation from tamponade physiology.
- Surgical resection curative.

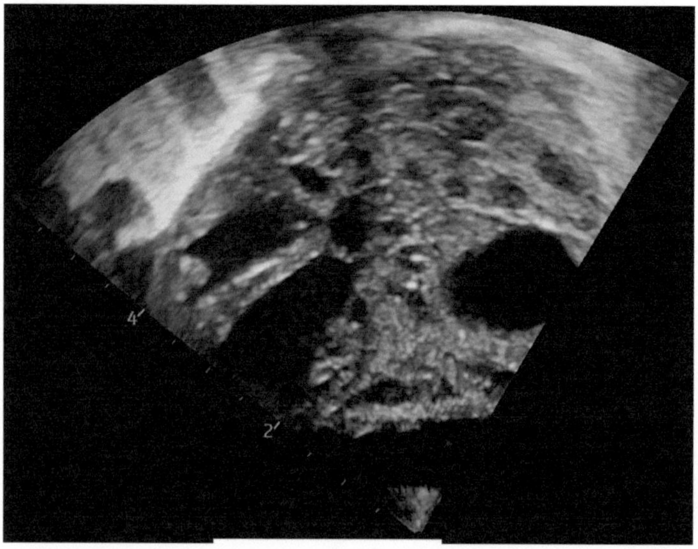

Fig. 4 Large pericardial teratoma bordering the left atrium and ventricle. Reproduced with permission from Dr. Christopher Lam

6.5 *Hemangiomas*

- Single tumors comprised of abnormal collection of blood vessels.
- May involve pericardium and myocardium.
- Surgical excision required only if clinically symptomatic and transplantation considered if extensive disease.

6.6 *Rare Tumors*

- Malignant tumors of the heart (predominantly rhabdomyosarcomas) are extremely rare, resistant to treatment and associated with poor prognosis.
- Metastatic tumors can originate from lymphomas, Wilm's tumors, and hepatomas.

6.7 *Indications for Intervention/Surgery*

- Hemodynamic compromise—due to obstruction to left ventricular inflow, outflow, or cavity volume.
- Cyanosis as a result of limitation to pulmonary blood flow.
- Tumor morphology—e.g. Fibroma, myxomas, teratomas.
- Large pericardial effusions.
- Intractable arrhythmia—unresponsive to medical management
- Transplantation considered if surgical resection not feasible.

Bibliography

1. Becker AE. Primary heart tumors in the pediatric age group: a review of salient pathologic features relevant for clinicians. Pediatr Cardiol. 2000;21(4):317–23.
2. Freedom RM, Lee K-J, MacDonald C, et al. Selected aspects of cardiac tumors in infancy and childhood. Pediatr Cardiol. 2000;21(4):299–316.
3. Isaacs H Jr. Fetal and neonatal cardiac tumors. Pediatric Cardiol. 2004;25(3):252–73.
4. Paraskevaidis JA, Michalakeas CA, Papadopoulos CH, Anastasiou-Nana M. Cardiac tumors (review article). Int Schol Res Netw (ISRN) Oncol. 2011.

Marfan Syndrome, Loeys-Dietz Syndrome and Related Aortopathies

Timothy J. Bradley

Abstract Marfan syndrome (MFS) and Loeys-Dietz syndrome (LDS) are connective tissue disorders associated with aortopathy in childhood. Childhood aortopathy can be associated with other syndromic conditions, either associated with connective tissue disorders like vascular Ehlers-Danlos syndrome (vEDS), or not, like arterial tortuosity syndrome (ATS), bicuspid aortic valve (BAV), or some types of familial thoracic aortic aneurysm and dissection (FTAAD). Family screening is key as early diagnosis and effective management can improve outcomes. MFS and LDS can be discriminated from other causes of aortopathy/arteriopathy in childhood by clinical assessment and genetic testing. Echocardiography, MRI and/or CT can be used for aortic surveillance. Medical therapy includes beta-blockers (BB) and/or angiotensin receptor blockers (ARB), with surgical intervention for aortic repair tailored to disease- and patient-specific factors. LDS is associated with need for heightened aortic surveillance, earlier introduction of medical therapy and increased risk of aortic dissection compared to MFS or other aortopathies. BB and ARB, when indicated, may both be of more benefit if started early, and in the setting of a malignant family history and/or rapid aortic root growth.

Keywords Marfan syndrome · Loeys-Dietz syndrome · Connective tissue disorder · Aortopathy

Abbreviations

AAo	Ascending aortic
AI	Aortic insufficiency
AoD	Aortic dissection
AoR	Aortic root
AoRz	Aortic root Z-score

T. J. Bradley (✉)
Department of Paediatrics, University of Saskatchewan, Jim Pattison Children's Hospital, Saskatchewan Health Authority, Saskatoon, SK, Canada
e-mail: tim.bradley@usask.ca

© The Author(s), under exclusive license to Springer Nature Switzerland AG 2024

A. I. Dipchand et al. (eds.), *Manual of Cardiac Care in Children*,
https://doi.org/10.1007/978-3-031-70973-9_45

ARB	Angiotensin receptor blocker
ATS	Arterial tortuosity syndrome
BAV	Bicuspid aortic valve
BB	Beta blocker
CoA	Coarctation of the aorta
EL	Ectopia lentis
FBN1	Fibrillin-1 gene
FTAAD	Familial thoracic aortic aneurysm and dissection
LDS	Loeys-Dietz syndrome
LV	Left ventricle
MFS	Marfan syndrome
MPA	Main pulmonary artery
MR	Mitral regurgitation
MVP	Mitral valve prolapse
PDA	Persistent ductus arteriosus
TAA	Thoracic aortic aneurysm
TAAD	Thoracic aortic aneurysm and dissection
TEE	Transesophageal echocardiogram
TGF-β	Transforming growth factor-beta
TR	Tricuspid regurgitation
TVP	Tricuspid valve prolapse
vEDS	Vascular Ehlers-Danlos syndrome

Key Points

- Family screening is key as early diagnosis, screening and management can modify/ improve outcomes.
- Marfan syndrome (MFS) and Loeys-Dietz syndrome (LDS) can be discriminated from other causes of aortopathy/arteriopathy in childhood by clinical assessment and genetic testing.
- Aortic surveillance with echocardiography, MRI and/or CT, medical therapy with BB and/or ARBs, and surgical indications for aortic repair are tailored to disease- and patient-specific factors.
- Need for aortic surveillance, medical therapy and risk of aortic dissection are usually increased in LDS vs. MFS vs. other related aortopathies.
- Initiation of medical therapy in children is usually determined by measurement of aortic root Z-score (AoRz) by echocardiography.
- In MFS, BB and ARB may both be of more benefit if started early when high-risk factors present, including rapid aortic growth $\geq$ 5 mm in 1 year or $\geq$ 3 mm/year in 2 consecutive years at any location, rapidly progressive aortic insufficiency (AI), and/or a malignant family history.

- In LDS, BB and ARB are often started earlier particularly with rapid aortic root growth and/or a malignant family history.
- Surgical therapy in children is usually determined by aortic root (AoR) or ascending aortic (AAo) dimensions by echocardiography, MRI or CT:
  - In MFS, AoR/AAo $\geq$ 50 mm
  - In LDS, AoR/AAo $\geq$ 40–50 mm, dependent on genetic variant
  - In other related aortopathies, surgical indications for aortic repair are tailored to disease- and patient-specific factors.

1 Importance of Screening in Aortopathies

- Acute aortic dissection (AoD) may be the first presentation; early diagnosis and effective family screening can save lives.
- Diagnosis in the index case is based on clinical findings, targeted imaging, and genetic testing tailored to the patient and family history of vascular events.
- Full clinical examination is ideally performed by a medical geneticist with expertise in connective tissue disorders and familial aortopathies prior to deciding which genetic test(s) to order.
- Cardiac screening with echocardiography should be performed initially in all first-degree relatives of patients with suspected familial aortopathies.
- Presence of causal genetic mutation: genetic counseling and testing is recommended for first-degree relatives; more extensive imaging in mutation carriers.
- No causal mutation identified: screening every 2–5 years is recommended for 'healthy' at-risk relatives until a diagnosis is established or ruled out.

2 Marfan Syndrome (MFS)

2.1 Epidemiology

- Prevalence ~ 1 in 5,000 population, common.
- Autosomal dominant, ~ 1/3 de novo.
- Mutations in fibrillin-1 gene (*FBN1*), encoding for fibrillin-1, a glycoprotein component of the extracellular microfibril.

2.2 Diagnosis

- Based on revised Ghent Criteria:
  - In the absence of family history:

1. AoRz ≥ 2 or aortic root dissection AND ectopia lentis (EL)
2. AoRz ≥ 2 or aortic root dissection AND *FBN1* mutation
3. AoRz ≥ 2 or aortic root dissection AND systemic score ≥ 7 (see below)
4. EL AND *FBN1* mutation

– In the presence of family history of MFS:

5. EL
6. Systemic score ≥ 7 (see below)
7. AoRz ≥ 2 if > 20 years/adult or ≥ 3 if < 20 years/child

- The systemic score (positive if ≥ 7 out of a total 20 points) is calculated as follows:

Points	Findings (each)
3	– Wrist AND thumb sign (for arachnodactyly/long fingers)
2	– Pectus carinatum (pigeon-shaped chest) – Hindfoot deformity (forefoot abduction and lowering of the midfoot) – Spontaneous pneumothorax – Dural ectasia (widening of the dural sac, usually in the lumbosacral region) – Protrusio acetabuli (displacement of femoral head)
1	– Wrist OR thumb sign – Pectus excavatum (funnel-shaped chest) OR chest asymmetry – Pes planus (flat feet) – Reduced upper segment/lower segment ratio AND increased arm/height ratio AND no severe scoliosis – Scoliosis OR thoracolumbar kyphosis – Reduced elbow extension – Facial features (3/5 of dolichocephaly [long face/skull], enophthalmos [deep set eyes], downslanting palpebral fissures, malar hypoplasia [shallow cheekbones], retrognathia [recessed lower jaw]) – Skin striae (otherwise unexplained stretch marks) – Myopia [nearsightedness] > 3 diopters – Mitral valve prolapse (MVP)

2.3 Cardiovascular Involvement

- Aortopathy
  - Aortic root dilatation/aneurysm (common).
  - Type A AoD (common adults, rarely in adolescents > 12 years).
  - Descending thoracic aortic aneurysm and type B AoD (adults only).
- Arterial involvement
  - Main pulmonary artery (MPA) dilatation/aneurysm is very common but dissection is very rare.
  - Arterial aneurysm/dissection (reported, but not greater than population risk).

- Valvulopathy
  - MVP/mitral regurgitation (MR) (very common).
  - Tricuspid valve prolapse (TVP)/tricuspid regurgitation (TR) (common).
  - AI (common with significant AoR dilatation).
- Myocardial involvement
  - Secondary myocardial dysfunction (reported with severe valvular disease/volume overload).
  - Primary cardiomyopathy (severe LV dysfunction in neonatal MFS, mild in some adult MFS).

2.4 *"Neonatal/Infantile" MFS*

- Early presentation in intractable heart failure due to severe MVP/MR and TVP/TR.
- Significant AoR dilatation and AI often also present.
- Associated with myocardial dysfunction, chest deformity, "infantile pulmonary emphysema" and other severe musculoskeletal features.
- Often fatal in the first year, even after valvular repair.

3 Loeys-Dietz Syndrome (LDS)

3.1 *Epidemiology*

- Prevalence unknown, less common than MFS.
- Autosomal dominant, significant proportion de novo.
- Types 1 and 2: *TGFBR1* and *TGFBR2* mutations encoding for transforming growth factor-beta (TGF-β) receptor 1 and 2 proteins.
- Type 3 (Osteoarthritis-Aneurysm syndrome): *SMAD3* mutations encoding for SMAD3 protein
- Type 4 and 5: *TGFB2* and *TGFB3* mutations, encoding for TGF-β ligand 2 and 3 proteins.
- LDS Types 3, 4 and 5 associated with less severe aortic/arterial phenotypes.

3.2 *Diagnosis*

- Classic triad: hypertelorism, bifid/broad uvula and/or cleft palate, early onset aortic aneurysm and generalized arterial tortuosity.
- Different features from MFS:

  - Absence of EL and tall stature
  - Presence of Chiari malformation, craniosynostosis, cervical spine instability, talipes equinovarus, thin translucent skin, atrophic scars, asthma/food allergy/eczema/allergic rhinitis, eosinophilic esophagitis, inflammatory bowel disease, constipation and failure to thrive.

- Overlapping features with MFS:
  - Arachnodactyly (less common).
  - Pectus carinatum, pectus excavatum or chest asymmetry.
  - Hindfoot deformity or pes planus.
  - Spontaneous pneumothorax.
  - Dural ectasia.
  - Scoliosis.
  - Skin striae.

3.3 Cardiovascular Involvement

- Aortopathy
  - Earlier onset aortic root aneurysm and type A AoD (particularly in *TGFBR1* and *TGFBR2* mutations)
- Descending thoracic aortic aneurysm (TAA) and type B AoD less common.
- Arterial involvement
  - MPA dilatation/aneurysm (common). MPA dissection (not reported).
  - Arterial aneurysm/dissection (earlier onset, reported in infancy).
- Valvulopathy
  - MVP, MR, TVP, TR (less common).
  - AI (common with significant AoR dilatation).
- Myocardial involvement: secondary myocardial dysfunction is rare.
- Associated lesions: Increased prevalence ASD, PDA, BAV.

4 Bicuspid Aortic Valve-Associated Aortopathy

4.1 Epidemiology

- BAV: most common congenital heart defect affecting ~ 1.3% of the population
- Associated with:
  - HLHS, CoA and some VSDs.

  - Genetic syndromes: Andersen-Tawil, DiGeorge/22q11 deletion, Noonan, LEOPARD, Turner syndromes, LDS and FTAAD-ACTA2.
  - Genetic mutations: NOTCH1 and GATA2.

4.2 Cardiovascular Involvement

- Increased risk (26%) at 25 years after initial diagnosis of aneurysm (when defined as AoR or AAo $\geq$ 45 mm); with incidence ~ 85 cases per 10,000 patient-years, which is 80 times greater than the general population.
- With 23% of these at 25 years already having undergone elective aortic repair; and an incidence of AoD in non-repaired BAV-aortopathy of ~ 3 cases per 10,000 patient-years (0.03%).

5 Familial Thoracic Aortic Aneurysm and Dissection (FTAAD)

5.1 Epidemiology

- TAA: ~ 10 per 100,000 person years.
- Acute AoD ~ 3 per 100,000 person years.
- Non-syndromic TAAD: affected first-degree relative in up to 20% = familial TAAD (FTAAD).
- 20–25% of FTAAD accounted for by mutations in *ACTA2*; *MFAP5*, *MYH11*; *MYLK*; *PRKG1*; *TGFBR1*; *TGFBR2*; *SMAD3;* *TGFB2*; *TGFB3*; *FBN1*.

5.2 Diagnosis

- Based on imaging, clinical assessment and genetic testing.
- TAAD is defined as:
  - Dilatation of the ascending thoracic aorta at the level of the sinuses of Valsalva (aortic root) or ascending aorta or both; and
  - Dissections of the thoracic aorta involving either type A ascending AoD or type B descending AoD.
- Certain genetic mutations can be associated with specific extracardiac features.

5.3 Cardiovascular Involvement

- All FTAAD: associated with aortic root/ascending aorta aneurysms and type A ascending AoD, with variable involvement of the descending aorta and type B AoD and arterial involvement.
- Certain genetic mutations can be associated with premature stroke, coronary artery and Moyamoya disease, PDA, BAV, MVP, atrial fibrillation, amongst others.

6 Vascular Ehlers-Danlos Syndrome (vEDS)

6.1 Epidemiology

- Prevalence ~ 1 in 100,000 population, rare.
- Autosomal dominant.
- Due to mutations in *COL3A1*, encoding for type 3 procollagen.

6.2 Diagnosis

- Based on four clinical criteria:
  - Easy bruising.
  - Thin skin with visible veins.
  - Characteristic facial features.
  - Rupture of arteries, uterus, or intestines.
- Other features include atrophic scars, clubfoot and/or congenital dislocation of the hips, recurrent joint subluxation or dislocation, inguinal hernia and pneumothorax.

6.3 Cardiovascular Involvement

- Aortic involvement is uncommon.
- Aneurysms, arteriovenous fistulae, dissection and/or rupture of medium-sized arteries.
- Intestinal and peripartum uterine rupture (associated with up to a 12% risk of death in pregnancy) secondary to arterial events.

7 Arterial Tortuosity Syndrome (ATS)

7.1 Epidemiology

- Very rare autosomal recessive disorder.
- Mutations in *SLC2A10*.
- May be lethal in infancy; milder forms may survive into adulthood.

7.2 Diagnosis

- Cardiovascular manifestations:
  - Widespread tortuosity of the aorta and medium-sized arteries with increased risk of aneurysms and dissections.
  - Focal stenosis of aorta and/or pulmonary arteries.
  - Dilations of large veins.
  - MVP/MR.
- Extracardiovascular manifestations include myopia, keratoconus (cone shaped cornea), characteristic facial features, high arched palate with dental crowding, arachnodactyly, camptodactyly, scoliosis, pectus excavatum or carinatum, joint laxity, knee/elbow contractures, muscular hypotonia, soft doughy skin, and inguinal/hiatal/diaphragmatic hernia.

8 Clinical Presentation of Aortopathies

- TAAs tend to be asymptomatic.
- AoD presentation is highly variable:
  - Sudden severe chest pain radiating to the back.
  - Features of myocardial infarction/stroke if coronary/cerebrovascular involvement.
  - Congestive heart failure if acute severe AI.
- AI usually progresses with aneurysmal dilatation of the aortic root.
- MVP may progress to severe MR, especially in females, by adolescence or acutely with a ruptured chord and a flail mitral leaflet usually in adults.
- TVP with or without TR is less likely to produce any complications.

9 Natural History/Survival

- MFS
  - Gradually progressive AoR dilatation that usually approaches elective surgical indications by age 20–40 years (rarely needed by adolescence).
  - AoD rarely occurs as young as 12 years old.
- LDS
  - Rapidly progressive AoR dilatation and arterial aneurysms that require early surgical intervention (particularly in *TGFBR1* and *TGFBR2* mutations).
  - AoD reported even in infancy, especially when associated with other severe syndromic features.
  - With minimal or no syndromic features, surgical indications are not usually met until mid-adulthood.
- BAV-aortopathy
  - Elective surgical indications may be reached by adolescence, but usually not until mid-adulthood.
- FTAAD
  - Variable presentation dependent on the underlying gene and family history.
- vEDS
  - Arterial complications are rare in childhood
  - Complications seen in 25% of affected individuals by age 20 years and > 80% by age 40 years, with a median age of death of 48 years.

10 Diagnostic Studies

10.1 ECG

- Usually normal.

10.2 Echocardiography

- Mainstay of aortic surveillance for monitoring proximal aortic dimensions (Fig. 1) and calculate AoRz and AAoz.
- Aortic arch, proximal head and neck branch, and MPA dimensions should also be recorded (Fig. 2) and z-scores calculated if enlarged.
- Assessment of valve function.

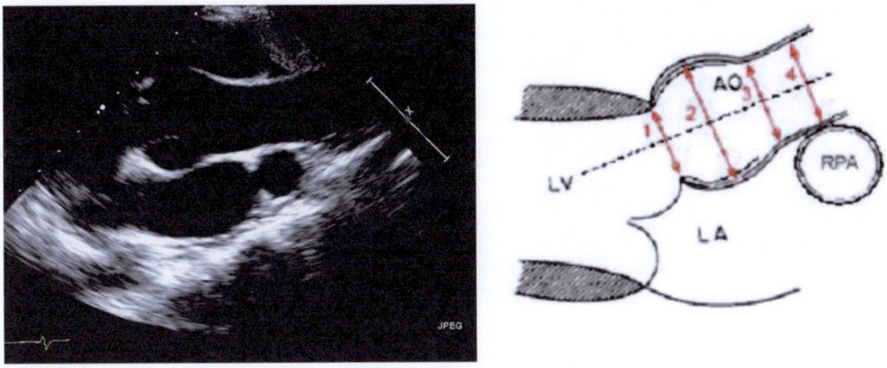

Fig. 1 Maximum aortic dimensions by TTE should be measured in peak systole at the levels of the (1) aortic annulus, (2) aortic root (AoR)/sinuses of Valsalva, (3) sinotubular junction and (4) ascending aortic (AAo) perpendicular to the right pulmonary artery (RPA), and the AoR and AAo Z-scores calculated

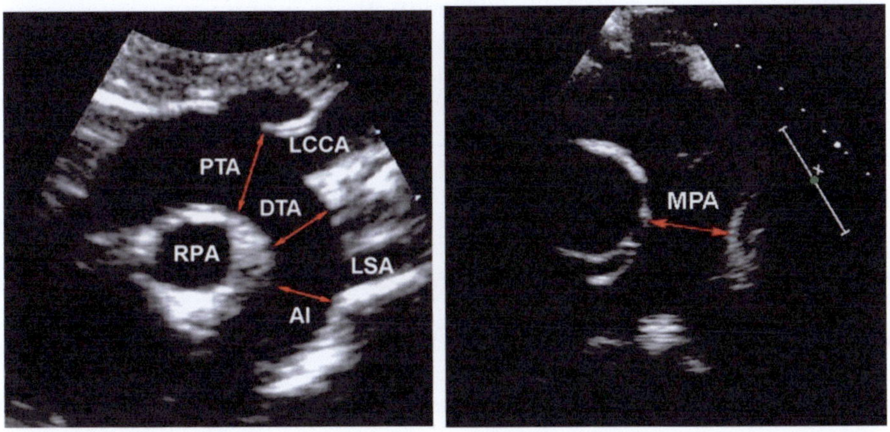

Fig. 2 Maximum dimensions in systole by TTE should be measured in peak systole at the levels of the proximal transverse arch (PTA), distal transverse arch (DTA), aortic isthmus (AI), main pulmonary artery (MPA) and the head and neck branch [right innominate artery, left common carotid artery (LCCA) and left subclavian artery (LSA)] and Z-scores should be calculated whenever thought to be enlarged

- Transesophageal echocardiography (TEE) can be used to detect acute AoD.

10.3 MRI and CT Imaging

- MRI/MRA of the entire aorta and arterial system if TTE imaging is inadequate or broader aortic or arterial disease is suspected.

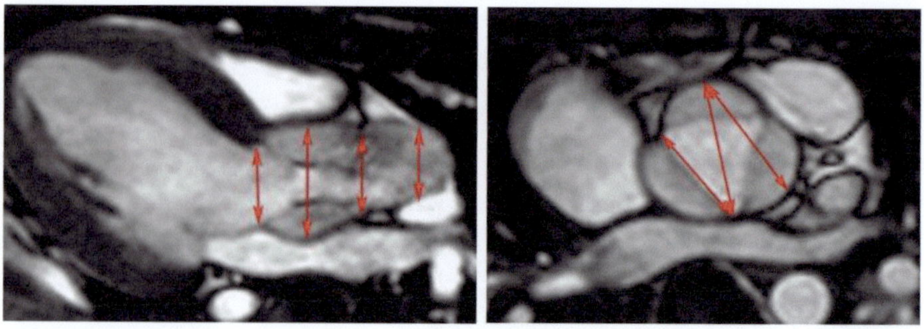

Fig. 3 Maximum aortic dimensions by MRI should be measured in peak systole in the equivalent long axis 3-chamber view at the levels of the aortic annulus, aortic root (AoR)/sinuses of Valsalva, sinotubular junction and ascending aortic (AAo) level, and widest commissure-commissure, cusp-commissure and cusp-cusp dimension measured in the orthogonal short axis view

- Aortic dimensions measured in an axis perpendicular to flow and compared to equivalent views by echocardiography (Fig. 3).
- Measurements routinely 2–4 mm more than echocardiography.
- Can document aortic/arterial tortuosity.
- CT/CTA preferred for acute AoD and peri-operative assessment.

11 Medical Therapy

- BBs reduce shearing stresses (lower dP/dt) on the aortic wall and reduce the risk of aortic dissection.
- ARBs attenuate TGFβ signaling, a signaling pathway heightened with deficiency of fibrillin-1.
- There is no role for angiotensin converting enzyme inhibitors and calcium channel blockers.
- In confirmed LDS, monotherapy or combination therapy is often started earlier with rapid aortic growth, progressive AI, or a malignant family history of aortic or arterial complications.
- BBs can be used in BAV-associated aortopathy and FTAAD with significant aortic dilatation and/or other risk factors for dissection; ARBs can also be used despite limited evidence (Table 1).

12 Medical Follow-Up

- Follow-up 6–12 months after initial assessment to determine the aortic growth rate.

Table 1 Medical therapy guidelines

	Child	Older adolescent/adult
MFS	Normal AoRz < 2—continue monitoring* Mildly dilated AoRz 2–3—consider medical therapy* Moderately dilated AoRz 3–4.5—start BB OR ARB Significantly dilated AoRz > 4.5—start BB AND ARB	Normal AoR < 35 mm**—continue monitoring* Mildly dilated AoR 35–40 mm**—consider medical therapy* Moderately dilated AoR 40–45 mm**—start BB OR ARB Significantly dilated AoR > 45 mm—start BB AND ARB
LDS	NormalAoRz/AAoz < 2—consider medical therapy* Mildly dilated AoRz/AAoz 2–3—start BB OR ARB* Moderately dilated AoRz/AAoz 3–4.5—start BB AND ARB Significantly dilated AoRz > 4.5—increase BB AND ARB doses	Normal AoR/AAo < 35 mm**—consider medical therapy* Mildly dilated AoR/AAo 35-40 mm**—start BB OR ARB* Moderately dilated AoR/AAo 40–45 mm**—start BB AND ARB Significantly dilated AoR > 45 mm—increase BB AND ARB doses
BAV	Normal AAoz < 2—continue monitoring* Mildly dilated AAoz 2–3—continue monitoring* Moderately dilated AAoz 3–4.5—consider medical therapy Significantly dilated AAoz > 4.5—start BB	Normal AAo < 35 mm**—continue monitoring* Mildly dilated AAo 35-40 mm**—continue monitoring* Moderately dilated AAo 40-45 mm**—consider medical therapy Significantly dilated AoR > 45 mm—start BB
FTAAD	Normal AoRz/AAoz < 2—continued monitoring* Mildly dilated AoRz/AAoz 2–3—consider medical therapy* Moderately dilated AoRz/AAoz 3–4.5—start BB Significantly dilated AoRz > 4.5—consider adding ARB	Normal AoR/AAo < 35 mm**—continue monitoring* Mildly dilated AoR/AAo 35–40 mm**—consider medical therapy* Moderately dilated AoR/AAo 40–45 mm**—start BB Significantly dilated AoR > 45 mm—consider adding ARB

* *Note 1* Medical therapy might be started earlier in the setting of rapid aortic growth ≥ 5 mm in 1 year or ≥ 3 mm/year in 2 consecutive years at any location, progressive AI, a malignant history of vascular events in the patient and/or other family members, and/or physician or patient preference
** *Note 2* AoR dimensions > 35 mm is considered dilated in most adults of normal stature, but may be up to 42 mm in adults of tall stature

- Exercise restrictions are mandatory, including the avoidance of heavy isometric exercise, competitive contact sports and activities involving sudden deceleration, particularly in high-risk patients with significant aortic dilatation.
- Management of pregnancy should occur in conjunction with a high-risk pregnancy clinic.

Table 2 Surgical indications for aortic repair

	Child*	Older adolescent/adult*
MFS	AoR/AAo $\geq$ 50 mm*	AoR/AAo/Arch/DAo/AbdAo $\geq$ 50 mm*
LDS	AoR/AAo $\geq$ 40–50 mm based on genetic variant*	AoR/AAo $\geq$ 40–50 mm based on genetic variant and Arch/DAo/AbdAo based on patient-specific factors*
BAV	AoR/AAo > 50–55 mm*	AoR/AAo > 50–55 mm*
FTAAD	AoR/AAo $\geq$ 45–50 mm based on genetic variant*	AoR/AAo $\geq$ 40–45 mm based on genetic variant and Arch/DAo/AbdAo based on patient-specific factors*
Turner syndrome	AoR/AAo size index > 25 mm/m^2	AoR/AAo size index > 25 mm/m^2

* Note 1: Surgical thresholds for aortic repair may be lowered in the setting of a malignant history of vascular events in the patient and/or other family members, with rapid aortic growth $\geq$ 5 mm in 1 year or $\geq$ 3 mm/year in 2 consecutive years, progressive AI, need for concomitant cardiac surgery, planned pregnancy, smaller stature, and/or physician or patient preference

13 Surgical Repair

- Aortic root replacement is based on AoRz and maximal aortic dimension thresholds (Table 2)
- Age, malignant family history, aortic growth, progressive AI, need for concomitant cardiac surgery, planned pregnancy, smaller stature, and surgeon or patient preference may all be indications for earlier surgery.

14 Surgical Strategy

- Valve sparing aortic root replacement is preferred.
- Ross procedure is contraindicated.
- Endovascular management is relatively contraindicated; may have a role in managing some descending thoracic and thoracoabdominal aortic aneurysms in other aortopathies.
- Aggressive surgical management of arterial aneurysmal disease in LDS is indicated, but usually reserved for life-threatening situations in vEDS due to increased risk of surgical complications.
- Aortic, mitral, tricuspid valve repair/replacement are as per standard indications.

15 Intensive Care Physiology and Management

- Important ICU considerations include:
  - Cervical spine instability in LDS.
  - Risk of pneumothorax in MFS, LDS, vEDS.
  - Sub-optimal respiratory physiology and mechanics due to pectus deformity, scoliosis and low muscle mass in MFS and LDS.
  - Once blood pressure is stable post-op, BB or ARB therapy should be restarted at ½ dose of one or other drug and can be gradually uptitrated to pre-op maintenance doses pre- and post-discharge.

Bibliography

1. Callewaert B, De Paepe A, Coucke P. Arterial Tortuosity Syndrome. In: Pagon RA, Adam MP, Ardinger HH, et al. editors. Seattle, WA: GeneReviews(R); 2014.
2. Isselbacher EM, Preventza O, Black JH 3rd, et al. 2022 ACC/AHA Guideline for the diagnosis and management of aortic disease: a report of the American Heart Association/American College of Cardiology joint committee on clinical practice guidelines. Circulation. 2022;146(24):e334–482.
3. Lacro RV, Dietz HC, Sleeper LA, et al. Atenolol versus losartan in children and young adults with Marfan's syndrome. N Engl J Med. 2014;371(22):2061–71.
4. Loeys BL, Dietz HC, Braverman AC, et al. The revised Ghent nosology for the Marfan syndrome. J Med Genet. 2010;47(7):476–85.
5. MacCarrick G, Black JH 3rd, Bowdin S, et al. Loeys-Dietz syndrome: a primer for diagnosis and management. Genet Med. 2014;16(8):576–87.
6. Michelena HI, Corte AD, Prakash SKA, et al. Bicuspid aortic valve aortopathy in adults: incidence, etiology, and clinical significance. Int J Cardiol. 2015;201:400–7.
7. Milewicz DM, Guo, D Regalado E. Thoracic aortic aneurysms and aortic dissections. In: Murray MF, Babyatsky MW, Giovanni MA, et al., editors. Clinical genomics: practical applications in adult patient care, 1st edn. McGraw Hill
8. Pepin M, Schwarze U, Superti-Furga A, Byers PH. Clinical and genetic features of Ehlers-Danlos syndrome type IV, the vascular type. N Engl J Med. 2000;342(10):673–80.
9. Pitcher A, Spata E, Emberson J, et al. Angiotensin receptor blockers and β blockers in Marfan syndrome: an individual patient data meta-analysis of randomised trials. Lancet. 2022;400(10355):822–31.

Approach to Genetic Evaluation in Children with Heart Disease

Laura Zahavich and Seema Mital

Abstract We describe the approach to the genetic evaluation of children with heart disease with a focus on congenital heart disease, cardiomyopathies, and inherited arrhythmias. Indications, types of genetic tests, yield of genetic tests, clinical utility of genetic test results, and importance of pre- and post-test counseling are described. The genetics of the subtypes of each condition and genetic-guided management or gene therapies are out of scope.

Keywords Genetics · Congenital heart disease · Cardiomyopathy · Channelopathy · Genetic counseling

Abbreviations

CHD	Congenital heart disease
CMA	Chromosome microarray analysis
CNV	Copy number variants
FISH	Fluorescent in situ hybridization
VUS	Variant of unknown significance
WES	Whole exome sequencing
WGS	Whole genome sequencing

L. Zahavich
Department of Genetic Counselling, Labatt Family Heart Centre, Hospital for Sick Children, University of Toronto, Toronto, ON, Canada

Department of Molecular Genetics, Labatt Family Heart Centre, Hospital for Sick Children, University of Toronto, Toronto, ON, Canada

L. Zahavich
e-mail: Laura.zahavich@sickkids.ca

S. Mital (✉)
Labatt Family Heart Centre, Department of Paediatrics, Hospital for Sick Children, University of Toronto, Toronto, ON, Canada
e-mail: Seema.mital@sickkids.ca

© The Author(s), under exclusive license to Springer Nature Switzerland AG 2024

A. I. Dipchand et al. (eds.), *Manual of Cardiac Care in Children*,
https://doi.org/10.1007/978-3-031-70973-9_46

Key Points

- Clinical genetic evaluation should be offered to affected individuals with cardiomyopathy, arrhythmic disorders, congenital heart disease (CHD) with a suspected genetic etiology (e.g., familial disease, suspected chromosomal or microdeletion syndromes), and some isolated CHD with strong genetic associations.
- For congenital heart defect patients, chromosomal microarray is the first line genetic test.
- For cardiomyopathies and channelopathies, multi-gene panel testing is the first line test for new diagnoses.
- A genetic diagnosis can aid in recurrence risk counseling, prenatal counseling, and genetic-guided therapies in some cases.
- A positive genetic finding in the proband can be used for genetic screening to identify asymptomatic family members at risk for developing cardiomyopathy or inherited arrhythmias.
- Genetic testing should be offered in the context of appropriate genetic counselling.

1 Glossary

- Pathogenic or likely pathogenic variant**:** A variant considered to be disease causing by the laboratory based on several criteria including the type of variant, rarity in ethnicity-matched control populations, conservation among species, replication in other affected individuals, predicted damaging, segregation with disease or de novo inheritance.
- Variant of uncertain significance (VUS): A variant where there is insufficient or conflicting evidence for the laboratory to classify as either benign or pathogenic. Should not be used for predictive testing of unaffected family members.
- Benign variant: A variant which does not appear to have a deleterious impact on gene function and/or is too frequent in the general population to be deemed pathogenic.
- Secondary findings: Disease-causing variants in genes unrelated to the primary condition but that may be associated with other medical conditions.

2 Introduction

- Understanding the genetic etiology of heart disease is important in the care of affected children and families.
- Clinical geneticists and genetic counsellors working closely with cardiologists are important in order to provide genetic services to patients.

3 Background

3.1 Congenital Heart Disease

- Congenital heart disease (CHD) has a complex etiology including genetic or environmental factors or gene-environment interactions.
- Occurs in conjunction with extra-cardiac congenital anomalies in ~ 25–40% of cases (i.e., syndromic).
- ~ 20% cases have a positive family history of CHD suggesting an inherited component.
- CHD is sporadic in the remainder, consistent with de novo variants, oligogenic inheritance, or non-genetic etiology.
- While most CHD is autosomal dominant, autosomal recessive or X-linked inheritance can also occur.
- In the absence of an identified genetic cause, recurrence risk is ~ 3–4% for most CHDs in subsequent offspring.
- Several hundred genes have been implicated in causing CHD.

3.2 Cardiomyopathies

- Cardiomyopathies are the most common cardiovascular genetic disorder.
- Cardiomyopathy is inherited in a third of cases and is sporadic in the remainder.
- While the majority are autosomal dominant, others have autosomal recessive or X-linked inheritance, or can occur due to mitochondrial defects.
- Over a hundred genes have been implicated in causing cardiomyopathies.

3.3 Channelopathies

- Channelopathies are heritable arrhythmic disorders with structurally normal hearts (e.g., long QT syndrome, Brugada syndrome, catecholaminergic polymorphic ventricular tachycardia).
- While the majority are autosomal dominant, others have autosomal recessive or X-linked inheritance.

Table 1 Components of a genetic evaluation

Components of evaluation	When to refer to Clinical Genetics and consider genetic testing?
3 generation family history	• Other first or second-degree relatives with CHD, cardiomyopathy, or birth defects • Any unexplained death (relevant for cardiomyopathy, channelopathy) • Neuromuscular disorder (relevant for cardiomyopathy) • Consanguinity • 2 or more pregnancy losses • One or more 2nd trimester or later miscarriages
Medical history and physical examination	• Dysmorphic facial features • Extra-cardiac congenital anomalies • Unexplained intrauterine growth restriction • Failure to thrive, short stature • Developmental delay, intellectual disability, mental retardation and/or abnormal neurological examination
Some isolated CHD	• Interrupted aortic arch, truncus arteriosus, Tetralogy of Fallot, Pulmonary atresia • Ventricular septal defect with arch anomaly • Isolated arch anomalies including right aortic arch • Supravalvar aortic stenosis • Hypoplastic left heart syndrome, bicuspid aortic valve • Heterotaxy/Isomerism
Recurrence risk counselling	• Parents and older children reaching adulthood and inquiring about offspring risk

4 Genetic Evaluation

- Genetic evaluation is an integral part of the medical evaluation of all patients with childhood onset heart disease especially CHD, cardiomyopathies and suspected channelopathies, as well. Table 1 describes the components of a genetic evaluation and when to refer to clinical genetics.
- When evaluating a family pedigree, consider mode of inheritance (i.e., X-linked, consanguinity) as well as phenotypes suggestive of systemic disease to guide test choices; where possible, attempts should be made to obtain records on family members.

5 Approach to Genetic Testing

- The aim of genetic testing is to identify the underlying etiology of the disease.

- Genetic testing for diagnosis should be offered to a phenotype-positive patient first.
- Genetic counseling should be offered prior to genetic testing to discuss risks and benefits of testing, as well as to aid in the interpretation and outcomes of positive and negative test results.
- A confirmed genetic diagnosis can aid in recurrence risk counseling for future pregnancies, prenatal counseling, and genetic-guided therapies in some cases.
- In the case of fetal onset heart disease, families should be offered a referral to a prenatal genetics clinic for discussion of options for invasive prenatal genetic testing.

5.1 *Cardiomyopathy and Channelopathies*

- Genetic testing should be offered to the affected proband first.
- A positive genetic test in a patient with cardiomyopathy or channelopathy can inform cascade testing of asymptomatic first-degree family members to identify those at risk for future disease.
- Cascade or predictive testing should be offered to family members only if a positive result is found on genetic testing of the affected proband or index patient. Figure 1 shows the approach to genetic testing for cardiomyopathy or channelopathy.
- Genotype-positive, phenotype-negative family members at risk for developing cardiomyopathy or arrhythmias require ongoing clinical screening. There are no activity restrictions, and no role currently for pre-emptive pharmacotherapy in phenotype-negative patients at risk for cardiomyopathy.
- Multi-gene cardiomyopathy panel testing is usually the first line test for an affected proband with cardiomyopathy.
- Yield on genetic testing is highest in hypertrophic and arrhythmogenic cardiomyopathies and lower in dilated, non-compaction and restrictive cardiomyopathies. Yield on genetic testing is over 50% in most types of channelopathies.
- Consider the yield on testing when choosing a gene panel. For hypertrophic cardiomyopathy, a targeted panel should be done first. For all other cardiomyopathies, an expanded cardiomyopathy panel can be used as the first line test. A targeted panel should be considered first for channelopathies.

5.2 *CHD*

- Chromosome microarray analysis (CMA) is usually the first line test for a patient with CHD and has replaced karyotype or Fluorescent in situ hybridization for the diagnosis of a microdeletion/microduplication syndrome.
- Single or multi-gene CHD panel testing may be offered in non-syndromic CHD cases.

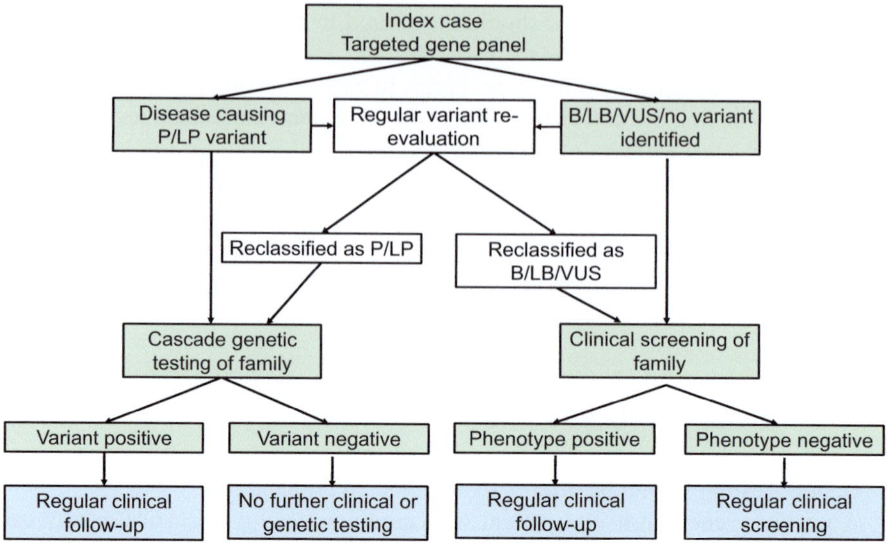

Fig. 1 Approach to genetic testing and family screening in cardiomyopathy or channelopathy*. The flowchart shows the approach to genetic testing of a cardiomyopathy or channelopathy proband and family members. P, pathogenic; LP, likely pathogenic; B, benign; LB, likely benign; VUS, variant of uncertain significance. *Reprinted from Circulation, Vol 142, Issue 25, Day SM, Ommen SR, Mital S,* et al., *2020 AHA/ACC HCM guidelines for the diagnosis and treatment for patients with hypertrophic cardiomyopathy, pp e558–e631, 2020, with permission from © American Heart Association Inc.*

- For CHD, the yield of genetic testing is highest in those with familial or syndromic disease although some isolated CHD lesions also have a strong heritable basis and may benefit from genetic testing (e.g., conotruncal malformations, supravalvar aortic stenosis, bicuspid aortic valve and left sided obstructive lesions, and heterotaxy/isomerism).
- Some CHD lesions with a genetic basis (e.g., left ventricular outflow tract lesions) can be associated with a spectrum of disease (e.g., bicuspid aortic valve, aortopathy). First-degree relatives should be offered echocardiographic screening for early detection of silent CHD.
- Given a higher recurrence risk in subsequent pregnancies, fetal echocardiographic screening should be offered to families with one or more affected children with CHD.

6 Principles of Genetic Counselling

6.1 Pre-test Counselling

- Should occur before ordering any genetic test and informed consent obtained from parents (assent from older children) for genetic testing.
- Discussion should include:
  - Reason for testing (e.g., confirm diagnosis, guide patient management, establish recurrence risk)
  - Type of test to be ordered (e.g., single or multi-gene panel, CMA, etc.) (Table 2)
  - Which conditions are being tested for and chances of secondary findings
  - Turnaround time to get test results
  - Risks (risk of genetic discrimination, loss of insurability, discovery of non-paternity).

6.2 Post-test Counselling

- If test result is positive i.e., detects a pathogenic or likely pathogenic variant in a relevant gene, it confirms the genetic basis for the disease and genetic counseling should include:
  - Recurrence risk counseling
  - Available options for cascade or predictive testing of other family members, if relevant
  - Options for prenatal and/or pre-implantation genetic diagnosis
  - Modification to patient management in cases of syndromic diagnosis
- If test result is negative i.e., no pathogenic or likely pathogenic variant is detected, a genetic cause cannot be ruled out. Whole exome or genome sequencing may be offered in selected cases. An empiric recurrence risk should be provided as well as recommendation for fetal echocardiogram in future pregnancies.
- If a VUS is detected, cascade testing of unaffected family members is not recommended, and standard clinical management and screening should continue. In some cases, parental testing of the VUS may be considered to assist with further variant interpretation e.g. a de novo finding may result in a VUS being upgraded a likely pathogenic or pathogenic variant.
- Families should be made aware that variant classification may change with time as new evidence emerges and this may change screening recommendation for family members. This variant re-interpretation is usually done by testing laboratories and/or geneticists or genetic counselors involved in patient follow-up.

Table 2 Types of genetic tests

Test	Format	Indications
Structural variants	**Cytogenetic testing**	
Karyotype	Profile of an individual's chromosome size, shape, and structure during cell division. Resolution = 5 Mb (e.g., 5 million nucleotides must be gained or lost to be visible as an abnormal karyotype on microscopy)	Any infant or child with the phenotype of a recognizable trisomy (e.g., trisomy 13,18, 21) or monosomy (e.g., 45X0 i.e. Turner syndrome) Suspected structural rearrangement
Fluorescent in situ hybridization (FISH)	Probe with fluorescence attaches to specific sequence if present. Can be done rapidly and detects submicroscopic deletions/duplications. Resolution ~ 35 kb	Any infant or child with the phenotype of a recognizable microdeletion syndrome if CMA not available
Chromosomal microarray (CMA)	Oligonucleotide array to detect presence or absence of chromosomal regions, microdeletions and microduplications across the genome	First line test for isolated complex CHD, multiple congenital anomalies, developmental delay, suspected deletion syndrome (e.g., 22q11.2 deletion, 7q11.23 deletion)
Sequence variants	**Sequencing**	
Targeted sequencing (single/multiple gene panel)	Test to detect changes in the sequence of nucleotides within a DNA molecule in a single gene or across multiple genes	Cardiomyopathies, inherited arrhythmogenic disorders and channelopathies, Marfan syndrome, RASopathies, familial congenital heart disease, heterotaxy/isomerism
Whole exome sequencing (WES)	Next generation sequencing to analyze coding regions (exons) of an individual's entire DNA sequence. Limited sensitivity to identify copy number variants	At least two of: (i) moderate to severe developmental delay, multisystem involvement, (ii) differential diagnosis requiring multiple panels, (iii) multiple affected family members, or (iv) consanguineous parents
Whole genome sequencing (WGS)	Analysis of an individual's entire DNA sequence including coding and non-coding regions, deep intronic variants, cryptic splice site variants, short structural variants and CNVs	At least two of: (i) moderate to severe developmental delay, multisystem involvement, (ii) differential diagnosis requiring multiple panels, (iii) multiple affected family members, or (iv) consanguineous parents

Table 3 Yield on genetic testing

Test	Methodology	Diagnostic Yield
Cardiomyopathy, arrhythmogenic cardiomyopathy	Sequencing	40–60%
Cardiomyopathy, dilated	Sequencing	10–15%
Cardiomyopathy, hypertrophic	Sequencing	30–50%
Channelopathy, Brugada syndrome	Sequencing	25–30%
Channelopathy, Catecholaminergic polymorphic ventricular tachycardia	Sequencing	55–65%
Channelopathy, long-QT syndrome	Sequencing	70–75%
Familial hypercholesterolemia	Sequencing	60–80%
Familial thoracic aortic aneurysm and dissection	Sequencing	25%
Congenital heart disease, syndromic	Sequencing and/or CMA	25–35% (Aneuploidy 14%, CNV 20%, Single gene 28%)
Congenital heart disease, non-syndromic	Sequencing and/or CMA	3–10% (CNV 5%, Single gene 5%)

Bibliography

1. Ackerman MJ, Priori SG, Willems S, et al. HRS/EHRA Expert Consensus Statement on the State of Genetic Testing for the Channelopathies and Cardiomyopathies. Heart Rhythm 2011;8(8):1308–1339
2. Fung A, Manlhiot C, Naik S, et al. Impact of prenatal risk factors on congenital heart disease in the current era. J Am Heart Assoc. 2013;2(3):e000064
3. Geng J, Picker J, Zheng Z, et al. Chromosome microarray testing for patients with congenital heart defects reveals novel disease causing loci ;and high diagnostic yield. BMC Genomics 2014;15(1):1127
4. Miller DT, Adam MP, Aradhya S, et al. Consensus statement: chromosomal microarray is a first-tier clinical diagnostic test for individuals with developmental disabilities or congenital anomalies. Am J Hum Genet. 2010;86(5):749–764
5. Musunuru K, Hershberger RE, Day SM, et al. Genetic Testing for Inherited Cardiovascular Diseases: A Scientific Statement from the American Heart Association. Circ Genom Precis Med. 2020;13(4):e000067
6. Ommen S, Mital S, Burke MA et al. AHA/ACC Guideline for the Diagnosis and Treatment of Patients with Hypertrophic Cardiomyopathy: A Report of the American College of Cardiology/American Heart Association Joint Committee on Clinical Practice Guidelines. Circulation 2020;142(25):e558–e631
7. Pierpont ME, Brueckner M, Chung WK, et al. Genetic Basis for Congenital Heart Disease: Revisited: A Scientific Statement from the American Heart Association. Circulation. 2018; 138(21):e653–e711
8. Song MS, Hu A, Dyamenahalli U et al. Extracardiac lesions and chromosomal abnormalities associated with major fetal heart defects: comparison of intrauterine, postnatal and postmortem diagnoses. Ultrasound Obstet Gynecol. 2009;33(5):552–559

Pulmonary Hypertension

Haley Christian and Andreea Dragulescu

Abstract Pulmonary arterial hypertension (PAH) in children carries a poor prognosis. There are multifactorial elements in pediatric pulmonary hypertensive vascular disease, including lung developmental abnormalities, genetic associations, pathological insults on a growing lung as well as other diseases and conditions. This chapter will focus on the most common presentations of pulmonary hypertension (PH) in children. The etiologic variety, clinical presentation and differences in outcomes require a unique, multidisciplinary approach to management.

Keywords Pulmonary hypertension · Pulmonary vascular disease · Vasoreactivity · Right heart failure · Lung transplantation

Abbreviations

ACD	Alveolar capillary dysplasia
BNP	B-type natriuretic peptide
BP	Blood pressure
BTT	Blalock Taussig Thomas
CHD	Congenital heart disease
ECMO	Extracorporeal membrane oxygenation
ERS	European respirology society
ESC	European cardiology society
FRC	Functional residual capacity
iNO	Inhaled nitric oxide

H. Christian
Department of Critical Care Medicine and Labatt Family Heart Centre, Hospital for Sick Children, University of Toronto, Toronto, ON, Canada
e-mail: Haley.christian@sickkids.ca

A. Dragulescu (✉)
Department of Paediatrics, Division of Cardiology, Labatt Family Heart Centre, Hospital for Sick Children, University of Toronto, Toronto, ON, Canada
e-mail: Andreea.dragulescu@sickkids.ca

© The Author(s), under exclusive license to Springer Nature Switzerland AG 2024

A. I. Dipchand et al. (eds.), *Manual of Cardiac Care in Children*,
https://doi.org/10.1007/978-3-031-70973-9_47

LV	Left ventricle
LVEDV	Left ventricular end diastolic volume
mPAP	Mean pulmonary artery pressure
PA	Pulmonary artery
PAH	Pulmonary arterial hypertension
PAP	Pulmonary artery pressure
PAPVC	Partial anomalous pulmonary venous connection
PAWP	Pulmonary arterial wedge pressure
PBF	Pulmonary blood flow
PDA	Persistent ductus arteriosus
PH	Pulmonary hypertension
PVOD	Pulmonary veno-occlusive disease
PVR	Pulmonary vascular resistance
PVRi	Pulmonary vascular resistance indexed
Qp	Pulmonary blood flow
Qs	Systemic blood flow
RA	Right atrium
RV	Right ventricle
RVEDP	Right ventricular end diastolic pressure
RVEF	Right ventricular ejection fraction
SaO2	Systemic arterial oxygen saturation
SVR	Systemic vascular resistance
V/Q	Ventilation/perfusion
VSD	Ventricular septal defect
WHO	World Health Organization
WU	Woods units

Key Points

- Pulmonary hypertension (PH) is the hemodynamic consequence of different mechanisms that affect the pulmonary circulation directly or indirectly, during fetal and postnatal periods, and resulting in elevated pulmonary pressures.
- The most prevalent etiologies in pediatric PH include idiopathic pulmonary arterial hypertention (PAH), PAH associated with congenital heart disease (CHD) and developmental lung diseases.
- PH associated with CHD represents highly heterogeneous subgroups.
- Given the diverse etiology on PH, a methodical and comprehensive diagnostic approach is essential for an accurate diagnosis and treatment plan.
- Management of PAH includes primarily pulmonary vasodilation therapies. In refractory PH with symptomatic heart failure and low cardiac output states, atrial septostomy, reversed Potts shunt and lung transplantation should be considered.

1 Definition

- The definition of PAH is based on invasive data, with a mean pulmonary artery pressure (mPAP) $\geq$ 20 mmHg at rest and pulmonary vascular resistance index (PVRi) $\geq$ 3WU*m2.
- Pulmonary arterial wedge pressure (PAWP), which measures the post-pulmonary capillary pressures, can be used to identify the anatomic source of the PAH.
  - A low PAWP ($\leq$15 mmHg) differentiates isolated pre-capillary PH from isolated post-capillary PH or combined pre- and post-capillary PH, both with PAWP > 15 mmHg.
- A standardized acute vasodilator testing is recommended to identify patients likely to respond to treatment, using oxygen and inhaled nitric oxide.
  - A positive test is defined by a decrease in mPAP by at least 10 mmHg with sustained cardiac output.
- Pulmonary arterial pressures (PAPs) are often reported in relation to systemic arterial pressures.
  - Normal PAPs are usually around 20% systemic.
  - PAH is a term generally applied to PAPs greater than 50% systemic.

2 Classification

- The clinical adult PH classification into 5 groups, updated in the last ESC/ERS guidelines, is also followed for pediatric PH, with some adaptations to include various cardiovascular and pulmonary diseases or specific pediatric conditions (Table 1).

3 Hemodynamic Principles

- From the fundamental axioms of fluid dynamics (conservation of mass, conservation of linear momentum and conservation of energy), we obtain principles that we can apply to cardiovascular hemodynamics:
- Resistance to flow through a tube is proportional to the length of the tube.
  - Example: a Blalock-Thomas-Taussig (BTT) shunt will provide higher resistance allowing better control of the pulmonary blood flow and protection of the pulmonary vasculature compared with a same diameter, but shorter persistent ductus arteriosus (PDA).
- Resistance to flow through a tube is exponentially inversely proportional to the radius of the tube or connection between cavities.

Table 1 Classification of Pulmonary Hypertension

Group 1. Pulmonary arterial hypertension • Idiopathic • Heritable • Associated with drugs and toxins • Associated with: – Connective tissue disease – HIV infection – Portal hypertension – ***Congenital heart disease (L-R shunts, Eisenmenger, postoperative PH)*** – Schistosomiasis • PAH with features of venous/capillary involvement • Persistent PH the of newborn
Group 2. PH associated with left heart disease • Heart failure • Valvular heart disease • ***Congenital/acquired cardiovascular conditions leading to post-capillary PH*** – Pulmonary vein stenosis – Cor triatriatum – Obstructed total anomalous pulmonary venous return – Mitral/aortic stenosis (including supra-/sub-valvar) – Coarctation of the aorta
Group 3. PH associated with lung diseases and/or hypoxia • Obstructive lung disease or emphysema • Restrictive lung disease • Lung disease with mixed restrictive/obstructive pattern • Hypoventilation syndromes • Hypoxia without lung disease (e.g. high altitude) • ***Developmental lung disorders (including bronchopulmonary dysplasia, congenital diaphragmatic hernia, Down Syndrome, alveolar capillary dysplasia, surfactant protein abnormalities, TBX4 mutations, pulmonary lymphangiectasia)***
Group 4. PH associated with pulmonary artery obstructions • Chronic thrombo-embolic PH or other pulmonary artery obstructions
Group 5. PH with unclear and/or multifactorial mechanisms • Haematological/systemic/metabolic disorders • ***Complex CHD (segmental PH, single ventricle, Scimitar Syndrome)*** • Chronic renal failure with or without haemodialysis • Pulmonary tumour thrombotic microangiopathy • Fibrosing mediastinitis

  - Example: pulmonary vasodilation (increased blood vessel radius) decreases pulmonary vascular resistance (PVR).

- The pressure gradient on either end of a flow resister (example a valve, stenotic vessel, or capillary bed) is proportional to the resistance to flow and the rate of flow.

- Example: the pressure gradient across a stenotic pulmonary vein increases as pulmonary blood flow increases, as occurs postnatally or with administration of pulmonary vasodilators or increased cardiac output.

- Pressure gradients are created by a resistor. If flow is through chambers or tubes that are separated by an unrestrictive connection, there will be no pressure gradient (i.e., chamber or tube pressures are equal).
  - Example: in an unrestrictive Ventricular Septal Defect (VSD), the pressure in the left ventricle (LV) and right ventricle (RV) are equal. So, in the absence of pulmonary valvar stenosis, the PAP will be, by definition, systemic. This alone does not infer small vessel PAH.
- Flow will always be directed proportionately towards the path of least resistance.
  - Example: in case of persistent fetal circulation in the newborn, with elevated PVR, there can be right to left systolic flow across a PDA.

4 Epidemiology

- Current epidemiological data is based on registry cohorts, and so potentially affected by selection bias.
- The estimated incidence of sustained PH in all categories in the US is 5–8 cases per million children per year with a prevalence of 26–33 per million children.
- The annual incident rate is higher when all "transient" PAH (i.e., persistent pulmonary hypertension of the newborn or repairable cardiac defect) cases are included:
  - 64 cases per million children (Dutch registry).
  - Transient PAH represented 82% of cases.
  - A third of the remaining cases had PH associated with developmental lung disease.
- PAH is a progressive pulmonary vascular disease that has poor prognosis and a median survival of < 3 years if untreated.
  - Predictors of outcome include diagnosis, WHO functional class, mPAP and PVRi.
  - PAH-targeted combination therapy is independently associated with improved transplant-free survival.

5 Diagnosis of PAH

5.1 Clinical Presentation

- In older children, shortness of breath, exercise intolerance, palpitations, syncopal or pre-syncopal episodes with exertion; more rarely hemoptysis
- Signs of right heart failure and/or low cardiac output state (distended jugular veins, abdominal distension, hepatomegaly, ascites, peripheral edema, prolonged capillary refill)
- Central, peripheral, or mixed cyanosis
- In the presence of a PDA: pre/post ductal saturation difference
- On cardiac auscultation: loud P2, systolic murmur of tricuspid regurgitation, diastolic murmur of pulmonary insufficiency

6 Investigations

6.1 ECG

- Right axis deviation, RV hypertrophy, arrhythmias

6.2 Chest X-ray

- Right atrium (RA), RV and pulmonary artery (PA) enlargement
- Decreased pulmonary blood flow: decreased vascularity (oligemic lung fields)
- Pulmonary edema/vascular congestion (in postcapillary PH): increased vascularity, bilateral diffuse interstitial patchy opacification (plethoric lung fields)

6.3 Echocardiogram

- Documents cardiac anatomy, identifies/rules out left sided lesions
- Estimates of pulmonary pressures:
  - Tricuspid regurgitation—peak velocity for estimation of RV systolic pressure in the absence of right ventricular outflow tract obstruction
  - Pulmonary insufficiency—peak early diastolic velocity for estimation of mPAP
- Presence and direction of shunts
  - Suprasystemic PH is associated with right to left shunting at the level of a VSD or PDA.

  - Elevated RVEDP secondary to high RV afterload and reduced right ventricular ejection fraction (RVEF) may promote right to left shunting through an atrial septal defect (ASD).
- RV size and function, RA size
  - PH is associated with RV hypertrophy, decreased RV systolic function, and increased RA size.
- LV size and function, septal curvature
  - PH is associated with septal flattening, or, in cases of suprasystemic PH, bowing of the ventricular septum into the LV.
  - PH is associated with decreased LV end diastolic volume (LVEDV).
- Presence of pericardial effusion

6.4 Cardiac Catheterization

- Right heart catheterization remains the gold standard for the definitive diagnosis and nature of PAH and provides useful data for risk stratification.
- It is important to calculate PVR and determine vasoreactivity (responsiveness to inhaled oxygen or nitric oxide).

7 Interpretation of Echo and Hemodynamic Data

- Care should be taken to understand the source and relevance of any measured value:
  - In the presence of an unrestrictive VSD, RVP will be systemic by definition. This does not infer elevated PVR.
  - A mPAP obtained in the context of low pulmonary blood flow (PBF) can be falsely reassuring. In other words, the PVR may be high, but this will only generate high mPAP if flow is also normal or high.

8 Additional Tests Part of a New PH Evaluation

- CTA chest can provide useful information related to lung disease and other specific diagnoses i.e., pulmonary embolism, alveolar capillary dysplasia (ACD), pulmonary veno-occlusive disease (PVOD)
- Serological markers, laboratory testing, liver ultrasound, lung function test, sleep study, genetic testing

- Invasive testing such as lung biopsy can also provide more definitive evidence of pathology such as ACD. Lung biopsy should be strongly considered for patients already undergoing surgical intervention for CHD when significant PAH or ACD is on the differential.

9 Treatment

- The treatment of PAH varies greatly with its etiology. In the presence of CHD, early diagnosis and "in window" treatment is essential for preventing early post-operative complications (PH crisis) as well as late development of PAH. This is particularly important in populations at higher risk, including premature babies or babies with Trisomy 21.
- The use of targeted PAH therapies in children is based mainly on expert opinion and adult data rather than evidence from pediatric clinical trials. The end goal of treatment is to improve survival and facilitate normal activities.
- Adjunctive therapy with diuretics, oxygen, anticoagulation and digoxin should be considered on an individual basis.
- Risk stratification will determine additional PAH specific therapy.
  - Important risk factors include WHO class III or IV, evidence of RV failure, BNP levels, and the presence of pericardial effusion.
  - Hemodynamic parameters that are associated with higher risk include mPAP/mSAP > 0.75, mRAP > 10 mmHg and PVRi > 20 WU·m^2.
- In lower risk patients, monotherapy with a PDE5 inhibitor (sildenafil, tadalafil) or an endothelin receptor antagonist (bosentan, ambrisentan) is recommended.
- Children with high risk and those deteriorating on monotherapy benefit from combination therapy.
- In high-risk patients, intravenous epoprostenol or treprostinil should be considered.
- It is important to consider early referral for lung transplantation and palliative bridges (atrial septostomy, reversed Potts) in deteriorating patients with high-risk features.

10 Indications for and Timing of Intervention/surgery

- Timing of catheter or surgical interventions in patients with PAH and CHD depends on the type of lesion and is discussed in the respective chapters.
  - Simple post-tricuspid shunt (VSD, PDA) with significant left to right shunt should ideally be performed within the first 6 months of life.

  - Simple pre-tricuspid shunts (ASD, partial anomalous pulmonary venous connection (PAPVC)) with significant shunt (Qp:Qs > 1.5) are usually done at preschool or school age.

- Patients with PAH-CHD and significant left to right shunt, congestive heart failure, and maintained SaO2 can be considered for closure in infancy.
- Out of window patients should undergo comprehensive assessment with right and left heart catheterization to determine operability and may require a period of PAH treatment (pulmonary vasodilator treatment and/or pulmonary arterial banding) followed by reassessment, before being considered for a high-risk surgery.

11 Critical Care Unit Management

- Especially in those with risk factors for PH, increased PVR can manifest in critically ill patients secondary to a variety of insults including cardiopulmonary bypass, infection, and severe systemic illness or shock.
- Management principles include supporting hemodynamics through reducing RV afterload and augmenting RV function.
- Pulmonary arterial line placement intraoperatively for continuous PAP monitoring post operatively can be a useful tool for patients at high risk of PH crisis.
- Central venous pressure via internal jugular lines or right atrial lines are more common, although indirect, markers of high PAP.

1) Reduce RV afterload:

  - Pulmonary vasodilation:

    Avoid hypoxia and increase FiO2.
    Aim for alkalosis via hyperventilation or bicarbonate administration (goal ph 7.4–7.5).
    Avoid exogenous catecholamines (via sedation/analgesia/paralysis/careful suctioning).
    Avoid hypothermia.
    Initiate inhaled nitric oxide (iNO).
    Systemic administration of pulmonary vasodilators can be useful to decrease PVR but in the context of pulmonary disease can also increase ventilation/perfusion (V/Q) mismatch. They can also cause systemic vasodilation and hypotension.

  - Lower mean airway pressure (MAP) by targeting functional residual capacity (FRC). This will minimize PVR by avoiding both atelectasis and pulmonary over-distension.

2) Support RV function

  - Inotropy (ie. epinephrine)

  - Increasing SVR, so long as the LV function is good, can improve RV function through mechanisms of ventricular interdependence. If the ventricular septum is bowing into the LV, a higher SVR will stent the septum back towards a more normal position which will improve LV preload.
  - Maintain coronary perfusion pressure.

12 Pulmonary Hypertensive Crisis

- Definition: sudden and dramatic increase in PVR with associated hemodynamic instability.
- The severe and acute increase in RV afterload can cause RV failure.
- The associated decrease in pulmonary blood flow and bowing of ventricular septum leftward affects LV preload and results in a sudden loss of cardiac output. In the presence of a residual shunt with potential right to left shunting (PDA, VSD, ASD), cardiac output may be preserved at the expense of systemic desaturation.
- Signs
  - Sudden onset
  - Associated with agitation/suctioning
  - Increased CVP/RAP/RVP, decreased systemic BP, tachycardia
  - Sudden decrease in end-tidal CO_2 (increased dead space ventilation)
  - Desaturation (in the presence of a right to left shunt)
- Acute Management
  - Lower PVR:

    Bag hyperventilate
    FiO_2 to 100%
    iNO at 20 ppm or greater
    Bolus HCO_3 (1 mmol/kg IV)
    Sedate and paralyze

  - Acutely support RV output

    Infusion $\pm$ bolus epinephrine
    Preload (volume)

  - If unable to rescue, consider extra-corporeal membrane oxygenation (ECMO).

13 Outcome

- In general, chronic PH represents a poor prognosis once the diagnosis is made.
- Prior to the availability of PAH targeted therapy, estimated median survival was ~ 3 years.

- With targeted treatment, the survival rate continues to improve with a current estimated 5 years survival rate ~ 70–75%.
- Patients with repaired CHD and PVOD have a lower survival than those with Eisenmenger Syndrome.

Bibliography

1. Berger RM, Beghetti M, Humpl T, et al. Clinical features of paediatric pulmonary hypertension: a registry study. Lancet. 2013;379(9815):537–46.
2. Hansmann G, Koestenberger M, Alastalo TP, et al. 2019 updated consensus statement on the diagnosis and treatment of pediatric pulmonary hypertension: the European pediatric pulmonary vascular disease network (EPPVDN), endorsed by AEPC, ESPR and ISHLT. J Heart Lung Transplant. 2019;38(9):879–901.
3. Humbert M, Kovacs G, Hoeper M, et al. 2022 ESC/ERS Guidelines for the diagnosis and treatment of pulmonary hypertension. Eur Heart J. 2022;43(38):3618–731.
4. Jone PN, Ivy DD, Hauck A, et al. Pulmonary hypertension in congenital heart disease: a scientific statement from the American Heart Association. Circ Heart Fail. 2023;16(7):e00080.
5. Li L, Jick S, Breitenstein S, et al. Pulmonary arterial hypertension in the USA: an epidemiological study in a large insured pediatric population. Pulm Circ. 2017;7(1):126–36.
6. Rosenzweig EB, Abman SH, Adatia I, et al. Paediatric pulmonary arterial hypertension: updates on definition, classification, diagnostics and management. Eur Respir J. 2019;53(1):1801916.
7. Zijlstra WMH, Douwes JM, Rosenzweig EB, et al. Survival differences in pediatric pulmonary arterial hypertension: clues to a better understanding of outcome and optimal treatment strategies. J Am Coll Cardiol. 2014;63(20):2159–69.

Anesthetic Management

Vannessa Chin

Abstract The anaesthetic management of the paediatric patient for cardiac surgery begins with a comprehensive preoperative assessment and optimization; this optimization involves a team approach, with input from the anaesthetist, cardiologist, cardiac surgeon and intensivist. This patient population may require multiple anaesthetics and the aim is to make each experience as atraumatic as possible for the patient and entire family; premedication is routine. Any special surgical considerations are clarified prior to anaesthetic induction. Intraoperative goals are to achieve an adequate level of anaesthesia, while maintaining haemodynamic stability, and adequate analgesia extending into the postoperative period, without respiratory compromise. The current widespread use of dexmedetomidine, and the multimodal approach to pain management, including regional anaesthesia, facilitate successful intraoperative extubation and seamless transition to ICU.

Keyword Paediatric cardiac anaesthesia

Abbreviations

ACE	Angiotensin converting enzyme
ACT	Activated coagulation time
AS	Aortic stenosis
BCPS	Bidirectional cavopulmonary shunt
BP	Blood pressure
BTT	Blalock Taussig Thomas
CHD	Congenital heart disease
CPAP	Continuous positive airway pressure
CPB	Cardiopulmonary bypass
CVP	Central venous pressure

V. Chin (✉)
Division of Paediatric Cardiac Anaesthesia, Department of Anaesthesia and Pain Medicine, The Hospital for Sick Children, University of Toronto, Toronto, ON, Canada
e-mail: Vannessa.chin@sickkids.ca

© The Author(s), under exclusive license to Springer Nature Switzerland AG 2024

A. I. Dipchand et al. (eds.), *Manual of Cardiac Care in Children*,
https://doi.org/10.1007/978-3-031-70973-9_48

DHCA	Deep hypothermic circulatory arrest
ECMO	Extracorporeal membrane oxygenation
ETT	Endotracheal tube
FFP	Fresh frozen plasma
HF	Heart failure
HLHS	Hypoplastic left heart syndrome
iNO	Inhaled nitric oxide
JET	Junctional ectopic tachycardia
LA	Left atrium
LAVVS	Left atrioventricualar valve stenosis
LIJV	Left internal jugular vein
LMWH	Low molecular weight heparin
LVOTO	Left ventricular outflow tract obstruction
MRSA	Methicillin resistant staphylococcus aureas
NiBP	Non-invasive blood pressure
NIRS	Near infrared spectroscopy
NPO	Nil per os
PEEP	Positive end expiratory pressure
PVR	Pulmonary vascular resistance
Qp	Pulmonary blood flow
Qs	Systemic blood flow
ROTEM	Rotational thromboelastometry
rVIIa	Recombinant factor VIIa
SVC	Superior vena cava
T21	Trisomy 21
TEE	Transesophageal echocardiogram
TOF	Tetralogy of Fallot
VAD	Ventricular assist device

Key Points

- Understand the anatomic, physiologic and psychosocial impact of congenital heart disease (CHD) for the child and family
- Account for other health issues and anomalies.
- Evaluate the haemodynamic and physiological impact of the planned procedure.
- Formulate an anaesthetic plan, including appropriate drugs, monitoring, special techniques and postoperative disposition of the patient.

1 Preoperative Assessment

- Understand the lesion and the proposed procedure

- Evaluate cardiac reserve and function
  - Heart failure (HF)
  - Cyanosis
  - Arrhythmia
  - Ischaemia
- Assess other anomalies and rule out intercurrent illness
- Evaluate medications, consider potential for drug interactions
  - Beta-blockers and anti-arrhythmic drugs should generally be continued
  - ACE inhibitors are generally withheld for pump cases
  - Coumadin can be withheld and converted to standard heparin (if clinically warranted). Rapid reversal in urgent/emergency situations with Vitamin K and human prothrombin complex or fresh frozeon plasma (FFP, see guidelines)
  - LMWH is withheld for 2 doses
  - ASA and clopidogrel are ideally withheld for a week and transitioned to LMWH or heparin infusion in high risk lesions
- Ascertain no adverse family/past medical history, e.g. bleeding, postoperative nausea and vomiting, allergy
- Ask about prior anaesthetic i.e. personal/family history of malignant hyperthermia or pseudocholinesterase deficiency, and pain experience where relevant
- Review CXR/echocardiogram/cardiac catheterization/head ultrasound/MRI etc.
- Review blood work, particularly as part of blood conservation strategy:
  - CBC, ferritin levels
  - Pre-operative iron therapy is routine, erythropoietin in special circumstances
- Evaluate the airway and assess appropriate sites for vascular access
- Preoperative anxiolysis is recommended for:
  - All children old enough to know that they are having heart surgery
  - Any child who will be upset by separation
  - Any child with a history of hypercyanotic spells (even if β-blocked).

2 Consent Discussion

- Premedication and NPO
- Vascular access and monitoring
- Pain management; consider patient controlled anesthesia for adolescents, regional anaesthesia
- Blood transfusion
- Early extubation/postoperative ventilation
- Risks and complications.

3 NPO and Premedication

- Routine NPO: Clear fluid (2 h), breast milk (4 h), formula (6 h), solids (8 h)
- Clear fluids should be encouraged in polycythaemic children until 2 h prior; or occasionally overnight or early morning admission for IV fluids
- Necessary oral medications should be given with a small amount of water.

3.1 Standard Premedication

- Midazolam 0.5–0.75 mg/kg po on call (syrup 3 mg/ml)
- Lorazepam 0.03–0.05 mg/kg sl one hour preoperatively (tablets).

3.2 Non-standard Premedication (Usually in Preop Area)

- Midazolam 0.3 mg/kg intranasal
- Dexmedetomidine 2–4 mcg/kg intranasal.

4 In the Operating Room

4.1 Monitoring

"Mechanical and electronic monitors are, at best, aids to vigilance."

- Standard non-invasive monitors
  - Pulse oximetry
  - ECG
  - NiBP (non-invasive blood pressure)
  - Temperature (nasopharyngeal/oesophageal and rectal)
  - End-tidal CO2
- NIRS (single forehead site for straightforward cases, bilateral for arch reconstruction, forehead and flank for single ventricle)
  - Pre-induction NIRS is recorded for baseline and trended (rather than absolute numbers) to guide management. Intermittent correlation with mixed venous saturations is recommended
  - Abrupt desaturations in NIRS can lead to early detection of SVC cannula obstruction. In arch reconstruction procedures, unilateral desaturation will prompt a check for aortic cannulation malposition.

- Invasive monitors depend on procedure:
  - Arterial pressure: quick ultrasound scan of radial/ulnar artery to ensure both present and pulsatile, larger vessel usually chosen for cannulation.

    R radial/ulnar artery for coartation repair and for cases with selective cerebral perfusion, L if right BTT shunt or aberrant right subclavian artery. Femoral arterial lines are avoided, especially in patients who will require multiple cardiac catheterizations, and brachial arterial lines (in our centre) are a last resort and should be removed as soon as possible. Rarely, both central (femoral) and peripheral (radial) arterial pressure monitoring are requested. For example, if a long pump run is anticipated and/or anticipated high vasopressor requirements, with potential dampening of the radial arterial line waveform and unreliable BP readings. Another example is potential residual arch gradient where direct BP measurement would be helpful; the surgeon is usually directly involved in this decision.
  - CVP, default is right internal jugular vein. Always scan both right and left neck prior to prepping and draping to ensure patency of the vessels. Be aware of rescue strategy for redo sternotomy or haemodynamic instability in infants; it may be preferable to use LIJV or subclavian if right neck cannulation for ECMO or CPB is likely.
  - Some centres avoid neck lines in single ventricle infants; alternatives include subclavian or femoral venous central lines or intracardiac lines.
- Check ultrasound results on repeat procedures for patency and size of groin and neck vessels
- Consider preoperative insertion of a cerebrospinal fluid drain in special cases: late coarctation, concerns about aortic dissection and spinal cord ischaemia. Neuromonitoring, including somatosensory and motor evoked potentials have been used by some centres to guide intraoperative haemodynamic management, and can also help set BP goals in the ICU postoperatively.

5 Induction of Anesthesia

- As with any major surgery, it is important to consider all the anaesthetic issues, including dosing of narcotics and sedatives and timing of extubation.
- Inhaled sevoflurane most frequently used if appropriate for haemodynamic goals
- Vascular access obtained at the earliest opportunity.
- Intravenous induction with topical analgesia if preferred by the patient as some dislike mask inductions; propofol, fentanyl, ketamine and midazolam in various combinations are commonly used.
- High dose fentanyl (30–50 μg/kg slowly) in neonates and patients with severely limited cardiac function.

- Remifentanil or Sufentanil infusions, combined with dexmedetomidine infusions, considered in OR extubation candidates.
- Rocuronium 1 mg/kg for muscle relaxation is routine.
- Dexmedetomidine is a short acting alpha-2 receptor agonist which inhibits central sympathetic outflow and reduces systemic norepinephrine release. This leads to improved haemodynamic stability and a favourable myocardial oxygen supply and demand balance. Its sympatholytic and anti-inflammatory properties may reduce the stress response to CPB. It has analgesic, anxiolytic and anti-delirium properties which make it an excellent option for OR extubation and transition to ICU.

6 Control of Airway and Appropriate Ventilation

- Cardiopulmonary interactions are clinically relevant in CHD e.g. Norwood procedure, Truncus arteriosus repair, Fontan procedure, late TOF
- Cardiac arrest risk from inappropriate ventilation is highest in Norwood and Truncus arteriosus: need to avoid high FiO_2 and hyperventilation (absolute or relative).
- Nasotracheal intubation in neonates and infants if prolonged postoperative course is anticipated, otherwise oral intubation is indicated.

7 Adjuvant Drugs

- Cefazolin
  - 30 mg/kg q4h (q6h for neonates), within 60 min of skin incision.
  - Vancomycin 15 mg/kg if β lactam allergic or if MRSA positive
- Tranexamic acid
  - For infants < / = 1 yr: 30 mg/kg bolus plus 16 mg/kg/hr.
  - For children > 1 yr: 10 mg/kg bolus plus 10 mg/kg/hr.
  - ½ dose may be repeated on initiation of CPB if an infusion is not used
- Benzodiazepines to prevent awareness (or inhaled sevoflurane/isoflurane). Dexmedetomidine may also be used
- Methylprednisolone
  - Intraoperative dosing for neonates/patients undergoing deep hypothermic circulatory arrest up to 30 mg/kg.
  - All heart transplant patients are consistently given 10–15 mg/kg on induction.

8 Surgical Time Out

- Prior to incision a surgical Time Out is completed to confirm the patient, procedure and surgical plan, proper positioning, availability and functionality of devices and/or implants, blood products, and administration of appropriate antibiotics.
- This involves confirming access to airway, lines and infusions.
- Any team member can highlight specific concerns or considerations relevant to patient care.

9 Maintenance of Anaesthesia and CPB

- Maintenance of anaesthesia using narcotics and sedatives is dictated by the patient's response to surgical stimulus, and haemodynamic robustness.
- Intraoperative Analgesia
  - Tailored to extubation plan—in OR vs early postop (<4 h) vs overnight intubation
  - Multimodal approach
- Infusions
  - Remifentanil 0.03–0.2 mcg/kg/min
  - Sufentanil 0.3–2 mcg/kg/hr
  - Dexmedetomidine 0.3–1 mcg/kg/hr
- Intravenous slow push
  - Ketamine 0.1–0.3 mg/kg
  - Hydromorphone 10–15 mcg/kg
  - Morphine 50–100 mcg/kg
  - Acetaminophen 10–15 mg/kg
  - Ketorolac 0.5 mg/kg if > 4 months, CPB < 2 ½ hrs, normal kidney function, no significant bleeding
- Regional analgesia/block
- Sternotomies:
  - Pecto-intercostal fascial plane block (aka superficial parasternal block)
  - Transversus thoracic muscle plane block (aka deep parasternal block)
- Thoracotomies:
  - Serratus anterior fascial plane block
  - Erector spinae plane block
- Inotropic support prior to CPB in elective procedures is unusual, except for mechanical support devices or transplants

- Heparin (400 units/kg) is given prior to cannulation for cardiopulmonary bypass (CPB)
- ACT and blood gas measurements are done 2.5 min after the heparin dose.
- Target ACT is 480 s
- Cannulation for CPB is often associated with haemodynamic fluctuations and occasionally with significant blood loss
  - May trigger hypercyanotic spells in TOF patients
  - Period of vigilance
  - Phenylephrine and volume should be administered as indicated.
  - Cardioversion may be required for arrhythmia (at this point internal paddles are used).

10 Establishing CPB

- Shared responsibility to confirm that CPB cannulas appropriately placed, connected and unclamped.
- As CPB is established watch for
  - Adequate perfusion via ECG, BP, NIRS
  - No SVC obstruction or cerebral congestion (i.e., high SVC), low cerebral NIRS
  - No issues with the pump
  - Turn off intravenous fluids
  - Discontinue ventilation once full CPB flows established; CPAP to lungs
- Therapeutic drug levels fall with dilution by the prime
  - Supplemental narcotic required
  - A minimum dose of vapour or sedative to avoid awareness
  - Repeat muscle relaxant is important if DHCA is contemplated and ice to the head
  - An additional bolus of tranexamic acid if an infusion is not running.

11 Weaning from CPB

- CPB weaned when repair completed and obvious suture deficiencies addressed
- The pleural spaces should be suctioned, if open
- The patency and positioning of the endotracheal tube is verified, and ventilation parameters ascertained with an appropriate FiO2
- ETT suctioned, especially after pulmonary artery surgery or concerns of pulmonary hypertension, or if inadequate lung expansion. Often prudent to establish baseline in cases of potential LA hypertension
- Nasopharyngeal Temperature > 35.5 C; key is to avoid hyperthermia

- Ensure adequate perfusion with sinus or paced rhythm
- Assess ventricular function and provide inotropic and/or vasopressor infusions, as needed, via relevant catheters
- Appropriate haematocrit and blood gases (this will vary depending on the lesion)
- Empty suction and Foley drainage
- TEE probe appropriately placed (care with oral ETT, small infants < 3 kg).

11.1 Monitor and Manage

- Haemodynamic status
  - Rate, rhythm
  - Preload, contractility (use echo as a guide), blood pressure
  - Oxygenation, ventilation, NIRS
- Effects of TEE
  - Tracheal compression with effects on tidal volume, airway pressure
  - Effects on BP which can be real or factitious—occasional compromise of LA filling
- Bleeding
  - Should go back to CPB circuit to allow for greater transfusions until protamine delivered
  - Modified ultrafiltration can also cause changes in preload but generally improves haemodynamics
- Direct pressure measurements may be made to confirm TEE findings (most commonly in the context of Tetralogy repair) or resolve uncertainty.
- Intracardiac samples can be taken to calculate Qp:Qs—preferable to have as low an FiO_2 as tolerated.

12 Post-CPB

- Protamine is given when:
  - Acceptable repair
  - Haemodynamically stable
  - Bleeding controllable
- Dose is determined by point-of care system
- Protamine reactions in children are very rare, but have been documented, so should still be cautious when administering.

12.1 Volume Replacement and Management of Bleeding

- Cell saved or modified ultrafiltered blood is transfused
- Bleeding is occasionally catastrophic so adequate resources appropriate for size are needed. Rapid infusion device may be needed for adolescents or young adults
- Hypovolaemia may not be tolerated well; but the same applies to rapid transfusion.

12.2 Post Operative Transfusion Therapy (Patients Who are not Bleeding Do not Need Blood Products)

- ACT post protamine administration to ensure adequate heparin reversal
- Rotational thromboelastometry (ROTEM) guided therapy as needed
- Platelets for count < 100,000 and/or ongoing bleeding: 10–15 mL/kg
- Cryoprecipitate/FFP/fibrinogen concentrate for fibrinogen < 1.5 g/L and ongoing bleeding
- Cell saved red blood cells have a hematocrit of 0.9 so polycythaemia is a hazard
- Human prothrombin complex and rarely recombinant factor VIIa (rVIIa) have both been used in persistent coagulopathic bleeding
- Consider 1/2 bolus dose of tranexamic acid for CPB runs > 2 1/2 hours.

12.3 Haemodynamic and Metabolic Therapy

- Glucose supplementation is sometimes needed for neonates and infants *(less common with Del Nido cardioplegia)*
- Calcium is frequently required after platelets and FFP
- Lactate levels usually fall after weaning from CPB if cardiac output is reasonable
- ABGs are frequently abnormal: atelectasis is common, and PEEP is helpful.

12.4 Haemodynamically Significant Pulmonary Hypertension

- At risk patients: hyperventilate and alkalinize the patient to pH 7.5 coming off
- Minimize atelectasis and make sure pleural spaces are empty
- FiO2 80%
- iNO 20 ppm
- Keep systemic BP up.

13 Commonly Used Inotropes and Vasoactive Drugs

- Epinephrine 0.02–0.2 μg/kg/min
- Norepinephrine 0.02–0.2 μg/kg/min
- Vasopressin 0.1–1 mu/kg/min has the advantage of not increasing myocardial O_2 consumption, unlike catecholamines, and does not increase PVR
- Milrinone 50 μg/kg as a bolus on CPB unless vasopressors were required on CPB or there is concern about residual lesions, (e.g., LVOTO including AS and arch, LAVVS). For these lesions, once all clear on echo, bolus 50 μg/kg over 20 min if haemodynamics permits. Infusion 0.5-1 μg/kg/min.
- Nitroprusside 0.5–6 mcg/kg/min for hypertension; a combination with low dose esmolol to offset tachycardia works well.

13.1 Antiarrhythmics (Rarely are Necessary)

- Amiodarone 5 mg/kg slow bolus plus infusion 5–15 μg/kg/min for incessant tachyarrhythmia
- Esmolol 500 μg/kg bolus plus infusion 50–300 μg/kg/min for tachyarrhythmia and blood pressure control if function allows
- Electrophysiology consult in the OR may be warranted.

14 Emergence and Transfer to CCCU

14.1 Indications and Considerations for OR Extubation

- Improves haemodynamics in right sided heart pathology, e.g. TOF (restrictive physiology), BCPS, Fontan, heart transplants, VADs
- May reduce sedation requirements and associated hypotension
- May reduce ICU length of stay.

14.2 Contra-Indications for OR Extubation

- Preexisting respiratory failure
- Airway issues (most commonly T21)
- Bleeding
- Haemodynamic instability including tachyarrhythmia (JET)
- Hypothermia < 35 °C
- Surgeon preference.

14.3 Transfer to CCCU

- Adequate analgesia especially if extubated
- Fluid hanging (or syringes for infants and smaller children) and blood products in cooler
- Invasive monitoring as in the OR
- Oxygen/air blender for respiratory support of HLHS and BTT shunt.

14.4 Handover

- Protocolized handover at SickKids is initiated by the Anaesthesia team, followed by the surgeon's description of the actual surgery performed. Patient remains under the care of the anaesthesia team until handover is complete.
- Transfer the patient to ICU monitors
- Establish adequate ventilation
- Standardized and organized handover to facilitate care
  - Name, weight, diagnosis, past medical history, allergies
  - Airway, vascular access, intraoperative course, residual lesions as identified by echo, optimal CVP, intravenous infusions, transfusions, and blood loss
  - Concerns and ongoing issues
  - Analgesia and antibiotics
  - Arrhythmia and pacemaker settings (if appropriate)
  - Most recent labs, peak and most recent lactate ± mixed venous saturation
- Goal is to relay any and all pertinent information to guide ICU management.

Acknowledgements The author would like to thank Dr. Helen Holtby MBBS, FRCPC for their contributions to this chapter.

Bibliography

1. Andropoulos DB, Stayer SA, Mossad EB, Miller-Hance WC, editors. Anesthesia for congenital heart disease. 3rd ed. London: Wiley-Blackwell Oxford; 2015.
2. Da Cruz EM, Ivy D, Jaggers J, editors. Pediatric and congenital cardiology, cardiac surgery and intensive care. 1st ed. London: Springer-Verlag; 2014.

Cardiovascular Perfusion

Lynn Crawford-Lean and Celeste Foreman

Abstract Cardiopulmonary bypass (CPB) in congenital heart disease offers particular challenges due to both the size and age-range of the patients as well as the spectrum of morphology in both arterial and venous arrangements, which can require specific cannulation strategies. Patients with cyanotic circulations need careful attention to Haematocrit management. CPB is very safe in children and the focus is on reducing the morbidity associated with pediatric surgery and CPB: the systemic inflammatory response, the effects of hypothermia, altered perfusion, hemodilution, acid-base management and embolization. Infants and neonates present additional challenges due to their small size, immature organ systems and altered physiology—they have a higher metabolic rate requiring higher pump flow rates per kg compared to an adult, and an impaired thermoregulatory response with greater dependence upon environmental temperature. Current perfusion management is characterised by extensive monitoring systems, smaller volume components and minimising inflammatory responses with techniques such as modified ultrafiltration.

Keywords Cardiopulmonary bypass · Perfusion · Heart–lung machine · Cardioplegia · Modified ultra-filtration: pH stat · Alpha-stat · Deep hypothermic circulatory arrest · Selective antegraded cerebral perfusion · Near infra-red spectroscopy

Abbreviations

ACT	Activated coagulation time
ASD	Atrial septal defect
BCPS	Bidirectional cavopulmonary shunt

L. Crawford-Lean · C. Foreman (✉)
Perfusion Services, Labatt Family Heart Centre, Hospital for Sick Children, Toronto, Ontario, Canada
e-mail: Celeste.foreman@sickkids.ca

L. Crawford-Lean
e-mail: Lynn.crawfordlean@sickkids.ca

© The Author(s), under exclusive license to Springer Nature Switzerland AG 2024

A. I. Dipchand et al. (eds.), *Manual of Cardiac Care in Children*,
https://doi.org/10.1007/978-3-031-70973-9_49

CaCl	Calcium chloride
CHD	Congenital heart disease
CPB	Cardiopulmonary bypass
CPS	Cardioplegia solution
CUF	Conventional ultrafiltration
DHCA	Deep hypothermic circulatory arrest
FP	Frozen plasma
HCT	Hematocrit
HLHS	Hypoplastic left heart syndrome
HLM	Heart–lung machine
iCal	Ionized calcium
MUF	Modified ultrafiltration
PLA A	Plasmalyte A
PRBC	Packed red blood cells
TAPVC	Total anomalous pulmonary venous connection
TOF	Tetralogy of Fallot
VSD	Ventricular septal defect

Key Points

- Cardiopulmonary bypass (CPB) is integral to all intra-cardiac surgery and extensive aortic arch surgery
- Congenital heart disease (CHD) offers specific challenges due to great variation in patient size, physiology and anatomy, often requiring specific cannulation strategies.
- Management is focused on minimising inflammatory response and high-fidelity monitoring systems to optimise end-organ function
- Cardioplegia protocols allow the heart to be safely arrested in diastole
- Deep hypothermic circulatory arrest (DHCA) may be needed for aortic arch surgery or for complex intracardiac surgery in neonates/small infants.
- Alpha-stat acid-base management is the most widely used.

1 Introduction

Cardiopulmonary bypass (CPB) is essential for any intra-cardiac surgery as well as most surgery on the aortic arch and is used in >90% of all index cardiac procedures. Modern pump systems and components have made CPB extremely safe, and the focus is now on minimising the inflammatory response and maximising monitoring systems to avoid end-organ injury/morbidity. Complex surgery, especially in neonates or involving the aortic arch may require periods of circulatory arrest or low flow which are made possible by using core cooling to moderate (28–32 °C) or deep (18–22 °C) hypothermia.

2 Heart–Lung Machine (HLM)

The following parameters are measured/monitored by the heart–lung machine and associated adjunct equipment:

- Arterial line pressure
- Blood flow (total pump flow and patient blood flow)
- Circuit venous, arterial, and heater/cooler water temperature
- Bypass, aortic cross-clamp, circulatory arrest, and other elapsed times
- Sweep gas flow (O_2 and CO_2), % isoflurane, FiO_2. These gases flow across the oxygenator to oxygenate the blood and clear away CO_2, the flowrate is referred to as the 'sweep'.
- Cardioplegia volumes, delivery pressure and temperature

The following servo-regulated alarms are engaged during bypass:

- Arterial and cardioplegia line pressure
- Low blood level detector
- Arterial and cardioplegia air emboli detector

Roller-pump designs are the most widely used HLM, but centrifugal pumps can be used.

3 Circuit Selection

- Choice of venous and arterial lines, boot and and oxygenator based on paediatric age group is summarized in Table 1.

Table 1 Line and equipment choices based on age

Circuit	Weight range	Venous line	Arterial line	Boot	Oxygenator
Newborn	Up to 8kg	1/4″	3/16″	1/4″ or 3/16″	Capiox FX05
Infant	8–11 kg	1/4″	1/4″	1/4″	Capiox FX05
Child	12–25 kg	3/8″	1/4″	3/8″	Capiox FX15/R30
Paediatric	25–65 Kg	3/8″	3/8″	3/8″ <35 kg 1/2″ >35kg	Capiox FX15/R30, FX25
Adolescent	>65Kg	1/2″	3/8″	1/2″	Capiox FX25

Table 2 Sample final prime components

Circuit	Newborn <8 kg	Infant 8–11 Kg	Child 12–25 Kg	Paediatric	Adolescent
Plasmalyte A	50 mls	50 mls	350–600 mls	600 mls	750 mls
PRBC	75 mls	75 mls	*	*	*
FP	75 mls	0–75 mls	0	0	0
25% albumin	20 mls	20–40 mls	60 mls	100 mls	100 mls
20% mannitol	0.25 g/kg	0.25 g/kg	0.25 g/kg	0.25 g/kg	0.25 g/kg
8.4% $NaHCO_3$	5 mEq	5 mEq	7–12 mEq	12–15 mmol	15–20 mmol
Sterile H_2O	25 mls	25 mls	0	0	0
Heparin	1000 iu	1200 iu	1400 iu	2400 iu	4000 iu
10% CaCl	50 mmol	30–50 mmol	20–50 mmol	0	0
Cefazolin	30 mg	34 mg	42 mg	90 mg	120 mg
Total prime volume (approx.)	250 mls	280 mls	350–600 mls	750 mls	1000 mls

* May require the addition of PRBC to ensure minimum hematocrit of 0.25 while on bypass

4 Bypass Circuit Priming

Each institution will have developed their own preferred crystalloid solutions. The following is the protocol used at the Hospital for Sick Children, Toronto (Table 2):

- Once assembled, the bypass circuit is primed with plasmalyte A (PLA A)
- Additional components are added with the goal of achieving a physiologic prime composition

  All primes include (unless contraindicated due to allergy, etc): PLA A, 8.4% $NaHCO_3$, 4 iu heparin/ ml of priming volume, 0.25 g mannitol/kg body weight, 30 mg cefazolin/250 mls of prime volume, 10% CaCl (to target iCal of 0.3–0.5 mmol/L in prime)

5 Cannulation

- Typical cannulation is an aortic/bicaval configuration
- Single venous cannulation may be used in the absence of an intra-atrial/ventricular communication, or if no plan to open the heart (eg aortic arch repair, aortic valve replacement)

- During DHCA, antegrade cerebral perfusion may be implemented via cannulation of the innominate artery or utilising a Goretex graft anatomosed to the innominate artery.
- In cases of interrupted aortic arch, two arterial inflows are required (one to ascending aorta, one via the ductus arteriosus. The duct must be snared around the cannula to prevent run-off into the lungs)
- In neonates with HLHS the ascending aorta is usually too small to cannulate. Arterial perfusion is either through a Goretex graft onto the innominate artery or direct cannulation of the ductus.

6 Conduct of bypass

6.1 Safety

- A 50-item pre-bypass safety checklist is completed following circuit assembly and priming, prior to the initiation of bypass (See Table 3)

6.2 Anticoagulation management

- Loading heparin doses: 450 iu/kg for patients <1 month of age; 400 iu/kg for all other patients
- Activated coagulation time (ACT) target for initiation and maintenance of bypass: >480 s
- In case of failure to achieve adequate ACT (eg. low antithrombin III), supplementary dose of 100–150 u heparin/kg is given
- 10 mls/kg frozen plasma (FP) administered to patients who do not achieve ACT > 400 s following loading dose and supplementary dose
- Prime dose: 4 IU heparin/ml of prime volume
- Heparin management while on bypass:

    ACT 400–500 s, 100 iu/kg bolus dose
    ACT <400s, 150 iu/kg bolus dose

- ACT measured q30 minutes or more frequently, as required

6.3 Hemodynamic Management

6.3.1 CPB Blood Flow Rate

- Neonates: up to 200 ml/kg/min

Table 3 Perfusion safety checklist

Patient/case assessment	•
Review patient chart and history including allergies	
Blood products checked and computer charting initiated	
ACT baseline performed	
Supplies and hardware inspection	
Perfusion supplies checked	
Sterile integrity of component packaging confirmed	
All clamps and holders secured	
Electrical components ad connectors checked	
Flashlight and hand cranks available (in event of total power loss)	
Clamps available (ten)	
Heater-cooler functioning and water level is full	
Integrity of gas lines and high-pressure gas hoses checked	
Oxygen flowmeter and blender functioning	
Vapouriser for anesthetic gas is in line and currently switched off	
System check	
Arterial pump-head calibrated to correct tubing size	
Fine calibration set for 1/4 and 3/8 inch tubing	
All pump heads (bypass pump and suckers) set to correct tubing size	
Cardioplegia module set to correct ratio (4:1 cardioplegia:blood for del Nido cardioplegia)	
Cardioplegia pump is stop linked to the arterial line	
Pressure transducers all zeroed, and pressure limits set	
Cardiotomy venous reservoir is vented	
All tubing is correctly mounted into the raceway on the pump heads	
All tubing connections are secured and cable-tied where necessary	
All one-way valves and stopcocks are correctly positioned	
Gas tubing with filter securely connected	
Gas exhaust port is unobstructed and scavenged with vacuum on	
Water lines primed and oxygenator checked for any water leakage	
Priming completed and all bubbles removed	
Priming of arterial filter complete	
Sampling ports ad pressure lines have been primed and bubble-free	
Cardioplegia primed, bubble-free and occlusion set	
Occlusion set on all pump-heads	
All temperature probes connected and functional	
Control panel checked. Bubble detector checked	
Low level alarm checked	
In-line continuous sensors calibrated, secured and functioning	

(continued)

Table 3 (continued)

Transonic flowsensor attached and zeroed	
Pre-initiation of bypass check	
All medications checked and added to the prime	
All rollerheads revolving in correct direction (counter-clockwise)	
Check suckers are all working	
Vent line open to gravity and checked	
Cardioplegia line connected and clamped	
Alarms operational and engaged (bubble alarm and level alarm)	
Heater-Cooler temperature set	
Manifold sampling lines off	
Arterial filter-line purge is closed	
Pump off and venous line clamped	
Arterial line occlusive—i.e. holds a constant positive pressure	
FiO_2 is set and gas is off	
Circuit lines kink-free and checked for connections	
ACT >480 s	

- Newborns: up to 150 ml/kg/min
- 7–10 kg: 100–120 ml/kg/min
- Over 10 kgs: BSA x 2.4–3.2 L/min/m^2
- Adolescents: BSA x 2.2–2.4 L/min/m^2 in a normothermic patient.
- Blood flow rate may be slightly decreased if hypothermia is employed.
- Blood flow rate recommendations are guidelines and will vary based on patient indicators of adequacy of perfusion such as venous saturation (>60%), cerebral saturation, pH, lactate etc.
- Selective antegrade cerebral perfusion blood flow rate is delivered at 35–50 mls/kg/min

6.3.2 Blood Pressure

- Mean arterial pressure (MAP) targets:

  0–6 months: 35–45 mmHg
  6 m–2 years: 40–50 mmHg
  2–12 years: 40–55 mmHg
  Over 12 years: 50–65 mmHg

- Central venous pressure (CVP) should be at or near zero on bypass

6.3.3 Near Infrared Spectroscopy (NIRS)

- NIRS is used increasingly to provide additional monitoring of brain and systemic perfusion:
- Baseline cerebral NIRS measurements performed during induction of anaesthesia.
- Cerebral and flank NIRS monitored during DHCA
- During CPB, cerebral NIRS should be maintained close to baseline with minimum acceptable drop of no more than 20%
- The following are considered to optimize cerebral NIRS while on bypass: aortic and/or SVC cannula position, hematocrit, blood flow rate, MAP, PaCO2, adequacy of anaesthesia and good probe contact

6.3.4 Blood Gas Management

- There are two different methods of pH management when cooling patients on CPB. 'Alpha stat' allows the pH to naturally increase during cooling, whereas 'pH stat' actively adds CO_2 to the blood to maintain normal pH. The latter promotes cerebral vasodilatation.
- Alpha stat blood gas management is utilized for most cases. Target pHa 7.40, $PaCO_2$ target 35–45 mmHg, PaO_2 120–150 mmHg at 37 C, regardless of patient core temperature i.e. temperature un-corrected
- Modified—pH stat blood gas management is used for DHCA. CO_2 titrated into sweep gas to achieve pHa 7.30, $PaCO_2$ 70–80 mmHg at 37C, which is the equivalent of pHa 7.45, $PaCO_2$ 25–35 mmHg at actual patient core temperature i.e. Temperature corrected
- Circuit arterial blood gas measurements are performed q30 minutes or more frequently as required
- Continuous in-line arterial blood gas/ potassium analysis and circuit venous hematocrit, hemoglobin and oxygen saturation are monitored using Terumo CDI550 Blood Monitor
- Cyanotic patients: bypass initiated using controlled reoxygenation at $PaO_2 < 100$–120 mmHg to minimize reperfusion oxidative injury
- Acyanotic patients: bypass is initiated at PaO_2 120–150 mmHg

6.3.5 Temperature Management

Each institution will have their own protocols according to preference. These are examples of what is used at the Hospital for Sick Children in Toronto:

- Nasopharyngeal and rectal temperatures are routinely used to monitor patient temperature
- Passively drift to 34 C—predominate method (e.g. VSD, ASD closures, BCPS, Fontan)

- Cool to 32 C—utilized for longer procedures (e.g. TOF repair, tricuspid atresia repair)
- Cool to 28 C—used to facilitate low flow requirements (e.g. TAPVC repair)
- Cool to 18 C—used for deep hypothermic circulatory arrest (e.g. Norwood, Arch repairs)
- All patients are rewarmed to a core temperature (rectal) of >35C prior to separation from bypass

6.3.6 Fluid Management, Blood Transfusion and Blood Conservation

- Minimum acceptable hematocrit on bypass is 25%
- Plasmalyte A, 25% albumin, 5% albumin, PRBC and FP are used for volume replacement, management of hematocrit, viscosity, colloid oncotic pressure, and supplementation of coagulation proteins
- If prime contains FP, 50–100 mls given immediately prior to aortic cross clamp removal to chelate calcium and reduce the risk of reperfusion induced "stone heart"; remainder of FP unit is transfused during rewarming phase
- Cardiotomy suction is utilized for all cases; blood salvage using cell saver also used for all redo cases and at request of surgeon
- Perioperative acute isovolemic hemodilution used on select patients deemed suitable by Anaesthesiologist; factors for suitability include baseline HCT, patient blood volume, expected transfusion requirements post-bypass, and cardiovascular status. Involves collection of volume of blood via central line, stored at room temperature to preserve platelet function and transfused post-bypass. Technique used to reduce allogeneic blood product exposure.

7 Hemoconcentration

- Ultrafiltration is commonly used as an adjunct to CPB. These are the parameters used at the Hospital for Sick Children, Toronto:
- Conventional ultrafiltration (CUF) is utilized throughout CPB to reverse the effects of deliberate hemodilution resulting from cardioplegia delivery, transfusion, volume administration, etc.
- Modified ultrafiltration (MUF) is utilized for all patients <15 Kg and all Fontan patients
- When utilized, the goal of MUF is to remove excess water and inflammatory mediators from the circulation following bypass. The result is an increased patient hematocrit, improved hemostasis, and early post-operative oxygenation and reduced ventilation requirements. Optimally performed for ~10–12 min following separation from bypass.

8 Cardioplegia

- A variety of different types of cardioplegia can be used according to institutional preference.
- There are two broad categories
  - 'extracellular' types have a biochemical composition similar to that of the extra-cellular fluid except for a high concentration of Potassium ± Lidocaine to prevent membrane depolarization (include 'St Thomas' solution and del Nido Cardioplegia)
  - 'intracellular 'types have a composition similar to the intra-cellular fluid consisting mainly of amino acids such as Histidine-Tryptophan-Ketoglutarate (e.g., Bretschneider solution and Custodiol®)
- At the Hospital for Sick Children, Toronto, the del Nido solution (Table 4) is preferred
- del Nido cardioplegia is delivered in a 1:4 blood to cardioplegia solution ratio.
- The temperature of the cardioplegia perfusate is cooled to 6 °C.
- Cardioplegia solution (CPS) is delivered cold with an initial arresting dose of 20–25 ml/kg to a maximum of one litre
- The patient may require subsequent doses of CPS, which is dosed at 10 ml/kg. Redosing occurs at 40 min interval or at discretion of surgeon

Table 4 del Nido formulation

Final composition of product compounded by pharmacy	del Nido Formulation Pharmacy adds to 1000 L Plasma-Lyte A: Potassium chloride: **26 mmol** Magnesium sulphate: **2 g** =8 mmol Final Concentration per 1000 mL
Na (mmol/L)	137.65
Cl (mmol/L)	121.90
K (mmol/L)	30.48
Mg (mmol/L)	9.34
Drugs added in or by perfusion	
Sodium bicarbonate 8.4% (Na 1 mmol/mL)	Add **13 mL** (13 mmol)
Mannitol 20 % (200 mg/mL)	Add **3.25 g (16.3mL)**
Lidocaine 1% (10 mg/mL)	Add **130mg (13mL)**

Managing the Complicated Post-operative Course

Luciana Rodriguez Guerineau and Oshri Zaulan

Abstract The key to successful management of any patient in the Cardiac Critical Care Unit (CCCU), particularly those who develop a more complicated post-operative course, is attention to detail and anticipation. Safe management of post-operative patients begins with an organized transition of care from the surgeons and anesthesiologists to the CCCU team. A detailed handover of the patient's pre and intraoperative course, including anesthetic, surgical aspects, echocardiographic findings and an overall impression from the operating room team of the salient physiological observations. The understanding of how specific lesions, operations, and types of cardiovascular physiology affect the postoperative course is a key element. Therefore, it is essential to know every aspect of the patient starting with the preoperative status, intraoperative issues, and postoperative concerns. There are also lesion-specific issues and common postoperative complications that the intensive care physician should be familiar with.

Keywords Cardiac surgery · Post-operative course · Cardiopulmonary bypass surgery · Children

Abbreviations

AKI	Acute kidney injury
ASD	Atrial septal defect
AV	Atrioventricular
AVRT	Atrioventricular re-entrant tachycardia
AVSD	Atrioventricular septal defect

L. R. Guerineau (✉) · O. Zaulan
Cardiac Critical, Department of Critical Care Medicine, Labatt Family Heart Centre, Hospital for Sick Children, Toronto, ON, Canada
e-mail: Luciana.rodriguezguerineai@sickkids.ca

O. Zaulan
e-mail: Oshri.zaulan@sickkids.ca

© The Author(s), under exclusive license to Springer Nature Switzerland AG 2024
A. I. Dipchand et al. (eds.), *Manual of Cardiac Care in Children*,
https://doi.org/10.1007/978-3-031-70973-9_50

AVV	Atrioventricular valve
CAPD	Cornell assessment of pediatric delerium
CCCU	Cardiac critical care unit
CFM	Cerebral function monitoring
CLABSI	Central line associated bloodstream infection
CO	Cardiac output
CVP	Central venous pressure
DO_2	Oxygen delivery
ECMO	Extracorporeal membrane oxygenation
FFP	Fresh frozen plasma
HF	Heart failure
iNO	Inhaled nitric oxide
LA	Left atrium
LCOS	Low cardiac output syndrome
LV	Left ventricle
NEC	Necrotizing enterocolitis
NG	Nasogastric
PA	Pulmonary artery
PICC	Peripherally inserted central catheter
PVR	Pulmonary vascular resistance
Qp	Pulmonary blood flow
Qs	Systemic blood flow
RA	Right atrium
ROTEM	Rotational thromboelastometry
RRT	Renal replacement therapy
RV	Right ventricle
RVSP	Right ventricular systolic pressure
SSI	Surgical site infection
SvO_2	Systemic venous oxygen saturation
SVR	Systemic vascular resistance
T21	Trisomy 21
TAPVC	Total anomalous pulmonary venous connection
TEG	Thromboelastography
TGA	Transposition of the great arteries
TOF	Tetralogy of fallot
TOF/PA	Tetralogy of fallot/Pulmonary atresia
UTI	Urinary tract infection
VAD	Ventricular assist device
VAP	Ventilator acquired pneumonia

Key Points

- Identifying patients at risk of a complicated post-operative course is imperative to anticipate problems and manage them preventatively or in a timely fashion.
- Understanding the underlying physiology, specific anatomic configuration, and residual lesions is paramount.
- Postoperative course may be complicated by hemodynamically significant residual lesions, ventricular dysfunction, suboptimal (competing) cardiopulmonary interactions, and end-organ injury.
- Adherence to basic critical care skills and safety bundles may minimize or prevent additional morbidity
- Families should be engaged and supported in patient centered care and their psychological and emotional needs considered

1 Overview

- Risk factors for a complicated postoperative course include preoperative, intraoperative, and postoperative factors (Fig. 1).
- Increased morbidity and mortality associated with related factors:
  - Patient: Prematurity, low weight (<2 kg), presence of genetic anomaly/ syndrome, other congenital malformations
  - Cardiac: High risk lesions (e.g. hypoplastic left heart syndrome, right atrial isomerism, obstructed pulmonary venous flow), ventricular dysfunction, previous cardiac surgery
  - Preoperative clinical state: Shock, existing end-organ injury (intracranial hemorrhage, necrotizing enterocolitis)
  - Intraoperative modifiers: increased cardiopulmonary bypass time and circulatory arrest times
  - Postoperative: Residual lesions, ventricular dysfunction, complications (e.g. arrhythmia, chylothorax, vocal cord dysfunction), feeding intolerance

2 General Postoperative Management

- Maximize oxygen delivery (DO_2) with an acceptable systemic perfusion pressure and, in cyanotic patients, saturation (Fig. 2).
- Maintain appropriate perfusion pressure—Hypotension is common and may be due to low cardiac output syndrome (LCOS) or low systemic vascular resistance (SVR).
- Ensure volume status and normal sinus rhythm.

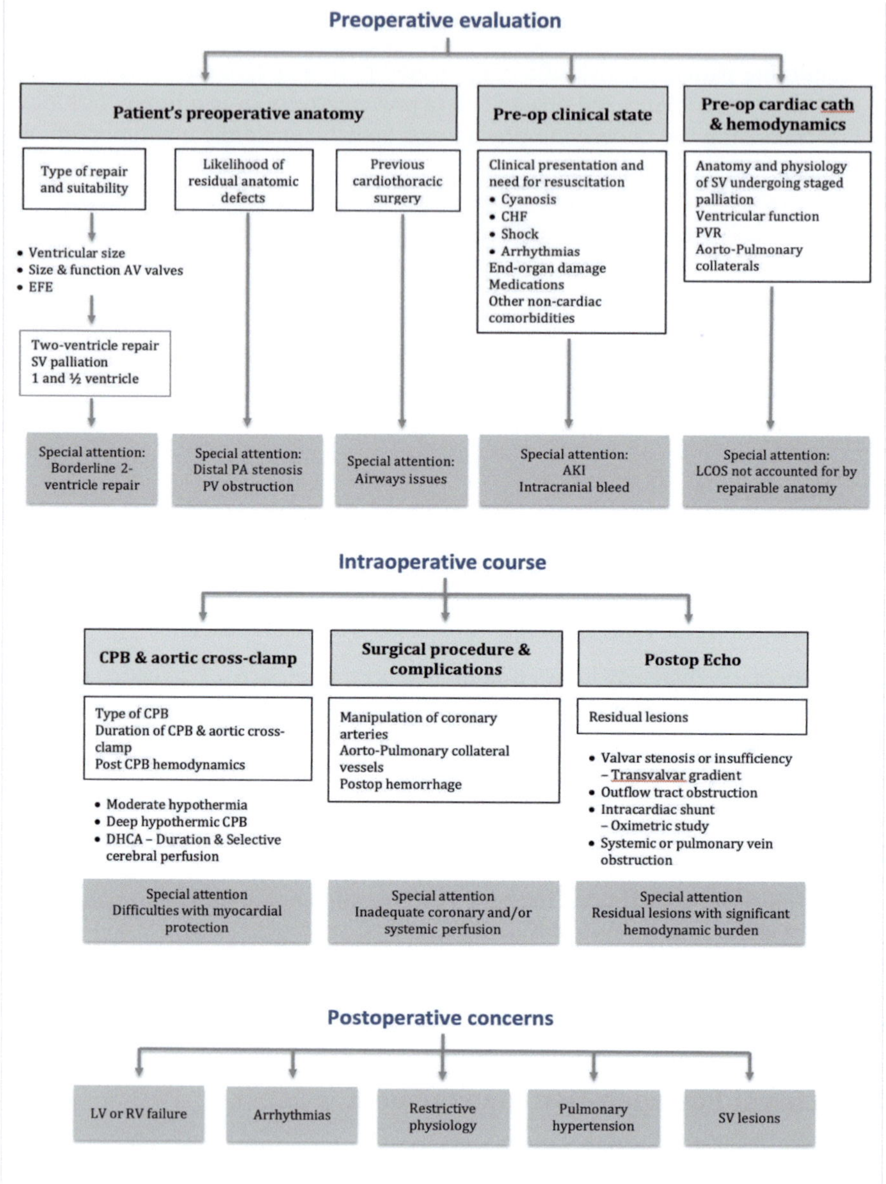

Fig. 1 Risk factors for a complicated postoperative course

$DO_2 = CO \times CaO_2$

$CO = \Delta P / SVR \rightarrow BP = CO \times SVR$

Determinants of CO (SV x HR)	Contractility Preload Afterload AV synchrony / Rhythm

Fig. 2 Common hemodynamic equations describing determinants for cardiac output and systemic oxygen delivery. CO—cardiac output; CaO_2—arterial oxygen content; ΔP—arterial pressure—central venous pressure; SVR—systemic vascular resistance; BP—blood pressure; SV—stroke volume. HR—heart rate

3 Postoperative LCOS

- Impaired DO_2 causing tissue hypoperfusion and lactic acidosis.
- It can lead to end-organ damage and failure.
- Signs of tissue hypoperfusion: tachycardia, cold extremities, prolonged capillary refill time, reduced urine output, metabolic acidosis, rising lactate, low SvO_2, hypotension.
- Causes of early postoperative LCOS include ventricular dysfunction, arrhythmia, hypovolemia, tamponade, pulmonary hypertension and residual lesions.
- May be multi-factorial and the causes may be inter-related.
- Treatment tailored to target the underlying aetiology and physiolgy (e.g. volume expansion for inadequate preload, inotropy for ventricular dysfunction).

4 Cardiac Tamponade

- Clinical diagnosis, echocardiogram confirmation if time permits. High suspicion if decrease in chest tube output, hypotension, and increase CVP.
- Localized collection behind the left atrium can present with tamponade physiology with low CVP
- Similar findings with tissue tamponade—mediastinal and myocardial swelling in absence of effusion
- Acute management includes fluid resuscitation and re-establishing chest tube patency
- Early reopening sternum prior to extremis or end-organ injury

5 Surgical Bleeding

- Mediastinal re-exploration strongly considered if sanguinous chest tube drainage >10 ml/kg/h over the first 2 h after admission or >4 ml/kg/h thereafter.
- Resuscitation can include volume expansion, packed red blood cells, platelets to address thrombocytopenia and dysfunction, and FFP, cryoprecipitate, and/or fibrinogen concentrate to reverse coagulopathy.

- Routine coagulation testing, ROTEM and/or TEG used to guide supplementation
- Avoid hypothermia, if possible
- Chest exploration required if hemodynamic instability.
- Activated factor VII is rarely required
- Blood gas analysis of chest tube drainage can be useful to identify arterial source.

6 Postoperative LV or Systemic Ventricular Failure

- Systolic dysfunction may be preexisting or secondary to poor myocardial protection (from cardioplegia), coronary ischemia, or residual lesions with increased pre/afterload
- Intraoperative imaging to identify intraoperatively or it may evolve secondary to inflammatory response.
- Postoperative echocardiography indicated if suspicion for evolving dysfunction, particularly in high risk lesions
- Treated with inotropy and afterload reduction (e.g. Milrinone, whenever possible)
- Additional afterload reduction with Phentolamine or nitroprusside and phentolamine if not hypotensive.
- Avoid excessive fluid resuscitation by following CVP
- Norepinephrine or arginine vasopressin limited to treatment of hypotension
- Maintaining strict calcium homeostasis prioritized in neonates (especially prematurity) given immature myocardial calcium handling.
- Stress dosing of steroids used for catecholamine resistant hypotension
- Intraoperative insertion of left atrial lines in high risk cases to monitor and guide fluid resuscitation

7 Postoperative RV Failure

- RV failure in patients with high RVSP or after right-sided surgery (TOF, TOF/PA, Ebstein's anomaly).
- RV systolic and diastolic dysfunction needs to be distinguished:
  - RV systolic dysfunction worsens with excessive volume and may require inotropic support and systemic vasoconstrictors.
  - RV diastolic dysfunction may require large amounts of volume, supranormal CVP, and worsens with inotropic-associated chronotropy
- LV dysfunction from RV dilation from interventricular septum leftward displacement, impairing LV filling and resultant LA hypertension—increases pulmonary pressures and worsens the RV function.
- Vasoconstrictors increase LV afterload, and end-diastolic pressure, reducing septal displacement and improve ventricular-ventricular interactions.

- Low-dose epinephrine for RV support
- Residual atrial communication can allow RA decompression to LA—to support systemic cardiac output and lower CVP at the expense of systemic desaturations. Degree of desaturation depends on RA pressure/poor RV compliance and size of ASD.
- In the absence of LV failure, negative pressure ventilation (spontaneous breathing) reduces RV afterload and improves pulmonary blood flow. Early extubation considered when appropriate.
- Reduction in PVR with oxygen, avoiding acidosis, and iNO if RV failure secondary to elevated pulmonary vascular reactivity.
- Important to exclude PA stenosis and/or pulmonary vein obstruction (e.g., following TAPVC repair).
- Maintaining AV synchrony with sinus or atrial rhythm will optimize cardiac output
- Evacuation of pleural effusions, reopening the sternum, and draining ascitescon-sidered if hypotension refractory to medical therapy.
- ECMO may be used as bridge to recovery.

8 Preoperative LCOS Not Accounted for by Repairable Anatomy

- Pre-existing systolic dysfunction and/or low cardiac output that does not result from reparable lesion (e.g., Coarctation, aortic stenosis) risk for worse function following CPB and cardioplegia.
- Mechanical circulatory support may be needed.

9 Postoperative Arrhythmias

- Common postoperative arrhythmias include junctional ectopic tachycardia, ectopic atrial tachycardia, re-entrant supraventricular tachycardia, and atrial flutter.
- Ventricular tachycardia rare and should prompt investigations to rule-out ischemia
- Heart block is also a common complication—usually transient (pacemaker required only if >7–10 days)
- Temporary atrial pacing wires helpful for diagnosis and treatment (AV synchrony in junctional ectopic tachycardia, overdrive pacing in AVRT, atrial flutter)
- Temporary ventricular pacing wires support ventricular and dual chamber pacing, as needed

10 Myocardial Ischemia

10.1 Myocardial Protection/Long Aortic Cross-Clamp Time

- Inadequate myocardial protection or long aortic cross-clamp time can lead to intraoperative ischemia and post-operative dysfunction.
- Myocardial recovery usually occurs within 5–7 days
- ECMO may be required as bridge to recovery—VAD insertion, heart transplant assessment and withdrawal of life-sustaining therapies is determined on an individual basis.

10.2 Inadequate Coronary Perfusion Postop

- Coronary artery surgery (e.g. TGA, Ross procedure, or Bentall procedure) can cause coronary artery distortion and compromise myocardial perfusion.
- Markers include increase coronary velocity on echo, regional wall abnormalities, ST segment changes on ECG, and ventricular arrhythmias.
- Concerns for ischemia should be immediately investigated by coronary angiography or cross sectional imaging

11 Hemodynamically Significant Residual Lesions

11.1 Tricuspid or Mitral Valve Dysfunction

- Residual stenosis or insufficiency following atrioventricular valve (AVV) repair, or pre-existing lesions unmasked after ASD closure (most commonly seen after AVSD repair).
- Volume overload from AVV regurgitation can lead to HF or LCOS.
- More symptomatic if the systemic AVV valve and ventricle is affected.
- Symptoms can be controlled with diuretics, positive pressure ventilation (for systemic AV valve lesions) or afterload reduction (including minimization of airway pressure for pulmonary ventricle AV valve lesions).
- Surgery considered if unable to wean from mechanical ventilation.
- AVV stenosis is associated with systemic (right-sided) or pulmonary (left-sided) venous hypertension and congestive symptoms. If severe, it can limit cardiac output.
- Surgery should be discussed early if medical management is necessary to maintain hemodynamics.
- In general, a mean AVV inflow gradient of less than 8 mmHg can be tolerated.

11.2 *Residual Systemic Ventricular Outflow Tract Obstruction*

- Residual obstruction can complicate surgeries to:
  - Relieve outflow obstruction (e.g., subaortic stenosis, aortic stenosis, supravalvar aortic stenosis)
  - Reconstruct the systemic outflow tract (Norwood operation) or the aortic arch (repair of hypoplastic aortic arch or coarctation).
  - Repair atrioventricular septal defect repair or after volume unloading of a single ventricle in who the systemic outflow tract is through a VSD or other potentially narrowed passage.
- Echocardiography can underestimate gradients if LCOS, severe systolic dysfunction, or systemic AVV regurgitation.
- Peak instantaneous gradients >50 mmHg (or lower if echo values unreliable) usually requires reintervention.
- Systemic vasodilation contraindicates due to risk of hypotension from an inability to increase the CO.
- For dynamic obstruction, chronotropic, inotropic, and afterload reduction agents should be avoided.

11.3 *Residual Left-to-Right Shunt*

- Due to patch leaks after repair of septal defects, unrecognized or untreated systemic to pulmonary artery shunts (e.g., aorto-pulmonary collaterals), or when intentionally left unrepaired
- Large shunts can cause pulmonary over-circulation, volume overload of the systemic ventricle, and HF.
- Atrial shunts are generally well tolerated unless a high-volume shunt from:
  - Mitral valve disease (stenosis/incompetence).
  - LV restrictive physiology (inadequate LV size or hypertrophy).
  - LV dysfunction
  - Residual LV outflow tract obstruction.
- Ventricular and arterial shunts have higher likelihood of pulmonary hypertension and congestive CHF, especially when the Qp:Qs is >2:1.
- Quantifying severity of shunt by cardiac MRI or catheterization required in clinically symptomatic patients
- Medical management includes diuretics, afterload reduction, avoiding further reduction in PVR (e.g. oxygen or hyperventilation), and positive pressure ventilation.

- Surgical repair or catheter occlusion for HF refractory to medical therapy or ventilation dependence; main pulmonary band may be necessary as staged approach.

12 Restrictive Physiology

- Diastolic dysfunction that limits ventricular filling at normal pressures
- Often encountered following surgery with:
  - Significant ventricular hypertrophy (TOF, outflow tract obstruction).
  - Hypoplastic ventricular (LV hypoplasia in biventricular repair of HLH variants or TAPVC).
- Retrograde congestion from atrial hypertension.
- Residual atrial communication:
  - Can maintain systemic CO with restrictive RV (increased cyanosis).
  - Reduce LA pressure and HF with restrictive LV physiology (at expense of increase pulmonary blood flow and possible marginal CO).
- Supportive management awaiting cardiac remodeling:
  - Maintaining optimal fluid status (drainage of effusions or ascites if needed)
  - Lusitropic agents (e.g., milrinone)
  - Adequate sedation and pain control.
- Severe RV restrictive may require creation of a residual ASD (if not present), delayed sternal closure/reopening, or ECMO.
- Severe restrictive LV physiology is more likely to be associated with prolonged HF.

13 Pulmonary Hypertension

- CPB can provoke pulmonary hypertension in patients with labile pulmonary vascular resistance (e.g. neonates, repair of pulmonary venous obstruction, mitral valve disease) or pre-existing elevated PVR (late presentation of VSD and AVSD, T21, TAPVC, Truncus arteriosus)
- A well-conditioned RV may tolerate even suprasystemic RV pressure and maintain CO.
- Unconditioned or failing RV may not tolerate even moderately elevated resistance.
- Pulmonary hypertension can cause cyanosis if there is a residual septal defect.
- If no shunt, may have acute RV failure and LCOS.
- Management of pulmonary hypertension described in Chap. 47.

14 Non-cardiac Complications

14.1 Airway Complications/Extubation Failure

- Extubation failure affects 7–8%
- The difficult airway should be identified prior to extubation for appropriate planning in case of failure.
- Upper airway obstruction treated with nebulized epinephrine, inhaled or systemic steroids, avoidance of agitation and use of non-invasive ventilation
- Nebulized epinephrine used with caution in patients with tachy-arrhythmias.
- Airway obstruction from vocal cord palsy may result from recurrent laryngeal nerve injury (left: aortic arch surgery, right: carotid surgery) or prolonged intubation injury.
- Extubation failure from:
  - Airway compression can occur secondary to dilated LA, reconstructed arch or dilated PA—aortic/PA—pexy may be required
  - Phrenic nerve injury and diaphragm palsy (neonates/infants > children)

15 Acute Kidney Injury (AKI)

- Preexisting AKI associated with postoperative morbidity
- Post-operative AKI is common, especially for those with prolonged LCOS or adverse hemodynamics (high venous pressure and/or low arterial pressure)
- Renal replacement therapy (RRT) may be required—peritoneal dialysis vs continuous renal replacement therapy.
- Role of early RRT unclear
- Peritoneum should be drained to prevent abdominal compartment syndrome and impaired renal perfusion.
- Limit exposure to nephrotoxic drugs.
- Careful attention to fluid balance including use of diuretics is critical.
- Peritoneal dialysis can be used for early fluid, electrolyte, and acid–base management, particularly for infants. Continuous RRT if concerns for intestinal integrity, older patients, or on ECMO.

16 Nutrition and Endocrinologic Complications

- Critical illness hyperglycemia is very common but tight glycemic control is not beneficial –target glucose 150–180 mg/dL.
- Preoperative malnutrition is common (up to 80%)—most likely in patients with cyanosis, large left-to-right shunts, and complex CHD.

  - Associated with a more complex postoperative recovery
  - Optimizing preoperative growth through increased caloric delivery (fortification, feeding tube) can reduce hospital length of stay, morbidity and mortality.

- Prolonged and difficult recoveries often complicated by poor growth and development
- Calories and macro/micronutrient delivery hindered by poor enteral feeds (often held for concerns of splanchnic hypoperfusion and risk of NEC), fluid restriction, and recurrent interventions.
- Enteral feeds promoted by feeding tubes (temporary NG vs gastrostomy tubes) and addressing intolerance

17 Infectious Complications

- Nosocomial infections most common complications and associated with increased morbidity
- Include surgical site infection (SSI), Central Line-associated Bloodstream Infection (CLABSI), Ventilator-Associated Pneumonia (VAP) and Urinary Tract Infection (UTI)
- Prevalence ranges between 10 and 30%
- CLABSI and infective endocarditis concerning, especially in setting of prosthetic material or dysplastic valves.
- SSI is most common infection and varies in severity from superficial wound infection to mediastinitis.

  - Organisms isolated from wound cultures: $\geq$2/3 of cases are Gram-positive bacteria (Staphylococcus aureus, coagulase-negative staphylococcus and Enterococcus species) and 1/4 are gram-negative bacteria (*Pseudomonas aeruginosa, Escherichia coli* and Enterobacter species)
  - Remaining cases are polymicrobial or fungal

- Prevention and antimicrobial stewardship are recommended

18 Neurological Complications/Comorbidities

- Prolonged ICU stay is associated with future developmental delays and learning problems.
- Causes unclear but ICU-related factors have been implicated—cerebral ischemia from LCOS, hypotension, hypoxemia, cardiac arrest, use of sedatives and anesthetics, and disruption of sleep cycles and sensory inputs
- Neuromonitoring (Cerebral function monitoring (CFM) or continuous EEG):

  - Used to evaluate for subclinical seizures following high-risk procedures (e.g., Norwood), neurologic injury (e.g., stroke), cardiac arrest, or ECMO.
  - Rule out a stroke if focal signs.

- Seizures can be a sign of a neurological from stroke (ischemic or hemorrhagic) or hypoxic ischemic injury
- Management should include antiepileptic medications, and consideration for continuous EEG, neuroimaging and neurology consultation

19 Delirium

- Associated with increased ICU morbidity
- Hyper or hypoactive subtypes
- Increase risk with benzodiazepine use, increase acuity and prolonged admission
- Followed by the Cornell Assessment of Pediatric Delerium (CAPD) score
- Reduction or elimination of contributing pharmacology is important
- Nonpharmacological treatment includes establishing normal sleep–wake cycles, normalizing routines and activities, reduction in ambient noise

20 Thrombosis

- Systemic venous and arterial thrombosis is common, particularly in small neonates/infants requiring prolonged access
- Risk is proportional to size of cannula relative vessel and inversely related to vessel flow
- Thrombosis of upper body veins may promote additional complications (sinus venous thrombosis, chylothorax)
- Ensuring vascular health is vital, especially for patients who will require repeated interventions (e.g., single ventricle patients)

  - Limit or avoid internal jugular access in smaller neonates
  - Consider early umbilical lines, PICC lines and intracardiac (right atrial) lines
  - Removal of lines as early as possible
  - Use of smallest caliber lines that are appropriate

Bibliography

1. Agus MS, Wypij D, Hirshberg EL, et al. Tight glycemic control in critically ill children. N Engl J Med. 2017;376(8):729–41.

2. Floh AA, Slicker J, Schwartz SM. Nutrition and mesenteric issues in pediatric cardiac critical care. Pediatr Crit Care Med. 2016;17:S243–9.
3. Hoffman TM, Wernovsky G, Atz AM, et al. Efficacy and safety of milrinone in preventing low cardiac output syndrome in infants and children after corrective surgery for congenital heart disease. Circulation. 2003;107(7):996–1002.
4. Penny DJ, Redington AN. Function of the left and right ventricles and the interactions between them. Pediatr Crit Care Med. 2016;17:S112–8.
5. Taylor RS, Shekerdemian LS. Avoidance of hospital-acquired infections in pediatric cardiac surgical patients. Pediatr Crit Care Med. 2016;17:S279–86.

Cardiac Critical Care Unit Surgical Procedures and Management

Myunghyun M. Lee and Fiona Perelini

Abstract Surgical procedures are a common occurrence in the cardiac intensive care unit. These interventions may be undertaken in response to an acute emergency or a component of routine care. Any surgical intervention carries increased risk and requires careful assessment, planning and management.

Keywords Cardiac surgical procedure · Cardiac critical care · Postoperative

Abbreviations

BP	Blood pressure
ECPR	ECMO cardiopulmonary resuscitation
ECMO	Extracorporeal membrane oxygenation
LV	Left ventricle
MPA	Main pulmonary artery
NIRS	Near infrared spectroscopy
PAB	Pulmonary artery band
PDA	Persistent ductus arteriosus
PRBC	Packed red blood cells
PVR	Pulmonary vascular resistance
Qp	Pulmonary blood flow
Qs	Systemic blood flow
SVR	Systemic vascular resistance
VAC	Vacuum assisted closure

M. M. Lee (✉)
Division of Cardiovascular Surgery, Labatt Family Heart Centre, Hospital for Sick Children, Toronto, ON, Canada
e-mail: Mike.lee@sickkids.ca

F. Perelini
Starship Children's Hospital, Auckland, New Zealand
e-mail: fionape@adhb.govt.nz

© The Author(s), under exclusive license to Springer Nature Switzerland AG 2024

A. I. Dipchand et al. (eds.), *Manual of Cardiac Care in Children*,
https://doi.org/10.1007/978-3-031-70973-9_51

Key Points

- Surgical procedures are common in the management of critically ill children with acquired or congenital heart disease
- Interventions may be in response to an acute emergency or a component of routine care
- A cardiac surgical emergency describes any acute hemodynamic alteration requiring immediate surgical intervention for patient stabilization

1 General Procedural Preparation

- Any surgical procedure in the intensive care unit is high risk and has the potential for serious complications.
- Preparation and planning prior to the procedure (if possible) is important.
- Delivery of appropriate anaesthetic, sedation, and analgesia provided by trained personnel (locally provided by critical care staff, anaesthiologists in other institutions).
- Timeout procedure to ensure entire team aware of plan and all considerations accounted for.

1.1 Patient

- Monitoring with ECG, oxygen saturation, BP monitoring (non-invasive or arterial), end-tidal CO_2

1.2 Environment

- Sterile environment
- Limit number of people if possible

1.3 Equipment

- Surgical equipment tray
- Head light
- Cautery
- External defibrillator

1.4 Personnel

- Cardiac surgical team—surgeon + fellow
- Intensive care team—intensivist, ICU fellow, bedside nurse, respiratory technician
- Cardiology—intra-operative echocardiogram may be required

1.5 Set-Up

- Appropriate anaesthetic monitoring tool on electronic medical record
- Anaesthetic and resuscitation drugs
- Volume—Crystalloid/Albumin
- Blood products—PRBC/coagulation factors (Blood available at the bedside if possible)
- Venous lines for access and monitoring—Ensure adequate venous access for medication and fluid delivery. Short bore peripheral IV access preferred for blood product delivery
- Pacing wires connected and tested prior to procedure (output and sensitivity thresholds) and pacemaker available (or connected)
- Prior to procedure review of recent blood gas/blood tests/CXR/echocardiogram (time permitting)
- External defibrillation and electrocautery pads placed
- Shoulder roll to displace chin away from sterile field
- Surgical dressings removed
- Surgical field prepared and draped using Betadine (fresh incision) or Chlorhexidine (healed incision)

2 Types of Surgical Interventions

- Surgical Emergencies—acute surgical interventions required for the immediate stabilization of a hemodynamic or respiratory emergency.
- Routine Surgical Interventions—planned procedures that are elements of routine perioperative management.
- Management of acute post-operative complications.

3 Potential Causes of Surgical Emergencies

- Critical hypoxia: critical reduction in systemic arterial oxygen tension and hypoxia due to a reduction to pulmonary blood flow in patients dependent on systemic-to-pulmonary connection

- Reduction in systemic cardiac output:
  - Caused by changes in preload, afterload, contractility, arrhythmia, and heart rate
  - Due to imbalance to pulmonary and systemic vascular resistance and blood flow with reduction in systemic perfusion

4 Specific Cardiac Surgical Emergency Procedures

4.1 Critical Hypoxia: Modified Blalock-Taussig-Thomas (BTT) Shunt Obstruction

- Caused by *in situ* thrombosis or external compression (eg. Large hematoma/seroma)
- Presents with severe hypoxia, elevated serum carbon dioxide, and low end tidal carbon dioxide
- Immediate medical management includes anticoagulation and raising systemic blood pressure and SVR to drive pulmonary blood flow
- Surgical aim: Achieve shunt patency and re-establish pulmonary blood flow
  - Median sternotomy
  - Sternal retractor and pericardial retraction
  - Potential factors contributing to BTT shunt obstruction may include proximal and distal anastomoses, conduit, inflow, and outflow. Only the anastomoses and conduit are surgically modifiable.
  - Immediate interventions including relief of external compression and/or evacuation of fluid collection, external "milking" of BTT shunt to disrupt in situ thrombosis and re-establish some forward flow, or cannulation onto ECMO.
  - Subsequent surgical options include shunt replacement (slower) or thrombectomy (faster) after appropriate proximal and distal vascular control achieved.

4.2 Critically Low Cardiac Output: Tissue Tamponade and Restrictive Filling

- Increased tissue edema, including myocardium and mediastinum, can compromise ventricular filling and impair cardiac output. Patients with ventricular hypertrophy and restrictive physiology are particularly vulnerable (Chap. 50).
- Improvement can be achieved by chest suspension or chest re-opening.

4.2.1 Chest Suspension

- Surgical aim: Reduce external cardiac compression effect of the closed thorax
- Chest suspension sutures may be pre-emptively placed for patients with elevated risk of ventricular dysfunction upon chest closure.
- Chest suspension sutures are connected to the overhead apparatus to "suspend" the patients by their sternum to increase their retrosternal space
- Maneuver is often performed as a first step for postoperative hemodynamic instability before committing to chest reopening, if hemodynamics permit.
- Procedural steps:
  - Sternal area with minimal retrosternal distance to heart or conduit selected for chest suspension
  - Double-loaded Prolene with each needle travelling deep to superficial through sternum and overlying subcutaneous and subcuticular tissues
  - Prolene tied as air-knot at subcuticular level and tied together at distal ends
  - Sternum closed using stainless steel wires
  - Overlying subcutaneous and subcuticular tissue closure
  - Surgical dressings
  - When indicated, silk string passed through suspension suture loop and secured to overhead apparatus using Kocher clamps with adjustable degree of chest suspension

5 Excessive Pulmonary Blood Flow/Pulmonary Over-Circulation

- Surgical aim: Restrict Pulmonary Blood flow and Increase Systemic Blood Flow
- Imbalance to systemic and pulmonary blood flow due to high pulmonary runoff lesion may complicate single ventricle heart disease or those with an aortic-to-pulmonary level shunt (PDA, surgical shunt, collateral)
- Clinical presentation with high saturations, pulmonary congestion, poor peripheral perfusion, and possibly myocardial ischemia and shock
- Medical management includes systemic afterload reduction, inotropy/volume to increase total cardiac output, optimising hemoglobin, intubation and hypoventilation to control respiration and elevated PVR.

5.1 Main Pulmonary Artery Band (PAB)

- PAB is fashioned as a 4 mm width strip from 3.5 mm polytetrafluoroethylene Gore-Tex graft opened longitudinally and applied to main pulmonary artery (MPA)

- Initial circumference is determined using Trusler formula and adjusted to the patient's hemodynamics and systemic saturations
- Trusler formula = 20 mm + 1 mm/kg in non-cyanotic lesions and 24 mm + 1 mm/kg in mixing lesions
- Adjustments are made to the MPA band circumference according to systemic saturations, cardiac output, intra-operative Qp:Qs calculation, and intraoperative echocardiogram.
  - Systemic saturations should be normal (>93%) in patients with non-cyanotic lesions and usually a target of 80% in room air is used in univentricular lesions.
  - Direct MPA pressure measurements may be required to adjust band tightness, aiming for mean MPA pressure of <20–25 mmHg. Intraoperative echocardiogram acceleration gradient >3 m/s.
- The addition or removal of hemoclips will reduce or increase the MPA band circumference
- Procedural steps:
  - Midline sternotomy
  - Pericardiotomy and suspension
  - MPA isolation
  - Additional dissection into branch pulmonary arteries as indicated
  - PAB placed circumferentially around MPA or branch pulmonary artery with PAB ends secured to each other using simple interrupted Prolene
  - PAB further tightened by placing additional interrupted Prolene more proximally under invasive or non-invasive pressure gradient guidance
  - Hemostasis
  - Team discussion on chest closure vs open chest protocol (described separately)
  - Surgical dressings

5.2 Bilateral Pulmonary Artery Band (PAB)—Single Ventricle with PDA Dependent Systemic Blood Flow

- Procedural steps:
  - PAB applied on left and right main branch pulmonary arteries.
  - PAB is fashioned as a 4 mm width strip from 3.5 mm polytetrafluoroethylene Gore-Tex graft opened longitudinally.
  - Branch pulmonary arteries are initially banded to 70–80% of normal branch pulmonary artery size.
  - PAB tightness is adjusted based on systemic saturations, hemodynamics and intraoperative echocardiogram.
  - Goal is to achieve improve systemic blood flow and balance Qp:Qs. Targets for band tightness include improved systemic blood pressure (MAP by 10 mmHg), saturations 75–85% in room air and improved central venous saturations/NIRS.

5.3 *Restriction of Modified BTT Shunt Flow*

- Adjustment of the modified BTT shunt diameter with clips or bands.
- Goal is to improve systemic blood flow and balance Qp:Qs.
- Target for modified BTT shunt diameter dependent on systemic saturations and improved systemic perfusion.
- Procedural steps:
  - Midline sternotomy approach
  - Sternal retractor and pericardial retraction sutures
  - Sequential placement of hemoclips to narrow the modified BTT shunt and reduce pulmonary flow until hemodynamic and saturation targets achieved.
  - Chest closure vs open chest protocol once ideal modified BTT shunt constriction achieved (described separately).

6 Extracorporeal Membrane Oxygenator (ECMO)

- Surgical aim: To maintain tissue oxygenation in setting of inadequate systemic artery oxygenation or low cardiac output refractory to medical therapy
- Peripheral cannulation—Preferred particularly if remote history of sternotomy or during ECPR
  - Neck cannulation (right carotid and internal jugular vessels accessed) is preferred for patients up to 15 kg of body weight
  - Femoral access for those above 15 kg
  - CXR and echocardiography to confirm cannulae positions
- Central cannulation if no history of sternotomy, early in postoperative course, or require higher flows:
  - Placement of cannulation purse strings on distal ascending aorta and right atrial free wall or appendage—may be placed intraoperatively in high-risk patients with open chest
  - Arterial and venous cannulae are placed in their respective cannulation sites and secured using Rummel tourniquets.
  - Consider left atrial vent placement via right superior pulmonary vein if inadequate LV decompression secondary to significant LV systolic dysfunction (alternative to balloon atrial septostomy if chest open).
  - May require partial or complete flow restriction through aorto-pulmonary shunt (e.g. BTT) if impaired systemic cardiac output despite higher flows; may clip PDA if ECMO in context of circular shunt
  - Goretex membrane (5 mm thickness) sutured to subcuticular tissue as per open chest protocol
  - Surgical dressing

7 Open Chest Protocol

- May be necessary to place sternal stent to secure additional space within the mediastinum
- Gore-Tex membrane (5 mm thickness) sutured to subcuticular tissue
- Surgical dressings

8 Chest Reopening and Exploration for Hemostasis

- Surgical aims
  - Indications: Persistent chest tube loss greater than 3–4 mL/kg/h that is refractory to medical therapy
  - Acute hemodynamic deterioration requiring direct cardiac resuscitation or central ECMO support.
  - Evacuation of hematoma or effusion to relieve cardiac tamponade
  - Improve cardiac preload by relieving tissue edema

9 Chest Closure

- Surgical indications: Resolution of physiological state that required chest to remain open. (e.g., low output state, tissue edema causing tamponade, arrhythmia, hemorrhage)
- Surgical considerations
  - Ensure all potential spaces/compartments (bilateral pleura) are drained
  - Gore-Tex membrane (1 mm thickness) placed within mediastinum as indicated for future re-entry
  - Suspension suture placed as indicated (described separately)
  - Sternum closed using stainless steel wires
  - Chest is initially approximated and physiology is observed
  - Overlying subcutaneous and subcuticular tissue closure
  - Surgical dressings

10 Vacuum Assisted Closure (VAC) Dressing Placement and Exchanges

- Surgical aim: Maintain surgical site infections clean and dry to promote wound healing by either secondary intention or primary closure.
- Procedural Steps:

- Clean infected site of interest using betadine and sterile equipment. Drape to establish sterile field.
- Keep sterile field to store VAC dressing components.
- Black foam fitted to cover the wound. Minimize contact with intact surrounding skin.
- Apply first layer of clear plastic film over the surrounding skin and the wound. Cut out a portion of the film above the black foam and apply the suction apparatus.
- Confirm tubing connections and initiate VAC therapy. Confirm complete seal.
- If significant leak exists, reinforce suspected areas of air leak until complete seal is obtained.
- For VAC dressing exchange, disconnect VAC suction and remove the old VAC dressing. Clean the site of interest using betadine. Follow remaining steps identical as above.

11 Chest Tube Insertion

- In setting of pleural effusion or pneumothorax
- Procedural Steps:
  - Ensure adequate sedation/analgesia. Intubation exclusively for this purpose is rarely required. Local analgesia recommended.
  - Sterile environment and collection of tube—usually inserted by Seldinger technique
  - Ultrasound guided to identify location and volume of infusion, and surrounding anatomy
  - Between Middle-and-Anterior axillary line and directed anteriorly for pneumothorax, and posterior deviated for effusion.
  - Inserted above the rib (usually 4–5th intercostal space) to avoid intercostal bundle (vein/artery/nerve)

12 Percutaneous Peritoneal Dialysis Insertion

- In setting of ascites with and without abdominal hypertension
- Procedural Steps:
  - Ensure adequate sedation/analgesia with/without muscle relaxation
  - Inserted by Seldinger technique under sterile conditions
  - Ultrasound guided to identify volume and pocket for insertion

Bibliography

1. Albus R, Trusler G, Izukawa T, Williams W. Pulmonary artery banding. J Thorac Cardiovasc Surg. 1984;88:645–53.
2. Davies RR, Piazarro C. Decision-making for surgery in the management of patients with univentricular heart. Front Pedatr. 2015;3(61):1–19.
3. Headrick AT, Qureshi AM, Ghanayem NS, et al. In-hospital morbidity and mortality after modified blalock-taussig-thomas shunts. Ann Thorac Surg. 2021;21:19677.
4. Honjo O, Haller C. Banding a systemic-to-pulmonary shunt to balance pulmonary blood flow. Oper Tech Thorac Cardiovasc Surg. 2018;22(3):157–72.
5. Ishii Y, Inamura N, Kayatani F, et al. Evaluation of bilateral pulmonary artery banding for initial palliation in single-ventricle neonates and infants: risk factors for mortality before the bidirectional Glenn procedure. Interact Cardiovasc Thorac Surg. 2014;19(5):807–11.
6. Mavroudis C, Backer CL, editors. Atlas of pediatric cardiac surgery. 1st ed. London: Springer; 2015.
7. Zhu S, Zhang G, You Q, et al. Sternal lifting increases the operating space in esophagectomy via mediastinoscopy: a prospective cohort study. J Thorac Dis. 2021;13(9):5546–55.

Analgesia and Sedation in the Cardiac Critical Care Unit

Seth B. Gray, Angie Thiessen, and Karen Wong

Abstract Ensuring patient comfort through delivery of adequate analgesia and sedation is paramount to administer proper critical care. Analgesia is provided using combination of acetaminophen (paracetamol), non-steroidal anti-inflammatory drugs, and/or opioid analogues. Sedation is commonly delivered using alpha-2-agonists, benzodiazepines, and opioids; alternative sedation adjuvants may be required. The depth of sedation is determined by the physiologic and treatment needs of the patient and must be balanced against the side effect profile experienced with higher doses. The effectiveness of analgesia and sedation are monitored regularly using validated age-specific scoring systems. Slow, protocolized weaning of sedation is required after prolonged exposure to minimize risk of withdrawal, which is assessed by withdrawal scores. Delirium often complicates the delivery and/or weaning of sedation and can be managed conservatively or with antipsychotic medications if clinically significant.

Keywords Analgesia · Sedation · Withdrawal · Delirium · Pain management

Abbreviations

CAP-D	Cornell assessment of pediatric delirium
FLACC-R	Revised face, legs, activity, cry, consolability scale
FPS-R	Revised faces pain scale
IV	Parenteral or intravenous

S. B. Gray (✉)
Division of Cardiac Critical Care Medicine, The Hospital for Sick Children, Toronto, ON, Canada
e-mail: seth.gray@sickkids.ca

A. Thiessen · K. Wong
Department of Pharmacy, The Hospital for Sick Children, Toronto, ON, Canada
e-mail: angie.thiessen@sickkids.ca

K. Wong
e-mail: Karen.wong@sickkids.ca

© The Author(s), under exclusive license to Springer Nature Switzerland AG 2024

A. I. Dipchand et al. (eds.), *Manual of Cardiac Care in Children*,
https://doi.org/10.1007/978-3-031-70973-9_52

NIPS	Neonatal infant pain scale
NSAIDS	Nonsteroidal anti-inflammatory drugs
PIPP-R	Revised premature infant pain profile
PO	Per os, enteral delivery
PR	Per rectum, rectal
PRN	Pro re nata, as needed
PWS	Pain word scale
RASS	Richmond agitation and sedation score
WAT-1	Withdrawal assessment tool

Key Points

- Comprehensive pain, sedation, withdrawal, and delirium management are essential components of cardiac intensive care
- Assessment of pain, sedation, withdrawal, and delirium should be completed and documented using standardized scoring scales
- Morphine is utilized as the opioid analgesic of choice, with Hydromorphone serving as an alternative
- Weaning protocols for opioids, benzodiazepines, and dexmedetomidine should be employed for patients at elevated risk for withdrawal
- Patients should be routinely screened for delirium, and non-pharmacologic interventions should be employed prior to pharmacologic interventions

1 Analgesia, Sedation, Withdrawal and Delirium in the Cardiac ICU

- Effective sedation, analgesia, delirium, and withdrawal management are essential components of high-quality pediatric cardiac intensive care. Routine assessment of both pain and sedation level is now recommended by the Pediatric Cardiac Intensive Care Society.
- Pain is commonly understood to be an unpleasant sensory and emotional experience associated with actual or potential tissue damage. Pain can be post-operative or associated with procedures, maintenance of medical devices (e.g., chest tubes, endotracheal tubes), wound care, or patient positioning.
- Sedation refers to the depression of awareness and limitation of response to external stimuli, and encompasses anxiolysis, amnesia, and analgesia. Sedation is often used to minimize the physiologic effects of pain and stress, tolerate procedures, invasive support or monitoring devices, promote patient-ventilator synchrony, and maintain patient safety.

- Delirium is an acute and fluctuating state of neurologic dysfunction characterized by altered awareness and cognition; it consists of three subtypes (hyperactive delirium, hypoactive delirium, and mixed).
- Withdrawal is defined as abnormal physical or psychological symptoms that occur with abrupt cessation of a drug.

2 Assessment of Analgesia, Sedation, Withdrawal and Delirium in the Cardiac ICU

- Careful history and clinical examination are essential to identify the etiology of pain or agitation
- Pain assessment can either be accomplished through self-report or observational scales
- Multiple pain scales are utilized in cardiac ICU and vary depending on patient age and cognitive stage of development
- Pain is evaluated and documented by nursing staff every 4 h and as needed (PRN).
- Sedation assessment is largely measured on level of arousal or consciousness.
- Sedation, withdrawal, and delirium are evaluated using a single scale and are recorded by nursing staff every 12 h and PRN.

3 Pain Assessment Scales

- **Premature Infant Pain Profile—Revised (PIPP-R)**
  - Preterm and full-term neonates
  - Scores range from 0 to 21
- **Neonatal Infant Pain Scale (NIPS)**
  - Full term neonates to 1 year of age
  - Scores range from 0 to 7. Score >3 indicates pain
- **FLACC-R (revised Face, Legs, Activity, Cry, Consolability) Scale**
  - 2 months to 7 years of age, or those with inability to communicate
  - Scores range from 0 to 10
- **Pain Word Scale (PWS)**
  - 3–7 years, or older children unable to use NRS scale
  - Scores include "none", "a little", "medium", "a lot"
- **Faces Pain Scale—Revised (FPS-R)**
  - 5–12 years of age
  - Patient self-selects a face, converted to a score of 0–10

- Scores range from mild pain (0–3), moderate pain (4–6), severe pain (7–10)

- **Numeric Rating Scale (NRS)**
  - 7 years and older
  - Scores range from mild pain (0–3), moderate pain (4–6), severe pain (7–10)

4 Sedation Assessment Scale

- **Richmond Agitation and Sedation Score (RASS)**
  - Infants to adults
  - Scores range from +4 to −5
  - Scores can be used as a goal to target sedative use

5 Withdrawal Assessment Scale

- **Withdrawal Assessment Tool (WAT-1)**
  - Infants to adults
  - Scores range from 0 to 12
  - Positive screen is a score ≥3. Interpretation is based on trend over time
  - Scoring should start on the first day of weaning opioids/benzodiazepines utilized for ≥5 days

6 Delirium Assessment Scale

- **Cornell Assessment of Pediatric Delirium (CAP-D)**
  - Newborn to 21 years of age
  - Scores range from 0 to 32.
  - Positive screen is a score ≥9

7 General Management Approaches for Analgesia and Sedation in Cardiac ICU

- Management should incorporate both non-pharmacological and pharmacological strategies.

- Non-pharmacologic strategies include ensuring age-appropriate communication, clustering cares, minimizing noise and stimulation, utilization of familiar caregivers at the bedside, maintaining day-night cycles and sleep promotion, and engaging child life specialists during procedures whenever possible.
- Pharmacologic strategies include the use of non-opioid analgesics, opioid analgesics, benzodiazepines, alpha-2 agonists, and other sedatives (i.e. chloral hydrate, ketamine, propofol).

8 Non-opioid Analgesics

8.1 Acetaminophen (Paracetamol)

- Analgesic and antipyretic effects
- Used for mild-moderate pain, or as an adjunctive therapy to opioids for moderate-severe pain
- Enteral (PO), parenteral (IV), and rectal (PR)
- Dosing
  - 15 mg/kg/dose every 6 h (similar across PO and IV formulations)
  - Consider decreasing the dose to 10 mg/kg/dose for those with mild hepatic impairment.
  - Does not require adjustment for renal dysfunction
  - Maximum dose: 75 mg/kg/day, or 4000 mg daily
- Onset
  - Analgesia: 5–10 min for IV, ~60 min for PO
  - Antipyretic: ~ 30 min
- Duration of effect
  - 4–6 h (both IV and PO formulation)
- Adverse effects: hepatotoxicity

8.2 Ibuprofen

- Non-steroidal anti-inflammatory drug (NSAID)
- Analgesic and antipyretic effects
- Used for mild-moderate pain, or as an adjunctive to opioid analgesia for moderate-severe pain
- Inhibit cyclooxygenase (COX) enzymes, which are involved in prostaglandin synthesis
- Approved for children >6 months of age and >5 kg

- Formulation: PO
- Dosing: 10 mg/kg/dose every 6 h, (maximum 40 mg/kg/day or 2400 mg/day)
- Onset: 30–60 min for analgesia, 60 min for antipyretic
- Duration of effect: 6–8 h
- Adverse effects: gastrointestinal disturbances, platelet dysfunction, renal impairment
- Contraindications: bleeding disorders, platelet dysfunction, gastric/duodenal/peptic ulcers, active GI bleeding, renal failure, postcardiac transplant

8.3 *Ketorolac*

- NSAID with analgesic and antipyretic effects
- Used for mild-moderate pain, or as an adjunctive to opioid analgesia for moderate-severe pain
- When used in combination with an opioid, has been demonstrated to have opioid-sparing effect allowing for lower dose of opioid use, improved pain relief, and reduced incidence of opioid side effects (respiratory depression, nausea/vomiting, ileus)
- Care should be taken to ensure adequate hemostasis has been obtained prior to administration in the post-operative patient
- Formulation: IV
- Dosing
  - 4 months–16 years: 0.5 mg/kg/dose (maximum 15 mg/dose) every 6 h
  - 16 years and older: 0.5 mg/kg/dose (maximum 30 mg/dose) every 6 h
- Onset of action: 30 min
- Adverse effects: gastrointestinal disturbances, platelet dysfunction, renal impairment
- Contraindications: <4 months of age, bleeding, renal impairment, post cardiac transplant

9 Opioid Analgesics

- Primarily used for their analgesic properties, although may also be used for sedation
- Analgesic effect occurs though activation of mu-, delta- and kappa- opioid receptors in the central and peripheral nervous systems
- Common side effects include respiratory depression, sedation, and dependence
- Analgesic dosing is based on patient weight and should be titrated to effect
- Care must be taken to prevent withdrawal when dosing is decreased
- Common opioids include Morphine, Hydromorphone, and Fentanyl.

Table 1 Common opioids utilized in the cardiac ICU

	Morphine	Hydromorphone	Fentanyl
Time for oral absorption	20 min (10–30)	30 min	N/A
Onset of effect	IV: 5–10 min PO: 30 min	IV: 5 min PO: 15–30 min	IV: 1–2 min
Analgesic duration of a single dose (IR)	IV/PO: 3–5 h	IV/PO: 3–4 h	IV: 0.5–1 h
Elimination half-life (median in hours)	Preterm: 10 h Neonate: 7.6 1–3 months: 6.2 3–6 months: 4.5 6 months–2.5 years: 2.9 Preschool: 1–2 Child: 1.3 Adult: 2–4	2–3 h	Neonate: 5 h 5 months–4.5 years: 2.4 5 months–14 years (long-term infusion): 21 Adult: 2–4
Equianalgesic dose	10 mg parenteral 30 mg oral	1.5 mg parenteral 7.5 mg oral	0.1–0.2 mg parenteral
SK dosage forms	Liquid, IR/SR tablet, ER capsule, injection	Liquid, IR tablet, CR capsule, injection	Injection, transdermal patch
Delivery	Intermittent IV, continuous IV infusion, intermittent PO or PR	Intermittent IV, continuous IV infusion, intermittent PO	Intermittent IV, continuous IV infusion

- At SickKids, Morphine is the standard opioid of choice. Hydromorphone is used as an alternative in patients with inadequate pain relief using morphine, or in those with unmanageable side effects. Fentanyl is often utilized for procedural anaesthesia and analgesia, as well as patients with hemodynamic instability or only requiring analgesia (ie trauma patients).
- When converting from one opioid to another, the equianalgesic dose should first be calculated (see Table 1) and then reduced by 30–50% due to incomplete cross-tolerance between opioids. Doses can then be titrated to effect.
- Management of opioid side effects is summarized in Table 2.

10 Alpha-2 Agonists

- Utilize the adenylyl cyclase and intracellular cAMP pathway
- Primarily used for their sedative and anxiolytic properties
- Common cardiac ICU options include Dexmedetomidine and Clonidine.

Table 2 Management of opioid side effects

Side effect	Preventative measures	Management
Respiratory depression		Naloxone reversal Partial: 5 mcg/kg IV every 2 min PRN Full: 10 mcg/kg IV every 2 min PRN
Pruritis	Use of synthetic opioid	Naloxone Low-dose infusion 0.25–1 mcg/kg/h IV intermittent 1 mcg/kg every 4–6 h Diphenhydramine, hydroxyzine
Nausea	Prevention of constipation	Ondansetron (follow QTc), dimenhydrinate, or diphenhydramine Metoclopramide Naloxone infusion (see above)
Constipation	Pre-emptive bowel regimen	Bowel regimen Naloxone infusion (see above)

10.1 Dexmedetomidine

- Analgesic and sedative properties
- Rapid onset and offset (half-life of distribution is 6 min). Elimination half-life is 2 h.
- Preserves respiratory drive and airway reflexes allowing for extubation
- Route: IV
- Dose:
  - Typically start at 0.5 mcg/kg/h, increase by 0.1–0.3 mcg/kg/h increments to a maximum dose of 2 mcg/kg/h
  - No loading dose
- Cardiopulmonary effects: bradycardia, hypotension
- Adverse effects: nausea, dry mouth
- Contraindications: severe bradycardia and hypotension
- Abrupt discontinuation can lead to rebound tachycardia

10.2 Clonidine

- Clinical onset in 60–90 min, elimination half-life 12–16 h
- Route: PO (IV formulation not universally available)
- Dose: 1–5 mc/kg/dose every 6 h PO
- Cardiopulmonary effects: hypotension and bradycardia
- Adverse effects: drowsiness and dry mouth
- Contraindications: severe bradycardia and hypotension
- Abrupt discontinuation may lead to rebound hypertension and tachycardia

11 Benzodiazepines

- Sedative medications that exert their mechanism of action through modulation of the GABAa receptor.
- Pharmacologic effects include sedation, anxiolysis, anticonvulsant, and anterograde amnesia.
- Common benzodiazepines used in the cardiac ICU include Midazolam (short duration), Lorazepam (medium duration), and Diazepam (long duration).
- A strong association exists with the use of benzodiazepines and the development of delirium in both pediatric and adult critically ill patients.
- Flumazenil is a competitive antagonist that can be used to reverse the GABAa receptor agonist effects (typical starting dose is 0.2 mg IV, with an effect within 2 min of administration).

11.1 Midazolam

- Considerations
  - Rapid onset (<5 min). Elimination half-life 1–4 h for bolus dose
  - Impaired metabolism in liver dysfunction, delayed elimination in renal impairment
  - High incidence of withdrawal after prolonged use
- Route: IV, PO, intranasal, SQ, IM
- Dose
  - IV: 0.05–0.1 mg/kg/dose every 30 min-2 h PRN (max 5 mg/dose)
  - Infusion: 1–6 mcg/kg/min
- Cardiopulmonary effects: hypotension, decreased SVR, apnea
- Contraindications: severe liver failure

11.2 Lorazepam

- Considerations
  - Onset of action: IV 1–2 min, peak in 15 min, duration 4–6 h
  - Elimination half-life 10–20 h (prolonged with hepatic dysfunction)
- Route: IV, PO, IM
- Dose: 0.05–0.1 mg/kg/dose every 2–6 h PRN (maximum dose 4 mg/dose)
- Cardiopulmonary effects: respiratory depression and apnea

11.3 Diazepam

- Considerations
  - Onset of action: 2–3 min, peak effects 15–30 min
  - Metabolized to active metabolites that have prolonged half-lives
- Route: IV, PO, PR
- Dose
  - IV: 0.1–0.2 mg/kg/dose every 6 h (max 5 mg/dose)
  - PO: 0.1–0.8 mg/kg/day divided every 4–8 h (max 5 mg/dose)
- Cardiopulmonary effects: transient decrease in blood pressure and cardiac output with IV administration
- Adverse effects: respiratory depression, apnea

12 Sedation and Analgesia Adjuncts

12.1 Ketamine

- Non-competitive antagonist at NMDA receptor that functions as a dissociative anesthetic. Opioid mu- and kappa-receptor agonist leads to its analgesic properties
- Can be used as an adjunct to opioids in acute pain to decrease total opioid doses
- Rapid onset (30 s if IV, 3–4 min with IM) and offset (5–10 min for IV, 15–20 min for IM)
- Route: IV, IM
- Dose
  - Intermittent IV: 0.5–2 mg/kg/dose
  - Infusion: start at 1 mcg/kg/min, titrate up to 5–10 mcg/kg/min
- Cardiopulmonary effects: tachycardia, hypertension, negative inotropy, bronchodilation
- Adverse effects: increase cerebral blood flow, cerebral metabolic rate, and intraocular pressure. Causes a dissociative state, hallucinations, and emergence delirium. Increased salivation and bronchorrhea.
- Considerations
  - Nystagmus can be used as a reliable sign of onset of action
  - Small doses of benzodiazepines may be utilized to counter the hallucinations and emergence delirium.
  - Preserves airway reflexes
  - Effective induction agent for procedures (e.g. intubation)

12.2 Propofol

- IV sedative often used for induction of anesthesia and procedural sedation
- Does not have analgesic properties
- Rapid onset (30 s), short duration (3–10 min), biphasic elimination (40 min for phase 1, 4–7 h for phase 2)
- Route: IV bolus, continuous infusion
- Dose: IV bolus 1 mg/kg/dose, infusions 20–100 mcg/kg/min
- Cardiopulmonary effects: hypotension, respiratory depression, negative inotropes, vasodilation
- Adverse effects: Propofol infusion syndrome—rare complication characterized with lactic acidosis, rhabdomyolysis, hyperkalemia, liver and renal dysfunction, and cardiovascular compromise associated with prolonged exposure. Monitor for lactic acidosis, hyperlipidemia, end-organ function, and electrolytes.

12.3 Chloral Hydrate

- Sedative drug that works via its metabolism by alcohol dehydrogenase to trichloroethanol (TCE), an alcohol
- Onset 15–30 min, duration 1–2 h in children (28–40 h in infants)
- Route: PO or PR
- Dose:
  - Neonate: 10–25 mg/kg every 6 h PO (titrate to 50 mg/kg/dose; maximum dose 1000 mg)
  - Sedation: Up to 80–100 mg/kg/single dose PO/PR (maximum single dose 2000 mg)
- Cardiopulmonary effects: arrhythmia, hypotension, decreased respiratory effort
- Adverse effects: gastric and esophageal irritation, direct hyperbilirubinemia
- Considerations
  - May accumulate in patients with liver dysfunction
  - May consider its use as a single dose sedative to support non-painful procedures or examinations, but caution against its repeated use as a sedative in critically ill infants and children

13 Common Approaches to Analgesia and Sedation Management Post-Cardiac Surgery

- Must be tailored to their underlying physiologic state and response.

- SickKids has created a 3-pathway system for routine post-cardiac surgery management based on expected duration of intubation, which includes sedation and analgesia management.

14 Green Pathway

- Patients admitted to the Cardiac ICU either extubated or anticipated to extubate within <12 h
- Goal is to achieve good analgesia with minimal effect on sedation and respiratory drive to facilitate early extubation
- Analgesia/Sedation Pathway
- Acetaminophen
  - IV Acetaminophen 15 mg/kg every 6 h × 1–2 doses, followed by PO 10 mg/kg every 4 h × 48 h, followed by 10 mg/kg every 4 h PRN
- NSAIDS: Ibuprofen or Ketorolac
  - If >4 months of age, bleeding <3 mL/kg/h. Avoid in renal impairment, bleeding disorder, ECMO, VAD, s/p heart transplant, stroke, on heparin
  - Ibuprofen: PO 10 mg/kg every 6 h PRN
  - Ketorolac: IV 15 mg/kg every 6 h PRN
- IV Morphine
  - Intermittent dosing 0.05–0.1 mg/kg every 30 min PRN
- Midazolam (if sedation required)
  - 0.05 mg/kg/dose every 4 h PRN

15 Yellow Pathway and Red Pathways

- Yellow Pathway = extubation anticipated within 12–24 h
- Red Pathway = extubation anticipated >24 h
- Goal: Need to achieve good analgesia and sedation to tolerate maintenance of devices, patient safety during prolonged recovery period
- Analgesia/Sedation Pathway
- Acetaminophen
  - IV Acetaminophen 15 mg/kg/dose every 6 h × 24 h, followed by PO Acetaminophen 15 mg/kg/dose every 6 h × 48 h, followed by PO Acetaminophen 15 mg/kg/dose every 6 h PRN
- NSAIDS: Ketorolac

  - If >4 months of age, bleeding <3 mL/kg/h. Avoid in renal impairment, bleeding disorder, ECMO, VAD, s/p heart transplant, stroke, on heparin
  - Ketorolac: IV 15 mg/kg every 6 h PRN × 48 h

- Morphine
  - Continuous infusion 10–40 mcg/kg/h
  - IV Intermittent: 0.1 mg/kg/dose every 30 min PRN × 24 h, followed by 0.1 mg/kg/dose every 2 h PRN

- Dexmedetomidine
  - IV Infusion 0.5–2 mcg/kg/h

- Lorazepam
  - IV 0.1 mg/kg/dose every 6 h PRN

16 Weaning and Withdrawal from Analgesia and Sedative Medications in the Cardiac ICU

- Risk for withdrawal exists when weaning opioids, alpha-2-agonists, and benzodiazepines after prolonged exposure.
- Patients are at risk for withdrawal from opioid infusions or regular opioid dosing after 5 days, dexmedetomidine infusions after 5 days, and benzodiazepine infusions or those requiring >3 doses per day × 5 days.
- Standardized weaning protocols minimize incidence and severity of sedation withdrawal (Fig. 1)

16.1 Opioid Withdrawal Symptoms

- Hypertension, fever, diarrhea, lacrimation, rhinorrhea, mydriasis, piloerection, tachypnea, yawning, nausea, vomiting, sweating, tachycardia, anxiety

16.2 Benzodiazepine Withdrawal Symptoms

- Confusion, hyperactive delirium, agitation, hallucinations, delusions, seizures, tremor, nausea, vomiting, sweating, tachycardia, anxiety

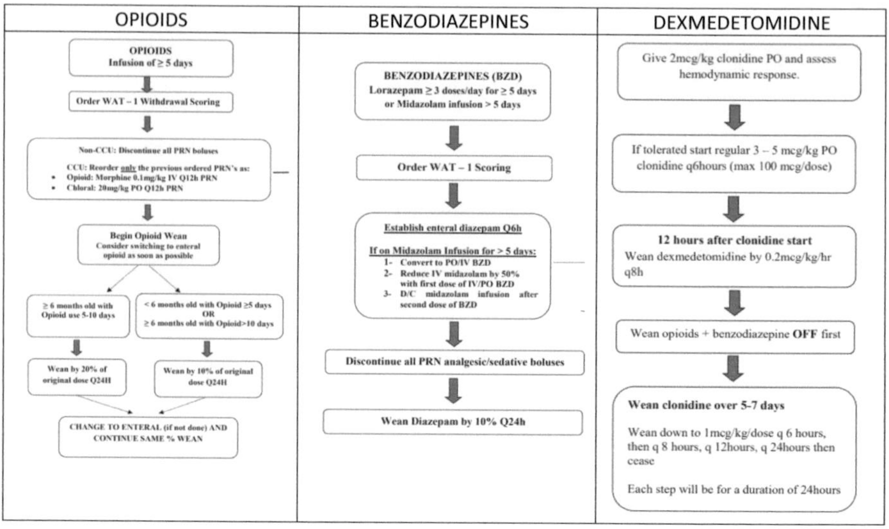

Fig. 1 Weaning algorithms for opioids, benzodiazepines, and dexmedetomidine

16.3 Alpha-2-Agonist Withdrawal Symptoms

- Rebound hypertension, tachycardia, agitation

17 Management of Delirium in the Cardiac ICU

- Delirium can complicate any cardiac critical care admission—early recognition, identification, and treatment is paramount
- Non-pharmacologic management consists of optimized management of underlying medical disease, with close attention paid to improving hemodynamics (hypoxia, hypotension), infection (e.g. urinary tract infections and peritonitis), metabolic abnormalities, and acute neurologic injury (e.g. stroke).
- Environmental modifications include promotion of circadian rhythm with lights on during day/lights off at night, bringing in familiar items from home, and family member presence and engagement at bedside.
- Management of iatrogenic sources of delirium include minimizing restraints, promoting mobilization, minimizing exposure to benzodiazepines and anticholinergics, and optimizing pain control.
- For patients refractory to non-pharmacologic delirium management, atypical antipsychotics can be utilized.
- Quetiapine is the standard for pharmacologic delirium management in the cardiac ICU (Table 3).

Table 3 Quetiapine dosing for delirium management

Age	Quetiapine dose
>2 months to <3 years	PO 0.125 mg/kg/dose once daily + 0.5–1 mg PO daily PRN, titrate to effect (Dose limit 0.5 mg/kg/day)
≥3 to <6 years	PO 3–6.25 mg PO once daily + 3–6.25 mg PO every 2 h PRN (Dose limit 25 mg/day)
≥6 to < 12 years	12.5 mg PO daily + 12.5 mg PO every 2 h PRN (Dose limit 50 mg/day)
≥12 years	25 mg PO daily + 25 mg PO every 2 h PRN (Dose limit 100 mg/day)

Bibliography

1. Hosokawa K, Shime N, Kato Y, et al. Dexmedetomidine sedation in children after cardiac surgery. Pediatr Crit Care Med. 2010;11(1):39–43.
2. Johnson PN, Miller JL, Hagemann TM. Sedation and analgesia in critically ill children. AACN Adv Crit Care. 2012;23(4):415–34.
3. Lucas SS, Nasr VG, Ng AJ, et al. Pediatric cardiac intensive care society 2014 consensus statement: pharmacotherapies in cardiac critical care: sedation, analgesia and muscle relaxant. Pediatr Crit Care Med. 2016;17:S3–15.
4. Moffett BS, Wann TI, Carberry KE, Mott AR. Safety of ketorolac in neonates and infants after cardiac surgery. Paediatr Anaesth. 2006;16(4):424–8.
5. Nasr VG, DiNardo JA. Sedation and analgesia in pediatric cardiac critical care. Pediatr Crit Care Med. 2016;17:S225–31.
6. Sessler CN, Gosnell MS, Grap MJ, et al. The richmond agitation-sedation scale: validity and reliability in adult intensive care unit patients. Am J Respir Crit Care Med. 2002;166(10):1338–44.
7. Smith HA, Boyd J, Fuchs DC, et al. Diagnosing delirium in critically ill children: validity and reliability of the pediatric confusion assessment method for the intensive care unit. Crit Care Med. 2011;39(1):150–7.

Nutrition in the Cardiac Critical Care Unit

Joann Herridge, Anna Tedesco-Bruce, and Alejandro A. Floh

Abstract Nutrition is an integral component of supportive care for children with congenital heart disease (CHD). Nutrition interventions aim to prevent or reduce malnutrition and growth impairment, which are associated with adverse outcomes. Adequacy of macro and micronutrient delivery is monitored, as well as feeding tolerance, biochemistry, and anthropometric measures to ensure adequate nutrients are provided in response to a patient's medical stability or growth requirements. Enteral nutrition is the preferred mode of nutrition delivery for acute and chronic conditions. Feeds are initiated within 24 hours of hospital and critical care admission, whenever possible, and escalated to meet a patient's metabolic demand. Feeds can be delivered by bolus or continuous basis, or via gastric and postpyloric routes for potentially improved tolerance. Parenteral nutrition is used as a supplemental or sole source of nutrition support in patients unable to receive enteral feeds. Alternative nutrition strategies exist for those with prematurity, necrotizing enterocolitis, chylothorax, gastrointestinal abnormalities, acute kidney injury or mechanical circulatory support.

Keywords Energy and protein requirements · Enteral nutrition · Feeding intolerance · Parenteral nutrition · Necrotizing enterocolitis · Chylothorax

Abbreviations

AKI	Acute kidney injury
AS	Aortic stenosis

J. Herridge · A. Tedesco-Bruce
Clinical Dietetics, Hospital for Sick Children, Toronto, ON, Canada
e-mail: joann.herridge@sickkids.ca

A. Tedesco-Bruce
e-mail: anna.tedesco-bruce@sickkids.ca

A. A. Floh (✉)
Division of Cardiac Critical Care Unit, Department of Critical Care Medicine, Labatt Family Heart Centre, The Hospital for Sick Children, University of Toronto, Toronto, ON, Canada
e-mail: alejandro.floh@sickkids.ca

© The Author(s), under exclusive license to Springer Nature Switzerland AG 2024

A. I. Dipchand et al. (eds.), *Manual of Cardiac Care in Children*,
https://doi.org/10.1007/978-3-031-70973-9_53

ASPEN	American society of parenteral and enteral nutrition
BMR	Basal metabolic rate
CHD	Congenital heart disease
DRI	Dietary reference intakes
ECMO	Extracorporeal membrane oxygenation
EER	Estimated energy requirements
EN	Enteral nutrition
ESPNIC	European society of pediatric and neonatal intensive care
GIR	Glucose infusion rate
HLHS	Hypoplastic left heart syndrome
IAA	Interrupted aortic arch
LCT	Long chain triglycerides
MCT	Medium chain triglycerides
NEC	Necrotizing enterocolitis
PDA	Persistent ductus arteriosus
PN	Parenteral nutrition
RDA	Recommended daily allowance
TEE	Total energy expenditure
WHO	World health organization

Key Points

- Growth monitoring
- Provision of nutrition support therapies, including enteral and parenteral nutrition
- Response to feeding intolerance
- Nutrition management of perioperative complications

1 Introduction

- Optimal nutrition is essential to improve outcomes for children with CHD
- Malnutrition occurs more often in infants with cyanosis, large left-to-right shunts, and complex CHD (up to 80%)
- Serial comprehensive nutritional assessments are completed to identify nutrient deficiencies and to optimize nutritional status
- Nutritional status can have a substantial impact on surgical outcomes and rate of recovery including hemodynamic stability, postoperative feeding tolerance, wound healing, shorter duration of mechanical ventilation and hospital admission

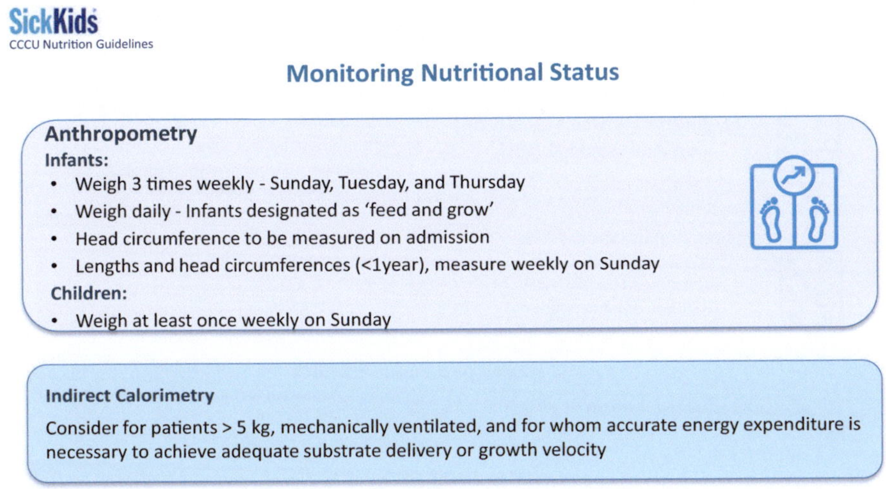

Fig. 1 CCCU nutrition monitoring

2 Growth

- Growth impairment is common in children with congenital and acquired heart disease (33–64%)
- Poor caloric intake, altered intestinal absorption, and increased energy expenditure leads to caloric deficiency
- Growth trajectory is monitored using World Health Organization (WHO) weight-for-age, length-for-age, weight-for-length, and head circumference Z scores
- Mid upper arm circumference measures are valuable in assessing growth
- Serial anthropometric measurements are crucial to ensuring adequate nutrition delivery during critical illness (Fig. 1)

3 Enteral Nutrition

- Enteral nutrition (EN) aids in maintaining normal gastrointestinal structure, lowers systemic inflammation, and boosts immunity
- The preferred route for nutrition delivery for all patients, including those who are critically ill
- Standardize nutrition algorithms improve caloric provision (Fig. 2)
- Goal is to introduce EN early (<24 hours following admission)
- To be initiated once hemodynamic stability is achieved, perfusion in adequate, and there is no concern for gastrointestinal injury, regardless of rate of inotropic and vasopressor infusions
- Efforts are made to optimize EN delivery and minimize feeding interruptions

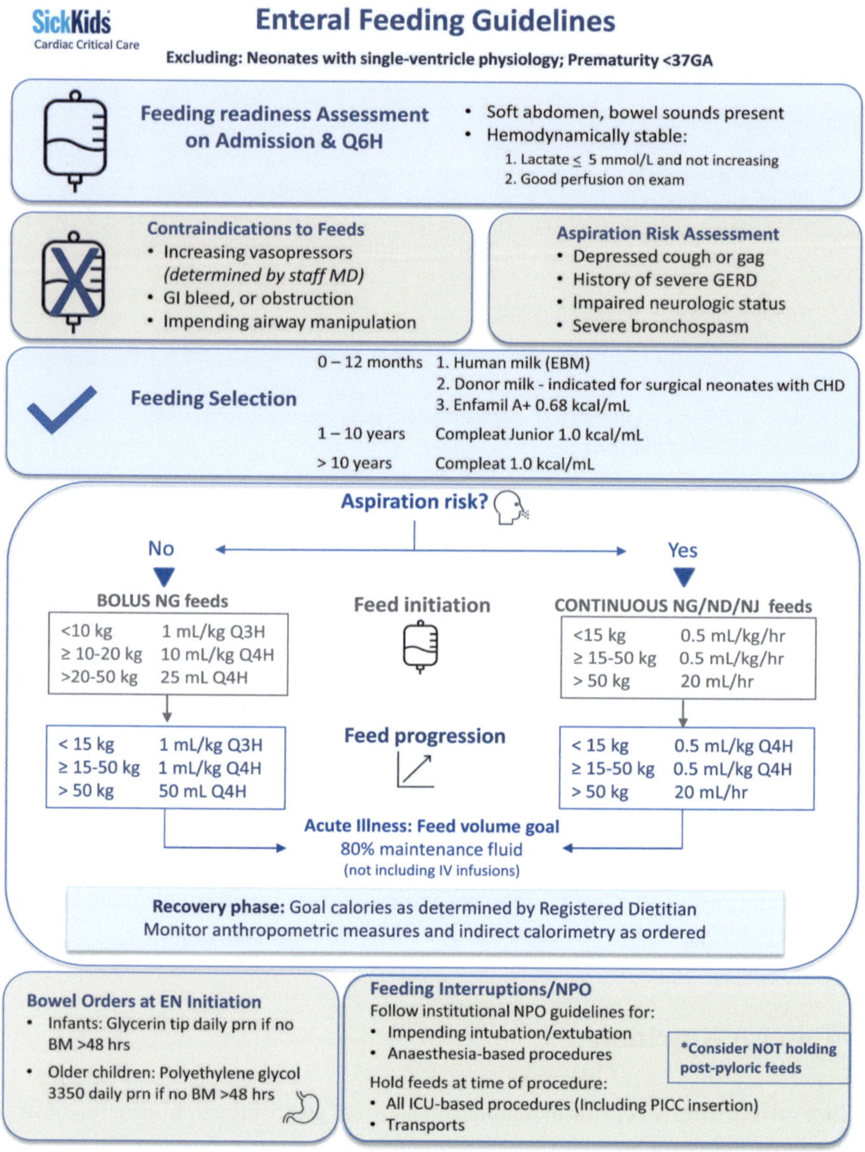

Fig. 2 CCCU Enteral feeding guidelines

- Held only prior to critical care procedures that may require airway manipulation/interventions – otherwise continue feeds in patients with secured airways undergoing procedures in the critical care unit
- Reduced or held temporarily during signs of feeding intolerance or medical instability (Fig. 3)

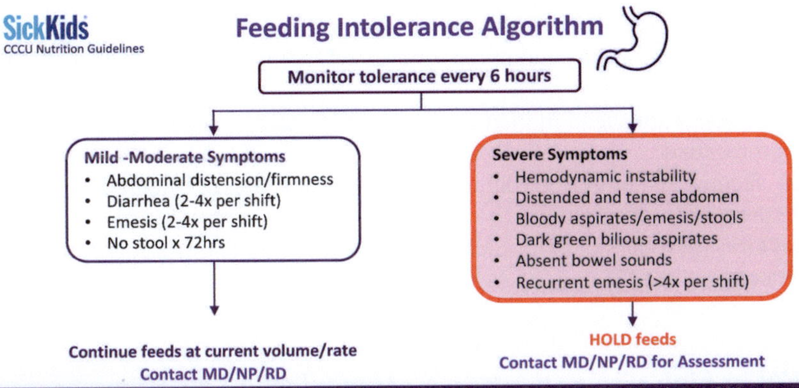

Suspicion of:	MD/NP/RD Initial Action	Continue monitoring tolerance Q6H: Symptoms improving	Continue monitoring tolerance Q6H: Symptoms persist or worsen
Constipation	• Continue feeding • Change bowel medication to scheduled dosing, and add a second agent	• Continue advancing feeds as per Enteral Feeding Guidelines	• Consider enema (for child /adolescent)
Diarrhea	• Assess for alternative diagnoses (i.e., withdrawal, medication reaction) • Re-evaluate bowel regime/prokinetic • Monitor for dehydration	• Continue advancing feeds as per Enteral Feeding Guidelines	• Consider decreasing feed volume by 50% or decreasing caloric density *(dilute prescribed feeds with Enfalyte, 1:1 ratio)* • Refer to Parenteral Nutrition Guidelines
Emesis, Nausea, Reflux	• Assess for alternative diagnoses (i.e., withdrawal, medication reaction) and reversible triggers (i.e., suctioning, cares) • Consider resuming previously tolerated feeds • Consider continuous NG or postpyloric feed • For nausea: Start ondansetron or dimenhydrinate • For reflux: Consider positioning, initiating or escalating anti-acid and/or prokinetic therapy	• Continue advancing feeds as per Enteral Feeding Guidelines	• Consider decreasing feed volume by 50% or decreasing caloric density *(After 5:00 p.m., dilute prescribed feeds with Enfalyte, 1:1 ratio)* • Refer to Parenteral Nutrition Guidelines
Ileus	• Hold feeds • NG to straight drainage • Consider starting a prokinetic • Re-evaluate pain & sedation medication(s)	Initiate feeds and advance as per Enteral Feeding guidelines • Restart at 50% of previous feeding volume if feeds held less than 24 hours • Start at beginning of Enteral Feeding Guidelines if feeds held greater than 24 hours	• Abdominal imaging • Consider General Surgery consult • Rule out Pancreatitis
Necrotizing Enterocolitis	• Hold feeds • Abdominal imaging • Antibiotics • Order abdominal girths Q12H • Consider General Surgery consult	• Once *npo* status discontinued: Restart feeds at beginning of Enteral Nutrition Guidelines	• Continue *npo* • General surgery consult • Refer to Parenteral Nutrition Guidelines • Reinitiate feeds according to surgical service
Cow's milk protein allergy	• Maternal elimination diet of all milk/soy containing foods • Transition from regular to hydrolyzed formula	• Continue on modified diet	• Transition to elemental formula • Consider alternate diagnoses (Infectious colitis) and GI consult

Fig. 3 CCCU Feeding intolerance algorithm

3.1 EN Source/Formula

- Human milk is promoted in the six months of life; donor human milk is the second best option and offered to critically ill neonates with CHD undergoing surgery in the first month of life

- Fortification of human milk with human milk fortifier or formula may be necessary for caloric delivery when patients have increased energy expenditure or are volume restricted
- Caloric density advanced in increments of ~0.1Kcal/mL (0.68 to >1.0 Kcal/mL) is recommended
- Bolus feeding is preferred but continuous feeds are considered if feeding intolerance and/or aspiration
- Postpyloric (nasoduodenal/nasojejunal) feeds are used to ensure delivery in the presence of severe feeding intolerance

3.2 EN in high-risk patients (e.g., Hypoplastic Left Heart, HLH)

- EN introduced in hemodynamically stable children – pre and postoperatively
- Feeds escalated slowly, as tolerated (Table 1)

4 Energy and Protein Requirements

- Caloric and protein delivery targets are designed to promote anabolism and to avoid over and underfeeding
- Energy expenditure fluctuates throughout all phases of illness and convalescence:
  - 34 to 70 kcals/kg/d in the immediate postoperative period following cardiopulmonary bypass surgery (24–72 hours)
  - Increase to 120–150 kcals/kg/d following surgery or between palliation interventions may be indicated
- Determination of energy expenditure by indirect calorimetry is the gold standard but not widely available
- Predictive equations can be used as an alternative to estimate energy consumption (WHO in acute presentation, Schofield for chronic patients) (Table 2)
- European Society of Pediatric and Neonatal Intensive Care (ESPNIC) recommends a minimum enteral protein delivery of 1.5 g/kg/d

Table 1 Feeding high risk subgroups: term single ventricle physiology infant

Timing	Feed schedule
Initiation	3 mL/feed q3h (or 1 mL/kg if weight >3kg)
At 24 hours	Increase 1 mL/kg/feed q6h x 4
At 48 hours	Increase 1 mL/kg/feed q3h
Initial goal feeds	10 mL/kg/feed q3h

Table 2 Predicted equations to determine estimated energy requirements for children

	Schofield	WHO
Indication	Applied for children receiving parenteral nutrition, ESPGHAN recommendations	Immediate postoperative (24–72 hrs)
Calculation	TEE (kcals/d), weight in kg **<3 yrs** Boys: (59.5 × wt.) – 30 Girls: (58.3 × wt.) – 31 **3–10 yrs** Boys: (22.7 × wt.) + 504 Girls: (20.3 × wt.) + 486	BMR (kcals/d), weight in kg **0–3 yrs** Male: (60.9 × wt.) – 54 Female: (61 × wt.) – 51 **3–10 yrs** Male: (22.7 × wt.) + 495 Female: (22.5 × wt.) + 499
Considerations		• BMR without added stress or activity factors, to be used. • AKI - aim for 120–130% BMR

AKI- Acute kidney injury, BMR – Basal Metabolic Rate; DRI – Dietary Reference Intake; EER – Estimated Energy Requirements; TEE – Total Energy Expenditure; WHO – World Health Organization; wt. – Weight; European Society of Gastroenterology, Hepatology and Nutrition (ESPGHAN)

Table 3 Protein recommendations

ASPEN		DRI	
Age	g/kg/d	Age	g/kg/d
0–2 yr	3–2	0–6 mo	1.52*
2–13 yr	2–1.5	7–12 mo	1.2+
13+	1.5	1–3 y	1.05+

* AI – Adequate Intake; ASPEN – American Society of Parenteral and Enteral

- American Society of Parenteral and Enteral Nutrition (ASPEN) recommends decreasing protein intake with increasing age (Table 3).
- Recommended protein delivery is higher in critical illness than the Dietary Reference Intakes (DRI) due to increased protein turnover

Nutrition; DRI – Dietary Reference Intake; +RDA – Recommended Daily Allowance

5 Parenteral Nutrition

- Parenteral nutrition (PN) is used for exclusive nutrition support or to supplement insufficient enteral intake
- Timing of PN initiation is based on patient age and medical diagnosis (Fig. 4)

SickKids
CCCU Nutrition Guidelines

Parenteral Nutrition Guidelines

Indications

Unable to provide minimum 50% of caloric goal by enteral nutrition:

- Premature neonate: Day 2 of life
- Term neonate: Day 3 of life
- Infants: Day 3 of life
- Children & adolescents: Day 7 of NPO

Special Considerations

Consider early initiation of PN:

- Metabolic disorders (as per metabolic team)
- Unable to establish adequate EN for burn patients
- Established PN dependence prior to admission
- Contraindications for EN

Lipid contraindications: Allergies to egg, soy, fish

Biochemical Monitoring

- Glucose, electrolytes, calcium, phosphate and magnesium, urea, creatinine (Monday & Thursday)
- Intralipid level (Monday & Thursday)
- Conjugated Bilirubin (Monday)

PN is evaluated daily in context of overall nutrition planning.
Changes will be guided by the Dietitian.

Macronutrient Recommendations

Macronutrient	Initial dose		Target dose
Amino acids (g/kg/d)*	Term infants 2m – 3y 3 – 18y	1.5 – 2.0 1.0 - 1.5 1.5 - 2.0	1.5 – 3 1.5 – 2.5 1.5 – 2.0
Lipids (g/kg/d)**	0.5 - 1.5		3
Glucose infusion rate (GIR)**	3 – 6 mg/kg/min		7 – 12 mg/kg/min

*Patients may require more protein to support growth and/or losses.
** Lipid and glucose targets are based on age.

PN Composition

- **Standard solutions** are available for peripheral and central access
- Custom solutions can be ordered between 10:00-14:00h (RD to guide)
- Lipid emulsion – SMOF 20%

Standard Solutions AA/Dextrose (g/L)

Indications for use by:	25/100	30/100	35/100	50/200
Weight	≤5.0 kg	≥5.0 kg	≥5.0 kg	≥5.0 kg
IV access	PIV or Central	PIV or Central	Central only	Central only

Weaning Parenteral Nutrition

- Provide adequate glucose source if PN is to be stopped abruptly
- Ensuring adequate energy and macronutrient delivery from EN, decrease PN accordingly
- Continuation of lipid emulsion may be required to promote growth

Fig. 4 CCCU Parenteral nutrition guidelines

- PN is available as standard stock solutions or can be prepared based on customized prescriptions
- PN solutions containing dextrose concentrations $\geq$10% require central access for delivery
- SMOFLipid® 20% can be used safely through either peripheral or central access

- PN therapy requires routine biochemical monitoring of macro and micronutrients

6 Nutrition Support Alternative Strategies and Controversies

- Randomized controlled trials are scarce and recommendations are largely limited to observational studies
- There is a lack of consensus pertaining to feeding management strategies in critically ill children
- Timing of PN initiation in critically ill children remains controversial with competing recommendations by governing bodies (ESPNIC suggests that PN be delayed up to one week while ASPEN recommends that PN should not begin within 24 hours of admission and supplemental PN should be individualized).

7 Complications and Considerations

7.1 Chylothorax

- Common complication following cardiac bypass surgery; multiple mechanisms including injury to thoracic duct or pulmonary lymphatics, or elevated venous pressures. Results in leakage of chyle into pleural cavities or pericardial space
- Volume increases with ingestion of long chain triglycerides (LCT) that are metabolized through the lymphatic system
- Diagnosed in patients with high chest tube output by identification of chylomicrons (if enterally fed) or high lymphocyte count (>80%) in pleural fluid
- Initial management is to transition to medium chain fatty acid formula (i.e., Portagen®, Monogen®) that bypass lymphatics.
- Alternatively, for infants receiving human milk, fat can be removed by a centrifuge and fortified
- A pre-existing cow's milk protein allergy requires an amino acid based formula (i.e., Vivonex Pediatric® containing a high MCT content or Tolerex®) that contains a low LCT content

8 Extracorporeal Membrane Oxygenation

- EN can safely be initiated and advanced following stabilization on ECMO
- Supplemental PN may be required if failure to achieve target EN due to frequent feeding interruptions or compromised gastrointestinal function

- There are no specific guidelines for nutrition delivery on ECMO. A protein intake target of 2–3 g/kg/d is generally used for neonatal and pediatric populations
- Caloric delivery guided by predictive equations, commonly WHO or Schofield equations, without applied stress factors

9 Gastroesophageal Reflux

- Common complication of heart failure and critical illness
- Can result in decreased nutrient delivery and/or absorption and oral aversion
- Medical treatment for symptomatic cases includes proton pump inhibitors, prokinetic agents, and conservative measures (elevation of head of bed or maintain upright position for 30 minutes following feeds)
- Severe cases may require continuous gastric feeds, transition to post-pyloric feeding, and/or instituting a hydrolyzed or free amino acid-based formula
- Feeds can be fortified to decrease feeding volume

10 Hypoglycemia/Hyperglycemia

- Intravenous dextrose infusions (i.e., dextrose 10%, D10W) is used to prevent hypoglycemia in neonates and infants that are *nil per os* (NPO)
- Target Glucose infusion rate (GIR) of 4–6 mg/kg/min
- Hyperglycemia (blood glucose level > 7 mmol/L or 126 mg/dL) following cardiac surgery is common and has been reported to be as high as 90% in the immediate postoperative period
- Glucose delivery is reduced with sustained blood glucose levels above 15 mmol/L (270 mg/dL)
- Use of insulin infusions is rare and used to address persistent hyperglycemia, unresponsive to changes in glucose delivery

11 Necrotizing Enterocolitis

- Necrotising enterocolitis (NEC) is characterized by intestinal inflammation, bacterial translocation, and possible epithelial necrosis
- Affects 3–7% of neonatal CHD admissions (cardiac NEC)
- Cardiac NEC is thought to result from inadequate intestinal hypoperfusion and splanchnic ischemia
- High risk lesions include those with systemic outflow tract obstructions (AS, IAA, HLHS), diastolic flow reversal (PDA dependent, aortic/truncal insufficiency, high pulmonary blood flow), and single ventricle physiology

Table 4 Feeding recommendations post NEC

Clinical status	Enteral feeding recommendation
Concern for heart failure or medical fragility	1mL/kg Q3H, no volume advancement
Weaning vasopressors Timing of feed advancement depends on dosing wean	Increase feeds 1mL/kg Q6H × 24–72 hours
Clinically stable as deemed by MD (de-escalating care, weaning inotropes, medications)	1mL/kg Q3H, increasing 1mL/kg Q6H x 24 hours; continue to increase 1mL/kg Q3H to goal volume feeds

- Despite numerous studies suggesting no association with feeds, concern for developing NEC often results in delaying EN initiation, slowing advancement, and interrupting enteral nutrition
- Disease is diagnosed and stratified according to Modified Bell's criteria
- Abdominal ultrasound has increased diagnostic sensitivity and commonly complements X-ray imaging
- Treated with cessation of enteral feeds and broad-spectrum antibiotics for a period of 7–10 days NPO, depending on the severity of NEC
- PN is initiated following diagnosis and safely advanced to goal energy and protein needs to support growth and recovery
- Following completion of NEC treatment, enteral feeds are slowly advanced depending on the child's clinical status. Recommended advancement guidelines are summarized in Table 4.

12 Renal Failure

- Acute kidney injury is characterized by severe catabolism with exaggerated metabolic derangements
- Early initiation of PN is indicated when EN delivery is suboptimal
- Estimated protein requirements during renal replacement therapy are 2–3 g/kg/d, to compensate for amino acid losses through the circuit
- Prolonged renal replacement requires increased carnitine and micronutrients (Vitamin A-E, selenium, zinc, manganese) supplementation

Bibliography

1. DiLauro S, Russell J, McCrindle BW, et al. Growth of cardiac infants with post-surgical chylothorax can be supported using modified fat breast milk with proactive nutrient-enrichment and advancement feeding protocols; an open-label trial. Clin Nutr ESPEN. 2020;38:19–27.

2. Floh AA, Nakada M, La Rotta G, et al. Systemic inflammation increases energy expenditure following pediatric cardiopulmonary bypass. Pediatr Crit Care. 2015;16(4):343–51.
3. Kelleher ST, McMahon CJ, James A. Necrotizing enterocolitis in children with congenital heart disease: a literature review. Pediatr Cardiol. 2021;42(8):1688–99.
4. Kumar SS, Maxvold N, Bunchman T, et al. Nutritional management in the critically ill child with acute kidney injury: a review. Pediatr Nephrol. 2017;32(4):589–601.
5. Mehta NM, Skillman HE, Irving SY, et al. Guidelines for the provision and assessment of nutrition support therapy in the pediatric critically Ill patient: society of critical care medicine and American society for parenteral and enteral nutrition. JPEN J Parenter Enteral Nutr. 2017;41(5):706–42.
6. Roebuck N, Fan CS, Floh A, et al. A comparative analysis of equations to estimate patient energy requirements following cardiopulmonary bypass for correction of congenital heart disease. JPEN J Parenter Enteral Nutr. 2020;44(3):444–53.
7. Salvatori G, De Rose DU, Massolo AC, et al. Current strategies to optimize nutrition and growth in newborns and infants with congenital heart disease: a narrative review. J Clin Med. 2022;26,11(7):1841.
8. Tume LN, Valla FV, Joosten K, et al. Nutritional support for children during critical illness: European Society of Pediatric and Neonatal Intensive Care (ESPNIC) metabolism, endocrine and nutrition section position statement and clinical recommendations. Intensive Care Med. 2020;46(3):411–25.
9. van Puffelen E, Hulst JM, Vanhorebeek I, et al. Outcomes of delaying parenteral nutrition for 1 week vs initiation within 24 hours among undernourished children in pediatric intensive care: a subanalysis of the PEPaNIC randomized clinical trial. JAMA Netw Open. 2018;1(5): e182668.
10. Zhang J, Cui YQ, Luo Y, et al. Assessment of energy and protein requirements in relation to nitrogen kinetics, nutrition, and clinical outcomes in infants receiving early enteral nutrition following cardiopulmonary bypass. JPEN J Parenter Enteral Nutr. 2021;45(3):553–66.

Anticoagulation

Leonardo R. Brandao

Abstract The coagulation system is a physiologic response to vessel injury to minimize blood losses by promotion of thrombus formation. Particularly in the venous vasculature, hemostasis is heavily influenced by stasis of blood flow, by local inflammatory response to the vessel wall to the injury, and by varying degrees of hypercoagulability states dependent on systemic vs local and/or disease vs therapy-induced factors. Pediatric patients undergoing or who have undergone cardiac interventions/surgeries are at high risk for thrombosis with venous thrombotic events in 19–40% of patients. Up to 28% of these are serious events. The identified risk factors for thrombotic events (TE) include mechanical valves, BTT shunts, and patients with single ventricle palliation physiology. Antiplatelet and anticoagulant agents act by inhibiting different steps of the formation of the platelet plug or the insoluble thrombus. Classes of agents include anticoagulants (unfractionated and low molecular weight heparin), oral vitamin K antagonists (warfarin), direct oral anticoagulants (DOACs), and antiplatelet agents (ASA, thienopyridines). The most common prophylactic and treatment algorithms are summarized in this chapter.

Keywords Anticoagulation · Heparin · Thrombotic event · Antiplatelet · DOAC

Abbreviations

AIS	Arterial ischemic stroke
aPTT	Activated partial thromboplastin time
APLA	Antiphospholipid antibody

The original version of the chapter has been revised: Spelling correction has been updated. A correction to this chapter can be found at
https://doi.org/10.1007/978-3-031-70973-9_57

L. R. Brandao (✉)
Division of Haematology/Oncology, Department of Paediatrics, Hospital for Sick Children, University of Toronto, Toronto, ON, Canada
e-mail: leonardo.brandao@sickkids.ca

© The Author(s), under exclusive license to Springer Nature Switzerland AG 2024, corrected publication 2025

A. I. Dipchand et al. (eds.), *Manual of Cardiac Care in Children*,
https://doi.org/10.1007/978-3-031-70973-9_54

ASA	Acetylsalicylic acid (aspirin)
AT	Antithrombin
BCPS	Bidirectional cavopulmonary shunt
BID	Twice a day
BTT	Blalock Taussig Thomas
CNS	Central nervous system
CPB	Cardiopulmonary bypass
CSVT	Cerebral sinus venous thrombosis
CVL	Central venous line
DTI	Direct thrombin inhibitor
DOAC	Direct oral anticoagulant
DVT	Deep vein thrombosis
ECLS	Extracorporeal life support
ECMO	Extracorporeal membrane oxygenation
FFP	Fresh frozen plasma
HIT	Heparin-induced thrombocytopenia
INR	International normalized ratio
IVC	Inferior vena cava
LMWH	Low molecular weight heparin
OVKA	Oral vitamin K antagonist
PE	Pulmonary embolism
PTS	Post-thrombotic syndrome
SC	Subcutaneous
SVC	Superior vena cava
TE	Thrombotic events
TID	Three times a day
UFH	Unfractionated heparin
VAD	Ventricular assist device
VTE	Venous thrombotic events

Key Points

- The coagulation system is a physiologic response to vessel injury, minimizing blood losses by promotion of thrombus formation.
- Pediatric patients undergoing or who have undergone cardiac surgery are at high risk for thrombosis with venous thrombotic events in 19–40% of patients. Up to 28% of these are serious events.
- Risk factors include vascular injury, foreign body material, stasis associated with low flow states or obstruction to blood flow (e.g. vascular access), and local and systemic inflammation.
- Thrombotic events (TE) are of particular concern in the setting of mechanical valves, BTT shunts, and in single ventricle palliation patients.

- Antiplatelet and anticoagulant agents act by inhibiting different steps of the formation of the platelet plug or the insoluble thrombus.
- Classes of agents include anticoagulants (unfractionated and low molecular weight heparin), oral vitamin K antagonists (warfarin), direct oral anticoagulants (DOACs), and antiplatelet agents (ASA, thienopyridines).
- The most common prophylactic and treatment algorithms are summarized in this chapter.
- Patients can be identified as low or high risk for the purposes of peri-procedural management of anticoagulation and/or reversal.

1 Hemostasis and the Coagulation System

- The coagulation system is a physiologic response to vessel injury, minimizing blood losses by the promotion of thrombus formation.
- The hemostatic response occurs in a stepwise manner, with vasoconstriction resulting from local cytokine release being followed by the formation of a platelet plug, which provides a platform for a more stable thrombus to ensue with the activation of the coagulation cascade.
- The platelet plug occurs in a sequential manner, as follows: platelet adhesion (platelet-vessel wall interaction), platelet activation (platelet format changes accompanied by the release of its internal contents), and platelet aggregation (platelet-platelet interaction). During each step, different platelet receptors expressed in the platelet membrane mediated this process.
- Activated platelets provide negatively charged phospholipid layers that foster the sequential activation of circulating coagulation factors, ultimately leading to the formation of a macroscopic insoluble thrombus.
- Antiplatelet and anticoagulant agents act by inhibiting different steps of the formation of the platelet plug or the insoluble thrombus, respectively (Figs. 1 and 2).

2 Who Should be Anticoagulated?

- Pediatric patients undergoing cardiac surgery are an especially high-risk group for thrombosis.
- Recommendations following interventional catheter procedures are summarized in Fig. 3.
- Up to 28% of TEs in the setting of pediatric cardiac disease are extremely serious events (e.g., cardio-embolic arterial ischemic stroke (AIS), cerebral sinus venous thrombosis (CSVT), pulmonary embolism (PE), superior vena cava (SVC) syndrome), either requiring thrombectomy/thrombolytic therapy, or leading to cardiopulmonary arrest or death.

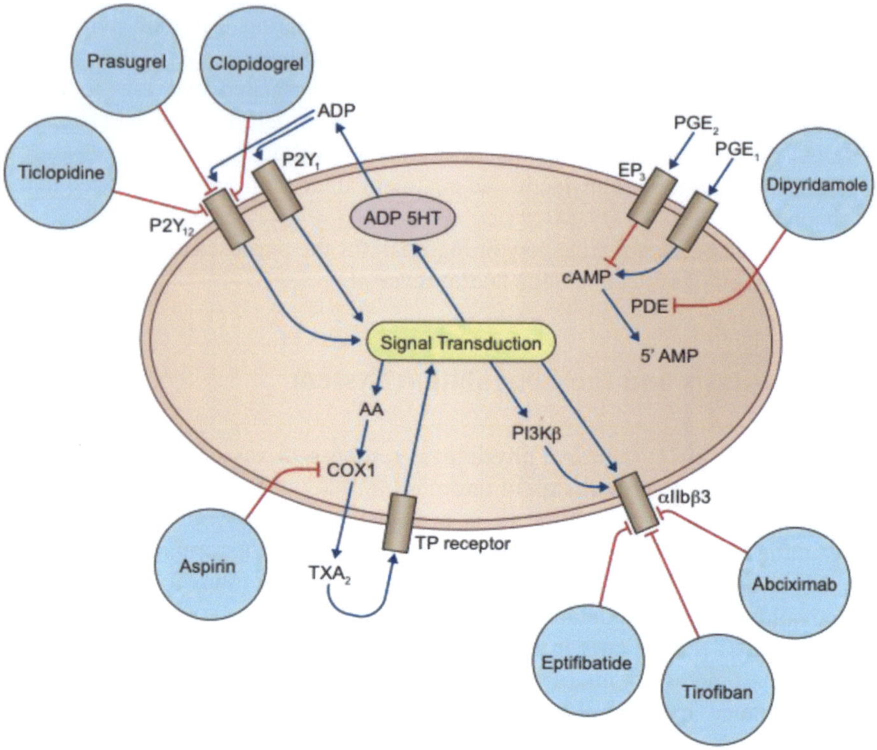

Fig. 1 Platelet receptors and inhibitors (simplified panel of platelet pathways)

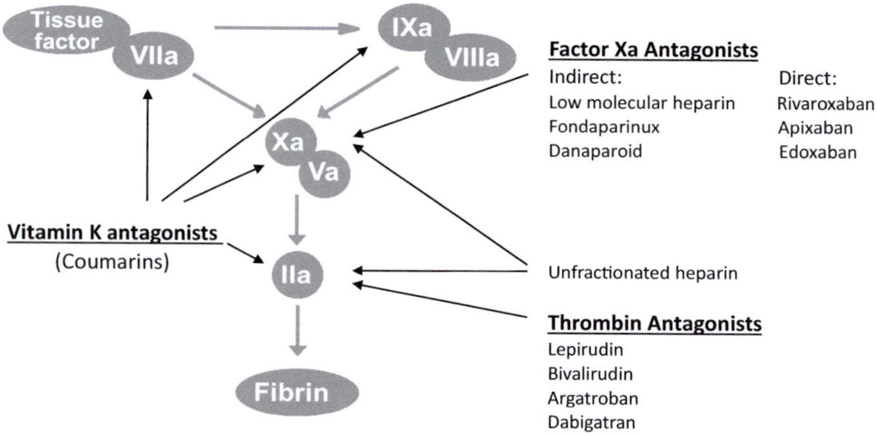

Fig. 2 Coagulation cascade and anticoagulants (simplified version)

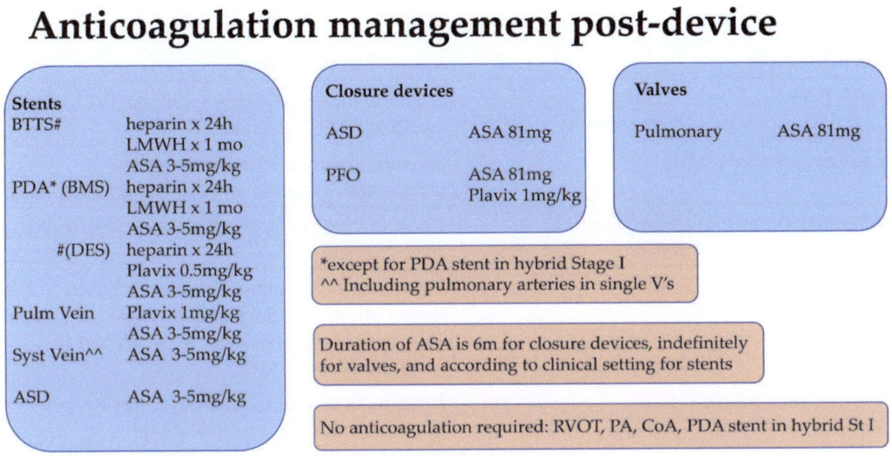

Fig. 3 Anticoagulation management post-device.

- Venous thrombotic events (VTE) in the setting of pediatric cardiac surgery is observed in 19–40% of patients with a 7% thrombosis-associated mortality, 15% recurrent VTE rate, and 8–30% post-thrombotic syndrome (PTS) frequency.
- Thrombosis risk factors: neonatal age, baseline oxygen saturation < 85%, previous thrombosis, heart transplantation, use of deep hypothermic circulatory arrest, longer cumulative time with central lines, and postoperative use of ECMO support.
- Thrombus' characteristics:
  - Location (e.g., intracardiac, pulmonary, brain, central venous are high risk locations; Table 1)
  - Cause (e.g., indwelling catheter-related thrombosis vs. non-catheter-related
  - Degree of occlusion (e.g., fully occlusive vs. non-occlusive)
  - Presence of symptoms (e.g., symptomatic vs. incidental).

3 Special TE Events in the Pediatric Cardiac Population

- Mechanical Valve Thrombosis
  - Can be obstructive, causing pulmonary edema, cardiogenic shock or systemic embolism; non-obstructive is more common, of which almost 50% are asymptomatic.
  - Current recommendations:

    In the presence of cardiovascular compromise, systemic thrombolytic therapy is the first line treatment.

Table 1 Thrombus location and clinical presentation

Intra-thoracic	**Clinical presentation**
SVC, IVC	Bilateral lower extremity swelling (IVC), facial swelling (SVC syndrome)
Cardiac chambers/valves	Asymptomatic, cardiac dysfunction, arrhythmia, systemic and pulmonary embolism
Pulmonary veins/pulmonary arteries	Cardiac /respiratory dysfunction (cyanosis > hypercapnea)
Aorta /intra-thoracic arteries	Decreased perfusion in lower extremities; potentially bilateral, discrepant upper and lower extremity blood pressures; hypertension (if renal artery is involved)
VAD/ECMO circuit	Visible circuit clots, circuit dysfunction, systemic embolism complications
Mechanical valves	Acute pulmonary edema, cardiogenic shock, systemic embolism
Extra-thoracic venous thrombosis	**Presentation**
CSVT	Seizures, neurological deficits
Cervical, upper extremity veins: internal/external jugular vein, brachiocephalic, subclavian vein	Upper extremity, facial swelling, catheter dysfunction
Intra-abdominal veins (portal, renal, umbilical)	Abdominal swelling, specific organ dysfunction, hepatic and/or splenomegaly
Lower extremity veins: iliac veins (common, internal, external), femoral vein (common, superficial)	Lower extremity swelling, catheter dysfunction, pulmonary embolism (rare)
Extra-thoracic arterial thrombosis	**Presentation**
Cerebral arterial (circle of Willis)	Seizures, neurological deficits
Cervical arteries: internal/external carotid artery	Seizures, neurological deficits
Lower extremity: iliac arteries, femoral arteries	Color change (pallor to purple black), decreased pulse, decreased temperature

Abbreviations: SVC, superior vena cava; IVC, inferior vena cava; VAD, ventricular assisted device; ECMO, extra-corporeal membrane oxygenation; CSVT, cerebral sinovenous thrombosis

Surgery is reserved for patients who have contraindication or who fail thrombolysis, or with impending cardiac arrest.

For the remaining cases, anticoagulation with unfractionated heparin (UFH) followed by oral vitamin K antagonist (OVKA) is recommended in association with frequent repeated echocardiographies to monitor for thrombus size.

- Blalock Taussig Thomas (BTT) shunt thrombosis
  - Occurs in up to 17% of children

- Presents with cyanosis if pulmonary blood flow is compromised often requiring immediate intervention.
- Options include: catheter-directed-thrombolysis, angioplasty with stenting, re-operation, and anticoagulation.

- TE after bidirectional cavopulmonary shunt (BCPS)
  - Occur in 28%; often associated with low BCPS flow state
  - Presents with cyanosis +/-.
  - Options: Catheter-directed-thrombolysis, angioplasty with stenting, re-operation, and anticoagulation
- TE after Fontan procedure:
  - Remain a major complication after Fontan surgery. Can occur any time after Fontan procedure, but often presents months to years later.
  - In general, in an acute presentation, aggressive antithrombotic strategy is recommended, including thrombolysis (local vs. systemic) and surgery
  - If chronic, anticoagulation should be discussed on a case-by-case basis
- Intracardiac thrombosis:
  - Can lead to pulmonary embolism (PE) and to arterial ischemic stroke (AIS).

4 Anticoagulants

- Heparinoids:
  - UFH
  - Low molecular weight heparin (LMWH) formulations (e.g., enoxaparin, tinzaparin, dalteparin).

4.1 Unfractionated Heparin (U FH)

4.1.1 Mechanism of action

- Glycosaminoglycan binds to the natural anticoagulant antithrombin (AT) via a pentasaccharide sequence. The heparin/AT complex inactivates thrombin (activated factor II [FIIa]) and FIXa, FXa and FXIa.
- Heparin catalyzes AT-mediated thrombin inhibition in a non-specific charge-dependent fashion to form a ternary heparin/AT/thrombin complex. In contrast, to catalyze FXa inhibition by AT, heparin needs only to bind to AT.

4.1.2 Laboratory monitoring

- UFH has a narrow therapeutic window. All children require daily monitoring.
- The inhibitory effect exerted by the UFH-AT complex over FIIa and FXa is monitored by
  - The prolongation of the coagulation test activated partial thromboplastin time (aPTT)
  - The activity against activated factor X (anti-Xa; heparin level).

4.1.3 Suggested Algorithm for UFH Administration in Children (Table 2)

- Prior to initiation: CBC and platelets, aPTT, international normalized ratio (INR), fibrinogen, and creatinine.
- Loading dose: 50–75 units/kg, IV, over 10 minutes (avoid boluses in neonates, patients with stroke, or when the perceived risk of bleeding is high)
- Maintenance dose: $\leq$ 1 year of age: 28 units/kg/hour >1 year of age: 20 units/kg/hour

4.2 Low Molecular Weight Heparin (LMWH)

- Shorter molecular length in comparison to UFH but with a similar mode of action to UFH (i.e., indirect Xa inhibitor via AT-mediated anticoagulation).
- Given by subcutaneous (SC) injections, either once or twice daily, and peak levels occur at around 2–4 hours after their administration.

Table 2 UFH dosing algorithm

aPTT (s)	Anti-Xa (units/mL)	Bolus (units/kg)	HOLD (minutes)	Rate change	Repeat aPTT
<50	<0.1	50	0	Increase 10%	4 hours
50–59	0.1–0.34	0	0	Increase 10%	4 hours
60–85	0.35–0.7	0	0	0	24 hours
86–95	0.71–0.89	0	0	Decrease 10%	4 hours
96–120	0.9–1.20	0	30	Decrease 10%	4 hours
> 120	>1.20	0	60	Decrease 10%	4 hours

4.3 *Suggested Algorithm for LMWH Administration in Children (Tables 3, 4 and 5)*

- Prior to initiation: CBC with platelets, aPTT, INR, fibrinogen, and creatinine.

Table 3 Low molecular weight (LMWH – Enoxaparin) dosing algorithm

	Age ≤ 2 months	Age > 2 months-18 years
Initial treatment dose	1.75 mg/kg/dose SC q12 h	1 mg/kg/dose SC q 12 h
Initial prophylactic dose	0.75 mg/kg/dose SC q12 h or 1.5 mg/kg/dose SC q24h	0.5 mg/kg/dose SC q12 h or 1 mg/kg/dose SC q24h
Maximum treatment dose	3 mg/Kg/dose SC q12 hrs	2 mg/Kg/dose SC q12 hrs
Maximum prophylactic dose		30 mg SC q 12hrs or 40 mg SC once daily

Table 4 Tinzaparin and Dalteparin Dosing Algorithms

Tinzaparin	Age 5–10 years	Age > 10 years
Initial treatment dose	175 units/Kg/dose SC daily	175 units/Kg/dose SC daily
Initial prophylactic dose	85 units/Kg/dose SC daily	87.5 units/Kg/dose SC daily
Maximum treatment dose	18,000 units/dose SC daily	18,000 units/dose SC daily
Maximum prophylactic dose	4,500 units/dose SC daily	4,500 units/dose SC daily
Dalteparin		
<12 months	150 U/Kg/dose q12 hrs	150 U/Kg/dose q24 hrs
1–12 years	125 U/Kg/dose q12 hrs	150 U/Kg/dose q24 hrs
13–18 years	100 U/Kg/dose q12 hrs	150 U/Kg/dose q24 hrs

Table 5 Low Molecular weight (LMWH – i.e., Enoxaparin) adjustment

Anti-Xa (units/kg)	HOLD	Dose change	Repeat anti-Xa
<0.35	No	Increase 25%	4 hours post next dose
0.35–0.49	No	Increase 10%	4 hours post next dose
0.5–1.0	No	0	1x/week; 4 hours post morning dose
1.01–1.5	No	Decrease 20%	4 hours post next dose
1.6-2.0	3 hours	Decrease 30%	Trough level prior to next dose; and then 4 hours post morning dose
>2.0	Yes (until level <0.5)	Decrease 40%	Trough level prior to next dose, until level <0.5, and then 4 hours post morning dose

Table 6 Warfarin loading doses (Day 2–4)

LOADING (days 2–4): if the INR is		
INR	1.1–1.3	Repeat initial loading dose
INR	1.4–3.0	50% of initial loading dose
INR	3.1–3.5	25% of initial loading dose
INR	>3.5	Hold until INR<3.5, then restart at 50% less than previous dose
MAINTENANCE oral anticoagulation guidelines		
INR	1.1–1.4	Increase by 20% of dose
INR	1.5–1.9	Increase by 10% of dose
INR	2.0–3.0	No change
INR	3.1–3.5	Decrease by 10% of dose
INR	>3.5	Hold until INR<3.5, then restart at 20% decreased dose

Loading dose: 0.2 mg/kg PO day; maximum 5 mg
0.1 mg/kg; with liver dysfunction, post-Fontan procedure, severe renal impairment

5 Oral Vitamin K Antagonists (OVKA)

- Warfarin (Coumadin) exerts its anticoagulant effect by interfering with the cyclic conversion of vitamin K to its reduced form (hydroquinone). Hydroquinone is an essential cofactor for γ-carboxylation of factor II (FII), FVII, FIX and FX, without which they cannot bind calcium and fail to promote thrombin formation.
- Its half-life is around 40 hours, with several recognized drug-drug/ drug-diet interactions that potentiate or inhibit its effect, requiring frequent dose adjustments and laboratory monitoring
- See Table 6 for loading doses and dose adjustments based on INR.
- See Table 7 for a comparison of the conventional anticoagulants in children.

6 Direct Oral Anticoagulants (DOACS)

- There are two classes of agents, direct thrombin (DTI, dabigatran) and direct factor Xa (apixaban, edoxaban, rivaroxaban) inhibitors.
- DOACs have a quick onset of action and are quite stable. Hence, they do not require laboratory monitoring.
- Pediatric treatment and prophylactic dosing regimens for DOACs are summarized in Tables 8, 9, 10 and 11.

Table 7 Conventional anticoagulants in Children

Mechanism of action	HEPARIN *(Anti-IIa and anti-Xa effect)*	LMWH *(Anti-Xa)*	OKVA *Vitamin K-dependent factors (FII, FVII, FIX, FX, PC, PS)*
Administration	IV, SC	SC	Oral
Half-life	30–60 min	10–12 hr	36–42 hr
Lab monitoring	aPTT, anti-Xa	Anti-Xa	PT, INR
Antidote	100% Protamine, FFP	~60% Protamine, FFP	Vitamin K, FFP, 3F-PCC, 4F-PCC
Bleeding risk	12.5%, (PICU: as high as 24%)	1.3% - 5.6%	12.5%; 0.5 – 3.2% pt-yr

Abbreviations: IIa, factor II activated; Xa, factor X activated; FII, factor II; FVII, factor VII; FIX, factor IX; FX, factor X; PC, protein C; PS, protein S; IV, intravenous; SC, subcutaneous; min, minutes; hr, hours; aPTT, activated partial thromboplastin time; INR, international normalized ratio; FFP, fresh frozen plasma; 4F-PCC, 4-factor prothrombin complex concentrate; 4F, 4-factor

Table 8 Rivaroxaban treatment dosing regimens for children

Bodyweight (kg)		Regimen			Total daily dose
Min	Max	OD	BID	TID	
2.6	<3			0.8 mg	2.4 mg
3	<4			0.9 mg	2.7 mg
4	<5			1.4 mg	4.2 mg
5	<6			1.6 mg	4.8 mg
6	<7			1.6 mg	4.8 mg
7	<8			1.8 mg	5.4 mg
8	<9			2.4 mg	7.2 mg
9	<10			2.8 mg	8.4 mg
10	<12			3.0 mg	9 mg
12	<30		5mg		10 mg
30	<50	15 mg			15 mg
>50		20 mg			20 mg

7 Antiplatelet Agents

- Salicylic Acid (e.g. aspirin/ASA)
- Thienopyridines (clopidrogel, ticlopidine, prasugrel, ticagrelor)
- Dipyridamole

Table 9 Dabigatran treatment dosing nomogram for children [Weight- and age-adjusted dosing (mg)]

	Age in years							
Weight (kg)	2.5 to <4	4 to <5	5 to <6	6 to <7	7 to <9	9 to <10	10 to <12	12 to < 18
≥91								330
81 to <91							330	330
71 to <81					330	330	330	330
61 to <71				330	330	330	330	300
51 to <61			300	300	300	300	300	260
41 to <51		260	260	260	260	260	260	220
31 to <41	190	190	190	190	190	190	190	185
26 to <31	180	180	180	180	180	180	180	150
21 to <26	180	180	180	180	180	180	180	150
16 to <21	140	140	140	140	140	140	140	125
13 to <16	140	140	140	140	140	140	140	
11 to <13	110	110	110	110	110			
9 to <11	80	80	80	80				
7 to <9	70							

Table 10 Rivaroxaban thromboprophylaxis in children Post-Fontan

Body weight (kg)	Twice a day dosing (mg or mL)*	Total daily dose (mg)**
7 to <8	1.1	2.2
8 to <10	1.6	3.2
10 to <12	1.7	3.4
12 to <20	2.0	4.0
20 to <30	2.5	5.0

* Oral suspension 0.1% (1 mg/mL)
** Equivalent to exposure of 10 mg once daily in adults

7.1 Aspirin (ASA)

- Irreversible inhibition of the cyclooxygenase enzyme preventing the formation of thromboxane A2 via the cyclo-oxyganase pathway. Effect lasts 5–7 days.
- Dose: 3–5 mg/Kg/day (taken daily or 3 times/week).

Table 11 Apixaban dosing nomogram for children (weight-based)

Weight range	Dose	Apixaban formulation*
3 to < 4 kg	0.2 mg twice daily	0.1 mg capsule
4 to < 5 kg	0.3 mg twice daily	0.1 mg capsule
5 to < 6 kg	0.5 mg twice daily	0.5 mg tablet
6 to < 9 kg	1 mg twice daily	0.5 mg tablet
9 to < 12 kg	1.5 mg twice daily	0.5 mg tablet
12 to < 18 kg	2 mg twice daily	0.5 mg tablet or 0.4 mg/mL oral solution
18 to < 25 kg	3 mg twice daily	0.5 mg tablet or 0.4 mg/mL oral solution
25 to < 35 kg	4 mg twice daily	0.5 mg tablet or 0.4 mg/mL oral solution
≥ 35 kg	5 mg twice daily	0.5 mg tablet or 0.4 mg/mL oral solution or 5 mg tablet

* Available formulations included 0.1 mg capsules or 0.5 mg tablets.
For children ≥ 5 years, available formulations included 0.5 mg tablets, 0.4 mg/mL oral solution, and 5 mg tablets (if body weight ≥ 35 kg)

7.2 Thienopyridines (Clopidrogel, Ticlopidine, Prasugrel, Ticagrelor)

- The thienopyridine are indirectly-acting platelet inhibitors where the active metabolites of the thienopyridine prodrugs covalently and irreversibly bind to the P2Y12 receptor during the entire lifespan of the platelet.
- First generation: ticlopidine; second generation: clopidrogel; third generation: prasugrel and ticagrelor.

7.3 Ticlopidine

- Effective inhibitor of platelet aggregation. Prodrug metabolized to an active form, which blocks the ADP receptor involved in GPIIb/IIIa receptor activation leading to platelet aggregation.
- Doses: 10 mg/Kg/day PO q12 hrs (maximum 250 mg/dose)

7.4 Clopidrogel (Table 12)

- Effect through an active metabolite that specifically and irreversibly modifies the ADP purinergic P2Y12 platelet receptor and through the subsequent ADP-mediated activation of the glycoprotein IIb/IIIa complex, thereby inhibiting platelet aggregation.
- Effects extend as long as 14 days after the last dose was given.

Table 12 Dosage of clopidrogel using 75 mg tablet

10 to <30 Kg	¼ tablet	18.75 mg
30 to < 50 Kg	½ tablet	37.5 mg
50 to < 70 Kg	¾ tablet	56.25 mg
< 70 Kg	1 tablet	75 mg

- Dose: 0–2 years: 0.20 mg/Kg/day PO; >2 years: 1 mg/Kg/day PO (adult doses 75 mg for $\geq$60 Kg adult)

7.5 *Prasugrel*

- Much more rapid and consistent inhibitory effect on platelet aggregation; specific, irreversible antagonist of the platelet ADP P2Y12 receptor.
- Pro-drug that must be converted to an active metabolite by the hepatic CYP system in order to exert antiplatelet activity.
- Distinct chemical structure permits conversion to its active metabolite with less dependence on CYP enzymes than clopidrogel.

7.6 *Ticagrelor and Cangrelor*

- High affinity ADP analogues that change the conformation of the P2Y12 receptor and therefore, result in reversible inhibition of the receptor without the need for any metabolic activation.

7.7 *Dipyridamole*

- Inhibition of adenosine deaminase and phosphodiesterase results in accumulation of adenosine and c-AMP, which causes a reduction in platelet aggregation in response to ADP.
- Effect lasts for only 12–24 h after the last dose was given.
- Frequently used as a second line antiplatelet agent or in combination with aspirin therapy.
- Dose in infants and children: 2–5 mg/Kg/day PO or IV TID. Dose limit 400 mg/day

Table 13 Level of thrombotic risk

High risk patient	Low risk patient
Congenital prothrombotic disorders	Old DVT
APLA +	Cardiomyopathy with no intracardiac thrombosis
Thrombus in the heart	Fontan with no intracardiac/ conduit thrombosis
Kawasaki disease with coronary aneurysms	Atrial fibrillation
Mechanical valves	Pulmonary stenosis
New DVT (< 5 weeks since diagnosis)	CVL prophylaxis
Stroke	
Stents	
BTT shunt	
Arterial thrombosis	
Pulmonary hypertension	
Fontan with prior intracardiac/conduit thrombosis	

Abbreviations: DVT deep vein thrombosis, APLA + antiphospholipd antibody positivity, CVL central venous line

8 Anticoagulation Management

8.1 Periprocedural (i.e., bridging)

- Anticoagulation may need to be held temporarily before or at the time of an invasive procedure.
- Patients may need to be "bridged" with short-term anticoagulation depending on their level of risk once anticoagulation is stopped.
- Table 13 categorizes patients into high risk versus low risk for the purposes of periprocedural anticoagulant management and determining the need for periprocedural bridging.

8.2 High Risk Patient

8.2.1 Periprocedural Protocol for High-Risk Patients on LMWH

- Hold LMWH for 12 hrs and start UFH 28 U/Kg/h (if the patient is < 1 year old) or 20 U/Kg/h (if the patient is > 1 year old). STOP UFH 4 hrs before an invasive procedure.

- Resume anticoagulant (AC) therapy with UFH at 4 to 6 hrs (non-CNS, non-intraocular, non- GI-tract; 12 to 24 hrs for remaining) and LMWH at 6-12 (or 12 to 24 hrs for CNS, intraocular, GI-tract) after invasive procedure, in consultation with surgery, provided hemostasis is achieved.

8.2.2 Periprocedural Protocol for High-Risk Patients on Warfarin

- Discontinue warfarin 72 hours prior to procedure.
- Give enoxaparin SC morning and night prior to procedure (last dose to be given 12 hrs prior to procedure).
- Obtain INR on day 2 following warfarin withdrawal and on morning of procedure; enoxaparin anti-Xa level on morning of procedure.
- Depending on the procedure, post-op initiate with enoxaparin and warfarin.
- Check INR 2 days after starting warfarin. If INR is in range, then enoxaparin can be discontinued.

8.3 Low Risk Patients

8.3.1 Periprocedural Protocol for Low-Risk Patient on LMWH

- Hold LMWH for 24 hours.
- Resume LMWH 6-12 hours after the procedure, in consultation with surgery, provided hemostasis is achieved.

8.3.2 Periprocedural Protocol for Low-Risk Patient on Warfarin

- Discontinue warfarin 72 hours prior to procedure.
- Measure INR on morning of the procedure.
- Depending on the procedure, post-op initiate with 1.5X maintenance dose of warfarin for 2 days. Resume maintenance dose. Repeat INR within 3–5 days of resuming maintenance dose.

8.4 Extracorporeal Life Support (ECLS)

- Initial UFH bolus of 50–100 U/Kg at the time of cannulation for ECLS, and then, UFH is continued as a continuous infusion during the ECLS course.
- Of note: some centres are moving towards bivalirudin infusions
- Table 14 summarizes the anticoagulation approach for common forms of circulatory mechanical support.

Table 14 Antithrombotic regimen for the common forms of circulatory mechanical support

	CPB	ECMO	VAD
Antithrombotic regimen	UFH during CPB. >1 year: bolus of 300 U/Kg. <1 year: bolus of 400 U/kg	Bolus of 75 U/Kg at cannulation followed by infusion at an initial rate of 10 U/Kg/h titrated to maintain ACT of 180–220 sec (primary target) and anti-Xa of 0.35–0.75 (secondary target).	UFH 8–48 h following implantation of VAD or bivalirudin, infusion starting at 0.3 mg/kg/hr Antiplatelet therapy (ASA) within 72 hr of VAD placement. Once clinically stable, switch from UFH/bivalirudin to therapeutic doses of LMWH (<1year) or VKA (>1 year) with target INR of 2.5–3.5 until transplanted or weaned from VAD support

9 Bleeding (For Anticoagulation in Children, in General)

- Major bleeding:
  - Clinically overt bleeding associated with a hemoglobin drop of at least 20 g L in a 24-hour period; > 20 ml/kg over a 24 hour period, or a transfusion requirement ≥10 ml/kg of PRBC over that same time period
  - Bleeding attributed to UFH treatment by the treating clinician that led to UFH being ceased
  - Bleeding within the retroperitoneal, pulmonary regions or located in the central nervous system
  - Bleeding requiring surgical intervention

9.1 Management of Life-Threatening Bleeding

- UFH: Stop UFH infusion and give protamine (14.15) (Table 15)
  - Maximum protamine dose is 50 mg. Infusion rate of 10 mg/mL solution should not exceed 5 mg/min. Hypersensitivity reactions to protamine sulfate may occur in patients with known hypersensitivity to fish or those previously exposed to protamine therapy or protamine-containing insulin.
- LMWH: Stop LMWH.
  - Protamine sulfate may be given. LMWH is not as readily reversed by protamine sulphate as UFH (around 40–60%). The dose of protamine is estimated according to the degree of reversal required and the time elapsed since the last LMWH dose was given.

Table 15 Protamine dosing algorithm for the reversal of UFH infusion

Time since last Heparin dose, (min)	Protamine dose
<30	1 mg/100 Units of heparin received
30–60	0.5–0.75 mg/100 Units of heparin received
60–120	0.375–0.5 mg/100 Units of heparin received
>120	0.25–0.375 mg/100 Units of heparin received

- Warfarin: Stop Warfarin.
  - Immediate reversal is achieved by using FFP 15 ml/Kg or PCC 25–50 U/Kg IV + I.V. vitamin K 5 mg (if they are unlikely to restart a VKA). In case of vitamin K infusion, it should be infused over, at least, 30 minutes to minimize the risk of anaphylactic reactions.

9.2 Management of Non-Life-Threatening Bleeding

- UFH: STOP UFH infusion. Within 2–4 h, reversal may be considered.
- LMWH: STOP LMWH. It will take 7–12 hours of the last dose of enoxaparin and 18–24 hr of the last dose of tinzaparin.
- Warfarin: slow reversal with ORAL or I.V. vitamin K 30 ug/Kg (1–2 mg). Oral vitamin K takes 24 hours to act, or 4 to 6 hours for I.V. vitamin K to commence its effect.

9.3 Classic Heparin-Induced Thrombocytopenia (HIT)

- Rare and paradoxical complication secondary to the use of heparinoids, when a hypercoagulable state ensues instead of bleeding due to the drug's effects.
- Immune-mediated prothrombotic state; antibodies directed against heparinoids paradoxically activate platelets, promoting thrombus formation.
- In the past, the quoted incidence of pediatric HIT was 1.5–2.3%, but it is now believed to be much lower.
- Characterized by moderate thrombocytopenia that occurs in a time-dependent manner to the FIRST exposure to heparin: 5–10 days after an initial heparin exposure or 1–3 days after re-exposure to heparin within the initial 100 days from the first exposure.
- Presentation:
  - Thrombocytopenia accompanied by the detection of platelet-activating anti-platelet factor 4 (PF4)/heparin antibodies.

- Associated with a tremendously increased risk of venous and arterial thrombosis.

- Complex diagnosis including:
  - Pre-screening: application of pre-test probability score (4T test; Thrombocytopenia, Timing, Thrombosis, oTher causes of thrombocytopenia). If low score (less or equal than 3), should not pursue laboratory investigation.
  - Screening: Immunoassays for anti-PF4/heparin antibodies (ELISA): has high sensitivity but poor specificity and can be detected in patients without HIT.
  - Confirmatory: Functional assay: the serotonin-release assay, which detects the platelet-activating effect of anti-PF4/heparin antibodies. It has >95% sensitivity and specificity for HIT.

9.4 Management

- Immediate discontinuation of all sources of heparin AND (Table 16)
- Initiation of an alternative (non-heparinoid) anticoagulant (Table 17), as follows:
  - Direct thrombin inhibitors: lepirudin, argatroban, bivalirudin.

    They directly bind to and inhibit thrombin

  - Direct FXa inhibitors: fondaparinux

    They work independently of AT and do not inhibit thrombin.

Table 16 Protamine dosing algorithm for the reversal of LMWH

Time since last LMWH	Protamine dose
Within 8 hrs	1 mg/100 Units (or 1 mg) of LMWH given in the last dose
More than 8 hours	0.5/100 Units (or 1 mg) of LMWH given in the last dose

Table 17 Non-heparinoid anticoagulation dosing regimens

Anticoagulant agent	Mode of administration	Dose	Monitoring test	Target range
Bivalirudin	I.V.	0.125 mg/Kg bolus, followed by 0.125 mg/Kg/h infusion	aPTT	60-85 sec
Argatroban	I.V.	0.75 μg/Kg/min	aPTT	60-85 sec
Fondaparinux	S.C.	0.1 mg/Kg once daily	Anti-Xa levels	0.5–1.0 IU/ml

Box 1: Anticoagulation and Antiplatelet Therapy following Cardiac Surgery.
All Norwood Procedures and BTT shunts

- When immediate post-operative bleeding has stopped (<2ml/kg/h for 2 consecutive hours) then start therapeutic heparin infusion.
- Aim for low level therapeutic heparinization (0.3–0.4 U/ml).
- Aspirin to be started (5mg/kg once daily) as soon as patient is tolerating enteral feeds.
- Heparin to continue until the third dose of aspirin has been given.
- Continue aspirin until Stage II (BCPS).

Bidirectional Cavopulmonary Shunt (BCPS)

- If there is no patching to the pulmonary arteries: no anticoagulation.
- Consider therapeutic heparinization if low BCPCS flows.
- If there is patching to pulmonary arteries: aspirin until Fontan completion (without heparin overlap unless it is a low flow BCPS as above).
- In all cases of bilateral BCPS: enoxaparin and then warfarin (when age and diet appropriate) until the time of Fontan completion. Target INR 2.5 (range 2–3) once using warfarin.

Fontan

- No need to give heparin in immediate post-op period.
- Overall approach is anticoagulation for at least 6 months postoperatively. Consider transitioning to aspirin indefinitely after 6 months regardless of initial anticoagulation strategy.
- Two potential approaches:

  Warfarin

    Start on day 2–4 (when tolerating enteral feeds).
    Target INR 2.5 (range 2–3).
    Start ASA when warfarin is discontinued and continue indefinitely.
    Consider Warfarin indefinitely for Y graft Fontan.

  DOAC (e.g. rivaroxaban, apixaban)

    Evolving experience showing at a minimum equipoise from a safety and efficacy perspective.
    Start on day 2–4 (when tolerating enteral feeds).
    No bloodwork or specific monitoring required.

Mechanical Valves

- Start heparin infusion on post-op day 1 and aim for low therapeutic range.
- Start warfarin day 2 (if tolerating enteral fees).

- Aim for INR 2.5 (2–3) for aortic valve and INR 3 (range 2.5–3.5) for mitral valve.

Melody Valves placed operatively in an AV valve position

- No need to give heparin in immediate post-op period.
- Give enoxaparin or warfarin (depending on age) for 3 months and then aspirin indefinitely

Bioprosthetic valves and RV-PA conduits

- No need to give heparin in immediate post-op period.
- Start aspirin once eating/drinking. Aspirin for 6 months.
- The pulmonary autograft used for aortic valve replacement in the Ross procedure does not require therapy.
- Homografts: no therapy required.

Metallic mitral valve rings (e.g. Cosgrove)

- Enoxaparin or warfarin for 3 months post procedure.

Bibliography

1. Avila ML, Shah V, Brandão LR. Systematic review on heparin- induced thrombocytopenia in children: a call to action. J Thromb Haemost. 2013;11(4):660–9.
2. Dahlbäck B. Blood coagulation. Lancet. 2000;355(9215):1627–32.
3. Garcia DA, Baglin TP, Weitz JI, Samana MM. Parenteral anticoagulants: Antithrombotic therapy and prevention of thrombosis, 9th ed: American College of Chest Physicians evidence-based clinical practice guidelines. Chest. 2012;141(2 Suppl):e24S–e43S
4. Manlhiot C, Menjak I, Brandão LR, et al. Risk, clinical features, and outcomes of thrombosis associated with pediatric cardiac surgery. Circulation. 2011;124(14):1511–9.
5. McCrindle B, et al. J Am Heart Assoc. 2021;10: e021765. https://doi.org/10.1161/JAHA.120.021765.
6. Monagle P, Chan AKC, Goldenberg NA, et al. Antithrombotic therapy in neonates and children: Antithrombotic therapy and prevention of thrombosis, 9th ed: American College of Chest Physicians evidence-based clinical practice guidelines. Chest. 2012;141(2 Suppl):e737S–e801S
7. Whitworth H, Amankwah EK, Betensky M, et al. Updated guidance for efficacy and safety outcomes for clinical trials in venous thromboembolism in children: communication from the ISTH SSC Subcommittee on pediatric and neonatal thrombosis and hemostasis. J Thromb Haemost. 2023;21(6):1666–73.
8. Whitworth H, Raffini L. Practical considerations for use of direct oral anticoagulants in children. Front Pediatr. 2022;10: 860369.

Cardiac Implantable Electronic Devices

Michael D. Fridman and Anica Bulic

Abstract Medical devices have revolutionized the care of individuals with heart disease. With the advent of new technologies and improving miniaturization, pediatric cardiologists are now able to enlist the help of myriad devices to monitor and treat a wide variety of bradyarrhythmias and tachyarrhythmias. The decisions for the type of device, implantation strategy, and monitoring/treatment parameters are often very complex in pediatrics, especially when the device needs are superimposed on congenital heart disease. Cardiologists are therefore required to balance many factors to allow for the treatment of smaller, more complex patients. For example, the needs of a patient with congenital complete heart block and a structurally normal heart are vastly different from one with ccTGA, complete heart block, and Fontan physiology. As the complexity of the pediatric and congenital cardiac population increases, more of these patients are requiring cardiac implantable electronic devices (CIEDs). Those involved in cardiac care must therefore ensure that they have a working knowledge of these systems and know when to reach out to their electrophysiology colleagues for help. In the following chapter, we will explore some of the basics of CIEDs including the major indications, types of devices, terminology used, and troubleshooting of common issues.

Keywords Cardiac implantable electronic devices · Pacemaker · Implantable cardioverter defibrillator · Cardiac resynchronization therapy · Pacing · Implantable loop recorder

M. D. Fridman
Section of Paediatric Cardiology, Department of Pediatrics, Alberta Children's Hospital, University of Calgary, Calgary, AB, Canada
e-mail: michael.fridman@albertahealthservices.ca

A. Bulic (✉)
Division of Pediatric Cardiology, Hospital for Sick Children, University of Toronto, Toronto, ON, Canada
e-mail: anica.bulic@sickkids.ca

© The Author(s), under exclusive license to Springer Nature Switzerland AG 2024

A. I. Dipchand et al. (eds.), *Manual of Cardiac Care in Children*,
https://doi.org/10.1007/978-3-031-70973-9_55

Abbreviations

AV	Atrioventricular
BPEG	British pacing and electrophysiology group
CCHB	Congenital complete heart block
ccTGA	Congenitally corrected transposition of the great arteries
CIED	Cardiac implantable electronic device
CRT	Cardiac resynchronization therapy
CRT-D	Cardiac resynchronization therapy - defibrillator
CRT-P	Cardiac resynchronization therapy - pacemaker
HRS	Heart rhythm society
ICD	Implantable cardiac defibrillator
ILR	Implantable loop recorder
LV	Left ventricle
NASPE	North American society for pacing and electrophysiology
PACES	Paediatric and congenital electrophysiology society
PFO	Persistent foramen ovale
PM	Pacemaker
PMT	Pacemaker mediated tachycardia
PVARP	Post-ventricular atrial refractory period
SVT	Supraventricular tachycardia
VF	Ventricular fibrillation
VT	Ventricular tachycardia

Key Points

- Implantatable loop recorders (ILRs) are useful tools for obtaining symptom-rhythm correlation but have no therapeutic modes.
- Pacemakers (PMs) and implantable cardiac defibrillators (ICDs) can be epicardial or transvenous as well as single- or dual-chamber.
- Cardiac implantable electronic devices (CIEDs) work exactly as programmed but this requires knowledge of troubleshooting to understand what a device is sensing, how it is interacting with the heart (e.g., undersensing, oversensing, loss of capture, impedance changes), and how to manage.
- Refer to the updated Paediatric and Congenital Electrophysiology Society (PACES)/Heart Rhythm Society (HRS) guidelines for specific recommendations on indications for device use.

1 Introduction

- Cardiac implantable electronic devices (CIEDs) have been a mainstay of therapy for patients with arrhythmias since the early 20th century.
- There have been enormous advances in arrhythmia management strategies, device evolution, and miniaturization to increase access for smaller patients.
- CIEDs are used to treat a myriad of diseases including, but not limited to, bradyarrhythmias, tachyarrhythmias, and cardiac dysfunction.
- In general, CIEDs fall into four major categories:

  – Implantable loop recorders (ILRs)

    Small, implantable devices that serve exclusively as heart rhythm monitors and have no therapeutic capabilities (e.g., cannot pace or defibrillate)
    Subcutaneous implantation anterior to the rib cage in a simple, day-procedure

  – Pacemakers (PMs)

    Implantable devices creating a circuit with the heart with the purpose of electrically stimulating the myocardium and triggering a mechanical event.
    Useful for bradyarrhythmias (e.g., complete heart block) and tachyarrhythmias amenable to overdrive pacing (e.g., atrial flutter).

  – Implantable cardioverter defibrillators (ICDs)

    Work like PMs with the addition of a high-voltage coil that can deliver a shock when tachyarrhythmias are detected (e.g., ventricular fibrillation).

  – Cardiac resynchronization therapy (CRT)

    Can be both pacemakers (CRT-P) and defibrillators (CRT-D) where multi-site ventricular pacing can be done to optimize mechanical contraction and improve ventricular function.
    Used to treat electromechanical dyssynchrony and heart failure

2 Indications

- PACES has published a comprehensive guideline on the indications for pediatric CIED implantation.
- The two most common scenarios for permanent pacing in children are congenital complete heart block (CCHB) and post-operative AV block.

- Class I permanent pacing indications for CCHB include symptomatic bradycardia; wide QRS escape rhythm, complex ventricular ectopy, or ventricular systolic dysfunction; and a mean ventricular rate of $\leq$ 50 bpm as seen on ambulatory monitoring (e.g., holter, telemetry) in neonates and infants.
- Class I permanent pacing indications in the post-operative setting include advanced 2nd or 3rd degree AV block that has not completely recovered by post-operative day 7–10, or late-onset advanced 2nd or 3rd degree AV block with a history of transient post-operative AV block.

• For a more extensive list of specific indications, please refer to the most recent PACES expert consensus guideline.

3 Device Types (Fig. 1)

• ILR

- Small recording device the size of a small thumb-drive (Fig. 1A)
- Sits subcutaneously to continuously monitor for tachycardia, bradycardia, and pauses based on programmed parameters
- Automatically sends alerts to the monitoring service when those parameters are met
- Can also be activated in real-time to record the rhythm during symptomatic episodes, which is especially useful in symptom-rhythm correlation for infrequent events
- Battery lasts ~3–4.5 years, depending on the model

• PM

- Can be temporary or permanent
- Can involve leads that are either:

  On the outer surface of the heart accessed via sternotomy, thoracotomy, or subxiphoid approach (epicardial)
  Implanted through systemic veins attached to the endocardial surface of heart (transvenous)

- Leadless PM: a relatively new technology where the entire system sits within the right ventricle.
- In general, transvenous systems are preferred over epicardial systems due to the less invasive implantation and improved lead longevity.
- Epicardial systems are usually indicated in patients <20 kg, with intracardiac shunts other than PFOs, and those with systemic venous anatomy that precludes transvenous lead implantation (e.g. stenosed/occluded subclavian vein)

  Single ventricle patients generally require epicardial systems due to risk of systemic thromboembolism from an intracardiac lead (Fig. 1B).

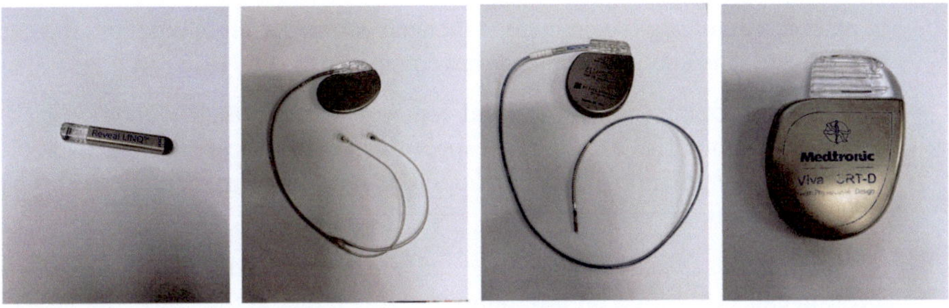

Fig. 1 Examples of different CIEDs, including an ILR (A), epicardial PPM (B), transvenous ICD (C), and CRT device (D). Reproduced with permission from Jessie Salway, Hospital for Sick Children

  - Decisions regarding epicardial vs transvenous, single- vs dual-chamber pacemakers, and pacing modes are ideally made in a shared decision-making model between the patient/family, treating cardiologist, and local electrophysiology team

- ICD and CRT devices also have pacing abilities but with a few key differences:
  - ICDs have a high-voltage coil that are able to deliver high-energy "shocks" to the heart in order to cardiovert/defibrillate VT/VF (Fig. 1C)
  - CRT devices have three leads (one atrial and two ventricular) to optimize both AV and interventricular electrical synchrony to improve mechanical contraction and ventricular systolic function (Fig. 1D)

4 Anatomy of a Device (Fig. 2)

- The "can" is the term for the device itself
  - Metallic object that contains the computer, battery, and header to connect to the lead
  - Vary in size from small (e.g., single-chamber devices requiring only one lead) to quite large (e.g., CRT-D devices requiring 3 leads including a high-output defibrillation coil).
- The lead is comprised of an insulated wire making an interface with the cardiac tissue.
  - Each lead has two poles which are used to complete the circuit.
  - Electrical circuits work by having electricity flow from higher electrical potential to lower potential from the cathode (negative pole) to the anode (positive pole).

- In an epicardial lead, the cathode is the lead coming straight out from the can to the heart. The anode is the lead that comes off the tine (Fig. 3A).

  Ideal positioning for an epicardial ventricular lead is the LV apex.
  Caution should be used with respect to intrathoracic lead bulk to avoid cardiac strangulation (e.g., lead looping around the heart) or coronary artery compression.

- In a transvenous system (Fig. 3B), the cathode is the tip of the lead. The anode's location can vary based on programming. It is either at the "ring," an area of metal just proximal to the tip, in a bipolar configuration, or in the can itself in a unipolar configuration.
- For an ICD, there is an additional defibrillation coil seen proximal to the ring for several centimeters of distance up the wire (Fig. 2B).

• Leadless pacemakers are small pacing systems implanted via femoral vein or right internal jugular with the advantage of not having any of the complications of transvenous leads.

  - The main drawback in the widespread use in children is that the delivery sheath is large (outer diameter 27 Fr). The most widely used leadless pacemaker is also not retrievable, which also lowers enthusiasm for pediatric implantation.
  - There may be a role for leadless pacemakers in those older and bigger adolescents with a low expected ventricular pacing burden or those who cannot have transvenous systems.

5 Basic Device Physics

• Electricity follows Ohm's Law, V = IR, where V is voltage in Volts, I is current in Amperes (a unit of charge or "Coulombs" per second), and R is resistance in Ohms.
• Voltage is the electrical potential difference down which electricity flows, similar to a pressure difference. The battery provides the potential difference, which then drives the current relative to resistance.
• For the same battery, a high-resistance circuit will result in very low current and a low-resistance circuit in very high current. This is important as battery drain depends on the amount of current used (more current use = faster battery depletion).
• In a bipolar circuit, the circuit moves from battery to cathode to the myocardium and to the anode and back to the battery. This generally involves the delivery of smaller amounts of energy to a more localized area for stimulation and senses a smaller area.

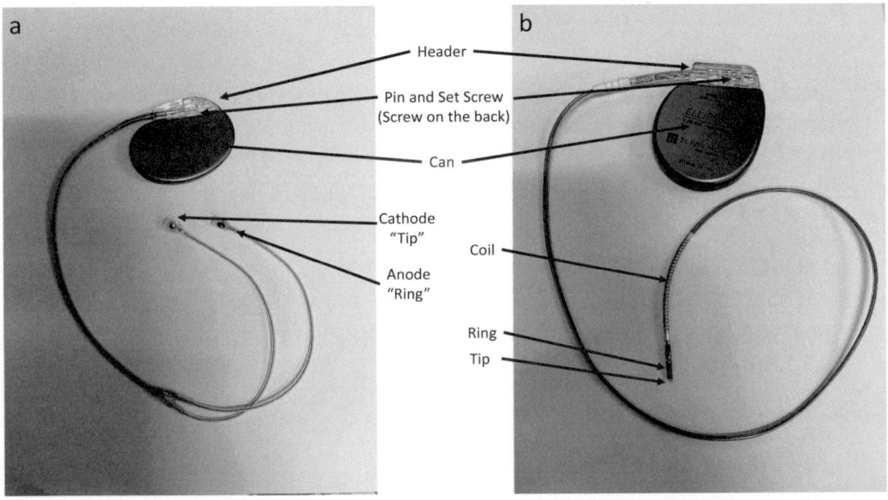

Fig. 2 The anatomy of a CIED. (A) An epicardial pacemaker. The cathode is equivalent to the "tip" electrode in a transvenous lead and is the wire going straight back to the device. The anode is equivalent to the "ring" electrode and is seen on x-ray slightly offset from the lead going back to the can. (B) A single-chamber transvenous ICD. Note the presence of the large "coil" which is used to deliver the shock when an arrhythmia is detected. Reproduced with permission from Jessie Salway, Hospital for Sick Children

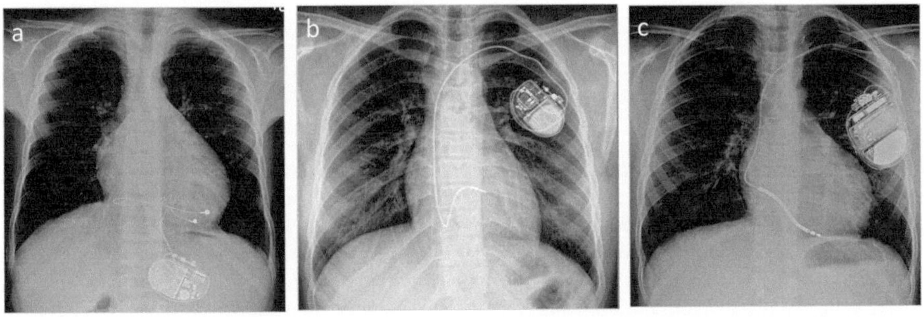

Fig. 3 X-ray examples of epicardial single chamber permanent pacemaker with electrodes on the LV apex (A), transvenous single chamber permanent pacemaker with the lead high in the RV septum (B), and transvenous single-chamber ICD with the lead embedded in the RV apex (C)

- In a unipolar configuration, the lead-heart interface is the cathode and the can itself is the anode. As there is much more fluid and body tissue between the lead and the can, the resistance is lower, so current drain is generally higher.

6 Pacemaker Modes

- PMs can be programmed in many ways and the PM mode is communicated by a 5-letter code based on the North American Society for Pacing and Electrophysiology (NASPE)/British Pacing and Electrophysiology Group (BPEG).
- Table 1 highlights the code and Table 2 outlines some of the most common modes used.
  - In children with CHB, both VVI and DDD modes are commonly used. Studies are ongoing to determine ideal pacing mode but strategies to minimize ventricular pacing should be employed alongside surveillance for pacing-induced cardiomyopathy.
- Pacing intervals are illustrated in Fig. 4.

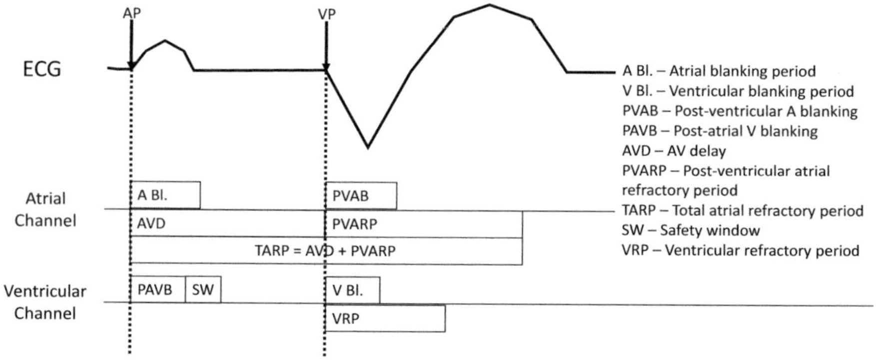

Fig. 4 Pacemaker intervals for dual chamber devices. Blanking periods are points where the pacemaker is not "listening." Refractory periods are still "listening" but do not react. TARP dictates upper rate limit as it is the shortest amount of time the pacemaker will allow between pacing cycles (Maximum Tracking Rate). The Safety Window is a sensitive period of time that will listen for activity. If activity is detected in the safety window, it will automatically pace (if ventricular safety pacing is turned on) to avoid underpacing (e.g. electromagnetic interference detected) or pacing on a T (if a PVC falls in the safety window). The lower rate limit is set on the device. The difference between the LRL and the TARP is the pacemaker's rate range

Table 1 NASPE/BPEG pacemaker code

I Paced chamber	II Sensed chamber	III Response to sensed event	IV Rate modulation	V Multisite pacing
O – None	O – None	O – None	O – None	O – None
A – Atrium	A – Atrium	I – Inhibit	R – Rate response	A – Atrium
V – Ventricle	V – Ventricle	T – Trigger		V – Ventricle
D – A + V	D – A + V	D – I + T		D – A + V

Table 2 Common pacemaker modes and indications in paediatrics

Mode	Description	Common indication
AAI	Atrial demand pacing with no rate modulation. Atrial pacing at set rate. If atrial event sensed, pacemaker inhibits.	Sinus bradycardia Overdrive pacing in JET, VT
VVI	Ventricular demand pacing with no rate modulation. Ventricular pacing at set rate. If ventricular event sensed, pacemaker inhibits.	Complete heart block Back-up pacing in high grade AV block, sinus pauses
DDD	Physiologic pacing with no rate modulation. Atrial pacing at set lower rate followed by AV delay then ventricular pacing. If atrial event sensed, V-pacing will trigger if no ventricular event seen within AV delay window.	Complete heart block
VVIR	Ventricular demand pacing with rate modulation. As above with VVI but rate varies with level of activity sensed by pacemaker accelerometer.	Complete heart block with inadequate chronotropic response (e.g. exercise intolerance)
DDDR	Physiologic pacing with rate modulation. As above with DDD but lower rate limit varies based on level of activity sensed by pacemaker accelerometer.	Complete heart block with sinus node dysfunction
VOO	Asynchronous ventricular pacing.	Complete heart block during surgery with electrocautery and *inadequate* intrinsic rate. Must watch for pacing on T-wave as pacemaker does not sense.
ODO	Sensing only. Effectively turns pacing off.	Complete heart block during surgery with electrocautery and *adequate* intrinsic rate.

7 Pacemaker Interrogation

- Every PM manufacturer and every device has its own interface but follow a basic approach to PM interrogation. Table 3 summarizes the terminology of an interrogation.
- Once the analyzer links to the device (usually through the "wand" or wirelessly via Bluetooth), several numbers are generated automatically.
- To be systematic, the PBL-STOP mnemonic (Table 4) allows for the end-user to get all the necessary information.

Table 3 CIED terminology

Term	Definition
Intrinsic rhythm	The underlying rhythm when not paced (e.g., complete heart block at X bpm with narrow-complex escape rhythm).
Battery voltage	The electrical potential a battery can generate. This deteriorates over time and manufacturers publish variables to identify when battery is nearing end of service.
Output	The energy delivered to the tissue from the pacemaker. Measured in milliamperes (mA) for temporary external pacemakers and Volts (V) for permanent pacemakers. Output in permanent pacemakers allows for adjustment of the pulse width (milliseconds) – the time over which the voltage is delivered.
Threshold	The minimum output required to reliably stimulate myocardial capture.
Loss of capture	Insufficient energy delivery to depolarize the myocardium. Seen on ECG as a pacing spike with no P wave or QRS following. Pacemaker "thinks" it delivered an appropriate pace and timing generally not affected
Sensitivity	The minimum amplitude (mV) of a wave that is "seen" by the pacemaker. Figure 5 shows the "fence" concept to help clarify. The higher the sensitivity, the lower the number, the greater the risk of over-sensing. The lower the sensitivity, the higher the number, the greater the risk of under-sensing.
Safety margin	Outputs: For permanent systems, generally 2x threshold or 3x pulse width. For temporary systems, as thresholds may rise quickly or be unpredictable, minimum of 10 mA Sensitivity: Usually 50% of the amplitude of the wave.
Impedance	The resistance of the pacemaker system in Ohms. Changes in impedance can help diagnose problems with the device
RRT/ERI	Recommended replacement time/ elective replacement index. A time recommended by the device manufacturer to schedule elective replacement of the generator. Usually indicates ~3–6 months of battery life remaining but this is only an estimate
EOL/EOS	End of life/end of service. Battery depleted and pacing function may be impaired or may stop completely.
Magnet mode	When a magnet is placed over the device, it will switch to asynchronous pacing at rates set by the manufacturer (AOO, VOO, DOO). The rate that is unmasked can help determine battery health remotely (e.g. with telephone transmitter)

8 Pacemaker Troubleshooting

- It is imperative that pacing leads, be they temporary or permanent, are checked after placement and before the chest is closed in the OR.
- Ensuring that leads have acceptable sensing ($\geq$ 7 mV) and thresholds ($\leq$ 1 V @ 0.5 ms) informs how the pacemakers are programmed and prolongs lead longevity.

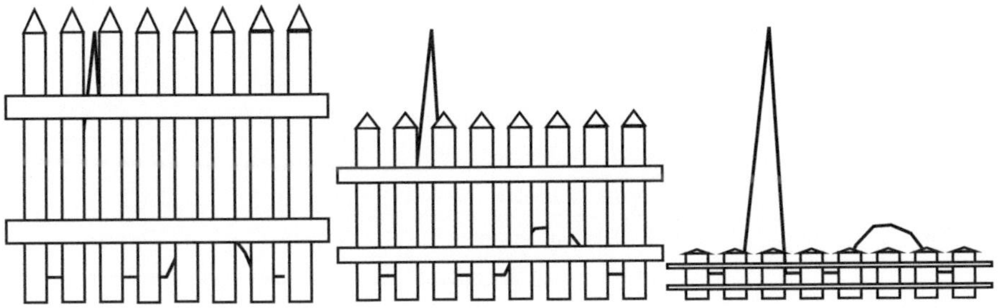

Fig. 5 The Fence concept for sensitivity

Table 4 Approach to the pacemaker interrogation

Mnemonic	Description	Example
P	Presenting rhythm and settings	Complete heart block with intrinsic rate at 45 bpm. Initially set to VVI 60 bpm
	Percent pacing	90% Ventricular pacing (VP).
B	Battery	Mean battery longevity estimated at 7 years before ERI.
L	Leads	Lead impedance: A lead 550 Ohms, V lead 600 Ohms. Stable trend line
S	Sensing	*Requires an intrinsic rhythm* Assesses amplitudes of P and R waves during intrinsic rhythm
T	Thresholds	*Testing should be done for each lead* Threshold testing of the V lead revealed a threshold of 1V at 0.4 ms.
O	Observations	One high-rate episode consistent with a 6-beat run of monomorphic VT
P	Program	Based on acquired information. Outputs optimized for adequate safety margin. Sensing optimized such that intrinsic P and QRS complexes are adequately sensed. Settings programmed into the device
	Print/Preserve/PDF	Print (or save to PDF) relevant testing and details of the interrogation for documentation and future review

Table 5 Differentiating aetiologies of pacemaker malfunction by threshold and impedance changes

Diagnosis	Threshold	Impedance
Lead dislodgement	Elevated	Normal
Lead insulation fracture	Elevated	Low
Lead conductor fracture	Elevated	High
Loose setscrew	Elevated	High
Battery depletion	Normal	Normal
Functional non-capture	Normal	Normal

Table 6 Potential causes of underpacing

Diagnosis	ECG finding
Loss of capture	Pacing spike with no subsequent P-wave or QRS complex.
Oversensing in AAI, VVI, DDI	No pacing spike where expected. Time from subsequent beat to see what is being sensed (eg. T-wave oversensing).
Upper Rate Behaviour	In DDD/DDDR, if sensed atrial rhythm faster than upper rate limit, PM will Wenckebach (prolong AV delay until non-conducted beat). If sufficiently fast, PM will enter 2:1 block.

8.1 Lead Impedance Changes

- As the PM and tissue create an electrical circuit, changes in lead impedance can result from systemic illnesses, myocardial disease, lead dislodgement or lead fracture (Table 5).
- Recognizing the significance of lead impedance trends can help identify lead issues and plan device revisions safely in advance.

8.2 Underpacing

- Heart rate slower than PM's lower rate. Potential causes are summarized in Table 6.

8.3 Overpacing

- Heart rate faster than expected for pacemaker settings. Potential causes are summarized in Table 7.

Table 7 Potential causes of overpacing

Diagnosis	ECG finding
Undersensing in AAI, VVI, DDI	Pacing spike comes earlier than expected. Time from early beat to see what is being sensed. Undersensing carries a risk of pacing on the P or T waves leading to tachyarrhythmias.
Pacemaker-mediated tachycardia (PMT)	In the presence of retrograde conduction of the P-wave (something more common in younger children), an atrial-tracking PM (e.g., DDD) will not be able to distinguish a sinus P-wave from retrograde P-wave resulting in an SVT with the PM acting as an antegrade accessory pathway. PMT algorithms are used to avoid this by extending the post-ventricular atrial refractory period (PVARP) after a set number of beats.

9 Advanced Topics in CIEDs

- In general, ICD and CRT devices (both CRT-P and CRT-D) are considered more complex and should have all troubleshooting and management coordinated with the local electrophysiology team.

9.1 Inactivation of an ICD

- All ICDs are designed to deliver up to 6 shocks for a single arrhythmia episode.
- ICD shock storm occurs when a patient is going in and out of an arrhythmia that continuously resets the device.
- ICDs may interpret electrocautery in the operating room as an arrhythmia and may deliver a shock.
- If an ICD needs to be inactivated, there are two main methods:
  - Device Programmer to inactivate the device through reprogramming
  - Placing a magnet over the device will turn off therapies
- Be careful when inactivating a device! An inactivated device means a patient is no longer protected. Always remember to review the device settings with the local electrophysiology team before discharge.

Bibliography

1. Aquilina O. A brief history of cardiac pacing. Images Paediatr Cardiol. 2006;8(2):17–81
2. Hongo RH, Goldschlager NF. Conduction disorders & cardiac pacing. In: Crawford M (ed) Current Diagnosis & Treatment: Cardiology 5th edn. McGraw-Hill, United States, 2017; pp 169–201

3. Shah MJ, Silka MJ, Silva S, et al. PACES expert consensus statement on the indications and management of cardiovascular implantable electronic devices in pediatric patients. Heart Rhythm. 2021;18(11):1888–924.

Extra Corporeal Life Support (ECLS) and Related Support Strategies

Cory Anderson, Mark Todd, and Haley Christian

Abstract Extracorporeal Membrane Oxygenation (ECMO) is a cornerstone of cardiac critical care, allowing for the cardiopulmonary support of tenuous physiology in the pre-operative, operative, and post-operative phases of managing patients with cardiac disease. ECMO support is characterized by complex interactions between dynamic patient physiology and biomedical engineering. This chapter will discuss the different modes of ECMO and their application in neonates and children with congenital and acquired heart disease. This chapter will also provide an overview of patient physiology while on ECMO, including the management of vasoactive medication, anticoagulation, and mechanical ventilation. An overview will be provided on common ECMO complications and methods for troubleshooting circuit dysfunction. Strategies for weaning ECMO and patient outcomes after ECMO are included. This chapter is not intended to be a comprehensive review, rather it should be used as a guide to understand and manage the patient and ECMO circuit at the bedside.

Keywords Extracorporeal life support · ECMO · Circuit · Anticoagulation management · Veno-arterial · Veno-venous

---

C. Anderson
Department of Paediatrics, Division of Critical Care Medicine, London Health Sciences Centre, Western University, London, ON, Canada
e-mail: cory.anderson@lhsc.on.ca

M. Todd
Department of Critical Care Medicine, Hospital for Sick Children, Toronto, ON, Canada

Department of Respiratory Medicine, Hospital for Sick Children, Toronto, ON, Canada

M. Todd
e-mail: Mark.todd@sickkids.ca

H. Christian (✉)
Department of Critical Care Medicine and Labatt Family Heart Centre, Hospital for Sick Children, Toronto, ON, Canada
e-mail: Haley.christian@sickkids.ca

Department of Pediatrics, University of Toronto, Toronto, ON, Canada

© The Author(s), under exclusive license to Springer Nature Switzerland AG 2024

A. I. Dipchand et al. (eds.), *Manual of Cardiac Care in Children*,
https://doi.org/10.1007/978-3-031-70973-9_56

Abbreviations

ACT	Activated coagulation time
BTT	Blalock Taussig Thomas
CPB	Cardiopulmonary bypass
CPR	Cardiopulmonary resuscitation
ECLS	Extracorporeal life support
ECMO	Extracorporeal membrane oxygenation
ECPR	ECMO cardiopulmonary resuscitation
INR	International normalized ratio
IVC	Inferior vena cava
LA	Left atrium
LV	Left ventricle
MAPCAs	Major aortopulmonary collaterals
MIS-C	Multisystem inflammatory syndrome in children
PDA	Persistent ductus arteriosus
PEEP	Positive end expiratory pressure
PIP	Peak inspiratory pressure
PVR	Pulmonary vascular resistance
RPM	Revolutions per minute
SVR	Systemic vascular resistance
VO_2	Oxygen consumption

1 The Extracorporeal Membrane Oxygenation (ECMO) Circuit: [Fig. 1])

- Involves two main functional components: an artificial membrane to support the pulmonary functions (oxygenation and CO_2 removal) and a pump to support the cardiac function[1].
- Pump: The circuit pump is most commonly a centrifugal pump created by fast-spinning motor or levitating magnet (occasionally can use a roller-pump).
- Membrane Oxygenator: performs gas exchange using countercurrent flows of blood and fresh gas through a hollow-fibre system
- Cannulas for vascular access:
  - Drainage cannula: removes blood from the patient, most often deoxygenated blood
  - Return cannula: returns oxygenated blood into either the venous or arterial system
  - Anatomical position of cannulas and flow direction of blood determines the configuration:

    VA – drainage from venous system and return to arterial system
    VV – drainage and return to venous system, generally peripheral cannulation

VA-A – drainage from venous and arterial (e.g., left atrial vent) system and return to arterial system
V-VA –drainage from venous system with return to both venous and arterial systems

- Cannulations may be central (via sternotomy) or peripheral (neck or femoral)
- Central cannulation:

  Direct venous cannulation of right atrium and aorta. Left atrium vented through separate cannula.
  Used primarily following cardiac surgery, high flow states (sepsis)

- Peripheral cannulation:

  Neck cannulation favoured for < 15 kg
  Femoral cannulation for > 15 kg but will depend on size and quality of vessels.
  Femoral Arterial cannulation preferably performed with a chimney graft to ensure perfusion to the distal limb (or a separate distal perfusion cannula)

- Cannula size are chosen based on patient's vessel size and the calculated flow required. Second venous cannula may have to be considered if inadequate drainage/flows.

• Heater exchanger system: to regulate blood temperature, which allows the system to maintain normothermia or mild hypothermia.
• Flow Probe: measures flow and can detect air bubbles in the circuit if equipped
• Pressure Monitors: transduces pressure pre-pump, post-pump/pre-oxygenator, and post oxygenator
• Heparin-coated circuit tubing and bridge: a specialized circuit can be used with a connection between return and drainage cannulas (bridge) that allows for circulation of blood through the circuit and for the isolation of the patient from circuit during weaning or emergency procedures

2 ECMO Indications

ECMO is a temporizing bridge to allow for definitive treatment, recovery, or transition to longer bridging support [Table 1].

ECMO is applied for:

1) Cardiac and cardiopulmonary failure

   a. Pre- or Post-operative stabilization (e.g., failure to wean CPB)
   b. Reversible imbalance of DO_2:VO_2 (e.g., myocarditis with cardiogenic shock)
   c. Myocardial failure (e.g., cardiomyopathy, intractable arrhythmias)
   d. To support a cardiac surgical procedure as an alternative to CPB (e.g. BTT shunt insertion)

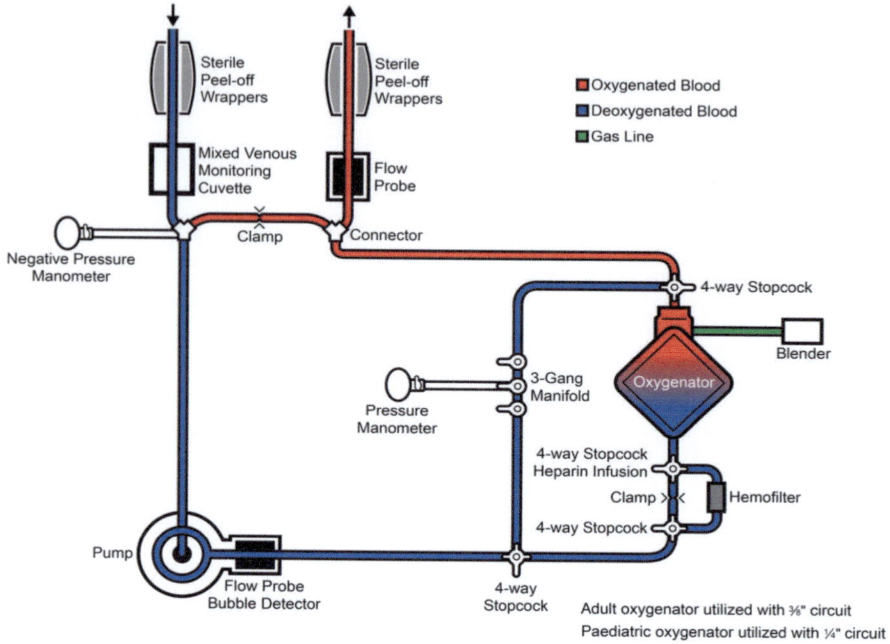

Fig. 1 The Extracorporeal Membrane Oxygenation (ECMO) circuit

Table 1 ECMO indications

Bridge to recovery anmd Therapies:	Bridge to decision	Bridge to organ replacement or transplant
Most frequent purpose for ECMO	Typically indicated in situations where time is needed to understand diagnoses, therapies, and prognosis (e.g., repairing a residual lesion)	Heart transplant candidates may be transitioned from ECMO to ventricular assist devices until transplant. Lung transplant candidates may be bridged to lung transplantation from ECMO

2) Oxygenation and ventilation failure
   a. Inadequate pulmonary blood flow (e.g., thrombosed BTT shunt)
   b. Severe lung parenchymal disease (e.g., pneumonia, and ARDS)
   c. Inadequate mixing for congenital heart with transposition physiology
   d. Meconium aspiration
3) Refractory cardiac arrest (ECPR)
   a. Witnessed in-hospital cardiac arrest refractory to conventional CPR (Table 2).

DO_2 – Oxygen delivery, VO_2 – Oxygen consumption.

Table 2 Goals of ECMO (Fig. 2)

Mode	VA-ECMO	VV-ECMO
Indication	• Cardiac or cardiopulmonary support • Refractory cardiac arrest (E-CPR)	Respiratory support: • Oxygenation support • Ventilation support
Main goals	1. Allow myocardial recovery: Maximize myocardial DO_2:VO_2 2. Optimize peripheral DO_2 to prevent end organ ischemia 3. Address important cardiac lesions	1. Provides adequate gas exchange 2. Supports tissue oxygenation 3. Decreases lung-injurious ventilation
Expected duration	Usual recovery in 3–7 days	7–10 days but may be up to 4–6 weeks
Frequency	75% of program volume (2/3 elective, 1/3 ECPR)	25% program volume

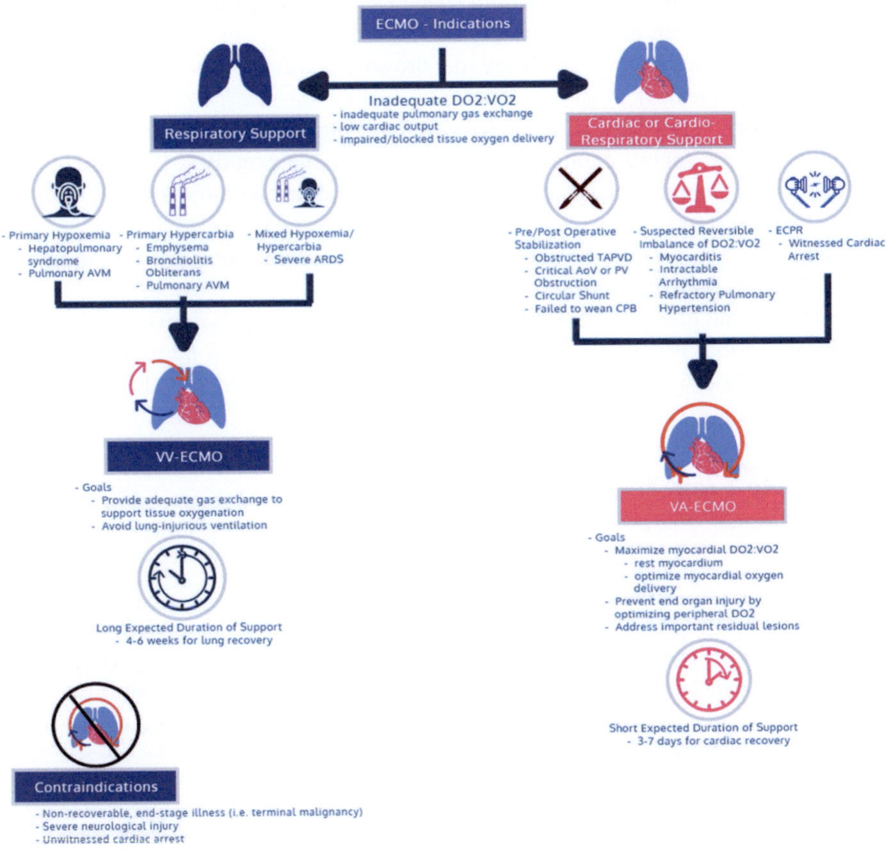

Fig. 2 ECMO Indications and Goals

3 Contraindications

- Irreversible disease with end-stage illness with or without multiorgan failure
- Severe irreversible neurologic injury
- Unwitnessed cardiac arrest
- Out-of-hospital cardiac arrest (relative contraindication)

4 ECMO Physiology

4.1 Flow Dynamics

- Continuous flow is driven by a pump (centrifugal pumps are used in the institution). Flow is dependent on pump speed (RPM) and resistance (summation of circuit, oxygenator, and patient).
- Pump generates a negative pressure that draws blood from venous reservoir (vena cava or right atrium)
- Negative pressures depend on size of cannulas, blood flow, venous reservoir (e.g. volume status, venous cannula position) – acceptable usually < 100 mmHg
- The patient's mean arterial blood pressure is dependent on pump flow and systemic vascular resistance.
- The pump does not adjust to changes in patient volume status (the volume of the reservoir) or patient afterload.
- Patient arterial line may be completely flat if ECMO circuit is delivering complete flow. Pulsatility is dependent on myocardial function, ventricular preload, and LV afterload. Return of pulsatility may be an indication of myocardial recovery.

4.2 Pump Flow Targets

Weight	Cardiac or cardiopulmonary support	Respiratory Support
< 10 kg	100–150 mL/kg/min (150–200 mL/kg/min for systemic to pulmonary shunt)	60–100 mL/kg/min
10–20 kg	Either mL/kg/min or flow indexed to cardiac index – typically highest that is reasonably achievable	
> 20 kg	Cardiac index 2.4–3.2 L/min/m^2	1.5–2.6 L/min/m^2

*Initial targets only – titrated to target adequate patient oxygen delivery.

4.3 Gas Exchange

- Dependent on gas flow: mixture of oxygen and air that flows through membrane.
- Flow Rate (called Sweep) set in L/min (or ml/min) initially set at 0.6 of ratio blood flow and titrated to desired patient P_aCO_2
- Fraction of device inlet oxygen (F_dO_2) is initially set at 0.5 and titrated to desired patient S_pO_2

4.4 Cardiac Lesions that Modify Physiology

- Increased blood flows (150–200 mL/kg/min) required for "run-off" lesions with aortic to pulmonary shunts, including:
  - Biventricular circulations with aorto-pulmonary connections (PDA, MAPCAs)
  - Single Ventricle Palliation Stage 1 with hybrid physiology, BTT or central shunts.
- Usual ECMO flows (100–150 mL/kg/min) required for Single ventricle palliations with:
  - Stage 1 with direct ventricle to artery connection
  - Stage 2 – May require 2 anatomical sites of venous return (individual cannulae for superior vena cava and right atrium) to ensure full decompression
  - Stage 3 – Generally cannulated SVC or IVC with tip close to junction of vena cava and Fontan baffle

    Cannulation of atrium possible if primary pump failure with low PVR

5 Managing the Patient on ECMO

5.1 Vasoactive Medications: Inotropes, Vasopressors and Pulmonary Vasodilators

- Vasopressors and dilators titrated to patient SVR to maintain adequate organ perfusion pressure and circuit flows (inverse relationship with higher SVR leading to lower flows)
- Inotropes weaned to minimize myocardial oxygen demand
- Monitor arterial pulsatility and signs of LA hypertension (pulmonary congestion/hemorrhage) → LA decompression if severe LV dysfunction via:
  - Direct LA cannulation
  - Balloon atrial septostomy (mostly if peripherally cannulated)
  - Impella device in adolescents
  - Percutaneous, trans-septal left atrial cannulas can be inserted in larger patients
  - Inotropic support and decreased SVR to maintain LV ejection

- Myocardial functional recovery unlikely if no pulsatility after > 7–10 days – consideration should be given to transition to another device or redirection of care
- Echocardiography unable to assess functional recovery while on full flows
- Focused echocardiography on low flow/no flow to assess ventricular recovery and residual cardiac lesions
- VV-ECMO: ECMO supports gas exchange with native cardiac output
  - Inotropic and vasoactive support titrated to maintain native systemic cardiac output and perfusion pressure
  - Increasing native cardiac output may worsen venous admixture and increase patient hypoxemia due to increased pulmonary venous hypoxemia

5.2 *Ventilation on ECMO*

- Main goal: minimize lung injurious ventilation and promote lung recruitment
  - VA ECMO: Institutional practice to use 'Rest' settings:

    Positive end expiratory pressure (PEEP) 10 cm H_2O, peak inspiratory pressure (PIP) < 20 cm H_2O, respiratory rate 10 breaths/min, FiO_2 < 0.3 (limited evidence of exact settings to use)
    Gas exchange occurs in circuit oxygenator and ventilator unnecessary for oxygenation or CO2 removal
  - VV ECMO: Settings individualized to support patient ventilation/oxygenation often accepting mild hypoxia and permissive hypercapnia

5.3 *Anticoagulation*

- ECMO circuit and oxygenator are prothrombotic and associated with thrombus in 40% and 15% of runs, respectively.
- Managing Anticoagulation:
  - Cannulation – Bolus 50 units/kg heparin given to patient
  - Maintenance – Unfractionated Heparin infusion 10–40 units/kg/h (Bivalirudin may be used as an alternative)

    Titrate to maintain Activated Clotting Time (ACT)160–180 s and Anti-Xa (Heparin assay) 0.35–0.75 units/mL [center and device specific]

      ACT is a complex measure of thrombosis and increased level does not exclude prothrombotic state

- Coagulation management should include:
  - Normalization of INR (consider replacing vit K (replace in all neonates)) and fibrinogen
  - Platelet count > 80–100,000/mL (depending on ACT and bleeding risk)
  - Trend D-dimer – increase may indicate consumptive coagulopathy or thrombosis
  - Plasma free hemoglobin – increase may indicate hemolysis and suggest clot burden
  - Surveillance of oxygenator function (increased transmembrane pressure, impaired gas exchange, lower flows) to monitor for thrombosis burden

5.4 *Complications (Table 3 and Fig. 3)*

- Acute neurologic complication (thrombus/hemorrhage) in 12–22%
  - Surveillance head ultrasounds conducted daily on neonates to rule out major hemorrhage/pathology
- Surgical bleeding
- End-organ injury

5.5 *ECMO Duration and Recovery*

- Myocardial recovery expected within 5–7 days of initial insult
- Ongoing ECMO requirement with good ventricular function should prompt further investigations (catheterization/CT) – re-evaluation of possible residual lesions or pathological physiologies (eg, diastolic dysfunction) driving support needs
- Coronary imaging (angiography/CT) is required immediately if concerns of myocardial ischemia (history, ST changes on ECG, ventricular arrhythmias), even with uncomplicated ECMO flows.

5.6 *Weaning/Discontinuation*

- VA-ECMO:
  - Consider reducing flows to 50% target and assess for functional recovery and gradual loading of systemic ventricle
  - If circuit includes a bridge can pursue a clamp trial off ECMO support:

Table 3 Troubleshooting: problems and solutions

Type	Problem		Solution
VA-ECMO	Myocardial Stun	Loss of LV output – may contribute to LA hypertension	Expected recovery: 1–3 days Monitor for LA hypertension and decompress left heart
	Differential Hypoxemia	Recovery of LV without lung recovery → delivery of deoxygenated perfusion to brain, coronaries (heart) and upper limbs	Ventilate, recruit, and oxygenate lungs to improve native function Increase ECMO Flow (out-compete native output) Consider change in ECMO configuration (i.e. V-VA)
VV-ECMO	Recirculation	Low effective flow due to drainage of oxygenated blood back through the pump	Echo/Chest X-Ray to assess cannula position → reposition if necessary Reduce RPMs/total flow if possible
	Venous Admixture	Excess deoxygenated blood mixing with oxygenated return from the circuit	Increase circuit flow Reduce systemic VO_2 → control fever, sedate/ neuromuscular blockade Transfuse RBCs to increase DO_2
Both VA and VV	Low Flow	Low Circuit Preload (more negative venous pressures)	Treat hypovolemia in patient Check drainage cannula for clot/kink Echo/X-ray for position → reposition/remove obstruction
		Poor Circuit Function	Check pump/oxygenator function → replace circuit if necessary
		High Circuit Afterload (increased pre/post membrane pressures)	Check return cannula for clot/kink Echo/X-ray for position → reposition/remove obstruction
	Hemolysis	Excess shear stress lyses RBCs	Optimize patient volume status Consider reducing RPMs Consider circuit change

(continued)

Table 3 (continued)

Type	Problem		Solution
	Coagulopathy	Systemic anticoagulation → increases bleeding risk	Assess for and correct coagulopathy (e.g., deficiency of vit K, fibrinogen, Antithrombin, VWF) Surgical exploration for refractory hemorrhage
		Inflammatory state → DIC, increased risk of emboli/stroke	Target therapeutic anticoagulation and treat source of inflammation (e.g., infection)
	Infection	Indwelling cannula and alterations of immune complexes from shear stress	Culture invasive devices and treat with antimicrobials
	Air Embolus	Entrainment of air into circuit → risk of ischemia (myocardial/ stroke)	De-air circuit Consider circuit change

Clamp for 5-minute intervals with 30 second flashes (unclamp) to test physiology and avoid thrombosis in cannulas (requires adequate circuit integrity and anticoagulation within target)
LA vent can be clamped first to determine impact of partial loading of LV

- Consider decannulation if:

  Functional recovery with acceptable haemodynamics/adequate oxygen delivery on reasonable levels of inotropic/vasoactive support
  Adequate gas exchange with non-injurious ventilatory settings

- Procedural Echocardiogram often completed to assess function and residual lesions

• VV-ECMO: gradually decrease gas flow until off – assess for functional recovery with adequate gas exchange through native lungs

6 Outcomes Following ECMO Runs

• VA-ECMO: Survival to Hospital Discharge varies between 43% (Neonates < 30 days) and 53% (children 1 month–17 years)

  - Improved survival for fulminant myocarditis 61–80%
  - Single Ventricle Patients and ECPR remain 35–43%
  - Multisystem Inflammatory Syndrome (MIS-C) 51%
  - Neonatal enteroviral myocarditis 33%

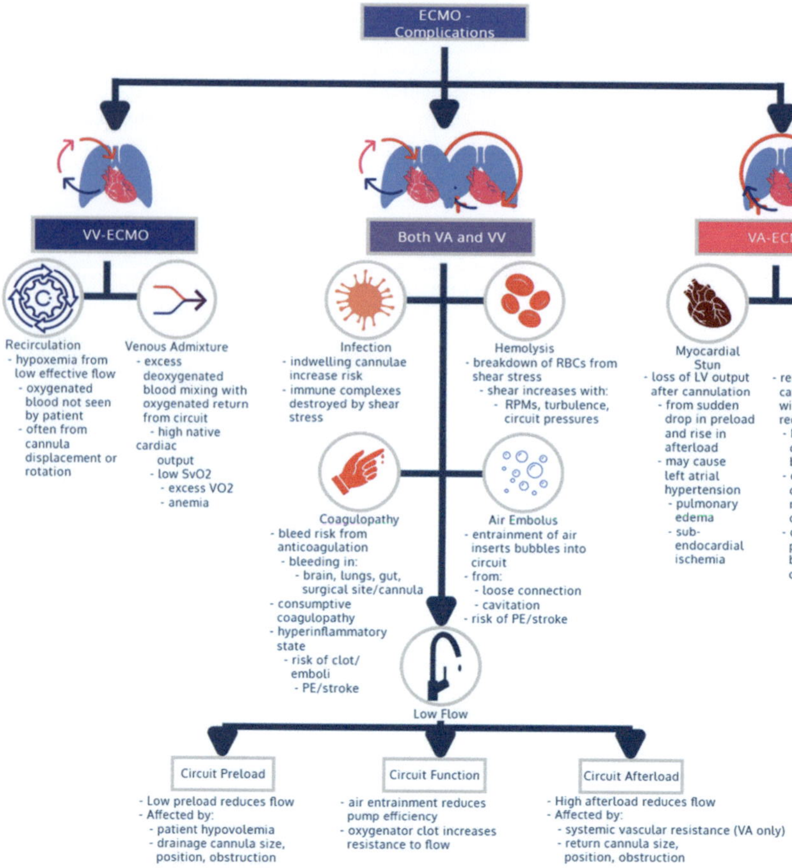

Fig. 3 ECMO Complications

  - Poor 5-year survival – complicated by Acute Neurologic Events (12–22%) and Developmental Disability 20–73%

- VA and VV-ECMO for Respiratory Disease
  - Neonates – hospital discharge 50–95% depending on primary diagnosis

    Presence of neurologic complications reduces survival by 50%
    Outcomes complicated by neurologic injury and renal impairment

  - Children – hospital discharge 50–70%

    Pre-ECMO ventilation > 2 weeks worsens survival to 50%
    VA-ECMO mode lower survival compared to VV-ECMO (50% vs 75%)

      5-year survival 42%.

Acknowledgements The authors would like to acknowledge Dr. Afrothite Kotsakis MD, MEd and Dr. Dr. Anne-Marie Guerguerian, MD, PhD for their contributions to this chapter.

Bibliography

1. Brogen TV, Annich G, Ellis WC et al (eds). ECMO specialist training manual, 4th ed. Extracorporeal Life Support Organization; 2018.
2. Fernando SM, Qureshi D, Tanuseputro P, et al. Long-term survival and costs following extracorporeal membrane oxygenation in critically ill children—Aa population-based cohort study. Crit Care. 2020;24(1):131.
3. M'Pembele R, Roth S, Metzger A, et al. Evaluation of clinical outcomes in patients treated with heparin or direct thrombin inhibitors during extracorporeal membrane oxygenation: a systematic review and meta-analysis. Thromb J. 2022;20(1):42.
4. MacLaren G, Brodie D, Lorusso R et al (eds). Extracorporeal life support: The ELSO red book, 6th ed. Extracorporeal Life Support Organization; 2022.
5. Extracorporeal Life Support Organization. ELSO registry data definitions 2022. https://www.elso.org/portals/0/files/pdf/elso%20registry%20data%20definitions%2005_17_22.pdf. Accessed 22 Dec 2022

Correction to: Anticoagulation

Leonardo R. Brandao

Correction to:
Chapter 54 in: A. I. Dipchand et al. (eds.), *Manual of Cardiac Care in Children*, https://doi.org/10.1007/978-3-031-70973-9_54

The original version of the chapter "Anticoagulation" was inadvertently published with incorrect spelling in Tables 11 and 13, which has now been updated. The chapter has been updated with the changes.

The updated version of this chapter can be found at
https://doi.org/10.1007/978-3-031-70973-9_54

© The Author(s), under exclusive license to Springer Nature Switzerland AG 2025

A. I. Dipchand et al. (eds.), *Manual of Cardiac Care in Children*,
https://doi.org/10.1007/978-3-031-70973-9_57

Appendix

Komail Nadeem, Meredith Ames and Winnie Seto

Abstract Pharmaceutical infusions are the cornerstone of delivering medical therapy for acutely ill children with cardiac disease. Broadly, infusions can be classified based on their clinical effect, including but not limited to (1) cardiac rhythm control, (2) sedation, analgesia and muscle relaxation, (3) cardiac output and blood pressure control, (4) fluid and electrolyte management, (5) anticoagulation and hemostasis. Infusion concentrations, delivery rate, and medication doses are usually weight-based. Care must also be taken to ensure appropriate compatibility between infusions running within a single catheter to avoid precipitation, catheter malfunction and adverse patient events.

Keywords Pharmaceutical infusions · Drug delivery · Drug compatibility

Intravenous Infusion Medications

Cardiac Rhythm Control

Sedation, Analgesia, and Muscle Relaxation

Drug	Usual start dose	Weight	Standard concentration	Rate based on start dose (mL/hr)	
Cisatracurium	0.3 mg/kg/hr	Rate < 2 mL/hr	20 mg/10 mL (undiluted)	0.15	X Wt
		Rate ≥ 2 mL/hr	100 mg/50 mL (undiluted)	0.15	X Wt

(continued)

K. Nadeem · M. Ames · W. Seto (✉)
Department of Pharmacy, The Hospital for Sick Children, Toronto, ON, Canada
e-mail: Winnie.seto@sickkids.ca

© The Editor(s) (if applicable) and The Author(s), under exclusive license to Springer Nature Switzerland AG 2024

A. I. Dipchand et al. (eds.), *Manual of Cardiac Care in Children*,
https://doi.org/10.1007/978-3-031-70973-9

(continued)

Drug	Usual start dose	Weight	Standard concentration	Rate based on start dose (mL/hr)	
DexmedeTOMIDine	0.5 mcg/kg/hr	< 10 kg	200 mcg/50 mL NS	0.125	X Wt
		10 to < 40 kg	400 mcg/50 mL NS	0.063	X Wt
		≥ 40 kg	800 mcg/50 mL NS	0.031	X Wt
FentaNYL	1 mcg/kg/hr	< 10 kg	1,000 mcg/50 mL NS, D5W	0.05	X Wt
		≥ 10 kg	2,500 mcg/50 mL (undiluted – contains NaCl)	0.02	X Wt
		PCA	1,000 mcg/50 mL NS, D5W	0.05	X Wt
			2,500 mcg/50 mL (undiluted – contains NaCl)	0.02	X Wt
HYDROmorphone	1 mcg/kg/hr	< 20 kg	0.5 mg/50 mL NS, D5W	0.1	X Wt
		≥ 20 kg	2 mg/50 mL NS, D5W	0.025	X Wt
			10 mg/50 mL NS, D5W	0.005	X Wt
		PCA	10 mg/50 mL NS, D5W	0.005	X Wt
			50 mg/50 mL NS	0.001	X Wt
KetAMINE	1 mcg/kg/min	All weights	100 mg/50 mL NS, D5W	0.03	X Wt
Midazolam	1 mcg/kg/min	< 20 kg	50 mg/50 mL NS, 0.45% NaCl, D5W	0.06	X Wt
		20 to < 40 kg	100 mg/50 mL NS, 0.45% NaCl, D5W	0.03	X Wt
		≥ 40 kg	250 mg/50 mL (undiluted – contains NaCl)	0.012	X Wt
Morphine	20 mcg/kg/hr	< 10 kg	5 mg/50 mL NS, D5W	0.2	X Wt
		10 to < 40 kg	10 mg/50 mL NS, D5W	0.1	X Wt
		≥ 40 kg	50 mg/50 mL NS, D5W	0.02	X Wt
		PCA	250 mg/50 mL NS	0.004	X Wt
Propofol	30 mcg/kg/min	All weights	500 mg/50 mL (undiluted)	0.18	X Wt

(continued)

(continued)

Drug	Usual start dose	Weight	Standard concentration	Rate based on start dose (mL/hr)	
		Rate > 15mL/hr	1,000 mg/100 mL (undiluted)	0.18	X Wt

Cardiac Output and Blood Pressure Control

Drug	Usual start dose	Weight	Standard concentration	Rate based on start dose (mL/ hr	
DOBUTamine	5 mcg/kg/min	< 10 kg	50 mg/50 mL	0.3	X Wt
		≥ 10 kg	250 mg/50 mL	0.06	X Wt
DOPamine CVL	5 mcg/kg/min	< 10 kg	40 mg/50 mL in D5W (800 mcg/ mL) (undiluted)	0.375	X Wt
		< 10 kg and > 4 mL/hr	200 mg/250 mL in D5W premix bag (800 mcg/ mL)	0.375	X Wt
		≥ 10 kg	160 mg/50 mL in D5W (3200 mcg/ mL) (undiluted)	0.094	X Wt
		≥ 10 kg and > 4 mL/hr	800 mg/250 mL in D5W premix bag (3200 mcg/ mL)	0.094	X Wt
Epinephrine CVL π Withdraw 40 mL (includes overfill volume and drug volume) from 250 mL IV bag prior to adding epinephrine Use epinephrine 1 mg/ mL	0.01 mcg/kg/ min	< 10 kg	0.1 mg/50 mL	0.3	X Wt
		10 to < 15 kg	0.25 mg/50 mL	0.12	X Wt
		≥ 15 kg	0.5 mg/50 mL	0.06	X Wt
	0.1 mcg/kg/ min	< 10 kg	1 mg/50 mL	0.3	X Wt
		10 to < 15 kg	2 mg/50 mL	0.15	X Wt
		≥ 15 kg	4 mg/50 mL	0.075	X Wt
		≥ 15 kg and > 4 mL/hr	20 mg/250 mL π	0.075	X Wt
Isoproterenol	0.01 mcg/kg/ min	< 20 kg	0.2 mg/50 mL NS, D5W, D10W	0.15	X Wt
		≥ 20 kg	0.4 mg/50 mL NS, D5W, D10W	0.075	X Wt
	0.05 mcg/kg/ min	< 10 kg	0.2 mg/50 mL NS, D5W, D10W	0.75	X Wt
		≥ 10 kg	0.4 mg/50 mL NS, D5W, D10W	0.375	X Wt

(continued)

(continued)

Drug		Usual start dose	Weight	Standard concentration	Rate based on start dose (mL/ hr	
Labetalol	PIV	1 mg/kg/hr	All weights	180 mg/50 mL NS, D5W	0.278	X Wt
			Rate > 15 mL/hr	900 mg/250 mL NS, D5W	0.278	X Wt
	CVL	1 mg/kg/hr	All weights	200 mg/40 mL (undiluted – contains dextrose)	0.2	X Wt
			Rate > 15 mL/hr	1,000mg/200 mL (undiluted – contains dextrose)	0.2	X Wt
Milrinone		0.5 mcg/kg/ min	< 10 kg	5 mg/50 mL NS, 0.45% NaCl, D5W	0.3	X Wt
			10 to < 50 kg	10 mg/50 mL NS, 0.45% NaCl, D5W	0.15	X Wt
			≥ 50 kg	40 mg/40 mL (undiluted – contains dextrose)	0.03	X Wt
NiCARdipine (Special Access)		0.5 mcg/kg/ min	All weights	20 mg/100 mL NS, 0.45% NaCl, D5W	0.15	X Wt
			Rate > 10 mL/hr	120 mg/250 mL NS, 0.45% NaCl, D5W	0.063	X Wt
Nitroglycerin		1 mcg/kg/min	< 5 kg	5 mg/50 mL NS, 0.45% NaCl, D5W	0.6	X Wt
			5 to < 15 kg	10 mg/50 mL NS, 0.45% NaCl, D5W	0.3	X Wt
			≥ 15 kg	50 mg/50 mL NS, 0.45% NaCl, D5W	0.06	X Wt
Nitroprusside		1 mcg/kg/min	< 10 kg	10 mg/50 mL NS, D5W	0.3	X Wt
			10 to < 40 kg	50 mg/50 mL NS, D5W	0.06	X Wt
			≥ 40 kg	200 mg/50 mL NS, D5W	0.015	X Wt

(continued)

(continued)

Drug	Usual start dose	Weight	Standard concentration	Rate based on start dose (mL/hr	
Norepinephrine CVL Ω Withdraw 40 mL (includes overfill volume and drug volume) from 250 mL IV bag prior to adding norepinephrine. Use norepinephrine 1 mg/mL (equivalent to 2 mg/mL of norepinephrine bitartrate).	0.01 mcg/kg/min	< 10 kg	0.1 mg/50 mL	0.3	X Wt
		10 to < 15 kg	0.25 mg/50 mL	0.12	X Wt
		≥ 15 kg	0.5 mg/50 mL	0.06	X Wt
	0.1 mcg/kg/min	< 10 kg	1 mg/50 mL	0.3	X Wt
		10 to < 15 kg	2 mg/50 mL	0.15	X Wt
		≥ 15 kg	4 mg/50 mL	0.075	X Wt
		≥ 15 kg and > 4 mL/hr	20 mg/250 mL Ω	0.075	X Wt
Phentolamine CVL	1 mcg/kg/min	< 5 kg	10 mg/50 mL NS	0.3	X Wt
		5 to < 20 kg	20 mg/50 mL NS	0.15	X Wt
		≥ 20 kg	50 mg/50 mL NS	0.06	X Wt
Phenylephrine CVL ¥ 0.1 mL of 10 mg/mL ampoule and 0.9 mL Sterile Water for Injection (SWI) = 1 mg/mL. Use this 1 mg/mL solution to prepare phenylephrine infusion.	0.01 mcg/kg/min	< 10 kg	0.1 mg/50 mL ¥	0.3	X Wt
		10 to < 15 kg	0.25 mg/50 mL ¥	0.12	X Wt
		≥ 15 kg	0.5 mg/50 mL	0.06	X Wt
	0.1 mcg/kg/min	< 5 kg	0.5 mg/50 mL	0.6	X Wt
		5 to < 10 kg	1 mg/50 mL	0.3	X Wt
		≥ 10 kg	2 mg/50 mL	0.15	X Wt
Vasopressin CVL φ Withdraw 21 mL (includes overfill volume and drug volume) from 250 mL IV bag prior to adding vasopressin	0.1 milliunit/kg/min =0.0001 unit/kg/min	< 10 kg	1 unit/50 mL NS, D5W	0.3	X Wt
		≥ 10 kg	4 units/50 mL NS, D5W	0.075	X Wt
		≥ 25 kg and > 4mL/hr	20 units/250 mL NS, D5W φ	0.075	X Wt

Fluid and Electrolytes Management

Drug	Usual start dose	Weight	Standard concentration	Rate based on start dose (mL/hr	
Bumetanide (Special Access)	1 mcg/kg/hr	All weights	1.25 mg/50 mL NS, 0.45% NS, D5W	0.04	X Wt

(continued)

(continued)

Drug		Usual start dose	Weight	Standard concentration	Rate based on start dose (mL/hr	
Calcium gluconate (use calcium gluconate 10%)	PIV	0.042 mmol Ca^{2+}/kg/hr	All weights	2.32 mmol/50 mL NS, D5W, D10W 23.2 mmol/500 mL NS, D5W, D10W	0.9	X Wt
	CVL	0.042 mmol Ca^{2+}/kg/hr	All weights	11.6 mmol/50 mL (undiluted)	0.18	X Wt
Furosemide		0.25 mg/kg/hr	< 10 kg	40 mg/50 mL NS, D5W, D10W	0.313	X Wt
			10 to < 40 kg	120 mg/50 mL NS, D5W, D10W	0.104	X Wt
			≥ 40 kg	250 mg/25 mL (undiluted)	0.025	X Wt
Potassium chloride CVL		High KCl IV infusion order	All weights	25 mmol/50 mL D5W/0.2% NaCl	Titrate	
Potassium phosphate (K^+)	PIV	0.042 mmol phosphate/kg/hr	All weights	6.75 mmol phosphate/250 mL 13.5 mmol phosphate/500 mL 20.25 mmol phosphate/750 mL (0.027 mmol phosphate/mL)	1.56	X Wt
	CVL	0.042 mmol phosphate/kg/hr	All weights	42.51 mmol phosphate/250 mL 84.99 mmol phosphate/500 mL 127.5 mmol phosphate/750 mL (0.17 mmol phosphate/mL)	0.25	X Wt

(continued)

(continued)

Drug		Usual start dose	Weight	Standard concentration	Rate based on start dose (mL/hr	
			Fluid-restricted AND CCU only	15 mmol phosphate/50 mL (0.3 mmol phosphate/mL)	0.14	X Wt
Sodium phosphate PIV	PIV	0.042 mmol phosphate/kg/hr	All weights	24.99 mmol phosphate/250 mL NS, D5W 50.01 mmol phosphate/500 mL NS, D5W 75 mmol phosphate/750 mL NS, D5W (0.1 mmol phosphate/mL)	0.42	X Wt
	CVL	0.042 mmol phosphate/kg/hr	All weights	75 mmol phosphate/250 mL NS, D5W 150 mmol phosphate/500 mL NS, D5W 225 mmol phosphate/750 mL NS, D5W (0.3 mmol phosphate/mL)	0.14	X Wt

Anticoagulation and Hemostasis

Drug	Usual start dose	Weight	Standard concentration	Rate based on start dose (mL/hr)	
Bivalirudin	0.05 mg/kg/hr	< 10 kg	50 mg/50 mL NS, D5W	0.05	X Wt
		10 to < 20 kg	100 mg/50 mL NS, D5W	0.025	X Wt
		≥ 20 kg	250 mg/50 mL NS, D5W	0.01	X Wt

(continued)

(continued)

Drug	Usual start dose	Weight	Standard concentration	Rate based on start dose (mL/hr)	
Heparin § Withdraw 45 mL (includes overfill volume and drug volume) from 250 mL IV bag prior to adding heparin. Use heparin 1,000 U/mL.	PROPHYLAXIS: 10 units/kg/hr	< 20 kg	5,000 units/50 mL	0.1	X Wt
		≥ 20 kg	10,000 units/50 mL	0.05	X Wt
	TREATMENT for ≤ 1 year old: 28 units/kg/hr	< 5 kg	2,500 units/50 mL	0.56	X Wt
		≥ 5 kg	5,000 units/50 mL	0.28	X Wt
	TREATMENT for > 1 year old: 20 units/kg/hr	< 20 kg	5,000 units/50 mL	0.2	X Wt
		≥ 20 kg	10,000 units/50 mL	0.1	X Wt
		Rate > 15 mL/hr	25,000 units/250 mL §	0.2	X Wt
		Fluid-restricted	30,000 units/50 mL	0.033	X Wt
Tranexamic acid	10 mg/kg/hr	All weights	100 mg/50 mL NS, D5W	5	X Wt

Other

Drug	Usual start dose	Weight	Standard concentration	Rate based on start dose (mL/hr)	
Alprostadil	0.01 mcg/kg/min	All weights	100 mcg/50 mL	0.3	X Wt
	0.1 mcg/kg/min or fluid-restricted	All weights	500 mcg/50 mL	0.06	X Wt
Insulin – Regular, Human (non-DKA) (HumuLIN R)	0.01 units/kg/hr	< 10 kg	2 units/50 mL (use diluted 10 units/mL HumuLIN R) NS, 0.45% NaCl, D5W	0.25	X Wt
		10 to < 40 kg	10 units/50 mL NS, 0.45% NaCl, D5W	0.05	X Wt
		≥ 40 kg	50 units/50 mL NS, 0.45% NaCl, D5W	0.01	X Wt
	0.1 units/kg/hr	All weights	25 units/250 mL NS, 0.45% NaCl, D5W	1	X Wt
		Fluid-restricted	50 units/50 mL NS, 0.45% NaCl, D5W	0.1	X Wt
Salbutamol	1 mcg/kg/min	All weights	50 mg/50 mL (undiluted)	0.06	X Wt
		Rate > 15mL/hr	100 mg/200 mL NS, D5W	0.12	X Wt

(continued)

(continued)

Drug	Usual start dose	Weight	Standard concentration	Rate based on start dose (mL/hr)	
		Rate > 15mL/hr AND fluid-restricted	100 mg/100 mL (undiluted)	0.06	X Wt

Index

© The Editor(s) (if applicable) and The Author(s), under exclusive license to Springer Nature Switzerland AG 2024
A. I. Dipchand et al. (eds.), *Manual of Cardiac Care in Children*, https://doi.org/10.1007/978-3-031-70973-9

MIX
Papier aus verantwortungsvollen Quellen
Paper from responsible sources
FSC® C105338

If you have any concerns about our products,
you can contact us on
ProductSafety@springernature.com

In case Publisher is established outside the EU,
the EU authorized representative is:
Springer Nature Customer Service Center GmbH
Europaplatz 3, 69115 Heidelberg, Germany

Printed by Libri Plureos GmbH
in Hamburg, Germany